Translational Approach to Heart Failure

Jozef Bartunek • Marc Vanderheyden
Editors

Translational Approach to Heart Failure

Springer

Editors
Jozef Bartunek
Cardiovascular Centre
OLV Hospital
Aalst, Belgium

Marc Vanderheyden
Cardiovascular Centre
OLV Hospital
Aalst, Belgium

ISBN 978-1-4614-7344-2 ISBN 978-1-4614-7345-9 (eBook)
DOI 10.1007/978-1-4614-7345-9
Springer New York Heidelberg Dordrecht London

Library of Congress Control Number: 2013940918

Printed on acid-free paper

Springer is part of Springer Science+Business Media (www.springer.com)

Foreword

The "Dirk Verheyden-foundation" wishes to add the following considerations and reflexions to this scientific foreword.

Young people suffering a heart failure are fighting so hard against this disease. Some win, some lose the fight. It would be a shame if we, healthy people, did not try to continue this battle on another field. That is why we founded the "Dirk Verheyden-foundation" in collaboration with the Cardiovascular Centre of the OLV Hospital in Aalst, Belgium.

With the possibilities we have, we succeeded to raise funds to enable the edition of this book about the experiences and findings of this resolute cardiovascular team.

It gives a sense to the loss of Dirk, our son, brother, friend, and we get a feeling of a resolute continuation of Dirk's struggle for life.

Our hope and wish is that this book will enable all the cardiac-research teams to get a flow of new findings, results, and experiences so that the progress towards an eventual ban of these cardiac failures can be reached or at least approached.

SUCCESS.

The "Dirk Verheyden-foundation."

Foreword

Preface

In memory of Dirk Verheyden, dedicated teacher and patient.

The heart failure pandemic is expanding at an alarming pace and has become a leading cause of morbidity and mortality in emerging and developed countries. The hallmark of this pathology is maladaptive ventricular remodeling that precipitates contractile dysfunction, and ultimately leads to the overt syndrome of congestive heart failure. The refined pathophysiological understanding of the heart failure syndrome as well as the surge of new technological advances led to innovative medical and interventional treatment strategies improving the outcome of heart failure patients. However the complex interplay between the clinical presentation and array of existing and emerging interventions requires a coordinated multidisciplinary "heart team" approach involving various specialists in the cardiovascular field including clinicians, interventionalists, surgeons, and cardiac intensivists.

The goal of this book is to provide with an overview of state-of-the-art management of heart failure. It presents a balanced mix of latest updates in the pathophysiology and clinical presentation of heart failure and its associated comorbidities. The topics cover burning clinical questions and challenges faced by the heart team. New medical and interventional therapies for chronic and acute heart failure are addressed by key opinion leaders bridging bench to bedside translation in science and technology towards the practical clinical application and guidance.

The book is divided into four parts. Part I, which aims to bridge pathophysiology of heart failure and its adoption in the clinical management, highlights the modern translational pathophysiology underlying systolic and diastolic heart failure as well as the latest advances in understanding the mechanisms of the cardiorenal syndrome. Ensuing chapter deals with practical guidance on the use of Doppler echocardiography as the most readily imaging tool to diagnose and monitor heart failure. Furthermore, clinical and pragmatic guidance on the methodical approach to a heart failure patient in the era of evidence-based guidelines is presented. The practical, evidence-based management of atrial fibrillation and life-threatening ventricular arrhythmias is further addressed in Part II. This part also provides with an up-to-date review of cardiac resynchronization therapy focusing on the cellular and molecular mechanisms underlying its improvements. In addition, the chapter on telemonitoring and sensor technologies gives a glimpse on their potential in the ambulatory management and therapeutic tailoring of the heart failure patient. Part III unravels issues related to the role of valvular or revascularization interventions. Mitral valve regurgitation in a heart failure is recognized as a novel "therapeutic target." Yet, the decision whether and how to intervene remains controversial. The contributors representing stakeholders of the multidisciplinary heart team including clinician, interventionalist, and surgeon will provide with a comprehensive views as well as pragmatic recommendations based on the available evidence and their respective clinical experience. This part will also reflect on the impact of recent clinical trials and controversies surrounding the surgical revascularization and ventricular reconstructive surgery. The final part is dedicated to end-stage heart failure. Cardiologists, intensive care physicians and surgeons share with the reader their opinion on the interventional and surgical management of acute or end-stage heart failure and emerging interventional techniques to reverse the vicious circle of heart failure progression. Readers will become familiar with the clinician-based immunosuppressive approach and management of the post-transplant patient. This part will also review current state-of-the-art in the mechanical support including the use of totally artificial heart as well as promise of novel cell-based interventions.

We want to express our deep gratitude and appreciation to all contributors who have done a commendable job in preparing their outstanding manuscripts. Their thoughtful, detailed, and yet pragmatic approach to each aspect of the heart failure syndrome enabled to reach a comprehensive synthesis of the truly multidisciplinary state-of-the-art management in the twenty-first century.

We wish to thank our many colleagues within the Cardiovascular Centre of the Onze Lieve Vrouw Hospital. Their wisdom and experience paralleled with a search for the continuous advances in patient-tailored management remain inspirational to us. This book is a "harvest" of the Aalst spirit uniquely merging excellence in clinical practice with patient-oriented clinical and translational research. We are also grateful to Mrs. Maggy Kuppens for her excellent and dedicated assistance in preparation of this book. Finally, we both remain indebted to our wives and children. Thanks to their unconditional support and patience, we keep expanding our professional horizons to better serve our patients.

It is our hope that with the current book the reader will be updated with the latest advances in the understanding, management, and treatment of heart failure integrating the multidisciplinary, interventional, and translational approach and yet emphasizing the need for the clinically relevant implementation in daily practice. *It is the patient not the syndrome that we should treat.*

This work has been granted by the Meijer Lavino Cardiac Research Foundation and Dirk Verheyden Fund.

Aalst, Belgium

Jozef Bartunek
Marc Vanderheyden

Contents

Contributors

Svend Aakhus Department of Cardiology and Institute for Surgical Research, Rikshospitalet, Oslo University Hospital, University of Oslo, Oslo, Norway

Jozef Bartunek Cardiovascular Centre, OLV Hospital, Aalst, Belgium

Atta Behfar Center for Regenerative Medicine and Division of Cardiovascular Diseases, Department of Medicine, Mayo Clinic, Rochester, MN, USA

Jerry Braun Department of Cardiothoracic Surgery, Leids Universitair Medisch Centrum, Leiden, The Netherlands

Dirk L. Brutsaert Center of Heart Failure and Cardiac Rehabilitation, AZ Middelheim, University of Antwerp, Antwerp, Belgium

Yong-Mei Cha Division of Cardiovascular Diseases, Department of Internal Medicine, Mayo Clinic College of Medicine, Rochester, MN, USA

Koen De Decker Department of Anesthesiology and Intensive Care, OLV Hospital, Aalst, Belgium

Marisa Di Donato Department Surgical and Medical Critical Care Medicine, University of Florence, Florence, Italy

Matthias Dupont Department of Cardiovascular Medicine, Heart and Vascular Institute, Cleveland Clinic, Cleveland, OH, USA

Caroline J.M. van Deursen Department of Physiology, Cardiovascular Research Institute Maastricht, University of Maastricht, Maastricht, The Netherlands

Martin Eisenberger Cardiovascular Centre, OLV Hospital, Aalst, Belgium

University of South Bohemia, Ceske Budejovice, Czech Republic

Mackram F. Eleid Division of Cardiovascular Diseases, Department of Internal Medicine, Mayo Clinic College of Medicine, Rochester, MN, USA

Peter Geelen Cardiovascular Centre, OLV Hospital, Aalst, Belgium

Marc Goethals Cardiovascular Centre, OLV Hospital, Aalst, Belgium

Roland Hetzer Deutsches Herzzentrum Berlin, Klinik Fur Herz-Thorax-und Gefäßchirurgie, Berlin, Germany

Gilles W. De Keulenaer Center of Heart Failure and Cardiac Rehabilitation, AZ Middelheim, University of Antwerp, Antwerp, Belgium

Robert J.M. Klautz Department of Cardiothoracic Surgery, Leids Universitair Medisch Centrum, Leiden, The Netherlands

Lars H. Lund Department of Medicine, Karolinska Institutet, Stockholm, Sweden

Department of Cardiology, Karolinska University Hospital, Stockholm, Sweden

David Messika-Zeitoun Department of Cardiology, AP-HP, Cardiovascular Division, Assistance Publique—Hôpitaux de Paris, Bichat Hospital, Paris, France

Wilfried Mullens Department of Cardiovascular Medicine, Heart and Vascular Institute, Cleveland Clinic, Cleveland, OH, USA

Lars B. van Middendorp Department of Physiology, Cardiovascular Research Institute Maastricht, University of Maastricht, Maastricht, The Netherlands

Anders Opdahl Department of Cardiology and Institute for Surgical Research, Rikshospitalet, Oslo University Hospital, University of Oslo, Oslo, Norway

Tom De Potter Cardiovascular Centre, OLV Hospital, Aalst, Belgium

Frits W. Prinzen Department of Physiology, Cardiovascular Research Institute Maastricht, University of Maastricht, Maastricht, The Netherlands

Martin Penicka Cardiovascular Centre, OLV Hospital, Aalst, Belgium

Frank Van Praet Department of Cardiovascular and Thoracic Surgery, OLV Hospital, Aalst, Belgium

Espen W. Remme Department of Cardiology and Institute for Surgical Research, Rikshospitalet, Oslo University Hospital, University of Oslo, Oslo, Norway

Vincent Segers Center of Heart Failure and Cardiac Rehabilitation, AZ Middelheim, University of Antwerp, Antwerp, Belgium

Win-Kuang Shen Division of Cardiovascular Diseases, Department of Internal Medicine, Mayo Clinic College of Medicine, Phoenix, AZ, USA

Helge Skulstad Department of Cardiology and Institute for Surgical Research, Rikshospitalet, Oslo University Hospital, University of Oslo, Oslo, Norway

Otto A. Smiseth Department of Cardiology and Institute for Surgical Research, Rikshospitalet, University of Oslo, Oslo University Hospital, Oslo, Norway

Christof Stamm Deutsches Herzzentrum Berlin, Klinik Fur Herz-Thorax-und Gefäßchirurgie, Berlin, Germany

Ivan Stankovic Department of Cardiovascular Diseases, University Hospital Gasthuisberg, Leuven, Belgium

W.H. Wilson Tang Department of Cardiovascular Medicine, Heart and Vascular Institute, Cleveland Clinic, Cleveland, OH, US

Andre Terzic Center for Regenerative Medicine and Division of Cardiovascular Diseases, Department of Medicine, Mayo Clinic, Rochester, MN, USA

Gabor Toth Cardiovascular Centre, OLV Hospital, Aalst, Belgium

Marc Vanderheyden Cardiovascular Centre, OLV Hospital, Aalst, Belgium

Sofie Verstreken Cardiovascular Centre, OLV Hospital, Aalst, Belgium

Jens-Uwe Voigt Department of Cardiovascular Diseases, University Hospital Gasthuisberg, Leuven, Belgium

Part I
Heart Failure: Back to Basics

Chapter 1
Pathophysiology of Heart Failure: Back to Basics

Gilles W. De Keulenaer, Vincent Segers, and Dirk L. Brutsaert

Abstract Basic mechanisms of chronic heart failure are reviewed. A central theme that cuts all the way through this review is that chronic heart failure is a problem of failing complexity, rather than a problem of the failure of a single unit (e.g., cell type) or processes (e.g., contractility). A brief paragraph introducing this central concept will precede the main text of this chapter.

Next, a definition of heart failure will be formulated, and the most common etiologies and symptoms of heart failure in clinical cardiology summarized. The progressive nature of chronic heart failure will then be described and its driving forces analyzed. Finally, indices of cardiac performance and heart failure will be summarized and placed into a conceptual frame. The chapter will end by scrutinizing the mechanisms of diastolic dysfunction and by formulating some future trends of heart failure research.

1 Introduction

Heart failure is a progressive clinical syndrome for which various definitions and pathophysiologic mechanisms have been proposed. Although cardiac pump dysfunction is an inherent pathophysiological mechanism of heart failure, many extracardiac dysfunctions contribute, especially when heart failure becomes chronic. Accordingly, in this multifactorial syndrome it is difficult to pinpoint the central pathophysiological mechanism. This complicates the introduction in heart failure of therapeutic strategies and of taxonomy, the latter being apparently attractive given the remarkable variability of how this syndrome clinically presents.

G.W. De Keulenaer (✉) • V. Segers • D.L. Brutsaert
Center of Heart Failure and Cardiac Rehabilitation, AZ Middelheim, University of Antwerp, Lindendreef 1, 2020 Antwerp, Belgium
e-mail: gilles.dekeulenaer@ua.ac.be

J. Bartunek and M. Vanderheyden (eds.), *Translational Approach to Heart Failure*, DOI 10.1007/978-1-4614-7345-9_1, © Springer Science+Business Media New York 2013

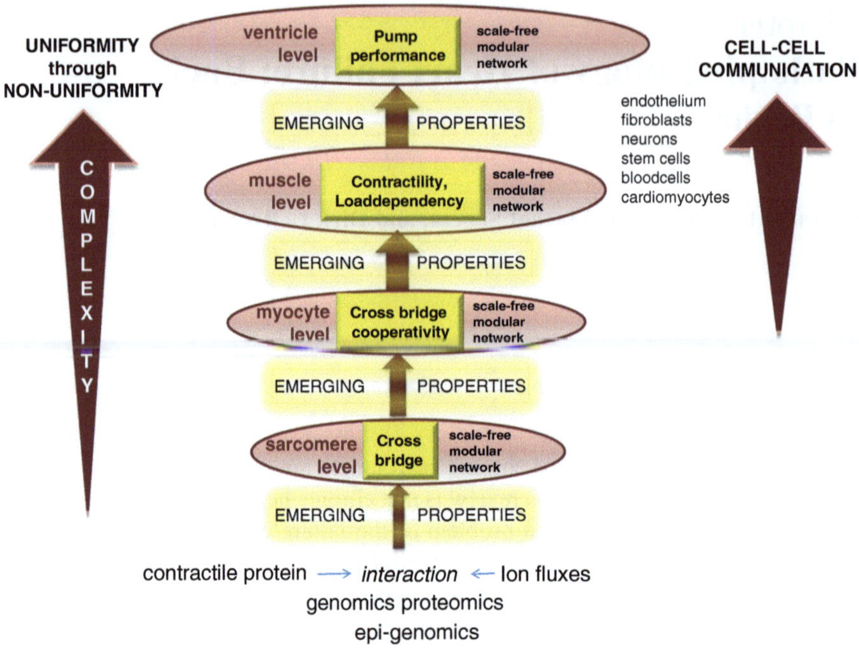

Fig. 1.1 The ventricle is a dissipative structure with emerging properties. Analogous to a dissipative structure, the heart grows as an ordered, self-organizing, optimizing pump, or super-system, through fluctuations, interactions and coherence of adjacent subsystems at each higher hierarchic scale, ranging from the subcellular modular networks (available through systems biology research) up to modular networks at the organ level and beyond. At each scale, emerging properties are added

Nevertheless, one may wonder what, if any, could be the central pathophysiologic aspect of heart failure? Could it be the maladaptive autoregulatory response upon ventricular dysfunction, involving hormones and paracrine factors, and the consecutive process of ventricular remodeling? Or should one perhaps look at lower structural/functional scales, e.g., impairment of cardiac muscle mechanical performance due either to failing excitation-contraction-relaxation coupling, or to disturbed cross-bridge cycling? Alternatively, could it be the repercussion of left ventricular dysfunction on the periphery including atria, the pulmonary circulation, the right ventricle, the kidneys, and skeletal muscles? Which of these phenomena is the most crucial, pernicious, irreversible?

These questions have no single answer as heart failure is the failure of a complex system; failure of a complex system cannot be reduced to the failure of a single process. The ventricle itself is a complex system, which means that its properties follow the scientific rules of complexity. These rules are characterized by mathematic phenomena like nonlinearity and self-organization, which provide the ventricle with all the properties of a "dissipative structure" [1–3]. This means that the ventricle behaves as a dynamic and self-organizing structure with emerging properties at each higher hierarchical scale of performance (Fig. 1.1).

From this perspective, *ventricular dysfunction and the heart failure syndrome are problems of failing complexity rather than the sum of failures of one or more components of the cardiovascular system.*

Application of scientific principles of "complex system behavior and failure" to the syndrome of chronic heart failure is unfortunately only in its infancy [4]. Heart failure is often described and subdivided from within a narrow oversimplified perspective, i.e., a single gene or gene product, a single cell type (e.g., the cardiomyocyte), a single parameter (e.g., left ventricular ejection fraction (LVEF)), a single functional aspect (e.g., contractility, filling), a single organ (e.g., the heart). In the next chapter, we discuss the pathophysiology of chronic heart failure avoiding the bias to such a narrow perspective. We also address some future perspectives and the need of introducing complex systems biology in the analysis of chronic heart failure.

2 Main Text

2.1 *Definition and Pathophysiology of Heart Failure*

Heart failure is a complex clinical syndrome characterized by fatigue and tissue congestion related to cardiac pump dysfunction. Cardiac pump dysfunction in heart failure may either impart impaired ventricular filling (predominantly diastolic pump dysfunction/failure) or impaired ventricular output (predominantly systolic pump dysfunction/failure), but it almost always consists of a combination of both impairments. There is currently insufficient evidence to subdivide heart failure in pathophysiological entities based on whether a diastolic or systolic impairment dominates, although this issue is currently still under debate [1, 5]. Subdivision of heart failure in distinct entities based on systolic/diastolic function ("systolic" and "diastolic" heart failure) is complicated by the fact that systolic and diastolic dysfunction nearly always coexist, that ventricular contraction and relaxation are physiologically coupled, and that there is no single criterion to precisely define a systolic or diastolic heart failure sub-entity. Most if not all heart failure indices show mere quantitative variations along the wide spectrum between predominantly concentric ("diastolic" heart failure) and eccentric ("systolic" heart failure) hypertrophy, and often follow a continuous linear relation when plotted against the patient's corresponding LVEF (Fig. 1.2) [6–9]. Cut-off values of these indices to introduce distinct heart failure sub-entities have been arbitrary. Hence, the connotations "diastolic" and "systolic" heart failure, or heart failure with a preserved (HFPEF) or reduced ejection fraction (HFREF), may have practical advantages in daily clinical medicine, but lack a conceptual basis.

Accordingly, heart failure emerges as a heterogeneous, but undividable spectrum of numerous overlapping phenotypes. Hence, at least from a pathophysiological

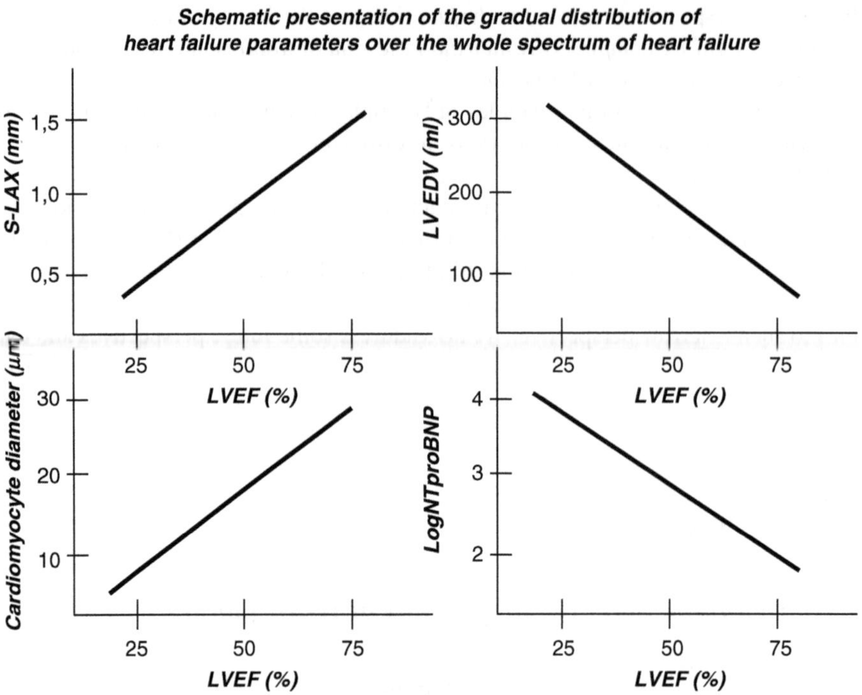

Fig. 1.2 Schematic presentation of the gradual distribution of heart failure parameters of the whole spectrum of disease. Opposite to a binary view on heart failure, most parameters of heart failure do not cluster in two groups ("low" and "high") when plotted against left ventricular ejection fraction (LVEF). Instead, they follow an uninterrupted linear relation over the whole spectrum of the syndrome (from low to high LVEF). *S-LAX* systolic long axis displacement of the mitral annulus, *LV EDV* left ventricular end diastolic volume, *LogNTproBNP* logarithm of the serum concentration of N-terminal brain natriuretic peptide. See text for references

perspective, it is artificial to subdivide heart failure in distinct disease entities. Heart failure's heterogeneity (e.g., forward and backward failure, systolic and diastolic failure, right and left ventricular failure) may, however, be accompanied by wide variations in prognosis and clinical responses to therapeutic (pharmacological and non-pharmacological) interventions. Thus, in daily clinical practice, medical management of heart failure should be individualized based on the specific phenotypic characteristics of the patient and the stage of the syndrome.

Key Points

- From a pathophysiological perspective chronic heart failure emerges as a heterogeneous, but individable spectrum of overlapping phenotypes.
- Surviving heart failure phenotypes in 2 or more so-called "disease entities" such as "HFNEF" and "HFPEF," "systolic" and "diastolic" heart failure, or "isch-

Table 1.1 Causes of heart failure

1. Cardiomyopathies
(a) Ischemic heart disease (infarction, stunning, hibernation)
(b) Genetic cardiomyopathy (dilated and hypertrophic)
(c) Infectious/inflammatory cardiomyopathy
(d) Metabolic cardiomyopathy (e.g., obesity, diabetes)
(e) Toxic cardiomyopathy (e.g., cancer drugs)
(f) Infiltrative cardiomyopathy (e.g., amyloidosis)
2. Myocardial overload
(a) Pressure overload (e.g., hypertension, aortic stenosis)
(b) Volume overload (e.g., mitral/aortic regurgitation)
3. Pericardial diseases
(a) Constrictive pericarditis
(b) Pericardial effusions (tamponade)
4. Electrical abnormalities
(a) Dyssynchrony
(b) Bradycardias
(c) Tachycardias

emic" and "non-ischemic" cardiomyopathy may have some clinical advantages in current clinical medicine, but this should be done carefully, and should never dominate pathophysiological research.

2.2 *Etiology of Heart Failure*

Heart failure may be the end stage of all forms of cardiovascular disease, and of many different risk factors, contributing to the heterogeneity of the syndrome. The causes of cardiac dysfunction leading to heart failure may be subdivided into whether they directly affect myocardial or ventricular function (e.g., ischemia, toxicity, gene dysfunction, metabolic dysfunction) or place an abnormal load on the myocardium (volume of pressure overload), resulting in impairment of ventricular function (Table 1.1). In most instances, the mechanisms of progression from cardiac insult to cardiac dysfunction and finally to the full-blown syndrome of heart failure are not well understood. *These mechanisms clearly surpass the structural and functional changes of the left ventricle and also involve a complex interaction of neuroendocrine, vascular, and other noncardiac processes.* Importantly, most currently available therapies of chronic heart failure target neuroendocrine and vascular processes, rather than the structural and functional changes of the ventricle per se. The complexity of pathophysiological processes in chronic heart failure seems common to most if not all causes of heart failure and contributes to the progressive character of the syndrome, to advancing symptoms and to premature death.

Key Point

- A list of etiological factors of heart failure in clinical cardiology is provided.

2.3 Symptoms of Heart Failure and Causes of Death

The major signs and symptoms of chronic heart failure are fatigue, exercise intolerance, breathlessness, and tissue edema. They may remain absent for a long period during disease development despite dysfunction of the heart first as a muscular and even as a hemodynamic pump. Once they develop, they may be present in different degrees and combinations. Consistent with the complexity of the heart failure syndrome, the origin of these signs and symptoms cannot linearly be explained by a single mechanism, although they somehow originate from dysfunction of the heart. Symptoms and signs of heart failure are the result of a combination of both cardiac and extra-cardiac dysfunctions of chronic heart failure.

Fatigue, particularly during exercise, is a common presenting symptom of chronic heart failure. It is often difficult to distinguish from breathlessness. The mechanism of fatigue is complex and poorly understood [10]; it clearly surpasses failure of the left ventricle as a hemodynamic pump (as it correlates poorly with LVEF). Impaired cardiac chronotropic reserve [11], muscle blood flow, deficient endothelial function [12], and disordered skeletal muscle structure and function have been involved [13].

Breathlessness is equally complex and poorly understood. It also surpasses mechanisms related to dysfunction of the ventricle as a muscular and hemodynamic pump; some studies showed correlations with left ventricular diastolic function, whereas other didn't [14]. Other heart failure-related, but extra-cardiac mechanisms, likely play a role including an exaggerated ventilatory response to exercise, resulting in an abnormally steep VE/VCO2 slope [15].

Tissue edema is related to the retention of salt and water in the kidneys, which on its turn is related to the activation of the renin-angiotensin-aldosteron system (RAAS), rather than to intrinsic dysfunction of the kidneys. To what extent RAAS activation is related to reduction in renal blood flow is, however, unclear.

Key Point

- Symptoms and signs of heart failure are not explained by dysfunction of a single process, but are the result of a complex interplay of mechanisms, both cardiac and extra-cardiac.

2.4 Progression of Chronic Heart Failure: Pathophysiology and Therapeutic Targets

The progressive nature of chronic heart failure has been the subject of intense research. Usually, its progression is explained by the vicious circle paradigm in which

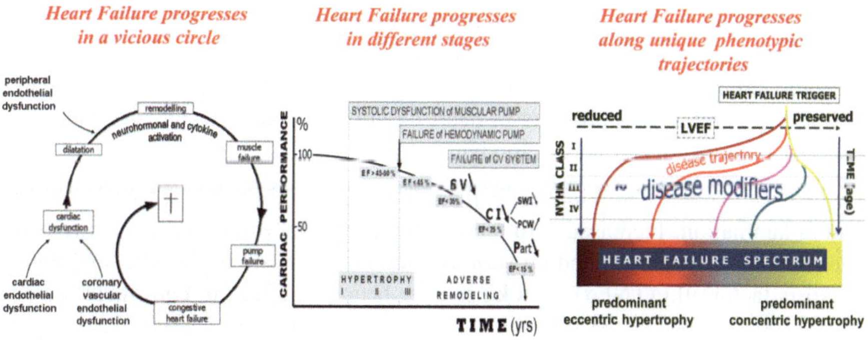

Fig. 1.3 Heart failure is a progressive disease. Each of the figures highlights a different aspect of the progression. In the vicious circle paradigm of heart failure (*left*), the pernicious, progressive, and irreversible character is emphasized as propelled by endothelial dysfunction, (mal) adaptive activation of neurohormones and cytokines. In the *middle* figure, the progressive nature of heart failure is equally emphasized, but focus is on the consecutive stages of failing cardiac performance, i.e., failure of the heart first as a muscular suction pump, then as a hemodynamic compression pump and finally of the whole cardiovascular system, with drop in stroke volume (SV), cardiac index (CI), and eventually of arterial blood pressure (Part). The spectrum paradigm of heart failure (*right*) visualizes how during heart failure progression each patient follows a unique disease trajectory. The trajectories depend on the relative contribution of the patient's traits and comorbidities (coined disease modifiers), are thus patient-specific, and hence create a spectrum of phenotypes throughout the entire population of heart failure patients

driving forces including hemodynamic disturbances, neurohormones, cytokines, and endothelial activation/dysfunction lead to successive failure of the heart as a muscular pump and hemodynamic pump, finally of the whole circulatory system. Within these progression, each patient follows its unique disease trajectory, in which LVEF remains preserved or gradually drops while symptoms develop (Fig. 1.3).

Hemodynamic disturbances. Ventricular pressure and volume overload (either directly related to the cause of heart failure, or indirectly induced by renal sodium/water retention and neurohormone-mediated vasoconstriction of arterioles) undoubtedly contribute to the progress of ventricular remodeling and heart failure, at least partly through effects of Laplace's law on ventricular wall stress. Therapeutic interventions aimed at reducing hemodynamic disturbances in heart failure (positive inotropes, diuretics, vasodilators) may reduce symptoms of heart failure. Their effects on mortality due to heart failure have, however, been disappointing [16–18].

Neurohormonal activation. Increased activity of the RAAS and of the symptathetic nervous system as well as activation of a wide variety of circulating and tissue hormonal systems are characteristic of the heart failure syndrome. These systems contribute importantly to the progression of ventricular remodeling and heart failure.

Therapeutic interventions aimed at reducing the activity of these systems (angiotensin converting enzyme inhibitors, angiotensin type I receptor antagonists, beta-1 receptor antagonists, and aldosterone receptor antagonists) have systematically reduced symptoms and mortality of heart failure, sometimes despite (temporarily) exacerbating the concomitant hemodynamic disturbances [19–22].

Cytokine activation. Cytokines are cell products released in response to tissue injury and inflammation. Increased serum concentrations of several cytokines have been shown in heart failure, including various interleukins (IL-6, IL-33, etc.) and tumor necrosis factor alfa (TNFα). Cytokines have been postulated to contribute to ventricular remodeling, but also to skeletal muscle wasting and cachexia. Therapeutic interventions directly targeting the effects of cytokines in heart failure have, however, not resulted in improved outcomes [23].

Endothelial activation/dysfunction. The endothelium in heart and vessels releases a number of local factors, both in rest and in response to a variety of stimuli, that exert effects on contractility, relaxation, passive stiffness, electrophysiology, survival and growth of cardiac and vascular cells [24]. In heart failure, the release of some of these factors is impaired, like nitric oxide, whereas the release of others is increased, like endothelin-1. Therapeutic interventions directly restoring the activity of one or more of these endothelial factors in heart failure have not yet resulted in a long-term survival benefit. There are promising preliminary data, however, with a recently discovered endothelial factor, neuregulin-1, which exerts cardioprotective and cardioregenerative effects [25]. Long-term studies still have to be performed.

Left ventricular remodeling. Although surpassing cardiac abnormalities, one of the key features of the heart failure syndrome is the pernicious process of cardiac remodeling (Fig. 1.4). This process is characterized by a progressive change in shape, volume, and muscle mass of the left ventricle, often accompanied by changes in shape and volume of the left atrium. Although ventricular remodeling is often assigned to be either eccentric (when left ventricular end diastolic volume increases) or concentric (when left ventricular walls thicken), eccentric and concentric remodeling often coexist, indicating that heart failure cannot be dichotomized into two distinct disease entities based on the ventricle's type of remodeling and its pathological architecture. *Ventricular dilatation* during cardiac remodeling has a potential hemodynamic advantage by preserving stroke volume without increasing contractility, but the disadvantage of this process is that it also augments ventricular wall stress (as defined by Laplace's law). Increased wall stress increases myocardial oxygen consumption and reprograms myocardial gene expression. *Ventricular wall thickening* has the advantage or normalizing wall stress when overcoming pressure overload, but it has the disadvantage of disturbing the relation between myocytes and microcapillaries [26]. Hence, ideally for a long term survival of chronic heart failure, a balanced spectrum of remodeling may be essential.

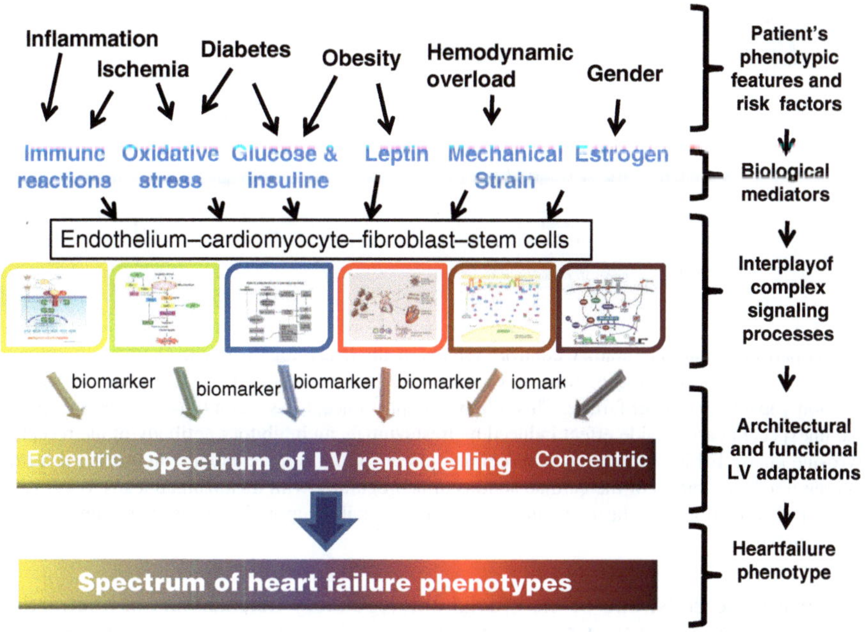

Fig. 1.4 Left ventricular remodeling results in a spectrum of cardiac phenotypes. Left ventricular remodeling is the result of an interplay of many complex processes in cardiac cells (endothelial cells, cardiomyocytes, fibroblasts, …). These processes are dependent on many mediators (reactive oxygen species, hyperglycemia, neurohormones, mechanical strain, sex hormones, etc.) whose contribution is dependent on the patient's phenotype and risk factors (e.g., gender, diabetes, coronary failure, and body mass index). Some mediators promote concentric remodeling (e.g., estrogens, leptin) whereas other promote eccentric remodeling (ischemia; inflammation, etc.). The relative contribution of each of the processes is unique for each patient, leading to a spectrum of cardiac phenotypes when a large group of patients is considered

Ventricular remodeling is the result of multiple interacting complex signaling processes, the contribution of which is linked to the patient's biological traits and comorbidities. Some of these signaling processes are linked to coronary failure, myocardial infection, or type 1 diabetes mellitus; these promote predominantly eccentric remodeling. Others, such as type 2 diabetes mellitus, obesity, hypertension, and female gender, instead tend to promote concentric remodeling [27–32]. The complex signaling processes triggered by each of the disease modifiers separately (or of their mediators, such as leptin, ischemia, hyperinsulinemia, and estrogen) are under intense investigation. In vivo, these complex signaling processes merge in qualitative and quantitative combinations, specific for each patient and leading to a spectrum of overlapping profiles of ventricular remodeling.

The cellular and subcellular processes during cardiac remodeling are extremely complex. Changes occur at the level of individual cardiomyocytes, fibroblasts, endothelial cells, purkinje fibers and cardiac stem cells, and also the communication

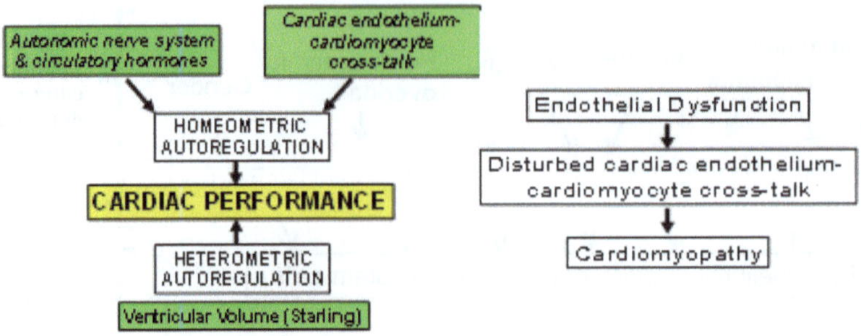

Fig. 1.5 Autoregulatory control systems of the heart. Cardiac endothelium-cardiomyocyte cross-talk is part of the autoregulatory control systems of the heart, together with the neurohormonal system and the Starling mechanism. Accordingly, cardiac endothelium dysfunction may lead to cardiomyopathy and heart failure. This relative simple concept has recently been underscored by the unexpected cardiac side effect induced by trastuzumab, an inhibitory antibody of the receptor tyrosine kinase ErbB2, which mediates cellular effects of the cardiac endothelium-derived factor neuregulin-1. Inhibition of the cardiac actions of neuregulin-1 with trastuzumab leads to left ventricular dysfunction and heart failure, which is reversible upon interrupting treatment with trastuzumab

between these cells, one of the crucial autoregulatory mechanisms of ventricular function is affected (Fig. 1.5) [33]. *Cardiomyocytes* undergo growth and apoptosis and receptor-signaling pathways of numerous hormonal and paracrine growth and survival factors (such as angiotensin II, endothelin-1, interleukin-6, IGF-1, and neuregulin-1) in the myocytes are activated. Essential myocyte functions like excitation-contraction-relaxation coupling [34] and adrenergic responsiveness [35] are disturbed. *Fibroblast* collagen synthesis is activated, but the release of enzymes for collagen degradation is also increased. Angiogenesis, controlled by *endothelial cells*, becomes impaired in the failing heart, contributing to maladaptive hypertrophy and transition to failure [26].

Cardiomyocyte renewal. The classical view on myocardial turnover and regeneration has been that cardiomyocytes are terminally differentiated cells and that no new cardiomyocytes are formed during adult life. This classical view has been challenged by recent data showing that new myocytes are formed during adulthood, both during normal aging and after myocardial injury. However, renewal of cardiomyocytes either by stem cells or cardiomyocyte division seems to be insufficient to repair myocardium and prevent heart failure after myocardial infarction. Stem cell biology has only recently been incorporated into the study of heart failure, and evidence of stem cell dysfunction as a part of heart failure pathophysiology is mounting. Development and progression of heart failure could be due in part to failure of cardiac stem cells; strategies that are focused on stem cell dysfunction might become available as a therapy in the future [36].

Key Points

- Chronic heart failure has a progressive nature, the mechanisms of which are still under investigation. Its driving forces provide therapeutic targets.

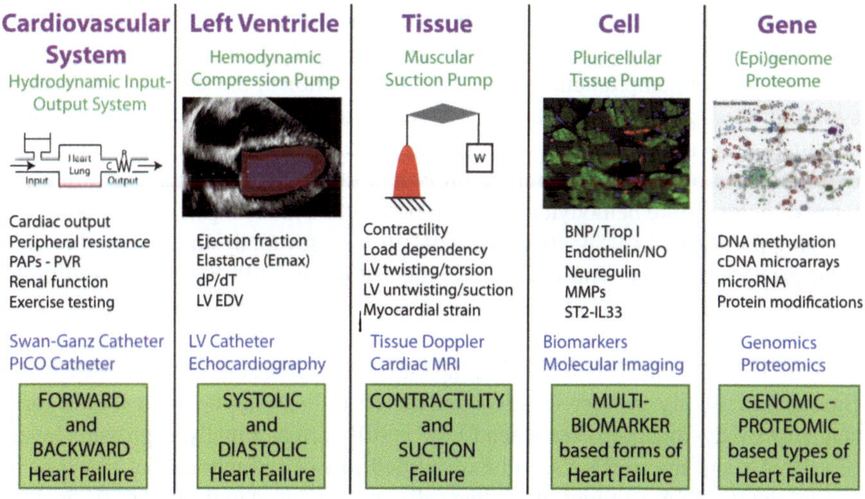

Fig. 1.6 Conceptual approaches to cardiac performance. The ventricle can be considered as part of a hydraulic input–output system with the ventricle as a *black box* (organism panel), as a hemodynamic compression pump with the cardiomyocytes as a *black box* (organ panel), as a muscular suction pump with the non-cardiomyocytes as a *black box* (tissue panel), as a pluricellular tissue pump with genes and proteins as *black box* (cell panel) or as the product of the individual's genome, epigenome, and proteome (gene panel). Within each panel-specific approach to cardiac performance, different phenotypes of heart failure can be proposed (forward and backward failure, systolic and diastolic heart failure, contractility and suction failure, multi-biomarker-based forms of heart failure, and perhaps in the future genomic-proteomic-based types of heart failure). While recording variables of cardiac function, they should be placed in their correct conceptual frame. *LV EDV* left ventricular end diastolic volume; *LA* left atrium, *BNP* brain natriuretic peptide, *TGF* tissue growth factor, *CRP* C-reactive protein, *MMP* matrix metallo-proteinase, *Tn-I* troponin-I, *SNP* single nucleotide polymorphism, *GWAS* genome wide association study

- Progression of heart failure is accompanied by structural and functional changes of the heart ("ventricular remodeling"), which result from multiple and interacting signaling processes.

2.5 *How to Measure Cardiac Performance in Heart Failure and Characterize the Syndrome?*

Diagnosis and follow-up of heart failure requires assessment of cardiac performance. Cardiac performance can be assessed at many different levels of the heart's functional complexity (Fig. 1.6), providing many possible performance indices and heart failure variables. Variables of heart failure may fit in a general circulatory context, like blood pressure and peripheral/pulmonary vascular resistance, which often receive large attention in the clinical setting of acute cardiac failure and circulatory shock. They do not reliably reflect the function of the pump, however, since they can be normal in advanced stages of pump dysfunction.

Parameters of pump function may reflect the function of the left ventricle (LV) as a *hemodynamic pump* (e.g., LVEF and LV end systolic elastance) or they may reflect the function of the LV as a *muscular pump* (e.g., myocardial segment strain, (un) twisting velocities). This differentiation is important since in some stages/phenotypes of heart failure hemodynamic pump parameters are still preserved, giving the false impression that LV function is normal, despite severe dysfunction of the muscular properties of the ventricle (e.g., in the setting of HFPEF, or in the setting of "low gradient aortic valve stenosis and a normal LVEF"). Next, serum biomarkers such as serum natriuretic peptides, metallo-proteinases, endothelin-1, and neuregulin-1 are indices of heart failure reflecting (secretory) processes of myocardial cells. Biomarkers usually are very sensitive parameters of heart failure, increased in early stages of LV dysfunction, even when LVEF is still normal. Finally, expression levels of mRNA's and micro-RNA's, to be quantified in isolated myocardial tissue or in serum, reflect DNA activities of cardiac cells and may used in the diagnosis or staging of heart failure, although this is still experimental to date.

Recording these variables of cardiac performance and heart failure gives a reliable picture of the severity and the stage of the disease in an individual patient. For example, measuring increased levels of serum natriuretic peptides, reduced left ventricular untwisting velocities but a normal LVEF indicates that heart failure has progressed up to the stage of dysfunction of the muscular pump, but that performance of the heart at a higher hierarchic level is still intact (often due to activation of compensatory processes which optimize the function of the hemodynamic pump, despite dysfunction of the heart at the level of the cardiac muscle and lower levels of complexity).

Interestingly, within each hierarchic level of cardiac dysfunction, different "clinical phenotypes" of the heart failure syndrome can be identified, which refers to with the above mentioned clinical heterogeneity of the syndrome. For example, when heart failure has progressed up to the most severe stage, i.e., failure of the heart as a hydrodynamic input–output system, it may clinically present as *forward or backward heart failure*. Similarly, when heart failure has progressed up to the level of the hemodynamic pump clinical phenotypes of predominant *systolic or diastolic heart failure* may be differentiated. Currently, there are attempts to define heart failure subtypes based on a *multi-biomarker panel*. None of these "phenotypes" of heart failure should be viewed as a distinct disease entity. They are mere variant clinical presentations in a spectrum of heterogeneous phenotypes, to which therapeutic interventions should be tailored.

Key Point

- All indices of cardiac performance and failure fall within a specific conceptual approach to cardiac performance.

2.6 Diastolic Dysfunction

Most if not all forms of heart failure, independently of LVEF, display a certain degree of diastolic dysfunction. In fact, in many clinical condition, i.p. ischemic heart disease and hypertrophic cardiomyopathy, relaxation and filling abnormalities occur long before contraction and ejection abnormalities.

Although often subject of misinterpretation, at least from the perspective of the heart as muscular pump, "true" diastole of the ventricle only starts after early rapid ventricular filling, and hence encompasses diastasis and the atrial contraction phase. Pressure fall during isovolumic relaxation in the pump (that fully completes at end systolic volumes) and the increase in pump volume during early rapid filling are strictu sensu still part of the contraction-relaxation cycle of the ventricular muscular "systole." Diastolic failure then refers to a disease process that shifts the end portion of the pressure–volume diagram inappropriately upward so that LV filling pressures are increased dysproportionally to the magnitude of LV dilatation (Fig. 1.7). The causes of such a shift can be subdivided into (Table 1.2):

1. Decrease in ventricular diastolic compliance (i.e., true diastolic failure)
2. Slow ventricular systolic relaxation (i.e., diastolic failure secondary to impaired systolic function of the muscular pump)
3. Inappropriate tachycardia (e.g., transient atrial fibrillation, supraventricular tachy-arrythmias) (i.e., diastolic failure secondary to inappropriate abbreviation of diastolic duration)
4. A combination of a, b, and c, as is usually the case.

Causes of impaired relaxation and/or compliance can be divided into (1) Factors intrinsic to the cardiomyocyte, (2) factors within the extracellular matrix (ECM) that surrounds the cardiomyocytes, and (3) factors that activate the production of neurohormones and paracrine substances.

Cardiomyocyte. Elements and processes intrinsic to the cardiomyocyte contributing to diastolic (dys)function have been summarized in Table 1.2. In general they relate to processes responsible for calcium removal from the myocyte cytosol (calcium homeostasis), to processes involved in cross-bridge detachment and to cytoskeletal functional elements. Changes in any of the processes and elements can lead to abnormalities in both active relaxation and passive stiffness.

1. *Calcium homeostasis.* Abnormal activity of SERCA2 has been implicated in the impaired relaxation in heart failure. SERCA2 activity declines in LV hypertrophy and heart failure by reduced gene and protein expression and by reduced phosphorylation of its inhibitory modulatory protein phospholamban (PLB) [37–40]. Conversely, experimental gene transfer with SERCA2a or a negative PLB mutant improves relaxation [41, 42]. It is as yet unclear at which stages of chronic heart failure SERCA2 activity becomes affected [43]. By all means, impaired SERCA2 activity is certainly not specific for HFPEF, as it will become more pronounced when global pump performance is reduced [37].

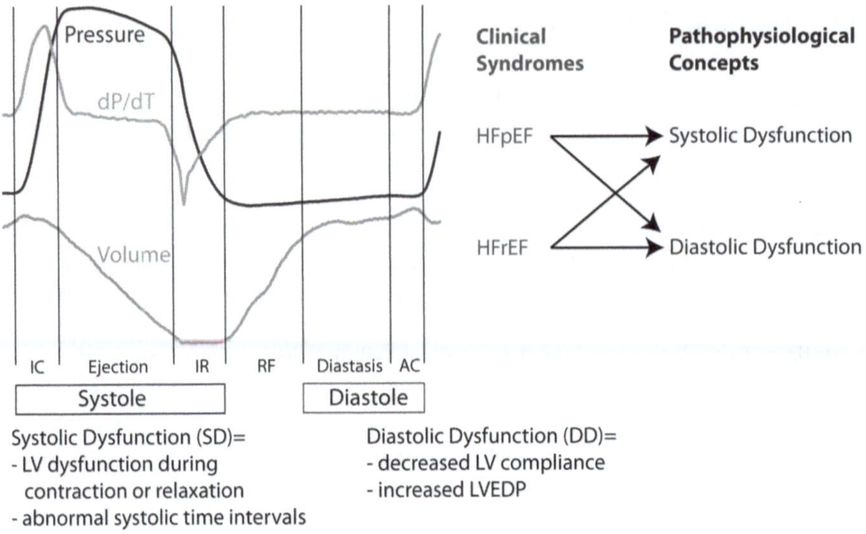

Fig. 1.7 Subdivision of the cardiac cycle from the perspective of the heart as a muscular pump. Taking into account that the heart is a muscle, "true" diastole of the ventricle only starts after early rapid ventricular filling, and hence encompasses diastasis and the atrial contraction phase. At normal rest heart rates, diastole usually lasts for approximately 50 % of the total time duration of the cardiac cycle. Pressure fall during isovolumic relaxation in the pump (that fully completes at end systolic volumes) and the increase in pump volume during early rapid filling are strictu sensu still part of the contraction-relaxation cycle of the ventricular muscular "systole." Diastolic failure then refers to a disease process that shifts the end portion of the pressure–volume diagram inappropriately upward so that LV filling pressures are increased dysproportionally to the magnitude of LV dilatation

Table 1.2 Mechanisms of diastolic dysfunction

Mechanisms of diastolic dysfunction

Inappropriate tachycardia	Impaired Load Dependence of Relaxation	Ventriculo-Arterial stiffening
Intermittent atrial fibrillation; atrial tachyarrhythmias	**- Excessive Load** ▪pressure-volume overload **- Impaired Inactivation** ▪calcium homeostasis ✓calcium overload ✓calcium transport (sarcolemma, SR) ✓modifying proteins (phospholamban, calmodulin) ▪myofilaments ✓Tn-C calcium binding ✓Tn-I phosphorylation ✓myofilament calcium sensitivity ✓Myosin Binding Protein C ▪energetics ✓ADP/ATP ratio ✓ADP and Pi concentration **- Excessive Non-uniformity of load or inactivation in space or time** **- Abnormal activity of RAAS, OS, ANP/BNP, cardiac endothelial system**	INTRACARDIAC: *Hypertrophy* **- Cytoskeletal abnormalities** ▪microtubules (tubulin) ▪intermediates filaments (desmin) ▪**Increased N2B/N2BA titin** ▪Nebuline **- Extracellular matrix** ▪fibrillar collagen ▪basement membrane proteins ▪proteoglycans ▪MMP/TIMP **- Abnormal activity of cardiac endothelial system (especially NO)** EXTRACARDIAL: *Arterial Stiffening* (reflected waves)

2. *Cross-bridge detachments*. Impaired relaxation and increased ventricular stiffness may result from slow or incomplete cross-bridge detachment.

   Abnormal cross-bridge detachment may result from reduced cAMP or cGMP-mediated phosphorylation of troponin-I, which increases calcium sensitivity of the myofibrils to calcium. Relaxation may also be impaired by alterations in the thick myofilaments as observed in genetic animal models [44], but whether this contributes to the development of relaxation disturbances in human heart failure is, however, still unknown.

   Cross-bridge detachment can also be disturbed by perturbations in loading (preload and afterload). Enhanced preload delays onset and rate of relaxation, an effect that may become particularly relevant during beta-adrenergic stimulation as the lusitropic effects of adrenergic stimulation in tachycardia may become blocked by this mechanism [45, 46]. Effects of loading on the timing and rate of relaxation are complex, and dependent on the timing of load [47, 48]. The importance of inappropriate loading has been reemphasized in studies demonstrating abnormal ventricular–arterial interaction due to a disproportionate cardiovascular stiffening in patient with HFPEF. Stiffening-induced imbalances of the ventricular–arterial load may exacerbate systemic afterload, i.e., arterial impedance and reflected waves, and hence affect onset and rate of LV relaxation [49].
3. *Cytoskeletal abnormalities*. Proteins within the sarcomere, other than the myofibrils that generate active force, contribute substantially to the stiffness of the cardiac muscle over the normal range of the sarcomere length (<2.2 μm). These molecules include titin, tubulin, and desmin, but most of the elastic force of the sarcomere is thought to reside in titin [50]. Interestingly, titin is subject of intense regulation, including isoform switching, calcium binding and phosphorylation, indicating that myocardial resting tension can be dynamically regulated.

   The two titin isoforms (N2B and N2BA) differ substantially in length and stiffness, with the N2B isoform being small and stiff. The distribution of these isoforms differs among species, heart chambers and disease states, and seems to track the corresponding variations in diastolic muscle stiffness [51]. Recent observations indicate that phosphorylation of titin may reverse the increased stiffness of cardiomyocytes in heart failure [52].

ECM. Changes in the structures within the ECM can also affect diastolic function (Fig. 1.2). The myocardial ECM is composed of three important constituents: (1) fibrillar protein, such as collagen type I, type III and elastin; (2) proteoglycans; and (3) basement membrane protein such as collagen type IV, laminin and fibronectin. It has been hypothesized that the most important component within the ECM that contributes to the development of diastolic dysfunction is fibrillar collagen (amount, geometry, distribution (especially as perimysial fibers), degree of cross-linking, ratio of collagen type I to III) [52–54]. Collagen synthesis is altered by load, both preload and afterload, by neurohormonal activation (e.g., the renin-angiotensin-aldosteron system- or RAAS—and the sympathic nervous systems), and by growth factors. Collagen degradation is under the control of proteolytic enzymes including matrix metallo-proteinases. Any change in the regulatory processes affecting collagen degradation and synthesis can thus alter diastolic function.

Several studies have made correlations between modifications of the collagen network and diastolic muscle stiffness, but usually with rather extreme collagen modifications only [54–56]. A direct linkage between fibrosis and stiffness is thus still controversial, especially since in some other studies, correlations between the amount of fibrosis and muscle stiffness was lacking. Hence, whether these inconsistencies point towards a role for the posttranslational structure of collagen rather than the amount of collagen, or instead indicate that titin plays a more important role than ECM in general, is still subject of debate [57].

Neurohormonal and cardiac endothelial activation. Both acutely and chronically, neurohormonal and cardiac endothelial activation and/or inhibition have been shown to alter diastolic function. Chronic activation of the RAAS has been shown to increase ECM fibrillar collagen. Inhibition of the RAAS prevents or reverses this increase. Generally but not consistently, these changes have been shown to affect ventricular stiffness. Acute activation of the cardiac endothelial system has been shown to alter relaxation and stiffness [58], most likely through the release of nitric oxide.

Key Points

- Diastolic dysfunction originates from a dysfunction at the level of cardiomyocytes, at the level of the ECM, or at the level of neurohormonal or paracrine systems.

3 Future Trends

Insights into the complex signaling cascades underlying ventricular remodeling and heart failure progression are rapidly expanding. Large-scale quantitative analyses of gene expression, including cDNA microarrays and proteomic analyses, have contributed to this progress. Interestingly, with each newly described cascade, novel biomarkers, and molecular targets for therapy emerge. There is a current trend to characterize and manage heart failure patients by the measurement of 1 or multiple biomarkers [59]. In clinical trials, this blind multimarker strategy may provide clinically useful and refreshing information. It surpasses patient selection based on LVEF alone. Moreover, it may personalize heart failure management and help to optimize current heart failure guidelines.

On the other hand, one may seriously question where this linear approach will eventually lead. It may be feared that adding still more biomarkers and other disease parameters in heart failure will never end, will add even more complexity and result in a reductionist search for perfection, and will fail to relaunch conceptual thinking about heart failure. Perhaps the time has come to envisage nonlinear integrative approaches already introduced in other fields of the life sciences that encounter

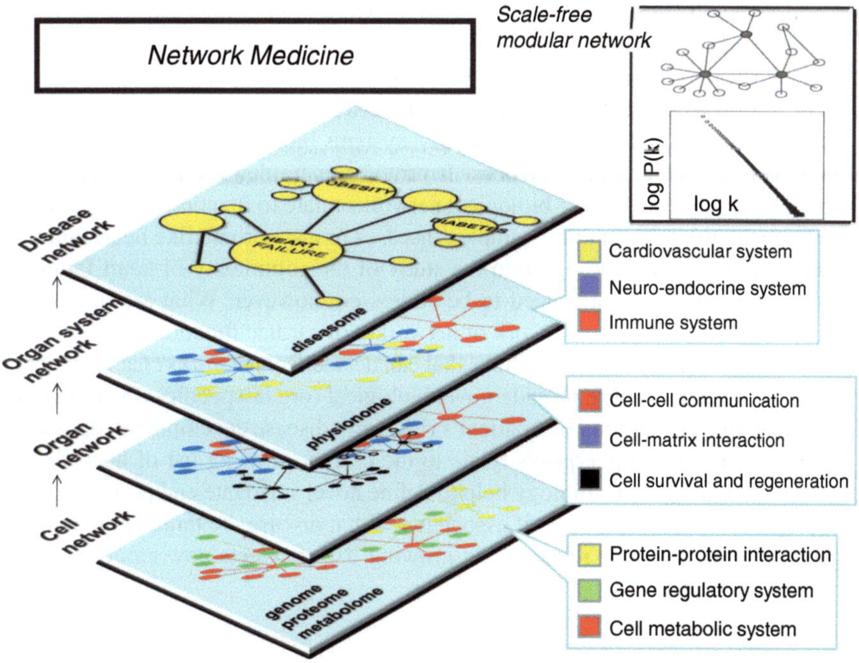

Fig. 1.8 Systems biology approach to medicine creates network medicine. Hypothetical scheme of network medicine with focus on the cardiovascular system and chronic heart failure. Biosciences are in transition from reductionist sciences to integrative sciences, i.e., a systems approach to biology. In this conceptually novel approach, physiology is not the result of traditional linear processes of structural and functional components (identified by genomic, proteomic, metabolomic sciences), but emerges from the interaction of scale-free modular biological networks composed by these components. Modular networks emerge at many different levels such as genes, transcripts, proteins, metabolites, organelles, cells, organs, and organ system

similar limits of reductionism and seek understanding from a myriad of validated bits of data [60].

Accordingly, life sciences, including heart failure sciences, encounter the limits inherent to linear reductionist approaches. Systems approaches to the complexity of the cardiovascular system are beginning to close this gap [4]. Systems biology seeks to provide a framework for the manner in which structural and functional components (as identified by, e.g., cDNA microarrays and proteomic analyses) interact in self-organizing modular biological networks. Networks, rather than the components themselves, create physiology and disease. Each node in a network represents a component (e.g., a gene, a transcript), and interconnecting nodes describe a typical architecture that is imposed by biological evolution and selection. Modular biological networks and clusters of interacting networks have been demonstrated to occur at different levels such as genes, transcripts, and proteins, but they probably also emerge at higher hierarchical levels, such as metabolites, organelles, cells, organs, and organ systems (Fig. 1.8). At each level, a network obtains new properties that are not predicted from the properties of the network at the lower level, referring to the aforementioned concept of emerging properties in a dissipative structure introduced by Prigogine and Strengers [3]. Hence, a network perspective to biology defines a disease as the failure of biological networks or as the failure to obtain a next-level emerging property. Accordingly, systems biology is not replacing but is complementing reductionist sciences. It provides a framework for analyzing the manner in which structures of biological networks relate to function. This process is a prerequisite to understanding complex diseases or a syndrome like heart failure.

Integrating systems biology into the study of the complexity of heart failure is timely. Many questions still need to be addressed, however. What are the crucial biological networks (in the network of networks) of cardiac function and heart failure, and where are the vulnerable hubs that can destabilize networks? Can a network perspective to heart failure provide novel biological (organ-specific) fingerprints of failure that allow prediction of a patient's risk, early disease development, or disease stage? How do these fingerprints relate to the current growing list of heart failure biomarkers? Can systems biology help to define novel surrogate end points for clinical trials? How can a network, if associated with a disease, be targeted pharmacologically? How does this relate to the growing list of targets now emerging from reductionist sciences?

References

1. De Keulenaer GW, Brutsaert DL (2011) Systolic and diastolic heart failure are overlapping phenotypes within the heart failure spectrum. Circulation 123:1996–2004
2. Brutsaert DL (2006) Cardiac dysfunction in heart failure: the cardiologist's love affair with time. Prog Cardiovasc Dis 49:157–181
3. Prigogine I, Strengers I (1979) La nouvelle alliance. Gallimard, Paris
4. Lusis AJ, Weiss JN (2010) Cardiovascular networks: systems-based approaches to cardiovascular disease. Circulation 121:157–170
5. Borlaug BA, Redfield MM (2011) Diastolic and systolic heart failure are distinct phenotypes within the heart failure spectrum. Circulation 123:2006–2013
6. Yip G, Wang M, Zhang Y, Fung JW, Ho PY, Sanderson JE (2002) Left ventricular long axis function in diastolic heart failure is reduced in both diastole and systole: time for a redefinition? Heart 87:121–125
7. De Keulenaer GW, Brutsaert DL (2009) The heart failure spectrum: time for a phenotype-oriented approach. Circulation 119:3044–3046
8. Chatterjee K, Massie B (2007) Systolic and diastolic heart failure: differences and similarities. J Card Fail 13:569–576
9. Januzzi JL, van Kimmenade R, Lainchbury J, Bayes-Genis A, Ordonez-Llanos J, Santalo-Bel M, Pinto YM, Richards M (2006) NT-proBNP testing for diagnosis and short-term prognosis in acute destabilized heart failure: an international pooled analysis of 1256 patients: the International Collaborative of NT-proBNP Study. Eur Heart J 27:330–337
10. Drexler H, Coats AJ (1996) Explaining fatigue in congestive heart failure. Annu Rev Med 47:241–256
11. Borlaug BA, Melenovsky V, Russell SD, Kessler K, Pacak K, Becker LC, Kass DA (2006) Impaired chronotropic and vasodilator reserves limit exercise capacity in patients with heart failure and a preserved ejection fraction. Circulation 14(114):2138–2147

12. Kubo SH, Rector TS, Bank AJ, Williams RE, Heifetz SM (1991) Endothelium-dependent vasodilation is attenuated in patients with heart failure. Circulation 84:1589–1596
13. Middlekauff HR (2010) Making the case for skeletal myopathy as the major limitation of exercise capacity in heart failure. Circ Heart Fail 3(4):537–546
14. Fukuta H, Little WC (2007) Contribution of systolic and diastolic abnormalities to heart failure with a normal and a reduced ejection fraction. Prog Cardiovasc Dis 49:229–240
15. Piepoli M, Clark AL, Volterrani M et al (1996) Contribution of muscle afferents to the hemodynamic, autonomic, and ventilatory responses to exercise in patients with chronic heart failure: effects of physical training. Circulation 93:940–952
16. Cohn JN, Archibald DG, Ziesche S, Franciosa JA, Harston WE, Tristani FE, Dunkman WB, Jacobs W, Francis GS, Flohr KH (1986) Effect of vasodilator therapy on mortality in chronic congestive heart failure. Results of a Veterans Administration Cooperative Study. N Engl J Med 314:1547–1552
17. DiBianco R, Shabetai R, Kostuk W, Moran J, Schlant RC, Wright R (1989) A comparison of oral milrinone, digoxin, and their combination in the treatment of patients with chronic heart failure. N Engl J Med 320(11):677–683
18. Packer M, Carver JR, Rodeheffer RJ, Ivanhoe RJ, DiBianco R, Zeldis SM, Hendrix GH, Bommer WJ, Elkayam U, Kukin ML (1991) Effect of oral milrinone on mortality in severe chronic heart failure. The PROMISE Study Research Group. N Engl J Med 325:1468–1475
19. The CONSENSUS Trial Study Group (1987) Effects of enalapril on mortality in severe congestive heart failure. Results of the Cooperative North Scandinavian Enalapril Survival Study (CONSENSUS). N Engl J Med 316(23):1429–1435
20. Cohn JN, Tognoni G, Valsartan Heart Failure Trial Investigators (2001) A randomized trial of the angiotensin-receptor blocker valsartan in chronic heart failure. N Engl J Med 345:1667–1675
21. Pitt B, Zannad F, Remme WJ, Cody R, Castaigne A, Perez A, Palensky J, Wittes J (1999) The effect of spironolactone on morbidity and mortality in patients with severe heart failure. Randomized Aldactone Evaluation Study Investigators. N Engl J Med 341:709–717
22. MERIT-HF Study Group (1999) Effects of metoprolol in chronic heart failure. Lancet 353:2001
23. Mann DL, McMurray JJ, Packer M, Swedberg K, Borer JS, Colucci WS, Djian J, Drexler H, Feldman A, Kober L, Krum H, Liu P, Nieminen M, Tavazzi L, van Veldhuisen DJ, Waldenstrom A, Warren M, Westheim A, Zannad F, Fleming T (2004) Targeted anticytokine therapy in patients with chronic heart failure: results of the randomized etanercept worldwide evaluation (RENEWAL). Circulation 109:1594–1602
24. Brutsaert DL (2003) Cardiac endothelial-myocardial signaling: its role in cardiac growth, contractile performance, and rhythmicity. Physiol Rev 83:59–115
25. Lemmens K, Doggen K, De Keulenaer GW (2007) Role of neuregulin-1/ErbB signaling in cardiovascular physiology and disease: implications for therapy of heart failure. Circulation 116:954–960
26. Tirziu D, Giordano FJ, Simons M (2010) Cell communications in the heart. Circulation 122:928–937
27. Piro M, Della Bona R, Abbate A, Biasucci LM, Crea F (2010) Sex-related differences in myocardial remodeling. J Am Coll Cardiol 55:1057–1065
28. Abel ED, Litwin SE, Sweeney G (2008) Cardiac remodeling in obesity. Physiol Rev 88:389–419
29. Cooper LT Jr (2009) Myocarditis. N Engl J Med 360:1526–1538
30. Turer AT, Hill JA (2010) Pathogenesis of myocardial ischemia-reperfusion injury and rationale for therapy. Am J Cardiol 106:360–368
31. Poornima IG, Parikh P, Shannon RP (2006) Diabetic cardiomyopathy: the search for a unifying hypothesis. Circ Res 98:596–605
32. Mudd J, Kass DA (2008) Tackling heart failure in the twenty-first century. Nature 451:919–928

33. De Keulenaer GW, Doggen K, Lemmens K (2010) The vulnerability of the heart as a pluricellular paracrine organ: lessons from unexpected triggers of heart failure in targeted ErbB2 anticancer therapy. Circ Res 106:35–46
34. Bers DM (2006) Altered cardiac myocyte Ca regulation in heart failure. Physiology (Bethesda) 21:380–387
35. Lefkowitz RJ, Rockman HA, Koch WJ (2000) Catecholamines, cardiac beta-adrenergic receptors, and heart failure. Circulation 101:1634–1637
36. Segers VF, Lee RT (2008) Stem-cell therapy for cardiac disease. Nature 451:937–942
37. Frank KF, Bolck B, Brixius K, Kranias EG, Schwinger RH (2002) Modulation of SERCA: implications for the failing human heart. Basic Res Cardiol 97(suppl 1):I72–I78
38. del Monte F, Harding SE, Dec GW, Gwathmey JK, Hajjar RJ (2002) Targeting phospholamban by gene transfer in human heart failure. Circulation 105:904–907
39. MacLennan DH, Kranias EG (2003) Phospholamban: a crucial regulator of cardiac contractility. Nat Rev Mol Cell Biol 4:566–577
40. Hasenfuss G, Pieske B (2002) Calcium cycling in congestive heart failure. J Mol Cell Cardiol 34:951–969
41. Miyamoto MI, del Monte F, Schmidt U, DiSalvo TS, Kang ZB, Matsui T, Guerrero JL, Gwathmey JK, Rosenzweig A, Hajjar RJ (2000) Adenoviral gene transfer of SERCA2a improves left-ventricular function in aortic-banded rats in transition to heart failure. Proc Natl Acad Sci U S A 97:793–798
42. Hoshijima M, Ikeda Y, Iwanaga Y, Minamisawa S, Date MO, Gu Y, Iwatate M, Li M, Wang L, Wilson JM, Wang Y, Ross J Jr, Chien KR (2002) Chronic suppression of heart-failure progression by a pseudophosphorylated mutant of phospholamban via in vivo cardiac rAAV gene delivery. Nat Med 8:864–871
43. Mercadier JJ (2000) Progression from cardiac hypertrophy to heart failure. In: Hosenpud D, Greenberg BH (eds) Congestive heart failure, 2nd edn. Lipincott Williams & Wilkins, Philadelphia, pp 83–100
44. Geisterfer-Lowrance AA, Christe M, Conner DA, Ingwall JS, Schoen FJ, Seidman CE, Seidman JG (1996) A mouse model of familial hypertrophic cardiomyopathy. Science 272:731–734
45. Paulus WJ, Bronzwaer JG, Felice H, Kishan N, Wellens F (1992) Deficient acceleration of left ventricular relaxation during exercise after heart transplantation. Circulation 86:1175–1185
46. Vantrimpont PJ, Felice H, Paulus WJ (1995) Does dobutamine prevent the rise in left ventricular filling pressures observed during exercise after heart transplantation? Eur Heart J 16:1300–1306
47. Brutsaert DL, Rademakers FE, Sys SU (1984) Triple control of relaxation: implications in cardiac disease. Circulation 69:190–196
48. Hori M, Inoue M, Kitakaze M, Tsujioka K, Ishida Y, Fukunami M, Nakajima S, Kitabatake A, Abe H (1985) Loading sequence is a major determinant of afterload-dependent relaxation in intact canine heart. Am J Physiol 249:H747–H754
49. Kawaguchi M, Hay I, Fetics B, Kass DA (2003) Combined ventricular systolic and arterial stiffening in patients with heart failure and preserved ejection fraction: implications for systolic and diastolic reserve limitations. Circulation 107:714–720
50. LeWinter MM, Granzier H (2010) Cardiac titin: a multifunctional giant. Circulation 121:2137–2145
51. Wu Y, Cazorla O, Labeit D et al (2000) Changes in titin and collagen underlie diastolic stiffness diversity of cardiac muscle. J Mol Cell Cardiol 32:2151–2162
52. Bishu K, Hamdani N, Mohammed S, Kruger M, Ohtani T, Ogut O, Brozovich F, Burnett J, Linke WW, Redfield MM (2011) Sildenafil and B-type natriuretic peptide acutely phosphorylate titin and improve diastolic distensibility in vivo. Circulation 124:2882–2891
53. Weber KT, Janicki JS, Pick R, Capasso J, Anversa P (1990) Myocardial fibrosis and pathologic hypertrophy in the rat with renovascular hypertension. Am J Cardiol 65:1G–7G

54. Kato S, Spinale FG, Tanaka R, Johnson W, Cooper G IV, Zile MR (1995) Inhibition of collagen cross-linking: effects on fibrillar collagen and ventricular diastolic function. Am J Physiol 269:H863–H868
55. Stroud JD, Baicu CF, Barnes MA, Spinale FG, Zile MR (2002) Viscoelastic properties of pressure overload hypertrophied myocardium: effect of serine protease treatment. Am J Physiol Heart Circ Physiol 282:H2324–H2335
56. Brower GL, Janicki JS (2001) Contribution of ventricular remodeling to pathogenesis of heart failure in rats. Am J Physiol Heart Circ Physiol 280:H674–H683
57. Kass DA, Bronzwaer JG, Paulus WJ (2004) What mechanisms underlie diastolic dysfunction in heart failure? Circ Res 94:1533–1542
58. Paulus WJ, Vantrimpont PJ, Shah AM (1995) Paracrine coronary endothelial control of left ventricular function in humans. Circulation 92:2119–2126
59. Blankenberg S, Zeller T, Saarela O, Havulinna AS, Kee F, Tunstall-Pedoe H, Kuulasmaa K, Yarnell J, Schnabel RB, Wild PS, Münzel TF, Lackner KJ, Tiret L, Evans A, Salomaa V, MORGAM Project (2010) Contribution of 30 biomarkers to 10-year cardiovascular risk estimation in 2 population cohorts: the MONICA, risk, genetics, archiving, and monograph (MORGAM) biomarker project. Circulation 121:2388–2397
60. Lander AD (2010) The edges of understanding. BMC Biol 8:40

Chapter 2
Heart Failure with Normal Left Ventricular Ejection Fraction: Basic Principles and Clinical Diagnostics

Otto A. Smiseth, Espen W. Remme, Anders Opdahl, Svend Aakhus, and Helge Skulstad

Abstract Heart failure with normal left ventricular (LV) ejection fraction (HF-NEF), sometimes named diastolic heart failure, is a common condition, most frequent in the elderly and is associated with arterial hypertension and LV hypertrophy. Prognosis is almost as severe as for heart failure with reduced EF, in part reflecting comorbidities. Because the heart failure diagnosis is based on relatively nonspecific symptoms and signs, it is important to apply objective measures of diastolic function when evaluating patients with potential HF-NEF. In the absence of invasive data, this is done by echocardiography to demonstrate signs of impaired relaxation, increased diastolic stiffness, or elevated LV filling pressure. The echocardiographic measures include transmitral, pulmonary venous, and intraventricular flow velocities and estimation of systolic pulmonary artery pressure from tricuspid regurgitation velocity. In addition, LV lengthening velocity by tissue Doppler should be measured. It is important to search for consistency between measures since no single variable provides sufficient diagnostic information. Treatment of HF-NEF is symptomatic, with similar drugs as in heart failure with reduced EF.

Keywords Heart failure • Diastolic function • Ejection fraction

1 Definition of Diastolic Heart Failure

Congestive heart failure is a clinical syndrome due to inability of the heart to provide adequate tissue blood flow. There is typically cardiac dilatation and reduced left ventricular (LV) ejection fraction (EF). Over the last two decades this concept

O.A. Smiseth (✉) • E.W. Remme • A. Opdahl • S. Aakhus • H. Skulstad
Department of Cardiology and Institute for Surgical Research, Rikshospitalet, University of Oslo, Oslo University Hospital, 0027, Oslo, Norway
e-mail: otto.smiseth@ous-hf.no

J. Bartunek and M. Vanderheyden (eds.), *Translational Approach to Heart Failure*,
DOI 10.1007/978-1-4614-7345-9_2, © Springer Science+Business Media New York 2013

has been challenged by studies which show that up to 50 % of patients with congestive heart failure have normal LV EF [1–5]. It appears that in most of these patients the heart failure is due to abnormal diastolic function [6]. But also other cardiac disorders may cause heart failure with normal EF, including right ventricular failure, valvular heart disease, and pericardial disease. When such disorders have been excluded and abnormal diastolic function is identified, the condition has been described as *diastolic heart failure* [7]. There has been some controversy, however, regarding the use of the name *diastolic heart failure* because the diagnostic methods to identify diastolic dysfunction have significant limitations and because the separation into systolic and diastolic heart failure is not that clear cut. Therefore, an alternative terminology which makes no assumptions regarding pathophysiology has been introduced, and patients are grouped into *heart failure with reduced ejection fraction* (*HF-REF*) when EF is <50 % and *heart failure with normal ejection fraction* (*HF-NEF*) when EF is ≥50 % [1]. None of the terminologies are perfect, and at the present time both *HF-NEF* and *diastolic heart failure* are in use.

Observations that patients with *HF-NEF* have reduced LV long-axis shortening during resting conditions [8], and may have attenuated increase in stroke volume during physical exercise [9], support the view that there is a problem with systolic function. Caution should be exerted, however, when using myocardial velocity or extent of shortening to measure systolic function, since reduction in these indices may reflect increased afterload rather than reduction in contractility. Furthermore, an attenuated increase in stroke volume during exercise may be due to impaired filling due to the stiff ventricle, and therefore insufficient increase in effective LV preload. In an attempt to resolve this issue Baicu et al. [10] studied a group of patients with HF-NEF and quantified LV systolic function by methods which accounted for loading conditions. They concluded that in their group of HF-NEF patients, LV systolic function and contractility were normal. Therefore, there appears to be a group of patients with essentially isolated diastolic heart failure, and this might include patients with LV hypertrophy secondary to arterial hypertension. There is reason to believe, however, that HF-NEF represents a spectrum of disturbances of LV function, spanning from patients with mildly reduced systolic function to those with essentially normal contractility. Because most patients with systolic heart failure have impairment of diastolic function, systolic, and diastolic heart failure should not be considered as entirely different disease entities. In diastolic heart failure, however, the pathophysiology is dominated by abnormal LV filling properties, while loss of contractile force dominates in systolic heart failure. The prognosis of patients with HF-NEF is almost as severe as for patients with heart failure and reduced ejection fraction [5, 11]. This may in part reflect an effect of comorbidities.

2 Pathophysiology of Diastolic Heart Failure

The underlying cardiac dysfunction in diastolic heart failure is slowing of LV relaxation and increased LV chamber stiffness which leads to elevated LV diastolic pressure [12]. The problems are aggravated during physical exercise, when compensatory

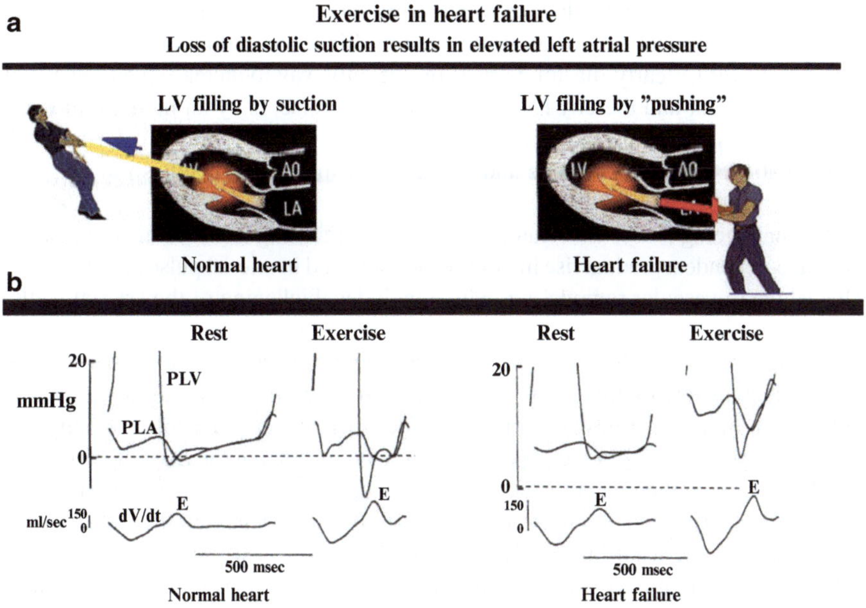

Fig. 2.1 Loss of diastolic suction in heart failure: *upper panels* illustrate the principle of diastolic suction which represents a force that "pulls" blood into the ventricle (*left panel*). During heart failure diastolic suction is lost and the ventricle fills because blood is "pushed" in from the left atrium (*right panel*). Smiseth, O.A. (2012). *Lower panels* are recording from an animal study showing in the *left panel* a normal heart in which left atrial pressure does not rise during exercise. This is due to markedly negative LV early-diastolic pressure which accounts for an increase in the transmitral pressure gradient. This negative LV pressure represents a suction force. During heart failure, shown in the *right panel*, there is no diastolic suction (early-diastolic pressure does not decrease) and transmitral flow increases due to elevation of left atrial pressure. *PLV* LV pressure; *PLA* left atrial pressure; d*V*/d*t* is time derivative of LV volume and *E* indicates peak early-diastolic transmitral flow rate. From H. Fukuta and W.C. Little. Diastolic Heart Failure, O.A. Smiseth and M. Tendera (Eds., Springer-Verlag London Limited 2008) [96]

mechanisms cause further elevation of LV end-diastolic pressure in an attempt to distend the stiff ventricle and thereby increase stroke volume by the Frank-Starling mechanism [13]. The resulting pulmonary congestion and the limited increase in stroke volume due to a stiff ventricle explain the exertional dyspnoea and fatigue in diastolic heart failure. This is in contrast to healthy individuals with a compliant ventricle and compliant arteries, who can increase cardiac output during exercise with minimal increase in filling pressure [13]. This principle is illustrated in Fig. 2.1 which shows that in the normal heart transmitral flow is increased during exercise by an increase in the transmitral pressure gradient with little or no rise in left atrial pressure (LAP). This is explained by a marked lowering of LV early-diastolic pressure to negative values and this represents a suction force which "pulls" blood into the ventricle. Therefore, increased filling during exercise in a normal heart is explained by diastolic suction. During heart failure, however, there is typically slowing of relaxation and reduction of restoring forces which lead to elevated early-diastolic pressure and loss of diastolic suction. Since the failing heart has lost its ability to lower LV early-diastolic pressure, the only way to increase the transmitral pressure gradient and thereby LV filling during exercise, is by an increase in LAP. This mechanism explains the elevation of pulmonary capillary pressure during exercise in patients with heart failure and the mechanisms is in principle similar in systolic and diastolic heart failure.

Normal ageing is also associated with arterial stiffening and is clinically evident as an age-dependent gradual rise in systolic pressure and in arterial pulse pressure [14]. This is due to vascular remodeling, which includes thickening of the arterial walls, particularly the intima, and increasing amount of collagen in the media. Therefore, the aging process further augments the problems that are due to hypertension. Ageing is associated with a shift in LV filling from early- to late-diastole. This is reflected in transmitral flow velocities as a decrease in early-diastolic velocity (*E*) and an increase in atrial-induced velocity (*A*), with reversal of the *E*/*A* velocity ratio. Similarly, LV lengthening velocities by tissue Doppler of the mitral annulus demonstrate an age-dependent decrease in peak early-diastolic lengthening velocity (e'), and an increase in atrial-induced lengthening velocity (a') with ageing. Therefore, elderly people often have a filling pattern that is typical for patients with impaired LV relaxation, as can be seen in early stages of many cardiac diseases and in LV hypertrophy. It is important, however, not to mix up *diastolic dysfunction* and *diastolic heart failure*, and it is not known if the age-related diastolic dysfunction identifies patients who are at increased risk of developing heart failure. In most cases the finding of diastolic dysfunction in patients with diabetes, hypertension or in the elderly has no clinical correlate, and is not associated with heart failure.

Systolic function in the healthy elderly appears normal since ejection fraction is similar to that in younger individuals. In the healthy elderly, however, there is reduced contribution from longitudinal shortening, which is balanced by an increase in circumferential shortening [15]. This shift may contribute to the age-dependent reduction in e'.

3 Etiology of Diastolic Heart Failure

The etiologies of diastolic heart failure include arterial hypertension, restrictive cardiomyopathy, cardiac amyloidosis, and hypertrophic cardiomyopathy. Myocardial ischemia may contribute to and precipitate diastolic heart failure. When HF-NEF occurs in patients with systolic hypertension, it is associated with LV hypertrophy, often in combination with coronary artery disease and/or diabetes mellitus [1, 16]. Each of the conditions are associated with variable degrees of structural remodeling and stiffening of the cardiovascular system. In hypertension there is thickening and deposition of collagen in the arterial walls, which lead to stiffening of the arterial system. This implies increased afterload for the left ventricle and serves as a stimulus to LV remodeling, resulting in concentric hypertrophy and increased LV diastolic stiffness. As suggested by animal studies, the increased LV stiffness is due to a combination of increased LV wall thickness and myocardial fibrosis [17]. The latter change appears to be due to activation of the renin-angiotensin-aldosterone system and different neurohormones [17]. In addition to the structural changes, arterial stiffening in hypertension leads to higher systolic LV wall stress, which results in slowing of LV relaxation [18].

It has been observed that a significant portion of HF-NEF subjects have chronotropic incompetence as indicated by blunted heart rate response to exercise, and it is likely that this mechanism contributes to their reduced exercise tolerance [19, 20].

4 Fundamental Problem: Relaxation and Stiffness

The two fundamental disturbances of LV function in diastolic heart failure are *slowing of relaxation* and *increased diastolic stiffness*. The slowing of relaxation results in loss of diastolic suction which in turn leads to elevation of LV early-diastolic pressure and compensatory increase in LAP in an attempt to maintain transmitral filling. Similarly, the increased passive elastic stiffness leads to a compensatory increase in LV end-diastolic pressure in an attempt to maintain LV preload and thereby stroke volume. This means that the primary disturbances are slowing of relaxation and increased diastolic stiffness and the elevated LV diastolic pressure represents a compensatory mechanism. Figure 2.1 illustrates how loss of diastolic suction in heart failure results in a compensatory increase in LV end-diastolic pressure during exercise.

In principle, slowing of LV relaxation and increased diastolic stiffness can be diagnosed clinically by invasive methods. Global LV relaxation can be quantified by measuring how rapidly LV pressure falls during isovolumic relaxation. This is measured as the time constant of LV isovolumic pressure fall (*tau*), and when *tau* is prolonged, it indicates slowing of global LV relaxation [21]. Measurement of *tau* requires high fidelity micromanometer-tipped catheters. There is, however, not sufficient data to support measurement of *tau* in a routine work up in patients with HF-NEF, and presently *tau* is measured only in research studies. Similarly, evaluation of LV diastolic stiffness by analyzing pressure-volume curves is done as part of research protocols, but has no role in clinical routine.

This implies that the two fundamental and most important measures of diastolic function are not available in routine clinical diagnostics. Instead we use LV end-diastolic pressure, which is actually a compensatory response, as indicator of diastolic dysfunction. Alternative explanations of elevated diastolic pressure, such as hypervolemia, can usually be easily identified. The most significant limitation of this approach is that invasive pressure is not available in most patients with HF-NEF. As will be explained in this chapter there are several echocardiographic measures which reflect abnormalities in relaxation, diastolic stiffness, and LV end-diastolic pressure. When these noninvasive methods are applied in combination it will often be possible to identify patients with diastolic heart failure.

5 How to Diagnose Diastolic Heart Failure by Noninvasive Methods

Patients with systolic and diastolic heart failure have similar symptoms and signs, and therefore clinical history and physical examination does not differentiate between the two conditions. For this reason and because the heart failure diagnosis is based on relatively nonspecific symptoms and signs, it is important to incorporate objective measures into the set of diagnostic criteria and to exclude alternative explanations, such as obesity and lung disease [22]. Therefore, in keeping with the recommendations from the European Study Group on Diastolic Heart Failure [7] we recommend that the diagnosis diastolic heart failure is restricted to patients in whom there is either invasive or noninvasive evidence of diastolic dysfunction.

The heart failure diagnosis is based on history, clinical examination, and on objective measures of cardiac dysfunction. Symptoms and signs include dyspnoea, tachypnea, cough, and abnormal auscultatory findings over the heart and lungs. There may also be secondary right-sided heart failure with distended neck veins and other signs of elevated central venous pressure. The symptoms and findings in diastolic heart failure, however, are similar to those of systolic heart failure. Therefore, additional diagnostic information is needed.

Since invasive studies are rarely available, the objective diagnostic evidence is most often limited to noninvasive data. The most important diagnostic information comes from Doppler echocardiography which allows comprehensive assessment of LV filling velocities by pulsed Doppler and LV lengthening velocities by tissue Doppler imaging (TDI). In addition echocardiography provides cardiac structural data which may be helpful. In the following text we will review the physiology of LV filling to provide a basis for interpretation of the diagnostic information provided by echocardiographic studies.

6 Transmitral Flow Velocities

Diastole is divided into four phases; i.e., isovolumic relaxation, rapid early filling, diastasis, and atrial-induced filling. During isovolumic relaxation LV pressure falls rapidly, the mitral valve is closed and no filling of the ventricle occurs. When ventricular pressure has declined to a level equal to atrial pressure, the mitral valve opens. As ventricular pressure subsequently declines more rapidly than atrial pressure, a gradient is established and the ventricle fills rapidly. During diastasis left atrial and left ventricular pressures almost equilibrate and transmitral flow occurs at a low rate. Subsequently, atrial contraction causes a brief increment in the transmitral pressure gradient and late-diastolic filling of the ventricle occurs (Fig. 2.2).

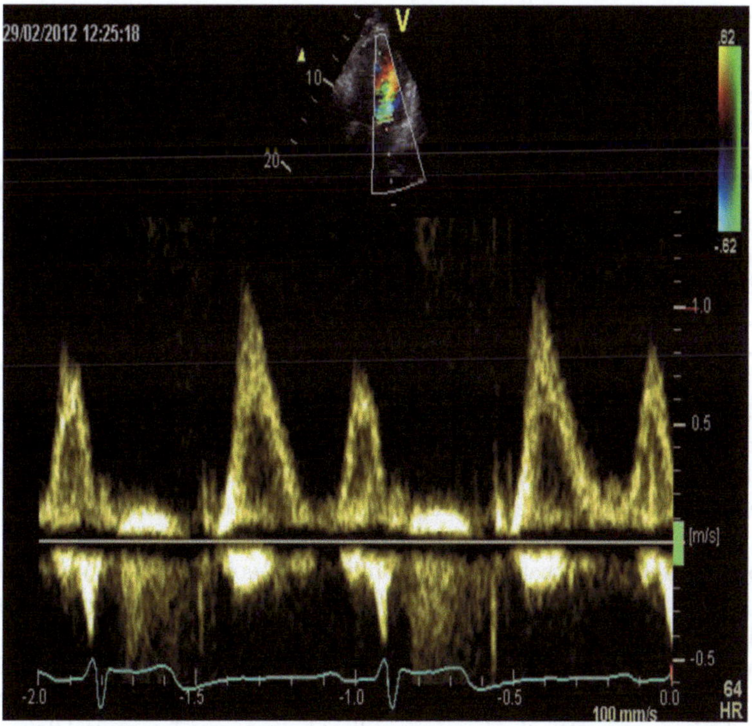

Fig. 2.2 Transmitral filling velocities in a normal heart

7 Isovolumic Relaxation

The isovolumic relaxation time (IVRT) is defined as the time interval between aortic valve closure and mitral valve opening, and can be measured by echocardiography. This time interval is determined by the decay rate of LV pressure, and therefore IVRT reflects the rate of LV relaxation. However, other determinants of valve movements will also influence IVRT, and this includes LV and LA pressures. For example, elevated LV systolic pressure will cause prolongation of IVRT since isovolumic relaxation starts from a higher pressure, while elevation of LAP will abbreviate IVRT due to premature opening of the mitral valve [23]. Therefore, IVRT as an index of LV relaxation is confounded by changes in LV systolic and LA pressure, and these variables need to be taken into account when using IVRT in the evaluation of diastolic function.

8 Early-Diastolic Filling

The transmitral pressure gradient refers to the difference between left atrial and LV pressure. The Bernoulli equation is used clinically to calculate transvalvular pressure gradients from Doppler flow velocities [24]. The Bernoulli equation consists of a *convective term* which relates the drop in pressure to the rise in kinetic energy as velocity increases due to narrowing at the valve orifice (convective acceleration), an *inertial term* which expresses the pressure drop needed to accelerate the mass of blood through the valve (local acceleration), and a *viscous term* which expresses the pressure loss because of viscous drag along the walls [25–27].

In mitral stenosis convective acceleration dominates, and the simplified Bernoulli equation ($\Delta P = 4\ v^2$) can be applied to calculate the transmitral gradient. In normal mitral valves, however, a relatively large volume of blood is contained within the valve, and a substantial fraction of the transmitral pressure gradient is needed to overcome inertia. Therefore, mitral velocity cannot be converted to pressure difference using the simplified Bernoulli equation, and the real pressure gradient is larger than predicted by the simplified Bernoulli equation. This is a systematic underestimation, and therefore peak transmitral filling rate correlates very well with the transmitral pressure gradient [28, 29]. Viscous friction is not important because the blood is in contact with the walls only briefly.

The inertial effect also accounts for the marked delay in peak velocity relative to peak gradient. This is illustrated in Fig. 2.3, which demonstrates that peak mitral flow velocity occurs when the pressure gradient is near zero. Transmitral flow velocity increases as long as there is a positive pressure gradient, i.e., an accelerating force. When the pressure gradient reverses, it represents a decelerating force, and causes velocity to decrease. This implies that timing of velocities cannot be used to define exact timing of gradient.

In spite of these limitations peak transmitral filling velocity is a very useful marker of peak mitral pressure gradient. For research studies color M-mode Doppler echocardiography represents a means to calculate the instantaneous transmitral pressure gradient by taking the inertial component into account [30, 31]. This methodology, however, is not needed in routine assessment of diastolic filling.

One should be aware of the confusion that may be created by using the terms *pressure gradient* and *pressure difference* interchangeably, as pressure gradient is pressure difference per distance (cm). In cardiology literature, however, it is customary to use gradient instead of pressure difference. In this chapter we will use the term pressure gradient, except when it is important to make the distinction. Due to regional pressure differences in the left ventricle during diastole (Fig. 2.4), the transmitral pressure difference may vary depending on catheter position, but this theoretical problem does not limit the use of transmitral filling velocities in a clinical context.

The peak early-diastolic transmitral pressure gradient is determined by rate of relaxation, by LV restoring forces (elastic recoil), by the diastolic pressure-volume relationship of the left ventricle and the left atrium, and by the operating pressure; e.g., slowing of relaxation leads to elevation of LV minimum diastolic pressure, and therefore tends to reduce the transmitral pressure gradient and E-velocity (Fig. 2.5).

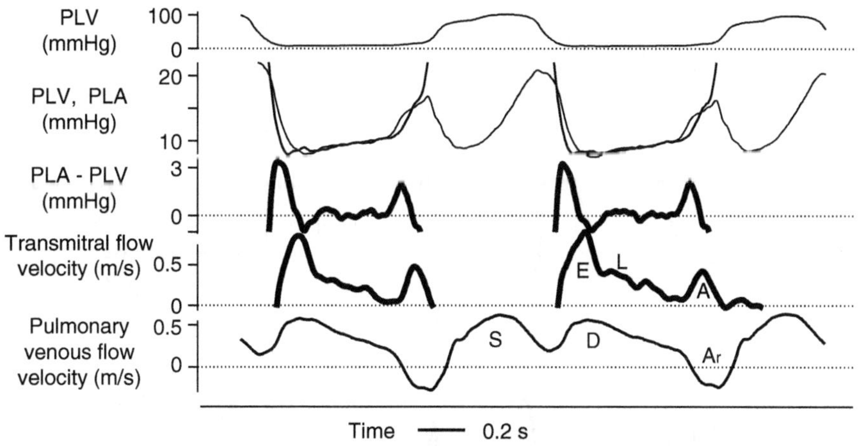

Fig. 2.3 Intraoperative measurements of left atrial and left ventricular filling in a patient with coronary artery disease. Left ventricular ejection fraction was normal. Recordings were done prior to cardiopulmonary bypass. Left atrial and LV pressures were measured with a single catheter with two pressure sensors 7 cm apart. Midway between the pressure sensors there was an electromagnetic velocity sensor that measured mitral blood flow velocity. Pressures were zero-referenced by comparison to pressure measured via a fluid-filled catheter in the left atrium. Pulmonary venous flow was measured by ultrasound transit-time from a flowprobe on the right lower pulmonary vein, and flow velocity was derived by dividing with the cross-section of the vein by transesophageal echocardiography. *PLV* left ventricular pressure; *PLA* left atrial pressure; *PLA-PLV* the atrioventricular pressure difference. *E* and *A* are transmitral early- and atrial-induced velocities; *L* mid-diastolic transmitral flow; *S* systolic velocity; *D* diastolic velocity; *Ar* atrial-induced reversed velocity. Modified from Smiseth and Thompson [97]

Since minimum diastolic pressure is dependent on end-systolic volume, changes in systolic function will modify the transmitral pressure gradient and hence the peak *E*-velocity. For instance, depression of systolic function with an increase in LV end-systolic volume leads to a higher minimum diastolic pressure, which tends to reduce peak early transmitral gradient and *E*-velocity. Improvement in systolic function with a reduction in end-systolic volume has the opposite effect. Changes in blood volume can markedly modify the transmitral pressure gradient. Furthermore, left atrial reservoir function and compliance determines how rapidly atrial pressure declines after onset of LV filling. This means that factors other than true changes in LV diastolic function can modify the peak *E*-wave.

9 Mid-Diastolic Filling

During diastasis left atrial and left ventricular pressures almost equilibrate and transmitral flow occurs at a low rate, i.e., the *L*-wave. The etiology and determinants of the *L*-wave are not entirely clear. As illustrated in Figs. 2.3 and 2.4, the *L*-wave does not appear to be the result of atrial emptying, since there is a steady rise in LAP

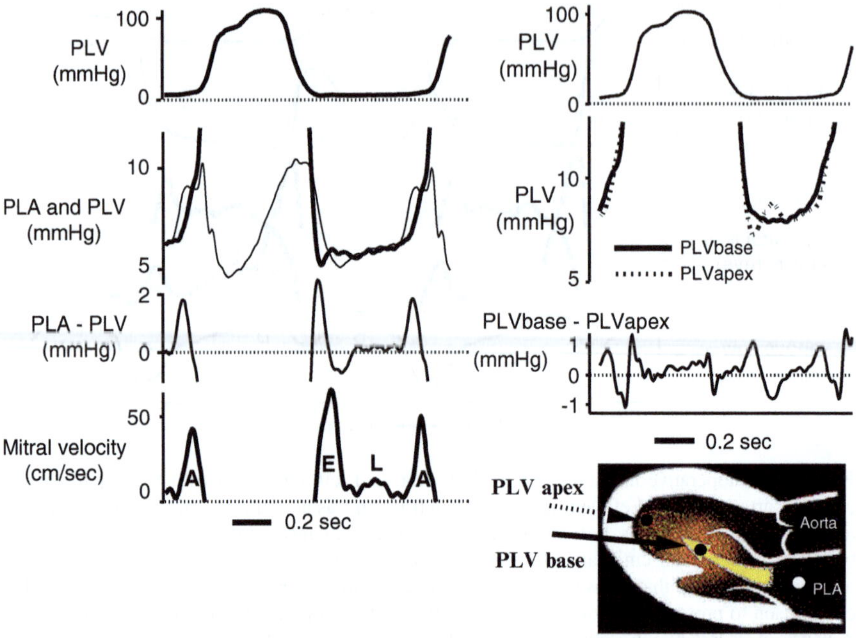

Fig. 2.4 Left atrial and intraventricular pressures recorded intraoperatively in a patient prior to coronary surgery. Recordings were obtained via a catheter with three micromanometers and an electromagnetic fluid velocity sensor (model SSD-827, Millar Instruments, Houston, TX, USA). The catheter was inserted via a pulmonary vein and was first advanced towards the LV apex, and pressures were recorded 4 cm apart (*right panel*). Then it was withdrawn such that the velocity sensor was near the mitral leaflet tips, and pressures were recorded 7 cm apart across the mitral valve (*left panel*). Across the mitral valve and inside the ventricle there is first a positive diastolic gradient which accounts for the early filling wave, and subsequently the gradient reverses and causes deceleration of flow. From Smiseth and Thompson 2000, reproduced with permission [97]

during diastasis, indicating increasing atrial volume. However, pulmonary venous flow continues throughout the period of diastasis, indicating that the *L*-wave is attributed entirely to pulmonary venous return. The transmitral pressure difference during the *L*-wave is very small, suggesting that transmitral flow during diastasis may be driven in part by the momentum of the blood which enters the atrium from the pulmonary veins.

10 Atrial-Induced Filling

The left atrium contracts in late-diastole and sets up a pressure gradient which causes the transmitral *A*-wave. As described for rapid early filling, there is flow acceleration when the gradient is positive, and deceleration when it reverses (Fig. 2.3).

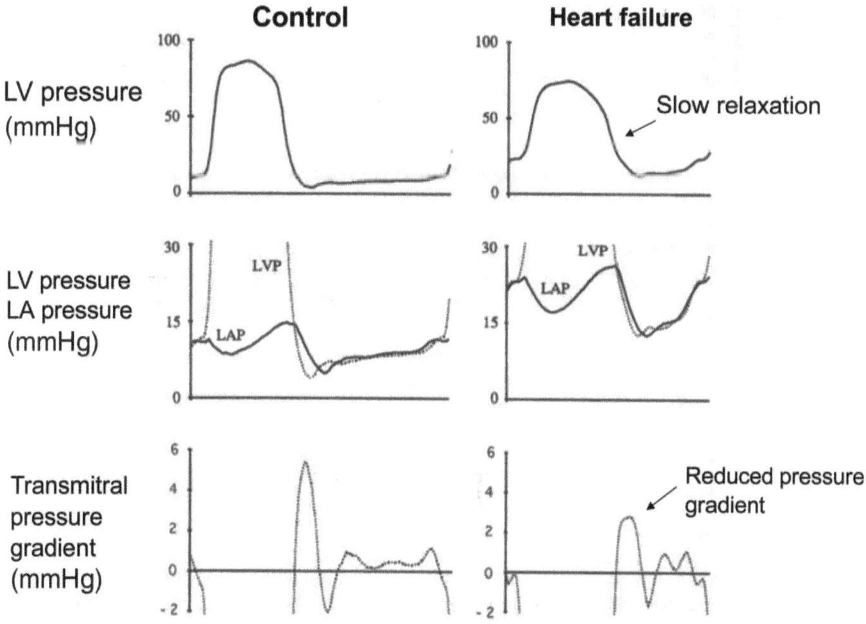

Fig. 2.5 Slowing of relaxation in heart failure causes a reduction in peak transmitral pressure gradient. Data from animal model of acute ischemic LV failure. Modified from Stugaard et al., 1994 with permission [56]

The transmitral *A*-velocity is determined by atrial function, LV function and loading conditions. In order to interpret measurements of transmitral *A*-velocity it is essential to understand the meaning of *LV chamber compliance*, since this variable is an important determinant of magnitude and duration of transmitral *A*-velocity.

Chamber compliance is the relationship between change in LV diastolic pressure and change in volume, and is determined by myocardial compliance and distensibility and by the extraventricular constraint exerted by pericardium and lungs. Furthermore, since the LV pressure-volume relationship is curvilinear, chamber compliance is a function of the operative LV diastolic pressure, and consequently is markedly load dependant. Therefore, a change in LV chamber compliance does not necessarily mean there has been a change in myocardial elastic properties, it may just be a change in loading conditions which moves the pressure-volume coordinate to a part of the curve which has different slope.

Figure 2.6 illustrates how an acute increase in LV diastolic pressure causes a marked decrease in atrial contribution and therefore an increase in the transmitral *E*/*A* ratio. The reduced atrial contribution was due to a reduction in chamber compliance, which represents an increase in afterload for the left atrium.

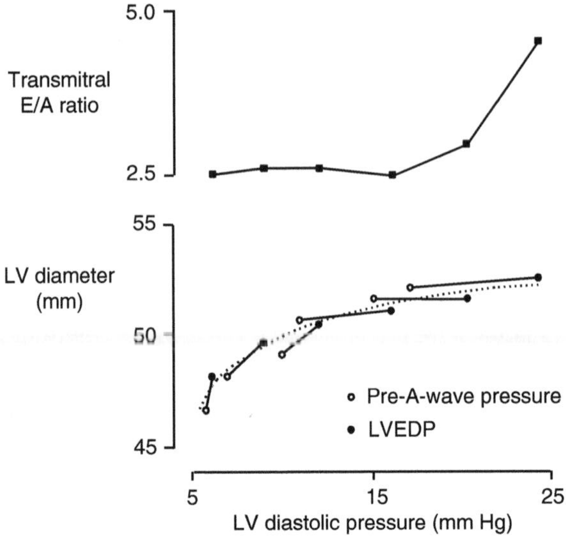

Fig. 2.6 Relationship between atrial contribution to LV filling and LV diastolic pressure: *upper panel* shows progressive rise in transmitral *E/A* velocity ratio at elevated LV diastolic pressures. *Lower panel* shows that atrial contribution to LV filling, measured as increase in LV short axis diameter during atrial contraction, is reduced when diastolic pressure is elevated. Pre-*A*-wave pressure is LV pressure prior to atrial contraction and LVEDP is LV end-diastolic pressure. From Myreng, Smiseth and Risoe, 1990 with permission [35]

11 Pulmonary Venous Flow Velocities

Assessment of pulmonary venous flow velocities by Doppler echocardiography represents an important "window" into the physiology of cardiac filling. Pulmonary flow velocities provide insights into left atrial as well as LV mechanical function. The pulmonary venous flow velocity has typically three phases, which includes a systolic wave (*S*-wave), a diastolic wave (*D*-wave) and a reversed flow wave during atrial contraction (*Ar*) (Fig. 2.7). Furthermore, as illustrated in Fig. 2.7, in many patients the systolic flow pulse has an early-systolic wave (S1) and a late systolic wave (S2). The S2 is usually the larger of the two waves. Figure 2.7 also demonstrates that the pulmonary venous flow trace looks like an approximately inverted LAP tracing, which means that flow accelerates when atrial pressure decreases, and vice versa. An exception to this is during mid/late systole, when flow accelerates while pressure is rising, and this will be discussed in more detail below.

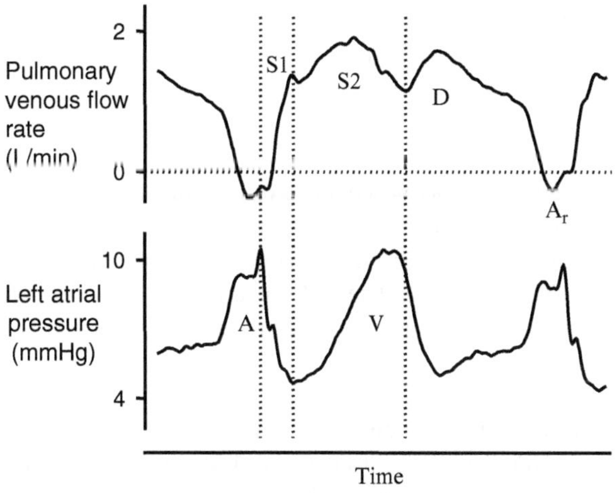

Fig. 2.7 Representative recording of pulmonary vein flow and left atrial pressure. Modified from Smiseth et al. [38], with permission. The recording was taken in a patient prior to cardiopulmonary bypass. The letters indicate the left atrial pressure waves and four pulmonary venous flow pulses, the A_r-wave during atrial contraction, the S1 (between *first* and *second vertical line*) and S2 (between *second* and *third vertical line*) waves during ventricular systole, and the *D*-wave in early diastole. Please note that during S2 both flow and pressure are rising, which is consistent with a forward going compression wave. However, during S1 and the other phases atrial pressure is falling when flow is rising. The latter is consistent with backward going expansion waves according to wave intensity analysis

12 Early- and Mid-Diastolic Pulmonary Venous Flow

The early-diastolic pulmonary venous flow is initiated by onset of transmitral filling, which leads to atrial emptying and a drop in LAP. This results in an increase in the pulmonary venous to LAP gradient. Therefore, the pulmonary venous *D*-wave corresponds to the transmitral early filling velocity, and the peak *D*-wave velocity is determined by many of the factors which determine peak early transmitral filling velocity [32]. Figure 2.3 illustrates the timings of pulmonary venous and mitral velocities. After the peak of the *D*-wave the pulmonary venous velocity decreases progressively, until atrial contraction causes marked flow deceleration.

13 Late-Diastolic Pulmonary Venous Flow

The reversed late-diastolic pulmonary venous flow (A_r) is caused by atrial contraction, and its magnitude and duration are determined by atrial systolic function, by atrial preload and by impedance to forward flow across the mitral valve and to retrograde flow into the pulmonary veins. Measurement of A_r in combination with transmitral flow, is of clinical interest for estimation of LV diastolic pressure [33, 34].

The relative amount of blood that moves forward or backward during atrial contraction depends on the relative compliance of the LV and the pulmonary veins. When atrial mean pressure is elevated, there is an accompanying decrease in LV chamber compliance. This is a consequence of the curvilinear relationship between LV diastolic pressure and volume. Therefore, at elevated LV diastolic pressure there is reduced atrial contribution to LV filling, which is reflected in a small and abbreviated transmitral *A*-velocity [35]. The pulmonary vasculature appears to be more compliant than the left ventricle. Thus, during atrial contraction some blood may flow retrogradely into the more compliant pulmonary veins instead of into the stiff LV. Markedly elevated preload is therefore associated with a large A_r, but a small and shortened transmitral *A*-velocity [33, 34]. This forms the basis for using the difference between duration of the transmitral *A*-wave and A_r as a clinical index of LV diastolic pressure, which is explained later in this chapter. This index functions best when atrial function is preserved and can generate a marked pressure rise in end-diastole.

Heart rate should be taken into account when using A_r to assess diastolic function [36]. Thus, at slow heart rates the pulmonary venous flow rate approaches zero prior to atrial contraction. Therefore, inertial forces are small, and atrial contraction most often results in flow reversal. During tachycardia, however, atrial contraction starts early in diastole when antegrade flow is substantial, and inertial forces are much stronger. Therefore, during tachycardia the A_r may be absent although left atrial mean pressure is markedly elevated [37]. Figures 2.8 and 2.9 illustrate the effect of pacing tachycardia on A_r in patients. The recordings were taken as part of an intra-operative study protocol with instrumentation as described previously [38]. Although this is an unphysiological situation it clearly shows that changes in A_r may be due to changes in heart rate. This means that heart rate should be taken into account when using pulmonary venous flow for noninvasive assessment of LV filling pressure.

14 Systolic Pulmonary Venous Flow

The etiology of the systolic pulmonary venous flow pulse (*S*) has been controversial [39–47]. One theory has been that the *S*-wave is caused by transpulmonary propagation of the right ventricular pressure pulse. The other theory has been the *S*-wave is caused by the early-systolic fall in LAP during atrial relaxation and descent of the *A–V* plane. The atrial pressure decay increases the pressure gradient between the pulmonary veins and left atrium which accelerates blood from the pulmonary veins. Differentiation between these two mechanisms has been possible by applying the principles of wave intensity analysis [38, 48]. This analysis indicates that the early-systolic flow wave (S1) is caused by atrial pressure decay (a backward going wave), while the mid/late systolic flow wave (S2) is caused predominantly by the right

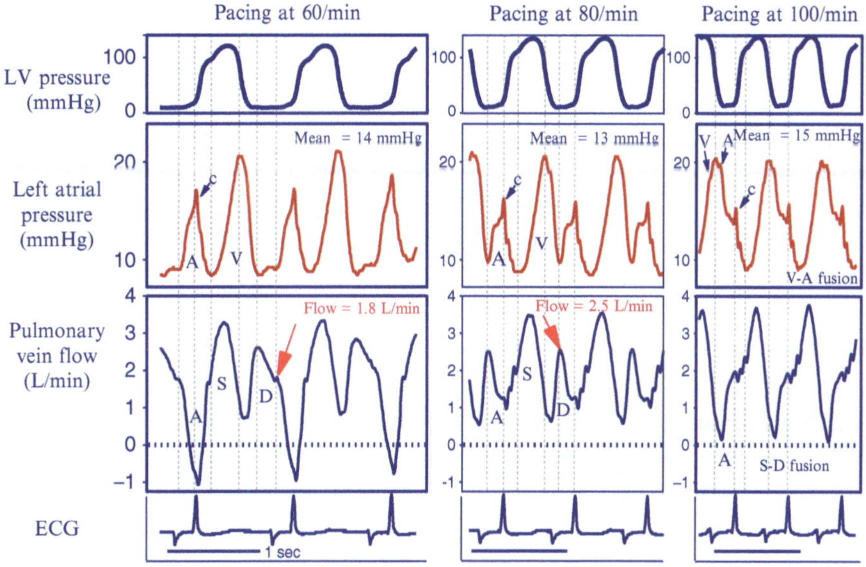

Fig. 2.8 Changes in pulmonary venous flow during atrial pacing. This protocol is part of an intra-operative study in a patient prior to cardiopulmonary bypass [38]. In this patient LV pressure is displayed for timing purposes. At 60/min there were two large antegrade flow waves, the *S*- and the *D*-wave, and a retrograde flow wave during atrial contraction. When pacing rate was increased from 60 to 80/min the *D*-wave was abbreviated and the A_r disappeared. Left atrial pressure was essentially unchanged during the different heart rates, with mean values ranging from 13 to 15 mmHg. Please note that antegrade flow at onset atrial contraction (arrow) is less at 60/min than at 80/min. Therefore, blood inertia, which is a force that must be overcome in order for atrial contraction to cause flow reversal, is larger at 80/min than at 60/min. During pacing at 100/min atrial contraction starts very early in diastole, and the pressure *A*-wave is superimposed on the *V*-wave. The *D*-wave can no longer be differentiated from the *S*-wave. The *dashed vertical lines* are provided to facilitate comparison of timing between pressure and flow traces

ventricular pressure pulse (a forward going wave). In addition, reflected waves may contribute to the pulmonary venous flow pattern, but do not appear to be of major importance.

As shown by the wave intensity analysis, the pulsations in the pulmonary venous flow trace throughout most of the heart cycle, i.e., diastole and early systole, are attributed to left-sided cardiac events [38]. The only phase when right-sided events dominate is mid and late systole. Another important point is that LV systolic function is a determinant of the systolic flow pulse since systolic descent of the AV-plane contributes to the *S*-wave both in the early and late phase of systole.

It has been suggested to use the pulmonary venous *S*/*D* ratio as a marker of LV diastolic pressure. This is based upon observations in patients with congestive heart failure who tend to have reduced magnitude of the *S*-wave [49, 50]. When LV diastolic pressure is elevated acutely, however, there is on the contrary an increase in the *S*-wave [38]. It is possible that the relationship between the *S*/*D* ratio and LV diastolic pressure in congestive heart failure reflects an association and not a causal

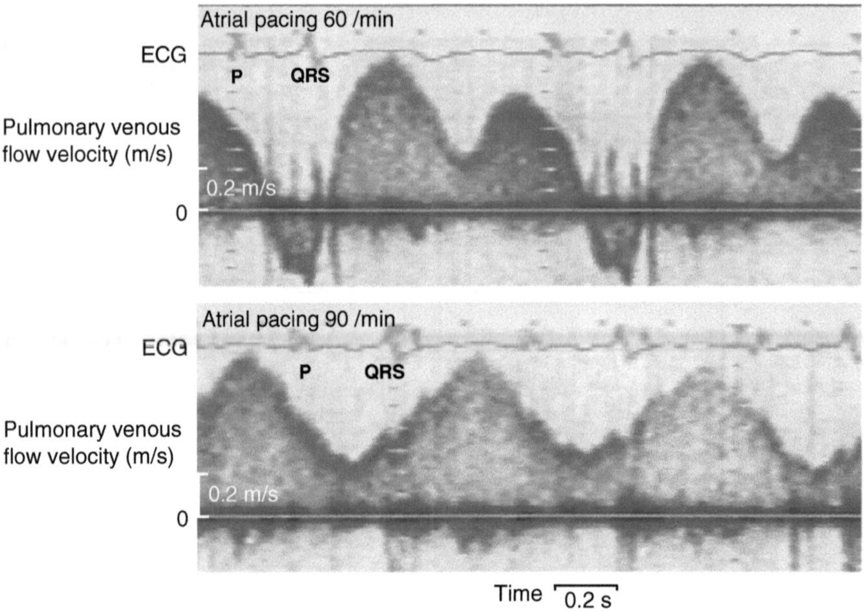

Fig. 2.9 Recording of pulmonary venous flow velocities by Doppler echocardiography. From same study as referred to in Fig. 2.8. When pacing rate was increased from 60 to 90/min the reversed flow wave during atrial contraction disappeared. Left atrial mean pressure was 10.5 and 9.0 mmHg at pacing rates 60 and 90/min, respectively

relationship. Possibly, reduced LV contractility in heart failure attenuates the *S*-wave by reducing systolic long-axis shortening, and hence the early-systolic fall in LAP. Furthermore, right ventricular contractility may be reduced and contribute to the reduction of the *S*-wave.

As demonstrated by Hunderi et al. [51], the deceleration time of systolic pulmonary venous flow (t_{dec}) reflects left atrial chamber compliance. Due to the curvilinearity of the atrial diastolic pressure-volume relationship, elevation of LAP leads to a decrease in LA chamber compliance and therefore a short t_{dec}. These principles explain why t_{dec} provides an estimate of atrial pressure.

It has been proposed to use the t_{dec} of pulmonary venous diastolic flow to estimate LAP [52]. Whereas this method is quite promising, it may be limited by tachycardia, which may markedly abbreviate or abolish the pulmonary venous diastolic flow wave.

In summary, the pulsations in pulmonary venous flow are attributed almost entirely to downstream events; i.e., the *D*-wave is caused by the decrease in LAP that results from LV relaxation, the A_r is caused by atrial systolic contraction, and the early-systolic flow wave is caused by the decrease in atrial pressure due to atrial relaxation and systolic descent of the mitral ring. The only exception is the mid-late systolic flow which is caused predominantly by an upstream event, i.e., forward propagation of the right ventricular systolic pulse.

The pulmonary venous velocity pattern is primarily a reflection of pressure oscillations in the left atrium, and therefore represents a noninvasive method for evaluating patients with potential diastolic dysfunction. It is important to be aware, however, that the pulmonary vein flow velocities are also influenced by left and right ventricular systolic function due to direct effects on the S-wave. The deceleration time for systolic pulmonary venous flow appears to be a marker of atrial compliance and pressure level.

15 Intraventricular Filling

Similar to transmitral filling, intraventricular filling has an early and an atrial-induced filling phase. In cardiac disease intraventricular filling may be disturbed, and the abnormal filling patterns have been introduced as markers of LV function and dysfunction (Fig. 2.10). However, assessing intraventricular filling is more complex than measuring flow velocities in blood vessels and across heart valves. This is due to the multitude of variables that determine intraventricular flow. Not only driving pressure, inertial forces, and viscous friction, but geometry, regional

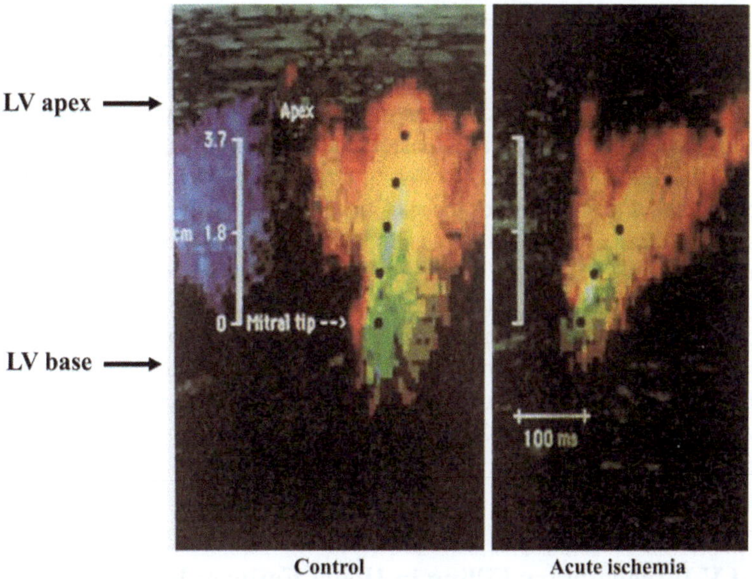

Fig. 2.10 Effect of acute myocardial ischemia on early-diastolic mitral-to-apical flow propagation: color M-mode Doppler recording of early-diastolic inflow in a patient treated for coronary artery (circumflex) stenosis. Images show recordings before and during balloon inflation. The *black dots* indicate peak velocities. Before balloon occlusion flow propagates rapidly towards the apex. During ischemia, however, there is a change in the flow image with apparent slowing of flow propagation. Modified from Stugaard et al. [56]

differences in function and asynchronies in contraction play major roles as well. Furthermore, flow occurs in multiple and rapidly changing directions, forming complex vortex patterns [53, 54]. It is therefore, difficult to relate measures of intraventricular flow to LV function. There is, however, a well defined intraventricular flow disturbance that has proven to be a marker of LV dysfunction, i.e., mitral-to-apical flow propagation or timing of early-diastolic apical filling. In this chapter we will discuss the mechanisms of mitral-to-apical flow propagation and how this variable may be related to diastolic function.

16 Intraventricular Pressure Gradients and Delayed Apical Filling

Similar to transmitral filling, normal LV intracavitary filling is dominated by an early wave and an atrial-induced wave. Most of the attention has been towards the early-diastolic filling wave as it has proven to change markedly during myocardial ischemia and LV failure [55, 56]. In the normal ventricle the early filling wave propagates rapidly towards the apex, and is driven by a pressure gradient between LV base and apex [57–60]. In LV dysfunction there is reduction of the gradient and therefore slowing of mitral-to-apical flow propagation [61, 62]. Nikolic et al. [62] demonstrated that the LV base-to-apex diastolic pressure gradient was related to the magnitude of LV restoring forces. Figure 2.4 illustrates intraventricular pressure gradients in a patient.

Since release of restoring forces and myocardial relaxation are assumed to contribute to the mitral-to-apical early-diastolic pressure gradient, the pressure gradient may be a marker of magnitude of restoring forces and relaxation rate. The notion is that blood is accelerated towards the apex in early diastole due to the pressure decay caused by release of restoring forces and relaxation. Doppler echocardiography represents a means to estimate the mitral-to-apical pressure gradient in patients [31, 59, 60, 63]. The analysis needed to calculate the intraventricular pressure gradient by Doppler, however, is complicated. Measurement of mitral-to-apical flow propagation may be an alternative method. Retardation of apical filling in LV dysfunction is consistent with loss of restoring forces and/or slowing of relaxation with a decreased pressure gradient [61]. Figure 2.10 shows slowing of flow propagation during acute myocardial ischemia.

17 LV Intracavitary Filling in Heart Failure: Role of Vortices

Experimental and model studies suggest that mitral-to-apical flow propagation is caused by two different mechanisms. In the normal ventricle blood propagates rapidly from the mitral tips towards the apex as if an entire column of blood moves towards the apex, attributed in part to the increased pressure gradient caused by release of restoring forces. This type of filling has been denoted column motion [36].

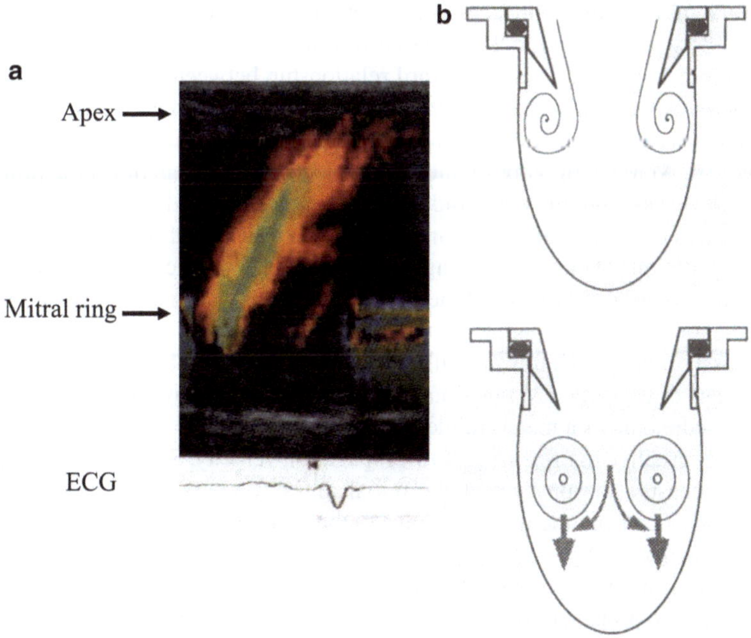

Fig. 2.11 Retarded LV apical filling and smoke ring vortices: (**a**) intraventricar filling by color M-mode Doppler in a patient with reduced LV ejection fraction. From Stugaard et al., 1994 with permission [98]. Please note that apical filling is markedly delayed relative to transmitral flow. (**b**) Schematic illustration of smoke ring vortices that propagate towards the apex. From Steen and Steen [36]. It seems that retarded apical filling in heart failure reflects slow propagation of vortices towards the apex

Thereafter, there is a phase of protracted filling which appears to represent smoke ring vortices that move slowly towards the apex [36, 64, 65]. In the normal ventricle the early rapid column motion dominates. In the failing ventricle and during severe myocardial ischemia the rapid column motion is reduced or lost and mitral-to-apical flow is attributed mainly to smoke ring vortices that move slowly towards the apex. Figure 2.10 illustrates the typical rapid early filling during baseline and a dominance of protracted filling during ischemia. Figure 2.11 illustrates schematically a proposed mechanism for the slow mitral-to-apical flow propagation in the failing ventricle; i.e., the smoke ring vortices which propagate from the mitral orifice towards the apex [36]. Therefore, when color M-mode Doppler is used to estimate mitral-to-apical flow propagation two different phenomena are quantified and this complicates interpretation of the findings.

The slow mitral-to-apical flow propagation in the failing ventricle is attributed to ring vortices that move slowly towards the apex, and the propagation velocity observed by color M-mode Doppler reflects how fast the vortex is moving towards the apex [36, 66]. Not only rate of LV relaxation, but also ventricular geometry and the ratio between mitral orifice size and LV cavity size influences vortex formation and mitral-to-apical flow propagation velocity [36, 67]. A relative reduction in the size of the mitral orifice enhances vortex formation, and causes slowing of mitral-to-apical flow propagation in the diseased ventricle.

Therefore, it is not a straightforward relationship between mitral-to-apical flow propagation velocity and LV diastolic function. This complicates the interpretation of intraventricular flow patterns and the use of intraventricular flow as a marker of dysfunction. Marked slowing of mitral-to-apical flow propagation is definitely a sign of LV disease, but the magnitude of flow propagation is determined by a number of factors other than diastolic function. The complexity of intraventricular flow and the limitations of current imaging techniques make it difficult to relate intraventricular flow patterns to LV wall function in a quantitative manner. This complexity limits the utility of assessing mitral-to-apical filling. Furthermore, in most patients with grossly abnormal intraventricular flow there are a number of other hemodynamic signs of impaired LV function, and assessment of intraventricular flow often becomes redundant as a means to identify dysfunction.

As an alternative to measuring flow propagation velocity, Stewart et al. [68] proposed to measure the product of the initial mitral-to-apical propagation velocity with the distance from the mitral annulus to the point where intraventricular velocity decelerates abruptly, and they named this product the strength of early filling. They showed that this product reflected diastolic dysfunction better than just the intraventricular propagation velocity. It remains to be determined how this new measure of intraventricular flow can be utilized clinically.

18 Left Ventricular Lengthening Velocities

During normal systole there is simultaneous longitudinal myocardial shortening, which causes the LV base to descend toward the apex whereas the apex is relatively stationary. During diastole there is myocardial lengthening during early-diastolic and during atrial-induced filling. The myocardial lengthening velocities, and in particular peak early-diastolic lengthening velocity, are very useful measures in the evaluation of diastolic function (Fig. 2.12).

The Doppler principle has traditionally been used to measure blood flow velocities, but may also be used to measure myocardial velocities. Separation between velocities in myocardium and blood is possible due to different signal amplitudes and Doppler frequencies. The myocardium is moving at much lower speed than blood, and therefore Doppler frequencies are lower. Furthermore, the amplitude of myocardial signals is much higher than for blood. These differences allow myocardial velocities to be separated from blood flow velocities by using filters which reject echoes that originate from the blood pool. Velocities can be recorded using color Doppler or pulsed Doppler mode. The most important measures from the velocity traces are peak systolic ejection velocity (s) and peak early-diastolic lengthening velocity (e'). It is important to be aware that the pulsed Doppler mode presents the peaks of the instantaneous velocity spectrum, while the color mode provides mean velocities. This implies that velocities measured by the 2D color method are

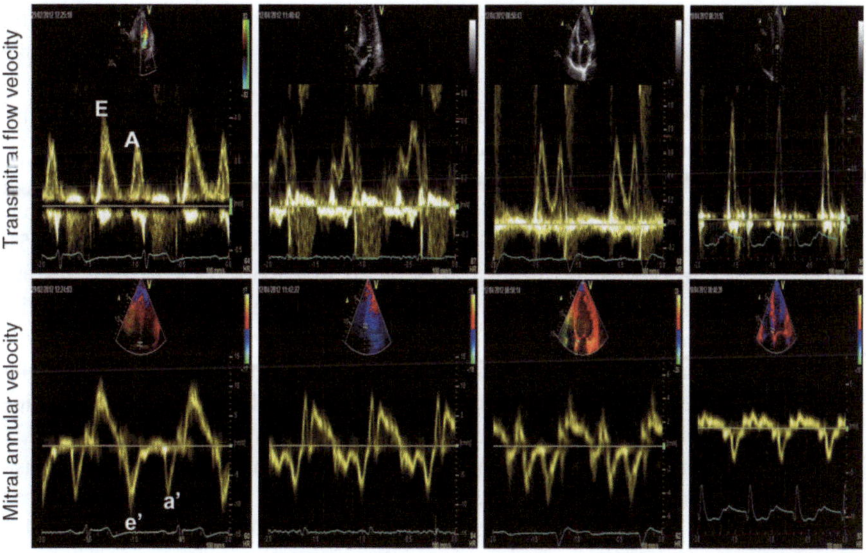

Fig. 2.12 Left ventricular filling patterns: the *upper panels* show transmitral velocities and the *lower panels* show pulsed wave TDI velocities from the septal part of the mitral annulus. The *left panels* are recordings from a normal control person. The mitral flow velocities in the *second panel* is a typical pattern of impaired relaxation, the next is a pseudonormalized pattern and the panel to the right is a typical pattern of restrictive filling. All three patterns are associated with reduced e' compared to the healthy individual. Importantly, the pseudonormalized trasmitral flow velocity pattern, which resembles that of a normal heart, is identified by the finding of reduced e'

lower than velocities by pulsed Doppler, typically about 25 % lower. When the ratio E/e' is used in the assessment of diastolic function the values in most cases refer to measurements by pulsed Doppler. More recently strain rate and strain have been introduced as clinical methods and may in principle be superior to TDI for evaluation of myocardial function [69, 70]. With regard to diastolic function, there are unresolved technical limitations of these modalities, and measures of strain rate and strain have no established role in clinical routine when evaluating diastolic function. Therefore, with the present state of the technologies, velocity imaging is the preferred methodology for assessing myocardial diastolic function [71]. One should be aware that in adults, e' velocity decreases with age; therefore, age-based normal values should be utilized when applying these measures of LV diastolic function in clinical practice.

Measurements of mitral annular velocities are done from apical views and velocities may be measured in several different planes. However, most often mitral annulus velocities are measured from an apical 4-chamber view and either the septal, the lateral or an average value of septal and lateral mitral annulus velocities are used. There are two main velocity waves that reflect early-diastolic (e') and atrial-induced (a') myocardial lengthening (Fig. 2.12). The e' wave is often followed by an oppositely directed wave of low amplitude (e'') during early diastasis, which reflects changes in geometry associated with redistribution of blood within the LV cavity. Similar to systolic velocities, diastolic velocities decrease progressively from base towards apex.

The magnitude of e' is closely related to myocardial relaxation as indicated by its correlation with the time constant of LV isovolumic relaxation [59, 60, 72–74]. In addition to relaxation, which reflects the decay rate of active fiber force, e' is determined by LV restoring forces which represent release of energy which is stored in the myocardium when the ventricle has contracted below its resting length [75]. During early diastole the restoring forces recoil the fibers back to their resting length, analogous to the recoil of a spring which has been compressed below its unstressed length. Restoring forces increase progressively when end-systolic volume is reduced and are therefore dependent on LV contractility. This illustrates the tight coupling between systolic shortening and diastolic lengthening and implies that e' is determined by systolic as well as diastolic function. Furthermore, since LV end-systolic volume is also a function of LV afterload, restoring forces will decrease when arterial systolic pressure is elevated.

In addition to LV relaxation and restoring forces e' is also determined by early-diastolic load, which is LV pressure at onset of filling [75]. Strictly speaking it is not LV intracavitary pressure, but LV transmural pressure (LV pressure minus pericardial pressure) which represents the distending force during filling [76]. Therefore, the early-diastolic transmural LV pressure represent the load that causes LV lengthening and it is named *LV lengthening load* [75]. In general, LV lengthening load will reflect changes in LV preload because changes in early-diastolic pressure are accompanied by changes in end-diastolic pressure. Thus, the three main determinants of e' are rate of relaxation, restoring forces, and lengthening load (Fig. 2.13). In addition, LV diastolic stiffness may modulate e'.

In the failing ventricle e' is much less load dependent than transmitral flow velocities, and when LV filling pressure becomes elevated in a failing ventricle, E increases more than e', and the E/e' ratio becomes elevated (Fig. 2.14). The relative load-independency of e' forms the basis for using the E/e' as a marker of elevated LV filling pressure.

19 Left Ventricular Twist: Untwisting Rate as Marker of Diastolic Dysfunction

During normal systole there is in addition to longitudinal and circumferential myocardial shortening, a twisting motion (torsion) of the ventricle. When viewed from LV apex toward base, there is systolic counterclockwise rotation of the apex and clockwise rotation of the base, and there is back-rotation in early diastole [77]. Because apex and base rotate in opposite directions, the ventricle is twisted about its long-axis. This pattern of contraction reflects the spiral orientation of myocardial fibers. Myocardial twist and twisting rate can be measured by speckle tracking echocardiography [78, 79].

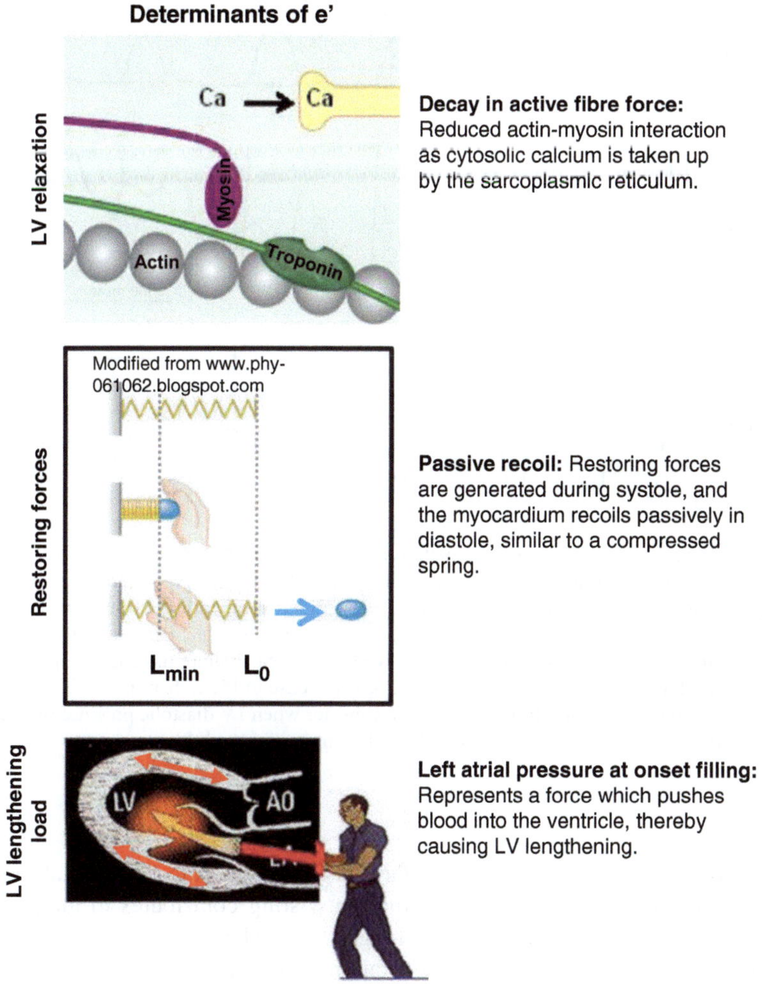

Fig. 2.13 Schematic illustration of the three independent determinants of e': *upper panel*: the LV relaxation rate is a measure of rate of decay of active fiber force, is coupled to calcium sequestration, and is a measure of diastolic function. *Middle panel*: restoring forces are illustrated by an elastic spring which is compressed to a dimension (L_{min}) which is less than its resting length (L_0) and it recoils back to its resting length when the compression is released. Similarly, when the LV contracts to a volume less than its unstressed resting volume it recoils back in early diastole when the myocardium relaxes. Restoring forces exert their effect in diastole, but are generated in systole, and therefore reflect systolic function. In the LV, restoring forces result in negative early-diastolic pressure which sucks blood into the ventricle. In the figure, the restoring force sets the blue bullet into motion analogous to blood that is moved from the left atrium into the LV. *Lower panel*: the LV lengthening load is the pressure in the LV at the time of mitral valve opening, and at this time LV pressure equals left atrial pressure. This is the pressure which forces (pushes) blood into the LV and thereby lengthens the ventricle

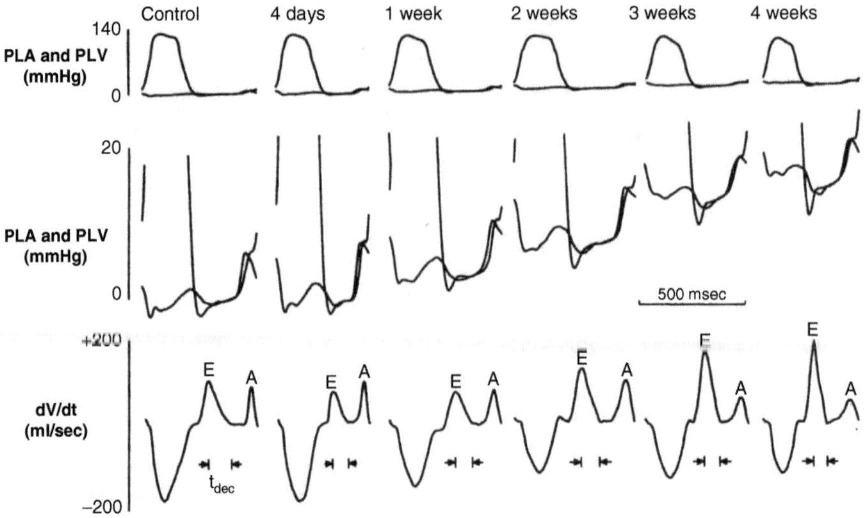

Fig. 2.14 Changes in transmitral flow pattern and relationship to transmitral pressure gradient during development of congestive heart failure in a dog model. The *left panel* shows analog recordings of left atrial and left ventricular pressures (PLA, PLV) along with the time derivative of LV volume (d*V*/d*t*). In diastole the latter measures transmitral filling rates. Peak early (*E*) and atrial-induced filling (*A*) are indicated. During the early phase of heart failure there is a drop in *E*. With more advanced heart failure, when there is a marked increase in PLA, there is tall *E* and small *A*. Furthermore, the deceleration time (t_{dec}) becomes shorter when LV diastolic pressure rises during progression of heart failure. From Ohno et al. 1994 with permission [29]

Left ventricular twist appears to play an important role for normal systolic function, and it has been speculated that untwisting contributes to the pressure decay during isolvomic relaxation, though a causal relationship has not been shown. Therefore, assessment of LV rotation represents an interesting approach for quantifying LV function. Left ventricular twist is calculated as the difference between apical and basal rotations. The early-diastolic untwist has previously been attributed to restoring forces [80]. However, as shown by Opdahl et al. [81] both restoring forces and relaxation rate are independent determinants of peak LV untwisting rate. In most cases peak untwisting rate seems to occur after mitral valve opening, and then LV early-diastolic pressure (lengthening load) is an additional determinant of LV untwisting rate. In this case, an increase in LAP leads to an increase in peak untwisting rate. The untwisting that occurs during isovolumic relaxation is determined by restoring forces and relaxation. Thus, maximal untwisting rate quantified prior to mitral valve opening may be a marker of restoring forces and relaxation rate independent of early-diastolic load [81]. Because restoring forces are generated by the degree of contraction in the previous systole, peak untwisting rate by definition is a function of systolic as well as of diastolic function.

Although peak untwisting rate is a promising measure of diastolic function, it has yet not been sufficiently validated in a clinical context to be recommended for routine application. In particular, there is need for more work on standardization of the methodology and definition of reference values for normality and disease.

20 Filling Patterns in Heart Failure

In the early stages of diastolic dysfunction there is typically slowing of LV relaxation, which causes a decrease in peak E-velocity and a compensatory increase in peak A-velocity [82, 83]. This shift in filling from early- to late-diastole, measured as a decrease in the E/A ratio, is described as a pattern of *impaired relaxation* (Fig. 2.12). As heart failure progresses and LAP becomes elevated, there is an increase of the early-diastolic transmitral pressure gradient, which increases peak E-velocity, and the E/A ratio may become normal. This is described as a *pseudonormalized* filling pattern. When heart failure progresses further, LAP may become markedly elevated and the early-diastolic transmitral pressure gradient increases, leading to supernormal peak E-velocity. Since elevation of LV diastolic pressure causes the ventricle to operate on a steeper portion of its pressure-volume curve, there will be a reduction of operative compliance, and therefore little further increase in LV volume during atrial contraction. This is measured as a small and abbreviated transmitral A-velocity. Furthermore, due to reduced LV chamber compliance the early transmitral flow decelerates rapidly [84, 85]. It has been shown that E-deceleration time is directly related to LV stiffness [84, 85]. This filling pattern with increased E/A ratio and short E-deceleration time is described as *restrictive physiology*. An additional feature of this filling pattern is abbreviated IVRT due to premature opening of the mitral valve caused by the elevated LAP. Since assessment of mitral flow velocities alone does not differentiate between pseudonormal and true normal filling, there is need for an additional technique. The best and easiest additional method is measurement of peak early-diastolic mitral annulus velocity (e'), which is reduced in patients with pseudonormalized filling. In patients with impaired relaxation and restrictive physiology there is also reduced e' (Fig. 2.3).

21 Estimation of LV Filling Pressure

A number of echocardiographic indices may be utilized to estimate LV end-diastolic or left atrial mean pressure and these methods are presented in a concencus document from the European Association on Echocardiography jointly with the American Society on Echocardiography [71]. In patients with heart failure and reduced EF the echocardiographic indices provide accurate diagnostic information which can be used to identify patients with elevated filling pressure. In patients with normal EF, however, the use of these indices is more challenging. The E/e' ratio, however, represents one of several approaches which may be of clinical value. It is recommended to use the average e' of septal and lateral mitral annulus recorded in an apical view, and a ratio <8 identifies patients with normal LV filling pressures, whereas an average ratio >15 indicates an increase in LV filling pressures. When the ratio is between 9 and 15, other measurements are essential. It is important to be aware that the values for E/e' ratios are based on e' recorded by pulsed TDI which gives peak velocities, and not by 2-D color mode which provides mean velocities which are lower.

Additional indices which are clinically useful include reversed pulmonary venous velocity and peak tricuspid regurgitation velocity. One advantage of considering the E/e' ratio, peak tricuspid regurgitation velocity, and reversed pulmonary venous flow during atrial contraction is that effects of normal ageing appear to be eliminated, and these indices become more reliable markers of elevated filling pressure. Figure 2.15 shows schematically relevant echocardiographic measures which may be of value when evaluating patients with HF-NEF. It is important to look for consistency between indices and not trust only one measure.

Provided signal quality is good, which is the case in approximately 25–30 % of patients with transthoracic imaging, the pulmonary venous reversed velocity during atrial contraction provides reliable information. If the duration of retrograde pulmonary venous flow exceeds antegrade transmitral flow with >30 ms, it is very likely that LV filling pressure is elevated [33, 71]. Furthermore, the peak value of reversed flow velocity increases along with elevation in LV filling pressure. The method has some limitations, including reduced atrial systolic function. Another very useful measure is estimation of pulmonary artery systolic pressure from peak tricuspid regurgitation velocity. This measure can be achieved in most patients and is part of almost every routine echocardiographic examination. Important limitations to this approach are lung disease and severe mitral regurgitation, but both these conditions can usually be sorted out. Systolic pulmonary artery pressure is estimated as the sum of the estimated right atrial pressure and the systolic tricuspidal pressure gradient. Provided there is no pulmonary vascular disease, an elevated pulmonary artery pressure is most likely a sign of elevated LAP.

21.1 CMR/Nuclear Methods/CT

Neither MRI, radionuclide-based methods, nor CT has a role in routine evaluation of patients with diastolic heart failure. There are exceptions such as constrictive pericarditis or pure myocardial diseases, which requires more comprehensive imaging.

22 Structural Changes

Increased left atrial volume may also be used as objective evidence of diastolic dysfunction. Furthermore, LV hypertrophy is consistent with impaired diastolic function and supports the diagnosis.

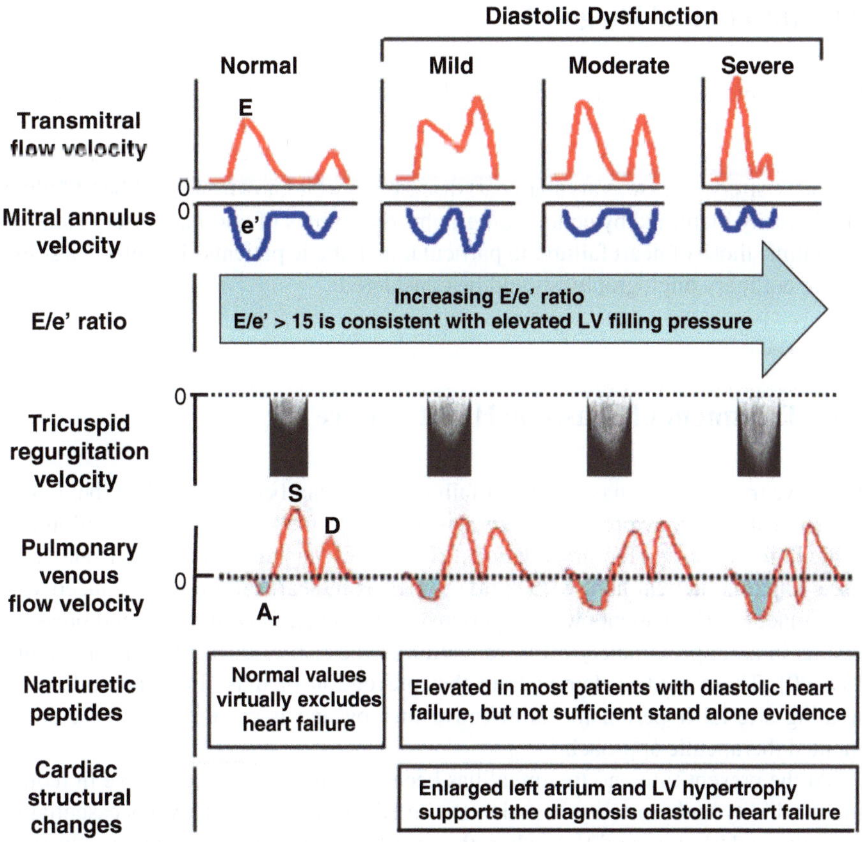

Fig. 2.15 Schematic representation of noninvasive methods to diagnose diastolic heart failure: diastolic dysfunction is supported by demonstration of abnormal transmitral and mitral ring velocities. Progression from mild to severe diastolic dysfunction is associated with increasing *E/e'* velocity ratio, and reflects increasing LV filling pressure; *E/e'* > 15 (average *e'* of septal and lateral annulus) supports filling pressure >15 mmHg, and *E/e'* < 8 supports normal filling pressure. For *E/e'* in the range 8–15, other indices should be used to estimate filling pressure. Systolic tricuspid regurgitation velocity increases progressively with increasing left atrial pressure. The pulmonary venous reversed *A*-wave (A_r) increases in magnitude and duration along with increasing LV end-diastolic pressure. Natriuretic peptides are used mainly to exclude heart failure, and have limited positive predictive value. Enlarged left atrium and LV hypertrophy supports the diagnosis diastolic heart failure

23 Blood Markers

Elevated BNP or NT-proBNP may be used to support the diagnosis diastolic heart failure, but is not considered sufficient stand-alone evidence for diastolic dysfunction [86, 87]. Natriuretic peptides are recommended mainly for the exclusion of the diagnosis, which is justified by its high negative predictive value for heart failure [88].

24 Differential Diagnosis

Since symptoms and signs of diastolic heart failure are relatively nonspecific it is important to exclude noncardiac etiologies, in particular lung disease. It is also important to exclude other cardiac disorders, such as valvular heart disease and coronary artery disease. Valvular heart disease is a well known cause of heart failure and is easily identified by echocardiography. Symptoms of coronary artery stenosis can mimic those of heart failure, in particular in diabetic patients. Therefore, a stress test or coronary angiography should be considered.

25 Treatment of Diastolic Heart Failure

Effective treatment of diastolic heart failure has yet not been established, but ongoing clinical trials may provide some answers. Due to the limited documentation it is difficult to give firm recommendations. At the present stage it seems reasonable to use symptomatic treatment with similar drugs as in heart failure with reduced systolic function. For patients with hypertension, however, lowering of blood pressure results in an approximately 50 % reduction in the risk of developing heart failure [89, 90]. These studies demonstrate that prevention of diastolic heart failure by treating arterial hypertension is effective therapy and is currently the best documented therapeutic approach.

At the present time, no treatment has been documented to be effective in reducing morbidity and mortality in patients with HF-NEF [91]. It is always essential to treat the underlying condition when that can be identified. In particular, adequate control of blood pressure in patients with hypertension is important. Diuretics can be used when there are signs and symptoms of congestion. Some smaller trials have demonstrated trends in favor of drug treatment in HF-NEF. However, as briefly reviewed in the following paragraph none of the larger mortality/morbidity trials have been able to demonstrate convincing effect of drug in the treatment of HF-NEF.

Angiotensin-converting enzyme (ACE) inhibitors and angiotensin-II receptor antagonists are potentially useful drugs for patients with HF-NEF, and both therapeutic principles have been studied. The response to ACE-inhibition was tested in the perindopril in elderly people with chronic heart failure (PEP-CHF) study, but failed to show reduction in the primary composite endpoint of death of heart failure hospitalization [92]. The angiotensin-II receptor antagonists candesartan and irbesartan have also been tested in HF-NEF populations. The candesartan in heart failure trial included different patient categories and also a group with heart failure NYHA class II-IV and ejection fraction higher than 40 % [93]. In this study cardiovascular death did not differ between groups, but fewer patients in the candesartan group than in the placebo group were admitted to hospital for CHF once or multiple times. A study which tested Irbesartan in heart failure with preserved systolic function (I-preserve) also failed to show reduction in the primary composite outcome of death or cardiovascular hospitalization [94]. In theory, reduced LV filling time due to impaired myocardial relaxation is a problem in patients with HF-NEF, in particular during exercise-induced tachycardia. Therefore, beta blockers which limit peak heart rate during physical exercise, might be beneficial. However, the Seniors Study which tested Nebivolol in patients with ejection fraction above 35 %, showed no significant change in neither systolic nor diastolic measures [95].

Some of the trials referred to above have limitations, in particular with regard to the diagnostic criteria for impaired LV diastolic function and they often represents patients with a wide range of etiologies. Therefore, there is need for trials which utilizes the most recent consensus on diagnostic criteria and takes into account that HF-NEF has different etiologies. With regard to studies on the effect of beta blockers, one should be aware that some patients with HF-NEF have chronotropic insufficiency and therefore beta blocker in theory may have a negative effect in this subgroup. Within a few years some of the ongoing trials of drug treatment in HF-NEF will be completed and hopefully will provide new insights into how to manage patients with HF-NEF.

26 Future Trends

The ultimate objective of all research on HF-NEF is to contribute to the development of better therapies which will not only relieve symptoms, but also improve prognosis in this patient group. To this end it will be increasingly important to gain more insight into the underlying mechanisms of HF-NEF. This includes understanding of the molecular mechanisms that account for slowing of myocardial relaxation and increase in passive elastic stiffness and cause the structural changes in myocardial microscopic architecture and myocardial hypertrophy which may be seen in patients with HF-NEF. Furthermore, since stiffening of the arterial wall may play an important role in the development of HF-NEF it is important to develop better methods to quantify the interaction between LV myocardium peripheral arteries.

The diagnostic criteria for LV diastolic dysfunction are undergoing continuous improvement by taking into account the most recent echocardiographic imaging modalities. It may be needed to expand the diagnostic modalities beyond echocardiography and to utilize cardiac magnetic resonance imaging to provide structural data and potentially positron emission tomography to gain insight into metabolic changes and myocardial energy utilization. It is also likely that a combination of functional imaging and blood biomarker will be useful. Future clinical studies on therapeutic interventions should utilize the most recent diagnostic criteria in order to study patients who have diastolic dysfunction by objective criteria. Furthermore, since HF-NEF has several different etiologies it is important that this is taken into account when designing clinical trials.

In most studies of HF-NEF the diagnostic work up has been done with patients in the resting state. This is not optimal since symptoms occur predominantly during physical exercise. Therefore, future studies on diagnostic methods should preferably include measurements during exercise. This is feasible by doing stress echocardiography during supine bicycling, and important measures are changes in cardiac output and LV filling pressure. One should search for signs of marked elevation of LV filling pressure and attenuated increase in stroke volume which is the characteristic response in HF-NEF. When imaging is optimal such data can be obtained and hopefully ongoing developments in cardiac imaging will make this feasible in most patients in clinical routine.

27 Summary

In summary, a diagnostic work up for patients with suspected diastolic heart failure can be done at low cost in almost every cardiology practice. When invasive data are not available, echocardiography is the preferred method to determine if there is LV diastolic dysfunction. In general practice, blood markers such as BNP may be used as the initial method, and when BNP is normal, it is very unlikely that the patient has any form of heart failure. Importantly, this does not mean that the patient has no heart disease, and it may be required to search for valve disease, coronary artery disease, or other cardiac disorders. When blood markers are elevated, however, heart failure is likely and the patient should be referred for echocardiography to define underlying pathology and to confirm the diagnosis.

28 Key Points About Heart Failure with Normal EF

- Prevalence and prognosis:
  - Accounts for approximately 50 % of all heart failure cases.
  - Prognosis almost as severe as for heart failure with reduced EF.
- Why evaluate diastolic function in heart failure patients with normal EF?
  - To confirm the diagnosis by showing abnormal diastolic function.
  - To estimate LV filling pressure.
  - To obtain prognostic information.
- What is the etiology of heart failure patients with normal EF?
  - Most patients have concentric LV hypertrophy due to arterial hypertension and increased arterial stiffness.
  - Coronary artery disease and diabetes mellitus have direct effects on myocardial function, leading to impairment of relaxation and increased diastolic stiffness.
  - Several cardiomyopathies have specific effects on diastolic function.
  - Many patients have mild reduction of systolic function in spite of normal EF.

- What is optimal treatment of heart failure patients with normal EF?
  - Objective data are very limited.
  - Symptomatic treatment with same drugs as in heart failure with reduced EF.
- How to diagnose heart failure with normal EF noninvasively?
  - Signs or symptoms of heart failure.
  - Measure LV EF.
  - Evidence of LV diastolic dysfunction by:

  Echocardiography

  - Signs of impaired relaxation and/or increased diastolic stiffness by combined assessment of transmitral and mitral ring velocities.
  - Signs of elevated LV filling pressure by measuring transmitral, pulmonary venous and intraventricular flow velocities, LV lengthening velocity and estimation of systolic pulmonary artery pressure from tricuspid regurgitation velocity. It is important to search for consistency between measures since no single variable provides sufficient diagnostic information.
  - Structural changes: LV hypertrophy or dilated left atrium.
  - Elevated BNP or NT-proBNP support heart failure. Normal values make the diagnosis of heart failure unlikely.

29 Sources for Further Information

Zile MR, Baicu CF, Gaasch WH. Diastolic heart failure—abnormalities in active relaxation and passive stiffness of the left ventricle. New England Journal of Medicine 2004 May 6;350(19):1953–9.

Yturralde RF, Gaasch WH. Diagnostic criteria for diastolic heart failure. Prog Cardiovasc Dis 2005;47:314–9.

Nagueh SF, Appleton CP, Gillebert TC, Marino PN, Oh JK, Smiseth OA, Waggoner AD, Flachskampf FA, Pellikka PA, Evangelisa A. Recommendations for the evaluation of left ventricular diastolic function by echocardiography. J Am Soc Echocardiogr 2009 Feb;22(2):107–33.

Mor-Avi V, Lang RM, Badano LP, Belohlavek M, Cardim NM, Derumeaux G, Galderisi M, Marwick T, Nagueh SF, Sengupta PP, Sicari R, Smiseth OA, Smulevitz B, Takeuchi M, Thomas JD, Vannan M, Voigt JU, Zamorano JL. Current and evolving echocardiographic techniques for the quantitative evaluation of cardiac mechanics: ASE/EAE consensus statement on methodology and indications endorsed by the Japanese Society of Echocardiography. Eur J Echocardiogr. 2011 Mar;12(3):167–205.

References

1. Bursi F, Weston SA, Redfield MM, Jacobsen SJ, Pakhomov S, Nkomo VT et al (2006) Systolic and diastolic heart failure in the community. JAMA 296(18):2209–2216
2. Vasan RS, Larson MG, Benjamin EJ, Evans JC, Reiss CK, Levy D (1999) Congestive heart failure in subjects with normal versus reduced left ventricular ejection fraction: prevalence and mortality in a population-based cohort. J Am Coll Cardiol 33(7):1948–1955
3. Senni M, Tribouilloy CM, Rodeheffer RJ, Jacobsen SJ, Evans JM, Bailey KR et al (1998) Congestive heart failure in the community: a study of all incident cases in Olmsted County, Minnesota, in 1991. Circulation 98(21):2282–2289
4. Yancy CW, Lopatin M, Stevenson LW, De MT, Fonarow GC (2006) Clinical presentation, management, and in-hospital outcomes of patients admitted with acute decompensated heart failure with preserved systolic function: a report from the Acute Decompensated Heart Failure National Registry (ADHERE) Database. J Am Coll Cardiol 47(1):76–84
5. Owan TE, Hodge DO, Herges RM, Jacobsen SJ, Roger VL, Redfield MM (2006) Trends in prevalence and outcome of heart failure with preserved ejection fraction. N Engl J Med 355(3):251–259
6. Oh JK, Hatle L, Tajik AJ, Little WC (2006) Diastolic heart failure can be diagnosed by comprehensive two-dimensional and Doppler echocardiography. J Am Coll Cardiol 47(3):500–506
7. Paulus WJ, Tschope C, Sanderson JE, Rusconi C, Flachskampf FA, Rademakers FE et al (2007) How to diagnose diastolic heart failure: a consensus statement on the diagnosis of heart failure with normal left ventricular ejection fraction by the Heart Failure and Echocardiography Associations of the European Society of Cardiology. Eur Heart J 28(20):2539–2550
8. Yu CM, Lin H, Yang H, Kong SL, Zhang Q, Lee SW (2002) Progression of systolic abnormalities in patients with "isolated" diastolic heart failure and diastolic dysfunction. Circulation 105(10):1195–1201
9. Tan YT, Wenzelburger F, Lee E, Heatlie G, Leyva F, Patel K et al (2009) The pathophysiology of heart failure with normal ejection fraction: exercise echocardiography reveals complex abnormalities of both systolic and diastolic ventricular function involving torsion, untwist, and longitudinal motion. J Am Coll Cardiol 54(1):36–46
10. Baicu CF, Zile MR, Aurigemma GP, Gaasch WH (2005) Left ventricular systolic performance, function, and contractility in patients with diastolic heart failure. Circulation 111(18): 2306–2312
11. Bhatia RS, Tu JV, Lee DS, Austin PC, Fang J, Haouzi A et al (2006) Outcome of heart failure with preserved ejection fraction in a population-based study. N Engl J Med 355(3):260–269
12. Zile MR, Baicu CF, Gaasch WH (2004) Diastolic heart failure—abnormalities in active relaxation and passive stiffness of the left ventricle. N Engl J Med 350(19):1953–1959
13. Kitzman DW, Higginbotham MB, Cobb FR, Sheikh KH, Sullivan MJ (1991) Exercise intolerance in patients with heart failure and preserved left ventricular systolic function: failure of the Frank-Starling mechanism. J Am Coll Cardiol 17(5):1065–1072
14. Chen CH, Nakayama M, Nevo E, Fetics BJ, Maughan WL, Kass DA (1998) Coupled systolic-ventricular and vascular stiffening with age: implications for pressure regulation and cardiac reserve in the elderly. J Am Coll Cardiol 32(5):1221–1227
15. Wandt B, Bojo L, Hatle L, Wranne B (1998) Left ventricular contraction pattern changes with age in normal adults. J Am Soc Echocardiogr 11(9):857–863
16. Gheorghiade M, Abraham WT, Albert NM, Greenberg BH, O'Connor CM, She L et al (2006) Systolic blood pressure at admission, clinical characteristics, and outcomes in patients hospitalized with acute heart failure. JAMA 296(18):2217–2226
17. Weber KT, Brilla CG (1991) Pathological hypertrophy and cardiac interstitium. Fibrosis and renin-angiotensin-aldosterone system. Circulation 83(6):1849–1865
18. Kawaguchi M, Hay I, Fetics B, Kass DA (2003) Combined ventricular systolic and arterial stiffening in patients with heart failure and preserved ejection fraction: implications for systolic and diastolic reserve limitations. Circulation 107(5):714–720

19. Borlaug BA, Melenovsky V, Russell SD, Kessler K, Pacak K, Becker LC et al (2006) Impaired chronotropic and vasodilator reserves limit exercise capacity in patients with heart failure and a preserved ejection fraction. Circulation 114(20):2138–2147
20. Brubaker PH, Joo KC, Stewart KP, Fray B, Moore B, Kitzman DW (2006) Chronotropic incompetence and its contribution to exercise intolerance in older heart failure patients. J Cardiopulm Rehabil 26(2):86–89
21. Weiss JL, Frederiksen JW, Weisfeldt ML (1976) Hemodynamic determinants of time-course of fall in canine left-ventricular pressure. J Clin Invest 58(3):751–760
22. Caruana L, Petrie MC, Davie AP, McMurray JJ (2000) Do patients with suspected heart failure and preserved left ventricular systolic function suffer from "diastolic heart failure" or from misdiagnosis? A prospective descriptive study. BMJ 321(7255):215–218
23. Myreng Y, Smiseth OA (1990) Assessment of left-ventricular relaxation by Doppler echocardiography—comparison of isovolumic relaxation-time and transmitral flow velocities with time constant of isovolumic relaxation. Circulation 81(1):260–266
24. Holen J, Aaslid R, Landmark K, Simonsen S (1976) Determination of pressure-gradient in mitral-stenosis with a non-invasive ultrasound Doppler technique. Acta Med Scand 199(6): 455–460
25. Yellin EL, Nikolic S, Frater RWM (1990) Left-ventricular filling dynamics and diastolic function. Prog Cardiovasc Dis 32(4):247–271
26. Thomas JD, Weyman AE (1989) Fluid-dynamics model of mitral-valve flow—description with in vitro validation. J Am Coll Cardiol 13(1):221–233
27. Nakatani S, Firstenberg MS, Greenberg NL, Vandervoort PM, Smedira NG, McCarthy PM et al (2001) Mitral inertance in humans: critical factor in Doppler estimation of transvalvular pressure gradients. Am J Physiol Heart Circ Physiol 280(3):H1340–H1345
28. Ishida Y, Meisner JS, Tsujioka K, Gallo JI, Yoran C, Frater RW et al (1986) Left ventricular filling dynamics: influence of left ventricular relaxation and left atrial pressure. Circulation 74(1):187–196
29. Ohno M, Cheng CP, Little WC (1994) Mechanism of altered patterns of left-ventricular filling during the development of congestive-heart-failure. Circulation 89(5):2241–2250
30. Greenberg NL, Vandervoort PM, Thomas JD (1996) Instantaneous diastolic transmitral pressure differences from color Doppler M mode echocardiography. Am J Physiol Heart Circ Physiol 271(4):H1267–H1276
31. Greenberg NL, Vandervoort PM, Firstenberg MS, Garcia MJ, Thomas JD (2001) Estimation of diastolic intraventricular pressure gradients by Doppler M-mode echocardiography. Am J Physiol Heart Circ Physiol 280(6):H2507–H2515
32. Nishimura RA, Abel MD, Hatle LK, Tajik AJ (1990) Relation of pulmonary vein to mitral flow velocities by transesophageal Doppler echocardiography. Effect of different loading conditions. Circulation 81(5):1488–1497
33. Rossvoll O, Hatle LK (1993) Pulmonary venous flow velocities recorded by transthoracic Doppler ultrasound: relation to left ventricular diastolic pressures. J Am Coll Cardiol 21(7):1687–1696
34. Appleton CP, Galloway JM, Gonzalez MS, Gaballa M, Basnight MA (1993) Estimation of left ventricular filling pressures using two-dimensional and Doppler echocardiography in adult patients with cardiac disease. Additional value of analyzing left atrial size, left atrial ejection fraction and the difference in duration of pulmonary venous and mitral flow velocity at atrial contraction. J Am Coll Cardiol 22(7):1972–1982
35. Myreng Y, Smiseth OA, Risoe C (1990) Left ventricular filling at elevated diastolic pressures: relationship between transmitral Doppler flow velocities and atrial contribution. Am Heart J 119(3 Pt 1):620–626
36. Steen T, Steen S (1994) Filling of a model left-ventricle studied by color M-mode Doppler. Cardiovasc Res 28(12):1821–1827
37. Steen T, Voss BM, Smiseth OA (1994) Influence of heart rate and left atrial pressure on pulmonary venous flow pattern in dogs. Am J Physiol 266(6 Pt 2):H2296–H2302

38. Smiseth OA, Thompson CR, Lohavanichbutr K, Ling H, Abel JG, Miyagishima RT et al (1999) The pulmonary venous systolic flow pulse—its origin and relationship to left atrial pressure. J Am Coll Cardiol 34(3):802–809
39. Guntheroth WG, Gould R, Butler J, Kinnen E (1974) Pulsatile flow in pulmonary artery, capillary, and vein in the dog. Cardiovasc Res 8(3):330–337
40. Morkin E, Collins JA, Goldman HS, Fishman AP (1965) Pattern of blood flow in pulmonary veins of dog. J Appl Physiol 20(6):1118–1128
41. Pinkerso AL (1967) Pulse-wave propagation through pulmonary vascular bed of dogs. Am J Physiol 213(2):450–454
42. Szidon JP, Ingram RH, Fishman AP (1968) Origin of pulmonary venous flow pulse. Am J Physiol 214(1):10–14
43. Morgan BC, Abel FL, Mullins GL, Guntheroth WG (1966) Flow patterns in cavae, pulmonary artery, pulmonary vein, and aorta in intact dogs. Am J Physiol 210(4):903–909
44. Rajagopalan B, Friend JA, Stallard T, Lee GDJ (1979) Blood-flow in pulmonary veins. 1. Studies in dog and man. Cardiovasc Res 13(12):667–676
45. Rajagopalan B, Friend JA, Stallard T, Lee GDJ (1979) Blood-flow in pulmonary veins. 2. Influence of events transmitted from the right and left sides of the heart. Cardiovasc Res 13(12):677–683
46. Keren G, Sherez J, Megidish R, Levitt B, Laniado S (1985) Pulmonary venous flow pattern—its relationship to cardiac dynamics—a pulsed Doppler Echocardiographic Study. Circulation 71(6):1105–1112
47. Barbier P, Solomon S, Schiller NB, Glantz SA (2000) Determinants of forward pulmonary vein flow—an open pericardium pig model. J Am Coll Cardiol 35(7):1947–1959
48. Parker KH, Jones CJH (1990) Forward and backward running waves in the arteries—analysis using the method of characteristics. J Biomech Eng 112(3):322–326
49. Kuecherer HF, Muhiudeen IA, Kusumoto FM, Lee E, Moulinier LE, Cahalan MK et al (1990) Estimation of mean left atrial pressure from transesophageal pulsed Doppler echocardiography of pulmonary venous flow. Circulation 82(4):1127–1139
50. Hofmann T, Keck A, Vaningen G, Simic O, Ostermeyer J, Meinertz T (1995) Simultaneous measurement of pulmonary venous flow by intravascular catheter Doppler velocimetry and transesophageal Doppler-echocardiography—relation to left atrial pressure and left atrial and left-ventricular function. J Am Coll Cardiol 26(1):239–249
51. Hunderi JO, Thompson CR, Smiseth OA (2006) Deceleration time of systolic pulmonary venous flow: a new clinical marker of left atrial pressure and compliance. J Appl Physiol 100(2):685–689
52. Kinnaird TD, Thompson CR, Munt BI (2001) The deceleration time of pulmonary venous diastolic flow is more accurate than the pulmonary artery occlusion pressure in predicting left atrial pressure (vol 37, pg 2025, 2001). J Am Coll Cardiol 38(2):586
53. Yellin EL, Peskin C, Yoran C, Koenigsberg M, Matsumoto M, Laniado S et al (1981) Mechanisms of mitral-valve motion during diastole. Am J Physiol 241(3):H389–H400
54. Meisner JS, Mcqueen DM, Ishida Y, Vetter HO, Bortolotti U, Strom JA et al (1985) Effects of timing of atrial systole on Lv-filling and mitral-valve closure—computer and dog studies. Am J Physiol 249(3):H604–H619
55. Brun P, Tribouilloy C, Duval AM, Iserin L, Meguira A, Pelle G et al (1992) Left-ventricular flow propagation during early filling is related to wall relaxation—a color M-mode Doppler analysis. J Am Coll Cardiol 20(2):420–432
56. Stugaard M, Smiseth OA, Risoe C, Ihlen H (1993) Intraventricular early diastolic filling during acute myocardial-ischemia—assessment by multigated color M-mode Doppler-echocardiography. Circulation 88(6):2705–2713
57. Ling D, Rankin JS, Edwards CH, Mchale PA, Anderson RW (1979) Regional diastolic mechanics of the left-ventricle in the conscious dog. Am J Physiol 236(2):H323–H330
58. Courtois M, Kovacs SJ, Ludbrook PA (1990) Physiological early diastolic intraventricular pressure-gradient is lost during acute myocardial-ischemia. Circulation 81(5):1688–1696

59. Firstenberg MS, Smedira NG, Greenberg NL, Prior DL, McCarthy PM, Garcia MJ et al (2001) Relationship between early diastolic intraventricular pressure gradients, an index of elastic recoil, and improvements in systolic and diastolic function. Circulation 104(12):I330–I335
60. Firstenberg MS, Greenberg NL, Main ML, Drinko JK, Odabashian JA, Thomas JD et al (2001) Determinants of diastolic myocardial tissue Doppler velocities: influences of relaxation and preload. J Appl Physiol 90(1):299–307
61. Steine K, Stugaard M, Smiseth OA (1999) Mechanisms of retarded apical filling in acute ischemic left ventricular failure. Circulation 99(15):2048–2054
62. Nikolic SD, Feneley MP, Pajaro OE, Rankin JS, Yellin EL (1995) Origin of regional pressure-gradients in the left-ventricle during early diastole. Am J Physiol Heart Circ Physiol 268(2):H550–H557
63. Yotti R, Bermejo J, Antoranz JC, Desco MM, Cortina C, Rojo-Alvarez JL et al (2005) A non-invasive method for assessing impaired diastolic suction in patients with dilated cardiomyopathy. Circulation 112(19):2921–2929
64. Beppu S, Izumi S, Miyatake K, Nagata S, Park YD, Sakakibara H et al (1988) Abnormal-blood pathways in left-ventricular cavity in acute myocardial-infarction—experimental-observations with special reference to regional wall motion abnormality and hemostasis. Circulation 78(1):157–164
65. Delemarre BJ, Bot H, Visser CA, Dunning AJ (1988) Pulsed Doppler echocardiographic description of a circular flow pattern in spontaneous left ventricular contrast. J Am Soc Echocardiogr 1(2):114–118
66. Vierendeels JA, Dick E, Verdonck PR (2002) Hydrodynamics of color M-mode Doppler flow wave propagation velocity V(p): a computer study. J Am Soc Echocardiogr 15(3):219–224
67. Hasegawa H, Little WC, Ohno M, Brucks S, Morimoto A, Cheng HJ et al (2003) Diastolic mitral annular velocity during the development of heart failure. J Am Coll Cardiol 41(9):1590–1597
68. Stewart KC, Kumar R, Charonko JJ, Ohara T, Vlachos PP, Little WC (2011) Evaluation of LV diastolic function from color M-mode echocardiography. JACC Cardiovasc Imaging 4(1):37–46
69. Urheim S, Edvardsen T, Torp H, Angelsen B, Smiseth OA (2000) Myocardial strain by Doppler echocardiography—validation of a new method to quantify regional myocardial function. Circulation 102(10):1158–1164
70. Amundsen BH, Helle-Valle T, Edvardsen T, Torp H, Crosby J, Lyseggen E et al (2006) Noninvasive myocardial strain measurement by speckle tracking echocardiography—validation against sonomicrometry and tagged magnetic resonance imaging. J Am Coll Cardiol 47(4):789–793
71. Nagueh SF, Appleton CP, Gillebert TC, Marino PN, Oh JK, Smiseth OA et al (2009) Recommendations for the evaluation of left ventricular diastolic function by echocardiography. J Am Soc Echocardiogr 22(2):107–133
72. Nagueh SF, Middleton KJ, Kopelen HA, Zoghbi WA, Quinones MA (1997) Doppler tissue imaging: a noninvasive technique for evaluation of left ventricular relaxation and estimation of filling pressures. J Am Coll Cardiol 30(6):1527–1533
73. Ommen SR, Nishimura RA, Appleton CP, Miller FA, Oh JK, Redfield MM et al (2000) Clinical utility of Doppler echocardiography and tissue Doppler imaging in the estimation of left ventricular filling pressures—a comparative simultaneous Doppler-Catheterization study. Circulation 102(15):1788–1794
74. Sohn DW, Chai IH, Lee DJ, Kim HC, Kim HS, Oh BH et al (1997) Assessment of mitral annulus velocity by Doppler tissue imaging in the evaluation of left ventricular diastolic function. J Am Coll Cardiol 30(2):474–480
75. Opdahl A, Remme EW, Helle-Valle T, Lyseggen E, Vartdal T, Pettersen E et al (2009) Determinants of left ventricular early-diastolic lengthening velocity: independent contributions from left ventricular relaxation, restoring forces, and lengthening load. Circulation 119(19):2578–2586
76. Smiseth OA, Frais MA, Kingma I, Smith ER, Tyberg JV (1985) Assessment of pericardial constraint in dogs. Circulation 71(1):158–164

77. Rademakers FE, Buchalter MB, Rogers WJ, Zerhouni EA, Weisfeldt ML, Weiss JL et al (1992) Dissociation between left-ventricular untwisting and filling—accentuation by catecholamines. Circulation 85(4):1572–1581
78. Notomi Y, Lysyansky P, Setser RM, Shiota T, Popović ZB, Martin-Miklovic MG, Weaver JA, Oryszak SJ, Greenberg NL, White RD, Thomas JD (2005) Measurement of ventricular torsion by two-dimensional ultrasound speckle tracking imaging. J Am Coll Cardiol 45(12): 2034–2041
79. Helle-Valle T, Crosby J, Edvardsen T, Lyseggen E, Amundsen BH, Smith HJ, Rosen BD, Lima JA, Torp H, Ihlen H, Smiseth OA (2005) New noninvasive method for assessment of left ventricular rotation: speckle tracking echocardiography. Circulation 112(20):3149–3156
80. Kroeker CAG, Tyberg JV, Beyar R (1995) Effects of load manipulations, heart-rate, and contractility on left-ventricular apical rotation—an experimental-study in anesthetized dogs. Circulation 92(1):130–141
81. Opdahl A, Remme EW, Helle-Valle T, Edvardsen T, Smiseth OA (2012) Myocardial relaxation, restoring forces, and early-diastolic load are independent determinants of left ventricular untwisting rate. Circulation 126(12):1441–1451
82. Appleton CP, Hatle LK, Popp RL (1988) Relation of transmitral flow velocity patterns to left ventricular diastolic function: new insights from a combined hemodynamic and Doppler echocardiographic study. J Am Coll Cardiol 12(2):426–440
83. Oh JK, Appleton CP, Hatle LK, Nishimura RA, Seward JB, Tajik AJ (1997) The noninvasive assessment of left ventricular diastolic function with two-dimensional and Doppler echocardiography. J Am Soc Echocardiogr 10(3):246–270
84. Flachskampf FA, Weyman AE, Guerrero JL, Thomas JD (1992) Calculation of atrioventricular compliance from the mitral flow profile—analytic and in vitro study. J Am Coll Cardiol 19(5):998–1004
85. Little WC, Ohno M, Kitzman DW, Thomas JD, Cheng CP (1995) Determination of left-ventricular chamber stiffness from the time for deceleration of early left-ventricular filling. Circulation 92(7):1933–1939
86. Maisel AS, Krishnaswamy P, Nowak RM, McCord J, Hollander JE, Duc P et al (2002) Rapid measurement of B-type natriuretic peptide in the emergency diagnosis of heart failure. N Engl J Med 347(3):161–167
87. Atisha D, Bhalla MA, Morrison LK, Felicio L, Clopton P, Gardetto N et al (2004) A prospective study in search of an optimal B-natriuretic peptide level to screen patients for cardiac dysfunction. Am Heart J 148(3):518–523
88. Zaphiriou A, Robb S, Murray-Thomas T, Mendez G, Fox K, McDonagh T et al (2005) The diagnostic accuracy of plasma BNP and NTproBNP in patients referred from primary care with suspected heart failure: results of the UK natriuretic peptide study. Eur J Heart Fail 7(4):537–541
89. Moser M, Hebert PR (1996) Prevention of disease progression, left ventricular hypertrophy and congestive heart failure in hypertension treatment trials. J Am Coll Cardiol 27(5): 1214–1218
90. Kostis JB, Davis BR, Cutler J, Grimm RH Jr, Berge KG, Cohen JD et al (1997) Prevention of heart failure by antihypertensive drug treatment in older persons with isolated systolic hypertension. SHEP Cooperative Research Group. JAMA 278(3):212–216
91. McMurray JJ, Adamopoulos S, Anker SD, Auricchio A, Bohm M, Dickstein K et al (2012) ESC Guidelines for the diagnosis and treatment of acute and chronic heart failure 2012: the task force for the diagnosis and treatment of acute and chronic heart failure 2012 of the European Society of Cardiology. Developed in collaboration with the Heart Failure Association (HFA) of the ESC. Eur Heart J 14(8):803–869
92. Cleland JGF, Tendera M, Adamus J, Freemantle N, Polonski L, Taylor J (2006) The perindopril in elderly people with chronic heart failure (PEP-CHF) study. Eur Heart J 27(19): 2338–2345
93. Yusuf S, Pfeffer MA, Swedberg K, Granger CB, Held P, McMurray JJ et al (2003) Effects of candesartan in patients with chronic heart failure and preserved left-ventricular ejection fraction: the CHARM-Preserved Trial. Lancet 362(9386):777–781

94. Massie BM, Carson PE, McMurray JJ, Komajda M, McKelvie R, Zile MR et al (2008) Irbesartan in patients with heart failure and preserved ejection fraction. N Engl J Med 359(23):2456–2467
95. Ghio S, Magrini G, Serio A, Klersy C, Fucilli A, Ronaszeki A et al (2006) Effects of nebivolol in elderly heart failure patients with or without systolic left ventricular dysfunction: results of the SENIORS echocardiographic substudy. Eur Heart J 27(5):562–568
96. Little WC, Fukuta H (1994) Modulation of diastolic dysfunction in the intact heart. In: Lorell B, Grossmann W (eds) Diastolic relaxation of the heart. Kluwer, Boston, pp 146–167
97. Smiseth OA, Thompson CR (2000) Atrioventricular filling dynamics, diastolic function and dysfunction. Heart Fail Rev 5(4):291–299
98. Stugaard M, Steen T, Lundervold A, Smiseth OA, Ihlen H (1994) Visual assessment of intra ventricular flow from colour M-mode Doppler images. Int J Card Imaging 10(4):279–287

Chapter 3
Cardiorenal Syndrome Revisited

Matthias Dupont, Wilfried Mullens, and W.H. Wilson Tang

Abstract Heart failure and renal dysfunction frequently coexist, and this combination has been labeled as the "cardiorenal syndrome" (CRS). This chapter highlights the epidemiology and prognostic significance of CRS before centering on the pathophysiology and treatment. The importance of neurohormonal changes and venous congestion in the development of the CRS will be extensively discussed. In addition, inflammation and oxidative stress have their significance in all types of the CRS. Neurohormonal blockade remains vital to prevent progressive cardiorenal disease. Many other aspects of prevention and treatment will be touched before revealing a glimpse on future treatments.

1 Introduction

Heart failure is a heterogenous syndrome with variable presentations and different underlying mechanisms. The syndrome converges in common signs and symptoms such as dyspnea, fatigue, and exercise intolerance. Although not specific and not invariably present, the tendency to develop congestion is perhaps the most striking feature of the heart failure syndrome [1]. This symptom is responsible for the huge burden in hospital admissions and costs. To maintain adequate control of volume status, proper functioning kidneys are vital, especially following aggressive diuretic therapy. Unfortunately, the coexistence of cardiac and renal disease is the rule rather than the exception. The concomitant impairment of both organs exceeds what is expected solely on the base of common etiologies such as diabetes and hypertension. This observation, together with the sometimes acute and dynamic changes in the function of both organs and recovery following their resolutions, gave rise to the conceptual

M. Dupont, M.D. • W. Mullens, M.D., Ph.D. • W.H.W. Tang, M.D. (✉)
Department of Cardiovascular Medicine, Heart and Vascular Institute, Cleveland Clinic,
9500 Euclid Avenue, J3-4, Cleveland, OH 44195, USA
e-mail: tangw@ccf.org

J. Bartunek and M. Vanderheyden (eds.), *Translational Approach to Heart Failure*,
DOI 10.1007/978-1-4614-7345-9_3, © Springer Science+Business Media New York 2013

term "cardiorenal syndrome (CRS)." This chapter will focus on the contemporary and evolving pathophysiologic insights of CRS, which are key to successful management and development of future renal-preserving therapies. Serving the purpose of this book, most attention will go to heart failure complicated by acute renal dysfunction (so-called CRS type 1) or chronic renal dysfunction (so-called CRS type 2).

2 Definition, Classification, and Scope of the Problem

2.1 Definition and Classification

The high prevalence of renal dysfunction in cardiac disease and vice versa has been recognized for decades as nephrologists saw their patients experiencing cardiac complications and as cardiologists were faced with patients developing progressive renal insufficiency. In the absence of a formal definition, physicians gradually started using the umbrella-term "cardiorenal syndrome" when they were faced with this situation. In its broadest context, CRS refers to any type of disorder of heart or kidney whereby acute or chronic dysfunction in one organ induces acute or chronic dysfunction in the other. In a stricter definition, but one often used in the heart failure setting, CRS describes a more restricted condition whereby attempts to relieve congestion in acute decompensated heart failure (ADHF) are limited by further decline in renal function (CRS type 1, see below). In the latter context, the term "worsening renal function (WRF)" is often used at the bedside as well. Although in general any decline in renal function is associated with excess mortality, WRF is commonly defined as a ≥0.3 mg/dL increase in serum creatinine in outcome studies [2, 3].

Recently, a classification scheme that divides CRS into five categories has been proposed, and has gradually found its way to everyday clinical practice (Fig. 3.1) [4]. This classification system recognizes the primary organ dysfunction (cardiac vs. renal) as well as the acute vs. chronic nature of the condition. To maintain uniformity with the renal literature, the severity of acute kidney injury in CRS type 1 or 3 could best be expressed using the RIFLE or AKIN criteria (Table 3.1) [5, 6].

2.2 Measuring Renal Function

Although well-functioning kidneys cover more than just proper filtration (e.g., tubular and endocrinologic functions), decline in glomerular filtration rate (GFR) has been considered the primary measure of kidney function by nephrologists. GFR is the product of filtration rate in single nephrons times the number of nephrons in both kidneys. Because glomerular hypertrophy or increased glomerular capillary

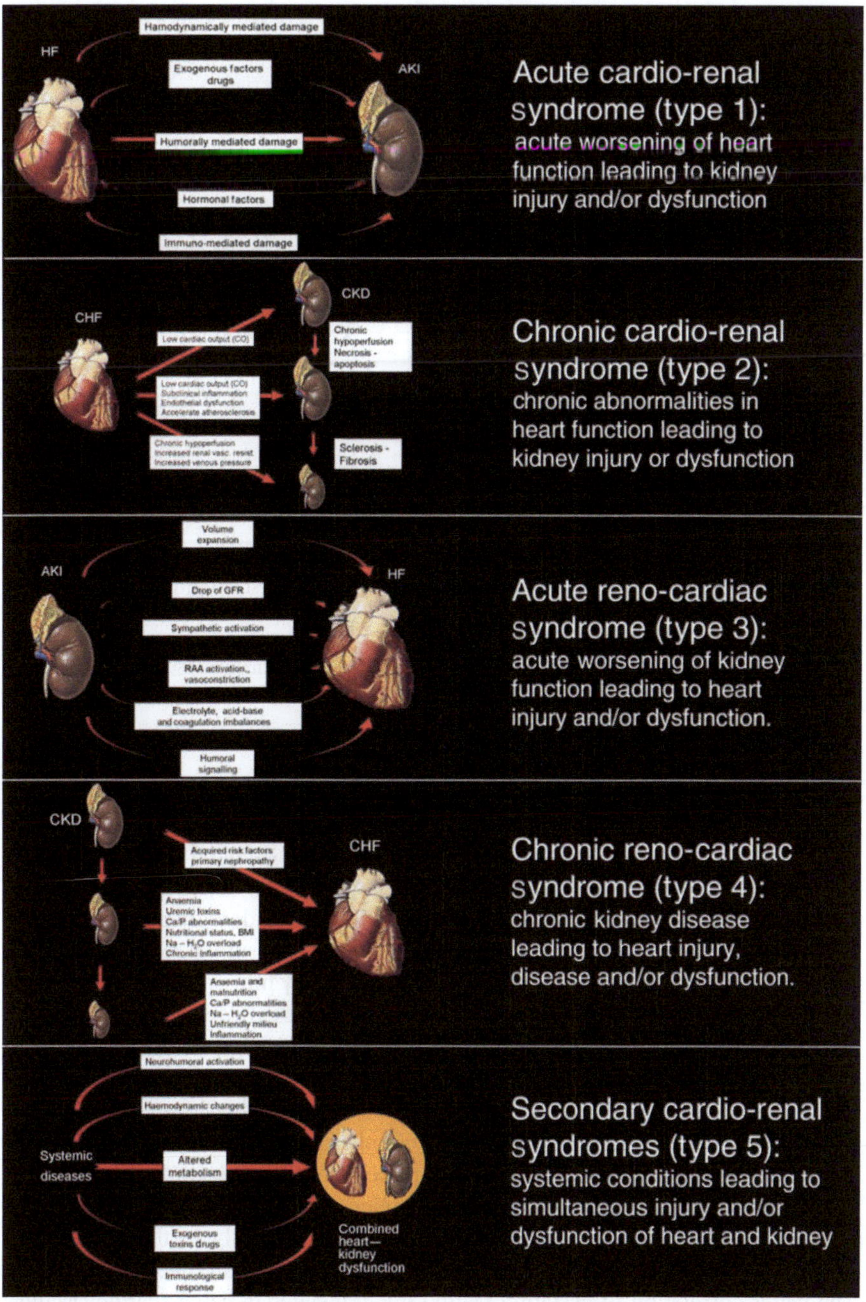

Fig. 3.1 Classification of the five subtypes of the cardiorenal syndrome. Classification as proposed by a consensus conference of the acute dialysis quality initiative. *HF* heart failure, *AKI* acute kidney injury, *CHF* chronic heart failure, *CKD* chronic kidney disease. (From Ronco et al. [4], personal courtesy of professor Ronco, with permission from the publisher)

Table 3.1 RIFLE and AKIN criteria for expressing the severity of acute kidney injury

Rifle category	Creat/GFR criteria	Urine output criteria	Creat criteria	Akin stage
Risk	↑ Creat × 1.5 GFR ↓ >25 %	UO ≤0.5 mL/kg/h × 6 h	↑ Creat × 1.5 ↑ Creat ≥0.3 mg/dL	Stage 1
Injury	↑ Creat × 2 GFR ↓ >50 %	UO ≤0.5 mL/kg/h × 12 h	↑ Creat × 2	Stage 2
Failure	↑ Creat × 3 GFR ↓ >75 % Creat ≥4 mg/dL with acute rise of ≥0.5 mg/dL	UO ≤0.3 mL/kg/h × 24 h Anuria × 12 h	↑ Creat × 3 Creat ≥4 mg/dL with acute rise of ≥0.5 mg/dL Renal replacement therapy	Stage 3
Loss	Persistent acute renal failure = complete loss of kidney function >4 weeks but ≤3 months	–	–	–
ESRD	Complete loss of kidney function ≥3 months	–	–	–

RIFLE and AKIN are two similar classification systems for acute kidney injury. Creatinine, GFR, or urine output is used. Patients are classified according to the worst criterion. The urine output criterion is the same for the two classification systems. The RIFLE classification has two outcome categories (loss and ESRD) as well

GFR glomerular filtration rate, *UO* urine output, *ESRD* end-stage renal disease

Source: Adapted from Bellomo et al. [5] and Mehta et al. [6]

pressure can compensate for loss in nephron number, substantial renal damage can remain unnoticed [7]. A second limitation encompasses our imperfect current tools to measure GFR. Due to both variable production, dependent on diet and muscle mass, and tubular secretion, creatinine is not an ideal measure of GFR [8]. Similar creatinine values can therefore reflect normal or severely impaired glomerular filtration depending on patient characteristics. Creatinine-based equations try to correct for this by incorporating determinants of muscle mass (age, gender, race, weight) in their formulas and many laboratories now automatically report estimated GFRs. These formulas were developed in patients with chronic kidney disease (CKD) and thus perform better in patients with GFR <60 mL/min/1.73 m^2.

Cystatin C has been considered to be a more ideal filtration marker because it is not secreted nor reabsorbed into the bloodstream and since its production is fairly constant and less dependent on other factors [9]. Especially in the higher GFR ranges (>60 mL/min/1.73 m^2), it has additional value over other measures of GFR. The better correlation of cystatin C with GFR translates in better (cardiovascular) risk prediction in the general as well as the heart failure population [10, 11]. Furthermore, both creatinine and cystatin C require some time to accumulate when GFR is declining.

2.3 *Epidemiology*

Data from the Acute Decompensated Heart Failure National Registry (ADHERE) reveal that only 9 % of the patients had an estimated GFR (eGFR) of ≥90 mL/min/1.73 m^2, a value that can be considered normal. Furthermore, 27 % had mild (eGFR 60–89 mL/min/1.73 m^2), 44 % moderate (eGFR 30–59 mL/min/1.73 m^2), 13 % severe (eGFR 15–29 mL/min/1.73 m^2) and 7 % end-stage renal failure (eGFR <15 mL/min/1.73 m^2 or on dialysis) [12]. As expected, the frequency of common risk factors such as diabetes mellitus, hypertension, and vascular disease increased with decreasing eGFR. Interestingly, lower left ventricular ejection fraction (LVEF) alone is not a risk factor for renal dysfunction, an important finding with the eye on the pathophysiology of the CRS.

CKD itself has repeatedly been identified as one of the major risk factors for WRF during treatment of ADHF, which has an incidence of 25–45 % [2, 13–15]. Other factors associated with WRF include diabetes mellitus, high blood pressure, older age, and a history of heart failure (but not impaired LVEF). In the majority of cases, WRF occurs within the first 3 days of hospitalization. Meanwhile, up to 44 % of patients with CKD die from cardiovascular disease, which is more than from renal failure itself [16]. The odds-ratios to die from cardiovascular disease are 10–20 times higher than in the matched general population. The risk not only stems from atherosclerotic disease, but also from heart failure (with preserved or decreased systolic function), which is present in roughly one in three dialysis patients [17].

Key Points

- The cardiorenal syndrome (CRS) is divided in five subtypes.
- CRS type 1 is also called worsening renal function (WRF) and often defined as a ≥0.3 mg/dL rise in serum creatinine.
- Cystatin C is a better marker of GFR especially in patients with higher GFR.
- The majority of heart failure patients have some degree of renal function limitation and approximately one third will develop WRF during treatment of ADHF.

3 Prognostic Importance in Heart Failure

3.1 *Chronic Renal Impairment*

The literature is unanimously about the prognostic value of chronic renal impairment in heart failure; it has consistently been identified as one of the strongest independent risk factors for mortality and is at least as powerful as most clinical variables such as New York Heart Association (NYHA) functional class and LVEF [12, 18–22]. Moreover, it is most predictive of death from heart failure progression, which suggests that adequacy of renal function is essential in the preservation of the compensated state in heart failure patients [18]. The risk becomes evident with eGFR ≤60 mL/min/1.73 m^2 [18]. The prognostic value of impaired renal function is as striking in heart failure with preserved ejection fraction (HFpEF) as in heart failure with reduced ejection fraction (HFrEF) [22]. In most studies creatinine or eGFR quantifies renal function. Although the correlation of GFR with blood urea nitrogen (BUN) is lower than with creatinine, eGFR, or cystatin C, there is evidence that the prognostic value of BUN is even higher [23–25]. Likely, this is explained by BUN levels being dependent on tubular reabsorption, which on itself is a function of neurohormonal upregulation [26]. Consistent with this observation, high BUN/creatinine ratios are worse than low ratios in subjects with impaired renal function (eGFR <60 mL/min/1.73 m^2). In fact the latter were not associated with excess mortality, suggesting that renal dysfunction without neurohormonal activation is more favorable [27]. In addition, it is well known that loop diuretics provoke neurohormonal activation through reduced sodium uptake via the sodium/potassium/2-chloride transporter in the macula densa. The combination of high BUN (as a surrogate for neurohormonal activation) and high-dose diuretics portends poor prognosis [28].

3.2 Worsening Renal Function

WRF has been associated with increased morbidity (length of stay in the hospital) and higher short- and long-term mortality as well. In some studies, WRF is even a stronger predictor as baseline renal function [2, 3, 13, 14]. However, it seems that the mechanism by which WRF occurs may directly influence its prognostic impact. If WRF is accompanied by vigorous diuresis resulting in hemoconcentration of red blood cells or proteins, prognosis is actually better, even when compared to patients without WRF [29]. Hemoconcentration was achieved with the use of larger doses of diuretics and accompanied by a greater decrease in filling pressures. Taken together, this underlines the significance of achieving proper decongestion during treatment of ADHF even at the cost of WRF (the majority of cases being transient and "prerenal azotemia" in nature). Similarly, when WRF is the consequence of the initiation of an angiotensin converting enzyme-inhibitor (ACE-I) or the result of treatment-induced hypotension, it is not detrimental [30]. In contrast, WRF portends poor prognosis in the setting of oliguria despite increasing diuretic dose. This again highlights the importance of the underlying mechanism by which WRF occurs. It also supports the idea that it is not WRF itself that leads to increased mortality, but rather the background (e.g., the underlying disease severity) on which it occurs.

Key Points

- Chronic renal impairment is uniformly associated with worse outcomes in heart failure patients.
- WRF, on the other hand, is most often but not always associated with worse outcomes, pointing towards different underlying pathophysiologic mechanisms.

4 Pathophysiology

The pathophysiology of the CRS is extremely complicated and still poorly understood. Changes in renal function, both GFR and tubular function, are the result of the complex interaction between hemodynamic and neurohormonal changes that are typical for cardiorenal disease progression. The general concept is that GFR may reflect the filtration rate in a single nephron times the number of functioning nephrons. Filtration in a single nephron is dependent on the pressure and oncotic gradients (filtration gradient) between the glomerular capillaries and Bowman's capsule. The pressures are function of different hemodynamic variables as shown in Fig. 3.2. Glomerular filtration pressure is dependent upon both the overall cardiac output and the difference in vasoactive states of the afferent and efferent arterioles. The pressure in Bowman's capsule (proximal tubular pressure) is influenced by venous congestion (see below) among other things. The glomerular filtrate will further be altered by secretion and reabsorption of electrolytes, water and different

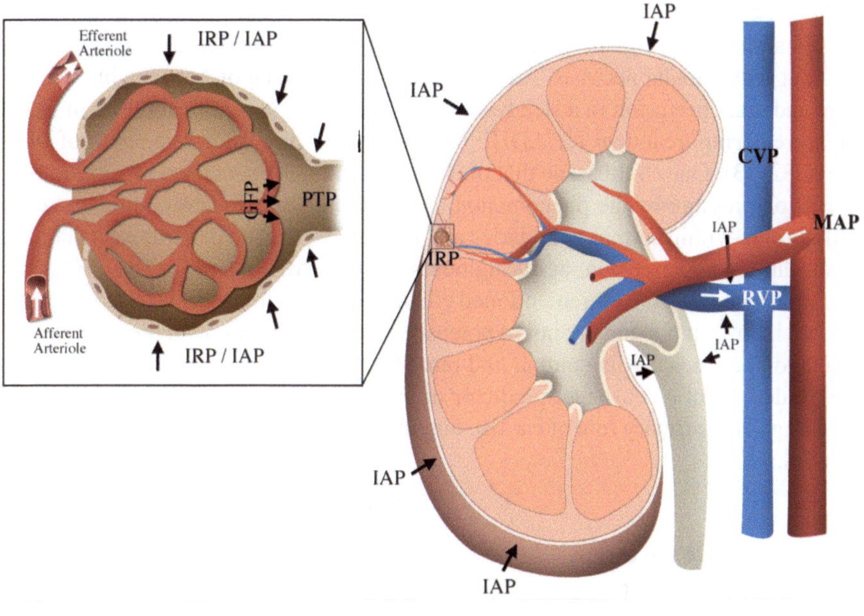

Fig. 3.2 Hemodynamic determinants of glomerular filtration rate (GFR). Apart from the total amount and quality of nephrons, GFR is dependent on multiple hemodynamic factors. The mechanical force driving fluid from the glomerular capillaries to the capsular space is the (renal) filtration gradient (FG) = glomerular filtration pressure (GFP)–proximal tubular pressure (PTP). PTP is dependent on interstitial renal pressure (IRP) and intra-abdominal pressure (IAP), both increased by venous congestion. GFP is dependent on renal blood flow = renal perfusion pressure (mean arterial pressure (MAP)–renal venous pressure (RVP))/renal vascular resistance. RVP is closely related to central venous pressure (CVP) and thus increased when venous congestion is present. GFP is further regulated by the complex interplay between afferent and efferent arteriolar vasoconstriction and vasodilatation. (From Dupont et al. [48])

metabolites. Although this tubular secretion and reabsorption will only slightly alter calculations of GFR (creatinine is secreted as well), it is crucial in the maintenance of volume homeostasis and of obvious importance in heart failure. Both renal hemodynamics and tubular function are governed by neurohormonal changes and autonomic modulation, inflammation, and oxidative stress. In what follows, the different factors influencing cardiorenal interactions are highlighted according to the current evidence and understanding. Somewhat artificially, different components are separated in hemodynamic, neurohormonal, inflammatory, and tubular factors.

4.1 Hemodynamic Factors

4.1.1 Cardiac Output and Blood Pressure

Traditionally, insufficient blood flow to the kidneys ("pre-renal") is considered the major determinant of both renal impairment and WRF in acute and chronic heart failure. There is no doubt that renal perfusion is important, given the well-known presentation of cardiogenic shock accompanied by acute renal insufficiency with or without acute tubular necrosis. Although there is no correlation between blood pressure and renal perfusion in a steady-state condition [31], a significant drop in blood pressure during treatment for ADHF has shown to evoke WRF as a result of ischemia [32, 33]. One could argue that the kidney is naturally protected to variations in perfusion pressure by the phenomenon of autoregulation. However, autoregulation only occurs within certain boundaries and is likely weakened in cardiovascular disease, chronic hypertension, or during treatment with ACE inhibitors [34–36].

Acknowledging the aforementioned clinical scenarios, most heart failure patients are not in low output and are not hypotensive. Large registries or studies do not find a relation between cardiac output and renal function [12, 37]. In addition, low cardiac index is not a consistent predictor of WRF [38–40]. These observations have challenged the primary role of cardiac output as the main driver of renal impairment in CRS.

4.1.2 Venous Congestion

Recent evidence suggests that venous congestion may be more contributory to the pathophysiology of renal impairment and WRF in the setting of CRS [37, 38]. Although the significance of these associations has only recently been demonstrated, the physiologic background was provided decades ago in mainly forgotten literature. As early as in 1931, Winton performed a series of elegant experiments on isolated mammalian kidneys whereby he influenced either the renal arterial or the renal venous pressure (RVP) [41]. It was shown that an increase in RVP provoked a marked decrease in urine output which was promptly reversed by normalization of the venous pressure. It was believed that the increase in venous pressure had two important effects; on the one hand it increased glomerular capillary (filtration) pressure which, on itself, should increase urine production. On the other hand however, by congestion of the tubular venules it increased the pressure in the renal tubules and Bowman's capsule similar to ureteral obstruction. The latter effect offsets the former with decreased glomerular filtration as the net effect. This theory also explains why ureteral obstruction, in addition to RVP elevation, does not further reduce urine output. In contrary, in the presence of ureteral obstruction, increase in venous pressure will augment urine output through an increase in glomerular capillary pressure. Although these experiments can be criticized for being not physiologic (the neurohormonal systems, mainly undiscovered at that time, is prevented to exert its effects in isolated kidneys), they provide a hemodynamic experiment in its purest form. Elevated RVPs not only evoke a decrease in GFR, but also increased tubular reabsorption of NaCl as nicely shown in animal experiments (intact dogs) [42, 43]. In some animals, sodium excretion and urine volume fell by more than 50 % despite an only minimal or absent decrease in creatinine clearance (and GFR). Interestingly, decreased GFR and decreased tubular reabsorption as a consequence of augmentations in RVP are only present in animals with volume expansion (as in heart failure) and not in hydropenic animals [44].

The exact mechanisms of decreased sodium excretion in the presence of venous congestion still need to be elucidated but the steep rise in renal interstitial pressure (as a consequence of an increase in RVP in already hypervolemic patients) is thought to play a role. Elevated interstitial pressures result in elevated tubular pressures, which slow down urine transit time and augment sodium reabsorption in the loop of Henle [44–46]. This mechanism may also provide a good alternative explanation for the sodium avidity in pathologies were the classic "arterial underfilling" hypothesis is less evident (such as cor pulmonale, constrictive pericarditis, and perhaps heart failure with preserved ejection fraction) [47].

In summary, the demonstration, in recent years, of the association between venous congestion and renal impairment provoked a paradigm shift towards congestion ("backward failure") and not cardiac output ("forward failure") as the main focus of our therapy. There are, in addition, many other good reasons to treat congestion; it causes symptoms, hospital admissions, costs, hepatic dysfunction, and anemia [48]. Nevertheless, the cardiorenal syndrome is definitely not explainable by one mechanism.

4.1.3 Intra-abdominal Pressure

Another hemodynamic contributor to the pathogenesis CRS involves the presence of raised intra-abdominal pressure (IAP), which is often in parallel to venous congestion and has been associated with the development and progression of WRF in the heart failure population [49, 50]. IAP refers to the pressure generated within the abdominal cavity, which can be considered a closed compartment with both rigid (costal arch, spine and pelvis) and flexible (abdominal wall and diaphragm) components. Therefore, the IAP is equally distributed throughout the whole abdomen in

Table 3.2 Different definitions concerning intra-abdominal pressure

Term	Abbreviation	Definition
Intra-abdominal pressure	IAP	• Steady-state pressure in abdominal cavity • Expressed in mmHg, transducer at mid-axillary line • Via the bladder, maximal instillation 25 mL saline • Measured at end-expiration • Normal value 5–7 mmHg
Intra-abdominal hypertension	IAH	• Repeated elevation of IAP ≥12 mmHg • Grade I: 12–15 mmHg • Grade II: 16–20 mmHg • Grade III: 21–25 mmHg • Grade IV: >25 mmHg
Abdominal compartment syndrome	ACS	• Sustained IAP >20 mmHg associated with new organ dysfunction • Primary: caused by pathologic process in abdominopelvic region • Secondary: Not caused by pathologic process in abdominopelvic region
Abdominal perfusion pressure (e.g., renal perfusion pressure)	APP	• MAP–RVP (renal venous pressure) • If CVP (central venous pressure) > IAP → RVP ≈ CVP • If CVP (central venous pressure) < IAP → RVP ≈ IAP
Filtration gradient	FG	• GFP (glomerular filtration pressure)–PTP (proximal tubular pressure) • Both pressures influenced by IAP

See also Fig. 3.2, adapted from Malbrain et al. [128]

agreement with Pascal's law. IAP may increase somewhat from anterior to posterior with a patient in the supine position due to gravity, and this likely explains why the kidneys in particular are vulnerable to intra-abdominal hypertension (IAH) [51]. The normal pressure in the abdominal cavity is <8 mmHg. Table 3.2 depicts different definitions of elevated IAPs.

The pathologic importance of increased IAP on renal function was first demonstrated by Bradley and Bradley in 1947 [49]. These authors showed that renal blood flow, GFR, urine production, and glucose reabsorption all decreased significantly after external pressure application in normal individuals. Water reabsorption was increased, leading to more concentrated urine. In more recent years, the pathophysiologic importance of elevated IAP has been described in critical illness and post-surgery [52]. The role of IAP in heart failure was demonstrated by the observation that elevated IAP is associated with impaired renal function and changes in IAP correlated better with changes in renal function than other hemodynamic variables [50]. In addition it was shown that mechanical fluid removal, by either paracentesis or ultrafiltration, can quickly decrease IAP and is accompanied by improvement in renal function [53]. Indeed, IAP may be transferred to both the renal veins and to the renal excretory system (ureter, tubules and Bowman's capsule) within an encapsulated organ. As a result, there is decrease in renal perfusion and filtration gradient associated with elevated IAP. In non-heart failure settings, renal perfusion pressure is often calculated as mean arterial pressure (MAP)−IAP instead of MAP−RVP. The reason is that in these circumstances IAP ≈ RVP. However in heart failure, central venous pressure (CVP), and so RVP, remain typically higher than the IAP.

There is another factor related to IAP that can play a role in the genesis of WRF during treatment of ADHF. Clinicians often rely on pressures (invasive or noninvasive) to guide their decongestive treatment. This builds on the premise that pressures represent intravascular volume. However, IAP is transdiaphragmatically transmitted and gives rise to elevation of all right- and left-sided filling pressures as read on pulmonary artery catheter tracings. The finding of elevated pressures therefore doesn't always correspond to increased intravascular volume. Inappropriate admission of diuretics can therefore create a real "pre-renal" state with WRF.

4.1.4 Renal Perfusion

Renal blood flow can mathematically be expressed as the ratio of renal perfusion pressure (estimated by the gradient between renal arterial and venous pressures) and renal vascular resistance. In the absence of renal artery stenosis, renal perfusion pressure can be estimated by the gradient between MAP and CVP.

The kidneys receive approximately 20 % of the cardiac output in normal subjects. When the (systolic) heart failure population as a whole is considered at steady state, this percentage remains the same [31]. In other words, despite the existence of autoregulation, renal blood flow decreases and renal vascular resistance increases proportionally to cardiac output and systemic vascular resistance, respectively. Whether the chronic impaired perfusion of the kidney contributes to the development of CKD is largely unknown at present. However, within the systolic heart failure population, flow to the kidney seemed somewhat spared as cardiac index drops further [31]. It is the pressure difference between the glomerular capillaries and Bowman's capsule that will ultimately determine GFR and these are influenced by other factors as well. This may also explain how it remains possible to have a perfectly normal GFR despite impaired renal perfusion. Although we know that renal blood flow is decreased in heart failure patients in steady state, it is unclear how renal perfusion evolves during treatment of ADHF. Unfortunately, there are currently no good ways to examine renal blood flow in a repeatable bedside fashion.

4.2 Neurohormonal Changes

The reciprocal connections between heart and kidneys in disease encompass more than just hemodynamics. Indeed, the striking common denominator in heart and kidney disease is the neurohormonal upregulation. Especially in advanced chronic disease (CRS types 2 and 4), it doesn't matter anymore what the primary disorder was. The result is neurohormonal upregulation, inflammation, and oxidative stress often leading to progressive disease in both organs via several positive feedback loops [54].

4.2.1 The Renin–Angiotensin–Aldosteron System (Fig. 3.3)

The renin–angiotensin–aldosteron system (RAAS) is one of the most studied pathways in both renal and cardiac disease and a major target of treatment. The present viewpoint is that the system serves as an acute (beneficial) defense against underperfusion of vital organs that becomes detrimental when chronically activated as in cardiovascular and renal disease [55]. The responsible stimulus for activation of the system is believed to be reduced "effective arterial volume" as sensed by the juxtaglomerular cells. The RAAS comprises both a systemic and a local tissue system. The negative effects of angiotensin II are multiple: volume retention (congestion) via aldosterone, vasoconstriction resulting in hypertension that increases LV afterload, LV hypertrophy, vascular hypertrophy, cell growth and proliferation, sympathetic nervous system activation, inflammation, and oxidative stress (see below) [56, 57]. Angiotensin II constricts efferent arterioles more than afferent arterioles thereby reducing renal blood flow while preserving glomerular filtration (increase in filtration fraction), an effect which has also shown to result in progressive renal dysfunction over time. It is clear that RAAS activation is a continuous drive for cardiorenal disease progression (CRS type 2 and 4).

4.2.2 The Sympathetic Nervous System

Cardiorenal disease is also characterized by excessive sympathetic activity. In heart failure its initial activation is supposed to result from baroreceptor activation whereas in kidney disease it has been found that the stimulus for sympathetic hyperactivity arises from the failing kidneys themselves [58]. Sympathetic stimulation of the kidneys is a well-known cause of renin release and angiotensin II stimulates the sympathetic nervous system, so these two systems constitute a positive feedback system. Similar to the RAAS system, is the initial sympathetic effect beneficial in terms that it provides inotropic support and preserves cardiac output. However, chronic and excessive activity leads to cardiomyocyte apoptosis, hypertrophy, beta-receptor insensitivity, proliferation of the wall of intrarenal blood vessels, inflammation, and oxidative stress [59–61]. Sudden excessive activation of the sympathetic nervous system can also cause a substantial (up to 800 mL) fluid shift from the splanchnic system to the effective circulation leading to ADHF [62]. Logically, sympathetic activation is another driver for progressive cardiorenal disease.

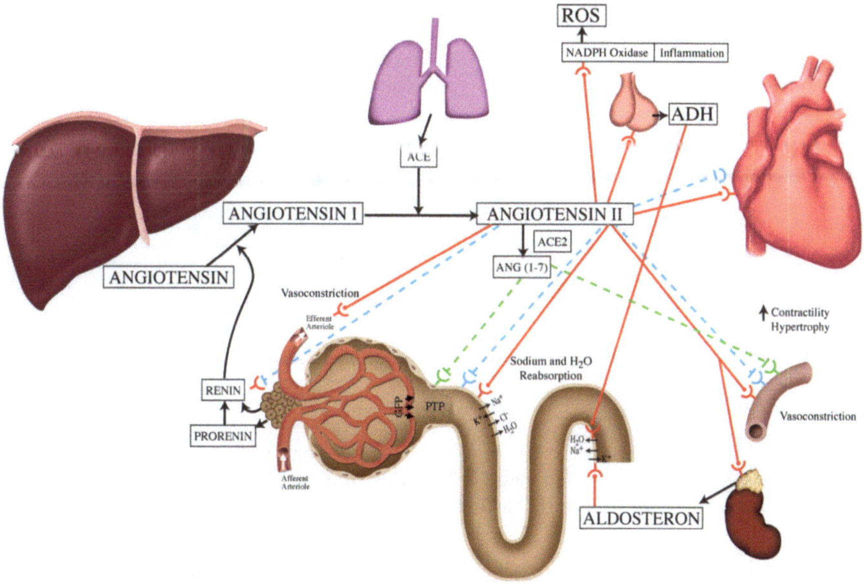

Fig. 3.3 The importance of the renin–angiotensin–aldosteron system (RAAS) in cardiorenal interactions. Prorenin and renin secretion is released by the juxtaglomerular cells following four different stimuli: a drop in renal perfusion pressure, lower Cl^- delivery to the macula densa, sympathetic nerve stimulation, and low angiotensin II concentration (negative feedback). Angiotensin (AT II) is the primary active product but some of its metabolites (AT III, AT IV, ang-(1–7)) have physiologic effects as well. Only the vasodilatory and natriuretic properties of ang-(1–7) are shown. Most effects of AT II are exerted via the AT_1-receptor (*red color*). However AT II exerts opposite effects (with unknown significance) via the AT_2-receptor (*blue color*). Receptors in green are specific for ang-(1–7). AT II constricts the efferent arteriole more than the afferent, causing an increase in filtration fraction. *ACE* angiotensin converting enzyme, *GFP* glomerular filtration pressure, *PTP* proximal tubular pressure, *ADH* antidiuretic hormone, *NADPH* nicotinamide adenine dinucleotide phosphate

4.3 *Inflammation and Oxidative Stress*

Both cardiac and renal disease is characterized by inflammation and oxidative stress [63, 64]. The involved pathways are multiple and complex but ultimately result in an imbalance between reactive oxygen species (ROS) and nitric oxide (NO) (skewed towards ROS) in addition to elevated levels of inflammatory cytokines [54]. As mentioned earlier, the RAAS and the sympathetic nervous system play a role in this. Angiotensin II will activate NADPH-oxidase resulting in the formation of ROS and will also induce chemotactic and adhesion molecules via the nuclear factor kappa B pathway [61]. Oxidative stress and inflammation have both been linked to further progression of heart failure and kidney disease partly by imposing damage on DNA, proteins, carbohydrates, and lipids. In the kidney, oxidative stress and inflammation can cause glomerular hemodynamic changes and enhanced sodium reabsorption in

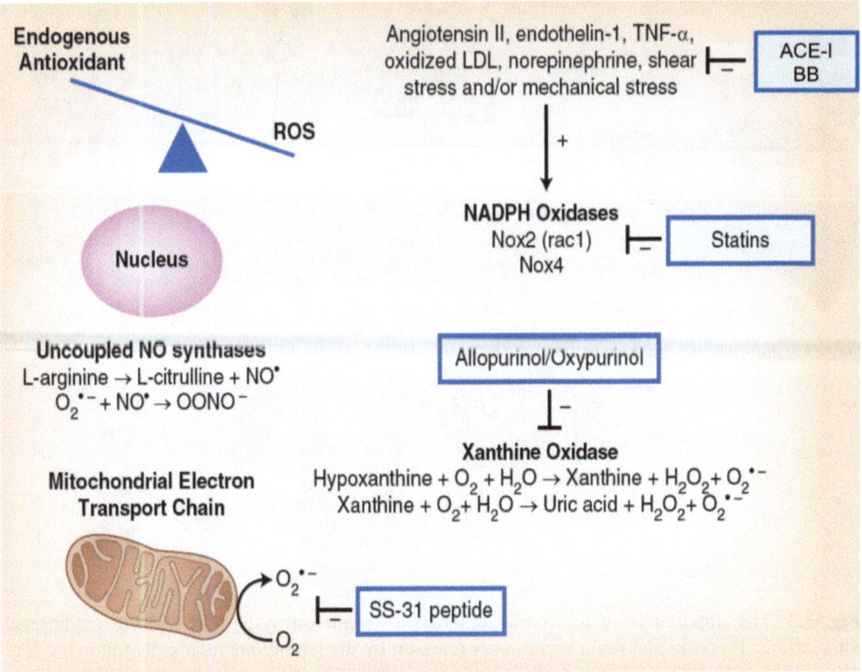

Fig. 3.4 Generation of reactive oxygen species (ROS) in the cardiorenal syndrome. Cardiac and renal dysfunction leads to (1) activation of NADPH-oxidases which come in different isoforms (Nox isoforms) (2) activation of Xanthine oxidase (3) uncoupling of NO synthase. Inhibitors of the pathways are depicted in *blue boxes*

the thick ascending limb [65–67]. Finally, positive feedback loops are again present because oxidative stress and inflammation activate each other, the RAAS and the sympathetic nervous system [68, 69]. The high prevalence of anemia in heart failure and renal disease is in part explained by the presence of inflammation and oxidative stress aside other causes such as renal impairment with absolute erythropoietin deficiency, hematinic deficiencies, plasma volume expansion, and certain drugs [70]. This has been labeled as the "cardiac-renal-anemia syndrome." As in the setting of anemia of chronic disease, anemia related to CRS is characterized by insufficient production or insensitivity to erythropoietin. A positive amplifying feedback loop is proposed because erythropoietin insensitivity disturbs the NO-ROS balance and modulates inflammation (Fig. 3.4) [70].

4.4 Renal Tubular Function

The kidney also has an important endocrinologic and a tubular function. Especially the latter is not without importance in heart failure. For instance to remove fluid in patients with ADHF, loop diuretics need to be excreted by the proximal tubular cells in order to reach the thick ascending limb where they inhibit the Na^+–K^+–$2Cl^-$ co-transporter. There are arguments that tubular injury is present in heart failure patients and is associated with a worse prognosis [71–73]. In addition, tubular injury seems to predict the occurrence of WRF during treatment for ADHF [74]. However, tubular injury is not as a dominant feature in WRF, as it is in other forms of acute kidney injury [75]. Tubular injury cannot be directly measured but is appreciated true elevated levels of biomarkers (NGAL, KIM-1, NAG) that specifically reflect tubular damage. The relative importance of this observation has not yet been fully disclosed, nor is there currently a specific treatment, but this is an active field of research.

Key Points

- The pathophysiology of the CRS is a combination of hemodynamic, neurohormonal, inflammatory, and tubular changes.
- Low blood pressure and venous congestion are more and more identified as the most important hemodynamic factors. Cardiac output seems less important than originally thought.
- The renin–angiotensin–aldosteron system and the sympathetic nervous system also play an important role and are grateful targets of therapy.
- Baseline renal tubular injury is present in heart failure patients, although it is not very dominant during WRF.

5 Prevention and Treatment

The above overview of the complex pathophysiologic mechanisms involved in CRS, highlights the challenges and difficulties of its treatment. From a hemodynamic standpoint, the punch line is to relieve, or better yet to avoid, congestion while at the same time maintaining renal perfusion. This concept is probably as old as the treatment of heart failure itself. However, the way to achieve this matters. Decongestion should ideally not be accompanied by evoking neurohormonal activation, inflammation, or oxidative stress, nor a decrease in filtration gradient in order to prevent acute deterioration of kidney function.

5.1 Sodium and Fluid Restriction

Although not rigorously tested in randomized clinical trials, salt and water restriction are essential to avoid congestion in heart failure patients. The typical recommended salt intake is 2–3 g daily. More salt intake, to a certain degree, usually can be overcome by diuretics. However, because loop diuretics may provoke neurohormonal activation and reduce GFR, this seems less appealing from a pathophysiological standpoint. Water restriction, typically less than 2 L per day, is reserved for advanced HF resistant to diuretics and when hyponatremia (<130 mEq/L) is present [1], although there have been controversies regarding the effectiveness of loop diuretic therapy in the setting of low sodium intake and hyponatremia in advanced heart failure.

5.2 *Neurohormonal Antagonists*

Activation of the RAAS and sympathetic nervous system are crucial in the progression of both cardiac and renal disease. Inhibition of these pathways with ACE inhibitors, angiotensin-receptor blockers (ARB), aldosterone receptor antagonists, and beta-adrenergic blockers are the mainstay of contemporary heart failure management. Out of all the treatments discussed in this section, they are the only ones with solid evidence. Yet, overzealous administration of these drugs may also induce unwanted adverse effects particularly when volume status is still fluctuating. An overview of all the trials done with these compounds falls outside the scope of this chapter. The bottom line is that every hear failure patient (NYHA II–IV) should be on these drugs if not contraindicated [76]. As mentioned before, small increases in creatinine after the start of RAAS antagonists are no reason to withheld these medications [30], but careful drug titration and monitoring are necessary to avoid unwanted consequences.

5.3 *Diuretics and Diuretic Resistance*

Diuretics are among the most widely used drugs in relieving congestion in the setting of HF, and are often crucial to control volume status in everyday management. The use of higher doses of loop diuretics has repeatedly been associated with higher mortality, although this might just reflect a sicker patient population or those with underlying renal impairment [40, 77–80]. In addition, WRF frequently develops after the administration of (high-dose) diuretics, especially in the presence of ACE inhibitors [81, 82]. Often this is attributed to overzealous diuresis leading to "intravascular underfilling." The reality is that most patients with HF still show signs of persistent congestion, and may still have elevated filling pressures at the time they develop WRF [38, 39]. Nevertheless, the use of a pulmonary artery catheter with careful monitoring of filling pressures failed to prevent WRF [83], which implies that the treatment itself may provoke further compromise.

The reasons why diuretics may be detrimental are complex. Loop diuretics may cause neurohormonal upregulation and an acute vasoconstrictor response [84, 85]. This is believed to be the consequence of decreased NaCl uptake by the macula densa following inhibition of the Na^{+}–K^{+}–$2Cl^{-}$ co-transporter that may ultimately lead to renin release by the juxtaglomerular apparatus, activation of the RAAS system and diminished renal blood flow. An acute decrease in GFR has repeatedly been documented after intravenous administration of diuretics, probably mediated by adenosine release [86, 87]. At the same time, neurohormonal activation will rapidly decrease when decongestion is achieved, counterbalancing the former effects [88]. Hence, diuretics can either preserve or even improve GFR by relieving congestion. These contrasting effects vary with individuals and situations and are difficult to predict, although baseline renal impairment (less "reserve") and a history of WRF (prior demonstration) are consistent risk factors.

Usually, WRF is also not accompanied by an "overzealous" diuresis but rather a decreased urine output. The term "diuretic resistance" highlights another aspect of the complex pharmacodynamics and pharmacokinetics of diuretic use. It refers to the situation whereby the administration of (high-dose) loop diuretics does not result in the expected diuresis. Although not required, it usually acts in concert with WRF and impaired natriuresis. One explanation for this phenomenon is hypertrophy of the distal tubules as a consequence of chronic use of loop diuretics. This form of diuretic resistance can sometimes be overcome by the addition of thiazides and/or aldosterone-antagonists ("sequential or total nephron blockade").

Another controversial treatment can be the administration of hypertonic saline and loop diuretics. This counterintuitive approach has demonstrated to increase diuretic response and decrease subsequent rehospitalizations [89, 90]. The mechanism is not fully explained but it is proposed that neurohormonal upregulation is blunted by delivery of higher concentrations of sodium chloride (and thus suppressed renin release) to the distale tubules, together with a possible osmotic effect [91]. However, this strategy is not widely adopted by clinicians, and likely applicable to a small subset of patients that are experiencing significant sodium depletion.

5.4 Inotropes

At first glance, inotropes seem a very reasonable therapy to treat or prevent CRS in severe heart failure. By augmenting "forward" cardiac output, the use of inotropic therapy may directly increase renal blood flow in proportion to the degree of increase in cardiac output [92]. However to date, no major trial with inotropes convincingly prevented CRS, nor demonstrated a mortality benefit. In fact, a routine strategy of short-term milrinone administration during hospitalization for ADHF was tested in the OPTIME-CHF trial. There was no benefit in terms of mortality, re-hospitalization, or length of stay (and even a hint of harm) even though the increase in BUN during hospitalization was slightly less in the milrinone group [24, 93].

There are physiologic arguments that dopamine could be a better inotropic choice to prevent WRF in the setting of cardiorenal compromise. Low-dose dopamine (2–5 μg/kg/min) demonstrated increased renal blood flow in animals, healthy humans, and stable heart failure patients [94–96]. Dopamine receptors are present in the renal vasculature (causing vasodilatation) and in the proximal convoluted tubule, medullary thick ascending limb, and collecting duct (causing natriuresis) [97]. However it is unsure whether these effects hold true when renal function is at risk or already impaired [98], or whether it is applicable to all patients. A recent meta-analysis (not specific to the HF population) failed to show any benefit of low-dose dopamine to prevent deterioration of renal function [99]. Encouraging on the other hand is a recent fairly small trial in ADHF, comparing high-dose diuretics vs. low-dose diuretics and low-dose dopamine. This trial demonstrated a significantly lower incidence of WRF in the dopamine group [100]. The controversy around inotropes in general and dopamine in particular thus continues, and the potential benefit of low-dose dopamine in CRS in the acute HF setting is currently being tested in an ongoing prospective clinical trial.

5.5 *Ultrafiltration*

Ultrafiltration, the mechanical removal of salt and fluid from the vasculature, is an alternative method to achieve decongestion with potential advantages. First and contrary to diuretics, it removes fluid and electrolytes in an isotonic way (hypotonic with diuretics). This should lead to less electrolyte disturbances and a lesser tendency for fluid re-accumulation. Second, ultrafiltration should not, or at least not to a similar degree, provoke neurohormonal upregulation [101]. Also important is that the technique of fluid removal, although still costly, becomes easier to apply in everyday clinical care by no longer requiring central venous access. One small and one bigger trial have directly compared diuretics with ultrafiltration [102, 103]. Important, none of these trials showed that WRF could be prevented with ultrafiltration. However, as mentioned earlier, WRF or CRS remain surrogate endpoints and are inferior to mortality, rehospitalization, length of hospital stay, or quality of life as endpoints. The aforementioned trials in addition to several small case series suggest less readmissions, more fluid removal and more improvement of dyspnea although the results are certainly not consistent [104–107]. In contrast, these data have yet to be replicated in larger cohorts or more advanced HF patients (i.e., those more likely to experience CRS). Several ongoing trials will hopefully reach a final judgment about the role of ultrafiltration in the management of ADHF.

5.6 *Novel Therapies with Conflicting Data*

5.6.1 Vasopressin Antagonists

Arginine vasopressine antagonists (“vaptans”) selectively block the V_2 receptors in the kidney, responsible for water retention. Initial results were promising in the sense that they resulted in additional fluid and weight loss with improved electrolyte balance and renal function. However, the large tolvaptan phase III trial

(EVEREST-trial), where tolvaptan was given on top of standard HF medication, had no incremental benefit on mortality, rehospitalization, or renal function [108]. Because tolvaptan causes more water than sodium loss, it can correct hyponatremia though. Severe, refractory hyponatremia therefore constitutes the primary indication for this drug class [109], and its clinical role in the management of CRS remains to be debated.

5.6.2 Adenosine Receptor Antagonists

Adenosine is increased in heart failure because of hypoxia and venous congestion [110]. Moreover, adenosine production is induced by treatment with diuretics. Through stimulation of the adenosine A1 receptor on the afferent arteriole, adenosine reduces renal blood flow and GFR and through stimulation of the same receptor on the proximal tubules, it increases sodium and water reabsorption. These effects were averted with the use of rolofylline, an A1 adenosine receptor antagonist, in initial studies, showing up to 50 % reduction of persistent WRF [86, 111]. However, once again, the large phase III trial (PROTECT) did not demonstrate prevention of WRF [112]. Off-target adverse effects (particularly seizures) have also precluded other compounds of this drug class to proceed to later phase investigations.

5.6.3 Natriuretic Peptides

B-type natriuretic peptide has vasodilatory properties and is part of the system that counterbalances the actions of the RAAS and sympathetic system. The use of nesiritide, recombinant human B-type natriuretic peptide, has evolved over the past decade. The controversies surrounding its safety and efficacy in the setting of ADHF have been enlightened by the results of the ASCEND-HF trial [113]. Early studies that led to its approval have demonstrated that nesiritide can provide effective incremental diuresis, improvement in dyspnea, and lowering of filling pressures in the setting of ADHF [114, 115]. However, there were serious doubts about its efficacy as compared to other vasodilators and in addition there were concerns about higher incidences of early death or WRF [116–118]. For these reasons, ASCEND-HF was conducted, and showed no detrimental effect of the drug (no more deaths or WRF) and showed a statistically significant but very small improvement of dyspnea [113]. Therefore, routine use of nesiritide was not recommended for the treatment of ADHF. Other vasodilators, with differential vasodilatory and natriuretic properties, are currently in clinical development, and may fine-tune their roles in CRS.

Key Points

- Avoiding congestion is crucial in preventing ADHF and CRS.
- Salt and fluid restriction and neurohormonal blockade are the cornerstones to achieve this goal.

- Diuretics are not essential, but often necessary to maintain the compensated state. They are associated with acute vasoconstriction and neurohormonal upregulation.
- Ultrafiltration is an alternative mode of salt and fluid removal with yet unclear effect on renal and overall outcomes.
- Vasopressin antagonists, adenosine receptor antagonists, and nesiritide failed to prevent WRF in large clinical trials.

6 Future Perspectives

The search for new pharmacologic or device strategies to treat or prevent CRS will continue, since CRS remains one of the most perplexing challenges for clinicians taking care of patients with HF. To achieve this, better understanding of the pathophysiology will be necessary, particularly with the help of more diagnostic tools. Table 3.3 gives a brief overview of areas of research with corresponding ongoing clinical trials in this area. A few new treatments strategies are worth highlighting.

The first is the metabolic aspects of CRS that has been overlooked. Because cardiorenal dysfunction is characterized by insensitivity to and/or absolute deficiency of erythropoietin, it makes sense to substitute this hormone. Moreover, as outlined before, anemia itself could enforce the progression of CRS. Iron substitution has a proven beneficial effect on exercise capacity and a phase II trial with darbepoetin alpha demonstrated some improvement in quality of life measures [119, 120]. In addition, a smaller trial even showed improvement in renal function [121]. However, some safety issues (thrombosis) have arisen as well [122]. RED-HF, an ongoing large phase III trial with darbepoetin alpha, is supposed to give the answer [123]. Other drug therapies evaluating the role of iron repletion are also promising, although its direct impact on CRS is not well examined.

The second is to examine the role of vasodilatory responses that can help modulate venous congestion and renoprotection. Relaxin is a naturally occurring peptide that modulates cardiovascular responses during pregnancy. It causes systemic and renal vasodilation and augmented arterial compliance, hence the interest for heart failure patients. A phase II trial in ADHF was promising in terms of dyspnea relief, although no significant effect on renal function was observed [124]. A large phase III trial is ongoing. Other chimeric natriuretic peptides as well as different administrative routes are also under evaluation.

The third is to identify opportunities in neurohormonal modulation that can provide benefits while reducing adverse consequences. Renin release by the juxtaglomerular apparatus is mediated by sympathetic stimulation. Recently, renal ablation (of the sympathetic nerves) has proven to be an effective treatment for therapy-resistant hypertension. The hope is that by decreasing activation of the RAAS, this will prove to be an effective treatment for the CRS as well [125]. Other strategies to modulate the autonomic system by vagal stimulation are also ongoing. Direct impact on CRS are not commonly assessed, although such strategies will likely provide an opportunity to better understand the intricate balance between the heart and the kidney in the setting of HF.

Table 3.3 Currently tested strategies in ADHF and CRS

Drug or device	Drug class	Proposed mechanism	ClinicalTrials.gov
Recombinant relaxin	Relaxin	Systemic and renal vasodilatation	NCT00520806 RELAX-AHF
Aliskiren	Renin inhibitor	Increase renal blood flow by inhibiting RAAS	NCT00881439 ARIANA-CHF-RD
LCZ696	Angiotensin II receptor/ neprilysin inhibitor (ARNI)	– Inhibit AT II-mediated vasoconstriction – Inhibit breakdown of natriuretic peptides by inhibiting neprilysin	NCT01035255 PARADIGM-HF
TRV120027	B-arrestin biased AT1R ligand	– Inhibit AT II-mediated vasoconstriction – Increase cardiomyocyte contractility – Increase RBF and GFR	NCT01444872
Cross-linked polyelectrolyte (CLP)	Non-absorbed polymers	Avoiding congestion by sequestering ions and fluid in the GI tract	NCT01265524
Vitamine D3	Vitamine D3	Prevention of RAAS activation by inhibiting renin transcription	NCT01092130 VitD-CHF
CXL-1020	Nitroxyl donor	Improve cardiomyocyte function and renal perfusion by enhancing sarcoplasmatic calcium cycling	NCT01096043
Pomegranate polyphenol extract	Antioxidant and anti-inflammatory	– Reduction of reactive oxygen species – Reduce inflammation	NCT01102140 ImPrOVE
Darbepoetin alpha	Erythropoetin	– Decrease anemia – Reduction of reactive oxygen species – Reduce inflammation	NCT00358215 RED-HF
Renal ablation	–	Decrease sympathetic activity	NCT01392196 SymplicityHF
Renal ablation	–	Decrease sympathetic activity	NCT01402726

7 Conclusion

Although much work has been done, several features of the CRS remain poorly understood. It is clear however, that renal dysfunction or WRF during treatment of ADHF has important prognostic implications and definitely identifies heart failure patients at increased risk for worse outcomes. Few treatment strategies have consistently provided opportunities for cardiorenal recovery. However, evolving insights have challenged the concept of a single mechanism, and even confronted the possibility that CRS can be induced by current treatment strategies. Clearly, hemodynamic changes perhaps play a more important role in the acute CRS subtypes (CRS 1 and 3). At the same time, neurohormonal, inflammatory, and oxidative changes are the common denominator in all subtypes of the CRS. This makes antagonism of these pathways of utmost importance and the best guarantee to prevent progressive organ failure (CRS subtypes 2 and 4). While old concepts have been revisited, newer technologies may overcome some of the bedside challenges and balancing current and future therapeutics will be the main quest for ongoing investigations.

8 Sources of Further Information

The CRS draws considerable attention of the cardiology community with an exponential rise in publications in recent years. We would advise the below-mentioned articles for more in-depth understanding.

- Definition and Epidemiology
  - Ronco et al. [4] to understand the current classification of CRS.
  - Gottlieb et al. [2] explains why a ≥0.3 mg/dL rise in serum creatinine was chosen to define WRF.
- Prognostic importance
  - Smith et al. [21] and Damman et al. [15] published important meta-analyses stressing the prognostic importance of CKD and WRF in heart failure.
- Pathophysiology
  - Francis et al. [85] published an often cited article explaining neurohormonal upregulation after lisdiuretic administration.
  - Mullens et al. [38] highlighted the role of venous congestion in WRF.
  - Testani et al. [29] identified a subgroup of patients with WRF without adverse outcomes, stressing the importance of different mechanisms leading to WRF.
- Treatment
  - Felker et al. [126] conducted a randomized trial of low vs. high-dose diuretic strategy showing no difference in outcomes despite a little more WRF in the high-dose arm.
  - Costanzo et al. [103] carried out a landmark trial investigating the role of ultrafiltration as an alternative for diuretics in the treatment of congestion.
  - O'Connor et al. [113] performed the largest randomized trial in ADHF patients, demonstrating the safety of nesiritide. However no significant benefit was shown.

- Reviews
  - Bongartz et al. [54].
  - Stevenson et al. [91].
  - Damman et al. [127].

References

1. Lindenfeld J et al (2010) HFSA 2010 comprehensive heart failure practice guideline. J Card Fail 16(6):e1–e194
2. Gottlieb SS et al (2002) The prognostic importance of different definitions of worsening renal function in congestive heart failure. J Card Fail 8(3):136–141
3. Smith GL et al (2003) Worsening renal function: what is a clinically meaningful change in creatinine during hospitalization with heart failure? J Card Fail 9(1):13–25
4. Ronco C et al (2010) Cardio-renal syndromes: report from the consensus conference of the acute dialysis quality initiative. Eur Heart J 31(6):703–711
5. Bellomo R et al (2004) Acute renal failure—definition, outcome measures, animal models, fluid therapy and information technology needs: the Second International Consensus Conference of the Acute Dialysis Quality Initiative (ADQI) Group. Crit Care 8(4):R204–R212
6. Mehta RL et al (2007) Acute Kidney Injury Network: report of an initiative to improve outcomes in acute kidney injury. Crit Care 11(2):R31
7. Stevens LA, Levey AS (2005) Measurement of kidney function. Med Clin North Am 89(3):457–473
8. Stevens LA et al (2006) Assessing kidney function–measured and estimated glomerular filtration rate. N Engl J Med 354(23):2473–2483
9. Coll E et al (2000) Serum cystatin C as a new marker for noninvasive estimation of glomerular filtration rate and as a marker for early renal impairment. Am J Kidney Dis 36(1):29–34
10. Shlipak MG et al (2005) Cystatin C and the risk of death and cardiovascular events among elderly persons. N Engl J Med 352(20):2049–2060
11. Shlipak MG et al (2005) Cystatin-C and mortality in elderly persons with heart failure. J Am Coll Cardiol 45(2):268–271
12. Heywood JT et al (2007) High prevalence of renal dysfunction and its impact on outcome in 118,465 patients hospitalized with acute decompensated heart failure: a report from the ADHERE database. J Card Fail 13(6):422–430
13. Forman DE et al (2004) Incidence, predictors at admission, and impact of worsening renal function among patients hospitalized with heart failure. J Am Coll Cardiol 43(1):61–67
14. Krumholz HM et al (2000) Correlates and impact on outcomes of worsening renal function in patients > or =65 years of age with heart failure. Am J Cardiol 85(9):1110–1113
15. Damman K et al (2007) Worsening renal function and prognosis in heart failure: systematic review and meta-analysis. J Card Fail 13(8):599–608
16. Tonelli M et al (2006) Chronic kidney disease and mortality risk: a systematic review. J Am Soc Nephrol 17(7):2034–2047
17. Harnett JD et al (1995) Congestive heart failure in dialysis patients: prevalence, incidence, prognosis and risk factors. Kidney Int 47(3):884–890
18. Dries DL et al (2000) The prognostic implications of renal insufficiency in asymptomatic and symptomatic patients with left ventricular systolic dysfunction. J Am Coll Cardiol 35(3):681–689
19. Hillege HL et al (2000) Renal function, neurohormonal activation, and survival in patients with chronic heart failure. Circulation 102(2):203–210

20. Mahon NG et al (2002) The prognostic value of estimated creatinine clearance alongside functional capacity in ambulatory patients with chronic congestive heart failure. J Am Coll Cardiol 40(6):1106–1113
21. Smith GL et al (2006) Renal impairment and outcomes in heart failure: systematic review and meta-analysis. J Am Coll Cardiol 47(10):1987–1996
22. Hillege HL et al (2006) Renal function as a predictor of outcome in a broad spectrum of patients with heart failure. Circulation 113(5):671–678
23. Cauthen CA et al (2008) Relation of blood urea nitrogen to long-term mortality in patients with heart failure. Am J Cardiol 101(11):1643–1647
24. Klein L et al (2008) Admission or changes in renal function during hospitalization for worsening heart failure predict postdischarge survival: results from the Outcomes of a Prospective Trial of Intravenous Milrinone for Exacerbations of Chronic Heart Failure (OPTIME-CHF). Circ Heart Fail 1(1):25–33
25. Fonarow GC et al (2005) Risk stratification for in-hospital mortality in acutely decompensated heart failure: classification and regression tree analysis. JAMA 293(5):572–580
26. Schrier RW (2008) Blood urea nitrogen and serum creatinine: not married in heart failure. Circ Heart Fail 1(1):2–5
27. Testani JM et al (2011) Influence of renal dysfunction phenotype on mortality in the setting of cardiac dysfunction: analysis of three randomized controlled trials. Eur J Heart Fail 13(11):1224–1230
28. Testani JM et al (2011) Interaction between loop diuretic-associated mortality and blood urea nitrogen concentration in chronic heart failure. J Am Coll Cardiol 58(4):375–382
29. Testani JM et al (2010) Potential effects of aggressive decongestion during the treatment of decompensated heart failure on renal function and survival. Circulation 122(3):265–272
30. Testani JM et al (2011) Prognostic importance of early worsening renal function following initiation of angiotensin converting enzyme inhibitor therapy in patients with cardiac dysfunction. Circ Heart Fail 4(6):685–691
31. Leithe ME et al (1984) Relationship between central hemodynamics and regional blood flow in normal subjects and in patients with congestive heart failure. Circulation 69(1):57–64
32. Testani JM et al (2011) Impact of changes in blood pressure during the treatment of acute decompensated heart failure on renal and clinical outcomes. Eur J Heart Fail 13(8):877–884
33. Voors AA et al (2011) Early drop in systolic blood pressure and worsening renal function in acute heart failure: renal results of Pre-RELAX-AHF. Eur J Heart Fail 13(9):961–967
34. Loutzenhiser R et al (2006) Renal autoregulation: new perspectives regarding the protective and regulatory roles of the underlying mechanisms. Am J Physiol Regul Integr Comp Physiol 290(5):R1153–R1167
35. Rea ME, Dunlap ME (2008) Renal hemodynamics in heart failure: implications for treatment. Curr Opin Nephrol Hypertens 17(1):87–92
36. Palmer BF (2002) Renal dysfunction complicating the treatment of hypertension. N Engl J Med 347(16):1256–1261
37. Damman K et al (2009) Increased central venous pressure is associated with impaired renal function and mortality in a broad spectrum of patients with cardiovascular disease. J Am Coll Cardiol 53(7):582–588
38. Mullens W et al (2009) Importance of venous congestion for worsening of renal function in advanced decompensated heart failure. J Am Coll Cardiol 53(7):589–596
39. Nohria A et al (2008) Cardiorenal interactions: insights from the ESCAPE trial. J Am Coll Cardiol 51(13):1268–1274
40. Butler J et al (2004) Relationship between heart failure treatment and development of worsening renal function among hospitalized patients. Am Heart J 147(2):331–338
41. Winton FR (1931) The influence of venous pressure on the isolated mammalian kidney. J Physiol 72(1):49–61
42. Hall PW III, Selkurt EE (1951) Effects of partial graded venous obstruction on electrolyte clearance by the dog's kidney. Am J Physiol 164(1):143–154

43. Wathen RL, Selkurt EE (1969) Intrarenal regulatory factors of salt excretion during renal venous pressure elevation. Am J Physiol 216(6):1517–1524
44. Burnett JC Jr, Knox FG (1980) Renal interstitial pressure and sodium excretion during renal vein constriction. Am J Physiol 238(4):F279–F282
45. Burnett JC Jr, Haas JA, Knox FG (1982) Segmental analysis of sodium reabsorption during renal vein constriction. Am J Physiol 243(1):F19–F22
46. Wencker D (2007) Acute cardio-renal syndrome: progression from congestive heart failure to congestive kidney failure. Curr Heart Fail Rep 4(3):134–138
47. Firth JD, Raine AE, Ledingham JG (1988) Raised venous pressure: a direct cause of renal sodium retention in oedema? Lancet 1(8593):1033–1035
48. Dupont M, Mullens W, Tang WH (2011) Impact of systemic venous congestion in heart failure. Curr Heart Fail Rep 8(4):233–241
49. Bradley SE, Bradley GP (1947) The effect of increased intra-abdominal pressure on renal function in man. J Clin Invest 26(5):1010–1022
50. Mullens W et al (2008) Elevated intra-abdominal pressure in acute decompensated heart failure: a potential contributor to worsening renal function? J Am Coll Cardiol 51(3):300–306
51. De Waele JJ et al (2011) Intra-abdominal hypertension and abdominal compartment syndrome. Am J Kidney Dis 57(1):159–169
52. Malbrain ML et al (2004) Prevalence of intra-abdominal hypertension in critically ill patients: a multicentre epidemiological study. Intensive Care Med 30(5):822–829
53. Mullens W et al (2008) Prompt reduction in intra-abdominal pressure following large-volume mechanical fluid removal improves renal insufficiency in refractory decompensated heart failure. J Card Fail 14(6):508–514
54. Bongartz LG et al (2005) The severe cardiorenal syndrome: 'Guyton revisited'. Eur Heart J 26(1):11–17
55. Warren DJ, Ferris TF (1970) Renin secretion in renal hypertension. Lancet 1(7639): 159–162
56. Atlas SA (2007) The renin-angiotensin aldosterone system: pathophysiological role and pharmacologic inhibition. J Manag Care Pharm 13(8 Suppl B):9–20
57. Griendling KK et al (1994) Angiotensin II stimulates NADH and NADPH oxidase activity in cultured vascular smooth muscle cells. Circ Res 74(6):1141–1148
58. Converse RL Jr et al (1992) Sympathetic overactivity in patients with chronic renal failure. N Engl J Med 327(27):1912–1918
59. Jackson G et al (2000) ABC of heart failure. Pathophysiology. BMJ 320(7228):167–170
60. Bleeke T et al (2004) Catecholamine-induced vascular wall growth is dependent on generation of reactive oxygen species. Circ Res 94(1):37–45
61. Prabhu SD et al (2000) beta-adrenergic blockade in developing heart failure: effects on myocardial inflammatory cytokines, nitric oxide, and remodeling. Circulation 101(17): 2103–2109
62. Fallick C, Sobotka PA, Dunlap ME (2011) Sympathetically mediated changes in capacitance: redistribution of the venous reservoir as a cause of decompensation. Circ Heart Fail 4(5):669–675
63. Heymes C et al (2003) Increased myocardial NADPH oxidase activity in human heart failure. J Am Coll Cardiol 41(12):2164–2171
64. Vallance P et al (1992) Accumulation of an endogenous inhibitor of nitric oxide synthesis in chronic renal failure. Lancet 339(8793):572–575
65. Sanchez-Lozada LG et al (2003) Glomerular hemodynamic changes associated with arteriolar lesions and tubulointerstitial inflammation. Kidney Int Suppl 86:S9–S14
66. Garvin JL, Ortiz PA (2003) The role of reactive oxygen species in the regulation of tubular function. Acta Physiol Scand 179(3):225–232
67. Juncos R, Garvin JL (2005) Superoxide enhances Na-K-2Cl cotransporter activity in the thick ascending limb. Am J Physiol Renal Physiol 288(5):F982–F987

68. Lin HH et al (2003) Hydrogen peroxide increases the activity of rat sympathetic preganglionic neurons in vivo and in vitro. Neuroscience 121(3):641–647
69. Katoh M et al (1998) Cardiac angiotensin II receptors are upregulated by long-term inhibition of nitric oxide synthesis in rats. Circ Res 83(7):743–751
70. Jie KE et al (2006) Erythropoietin and the cardiorenal syndrome: cellular mechanisms on the cardiorenal connectors. Am J Physiol Renal Physiol 291(5):F932–F944
71. Damman K et al (2008) Urinary neutrophil gelatinase associated lipocalin (NGAL), a marker of tubular damage, is increased in patients with chronic heart failure. Eur J Heart Fail 10(10):997–1000
72. Damman K et al (2010) Tubular damage in chronic systolic heart failure is associated with reduced survival independent of glomerular filtration rate. Heart 96(16):1297–1302
73. Maisel AS et al (2011) Prognostic utility of plasma neutrophil gelatinase-associated lipocalin in patients with acute heart failure: the NGAL EvaLuation Along with B-type NaTriuretic Peptide in acutely decompensated heart failure (GALLANT) trial. Eur J Heart Fail 13(8):846–851
74. Aghel A et al (2010) Serum neutrophil gelatinase-associated lipocalin (NGAL) in predicting worsening renal function in acute decompensated heart failure. J Card Fail 16(1):49–54
75. Dupont M et al (2012) Lack of significant renal tubular injury despite acute kidney injury in acute decompensated heart failure. Eur J Heart Fail 14(6):597–604
76. Zannad F et al (2011) Eplerenone in patients with systolic heart failure and mild symptoms. N Engl J Med 364(1):11–21
77. Eshaghian S, Horwich TB, Fonarow GC (2006) Relation of loop diuretic dose to mortality in advanced heart failure. Am J Cardiol 97(12):1759–1764
78. Philbin EF et al (1997) Association between diuretic use, clinical response, and death in acute heart failure. Am J Cardiol 80(4):519–522
79. Neuberg GW et al (2002) Diuretic resistance predicts mortality in patients with advanced heart failure. Am Heart J 144(1):31–38
80. Peacock WF et al (2009) Impact of intravenous loop diuretics on outcomes of patients hospitalized with acute decompensated heart failure: insights from the ADHERE registry. Cardiology 113(1):12–19
81. Weinfeld MS, Chertow GM, Stevenson LW (1999) Aggravated renal dysfunction during intensive therapy for advanced chronic heart failure. Am Heart J 138(2 Pt 1):285–290
82. Knight EL et al (1999) Predictors of decreased renal function in patients with heart failure during angiotensin-converting enzyme inhibitor therapy: results from the studies of left ventricular dysfunction (SOLVD). Am Heart J 138(5 Pt 1):849–855
83. Binanay C et al (2005) Evaluation study of congestive heart failure and pulmonary artery catheterization effectiveness: the ESCAPE trial. JAMA 294(13):1625–1633
84. Francis GS et al (1985) Acute vasoconstrictor response to intravenous furosemide in patients with chronic congestive heart failure. Activation of the neurohumoral axis. Ann Intern Med 103(1):1–6
85. Francis GS et al (1990) Comparison of neuroendocrine activation in patients with left ventricular dysfunction with and without congestive heart failure. A substudy of the Studies of Left Ventricular Dysfunction (SOLVD). Circulation 82(5):1724–1729
86. Gottlieb SS et al (2002) BG9719 (CVT-124), an A1 adenosine receptor antagonist, protects against the decline in renal function observed with diuretic therapy. Circulation 105(11): 1348–1353
87. Tenstad O, Williamson HE (1995) Effect of furosemide on local and zonal glomerular filtration rate in the rat kidney. Acta Physiol Scand 155(1):99–107
88. Johnson W et al (2002) Neurohormonal activation rapidly decreases after intravenous therapy with diuretics and vasodilators for class IV heart failure. J Am Coll Cardiol 39(10): 1623–1629
89. Paterna S et al (2005) Changes in brain natriuretic peptide levels and bioelectrical impedance measurements after treatment with high-dose furosemide and hypertonic saline solution versus

high-dose furosemide alone in refractory congestive heart failure: a double-blind study. J Am Coll Cardiol 45(12):1997–2003
90. Paterna S et al (2011) Short-term effects of hypertonic saline solution in acute heart failure and long-term effects of a moderate sodium restriction in patients with compensated heart failure with New York Heart Association class III (Class C) (SMAC-HF Study). Am J Med Sci 342(1):27–37
91. Stevenson LW, Nohria A, Mielniczuk L (2005) Torrent or torment from the tubules? Challenge of the cardiorenal connections. J Am Coll Cardiol 45(12):2004–2007
92. Drexler H et al (1987) Central and regional vascular hemodynamics following intravenous milrinone in the conscious rat: comparison with dobutamine. J Cardiovasc Pharmacol 9(5):563–569
93. Cuffe MS et al (2002) Short-term intravenous milrinone for acute exacerbation of chronic heart failure: a randomized controlled trial. JAMA 287(12):1541–1547
94. McDonald RH Jr et al (1964) Effect of dopamine in man: augmentation of sodium excretion, glomerular filtration rate, and renal plasma flow. J Clin Invest 43:1116–1124
95. McNay JL, McDonald RH Jr, Goldberg LI (1965) Direct renal vasodilatation produced by dopamine in the dog. Circ Res 16:510–517
96. Elkayam U et al (2008) Renal vasodilatory action of dopamine in patients with heart failure: magnitude of effect and site of action. Circulation 117(2):200–205
97. Satoh T, Ominato M, Katz AI (1995) Different mechanisms of renal Na-K-ATPase regulation by dopamine in the proximal and distal nephron. Hypertens Res 18(Suppl 1):S137–S140
98. Lauschke A et al (2006) 'Low-dose' dopamine worsens renal perfusion in patients with acute renal failure. Kidney Int 69(9):1669–1674
99. Marik PE (2002) Low-dose dopamine: a systematic review. Intensive Care Med 28(7): 877–883
100. Giamouzis G et al (2010) Impact of dopamine infusion on renal function in hospitalized heart failure patients: results of the Dopamine in Acute Decompensated Heart Failure (DAD-HF) Trial. J Card Fail 16(12):922–930
101. Forslund T et al (1992) Hormonal changes in patients with severe chronic congestive heart failure treated by ultrafiltration. Nephrol Dial Transplant 7(4):306–310
102. Bart BA et al (2005) Ultrafiltration versus usual care for hospitalized patients with heart failure: the Relief for Acutely Fluid-Overloaded Patients With Decompensated Congestive Heart Failure (RAPID-CHF) trial. J Am Coll Cardiol 46(11):2043–2046
103. Costanzo MR et al (2007) Ultrafiltration versus intravenous diuretics for patients hospitalized for acute decompensated heart failure. J Am Coll Cardiol 49(6):675–683
104. Jaski BE et al (2003) Peripherally inserted veno-venous ultrafiltration for rapid treatment of volume overloaded patients. J Card Fail 9(3):227–231
105. Costanzo MR et al (2005) Early ultrafiltration in patients with decompensated heart failure and diuretic resistance. J Am Coll Cardiol 46(11):2047–2051
106. Liang KV et al (2006) Use of a novel ultrafiltration device as a treatment strategy for diuretic resistant, refractory heart failure: initial clinical experience in a single center. J Card Fail 12(9):707–714
107. Agostoni P et al (1994) Sustained improvement in functional capacity after removal of body fluid with isolated ultrafiltration in chronic cardiac insufficiency: failure of furosemide to provide the same result. Am J Med 96(3):191–199
108. Konstam MA et al (2007) Effects of oral tolvaptan in patients hospitalized for worsening heart failure: the EVEREST Outcome Trial. JAMA 297(12):1319–1331
109. Aronson D et al (2011) Short- and long-term treatment of dilutional hyponatraemia with satavaptan, a selective arginine vasopressin V2-receptor antagonist: the DILIPO study. Eur J Heart Fail 13(3):327–336
110. Funaya H et al (1997) Plasma adenosine levels increase in patients with chronic heart failure. Circulation 95(6):1363–1365

111. Cotter G et al (2008) The PROTECT pilot study: a randomized, placebo-controlled, dose-finding study of the adenosine A1 receptor antagonist rolofylline in patients with acute heart failure and renal impairment. J Card Fail 14(8):631–640
112. Voors AA et al (2011) Effects of the adenosine A1 receptor antagonist rolofylline on renal function in patients with acute heart failure and renal dysfunction: results from PROTECT (Placebo-Controlled Randomized Study of the Selective Adenosine A1 Receptor Antagonist Rolofylline for Patients Hospitalized with Acute Decompensated Heart Failure and Volume Overload to Assess Treatment Effect on Congestion and Renal Function). J Am Coll Cardiol 57(19):1899–1907
113. O'Connor CM et al (2011) Effect of nesiritide in patients with acute decompensated heart failure. N Engl J Med 365(1):32–43
114. Colucci WS et al (2000) Intravenous nesiritide, a natriuretic peptide, in the treatment of decompensated congestive heart failure. Nesiritide Study Group. N Engl J Med 343(4):246–253
115. Clarkson PB et al (1995) Brain natriuretic peptide: effect on left ventricular filling patterns in healthy subjects. Clin Sci (Lond) 88(2):159–164
116. Sackner-Bernstein JD, Skopicki HA, Aaronson KD (2005) Risk of worsening renal function with nesiritide in patients with acutely decompensated heart failure. Circulation 111(12):1487–1491
117. Sackner-Bernstein JD et al (2005) Short-term risk of death after treatment with nesiritide for decompensated heart failure: a pooled analysis of randomized controlled trials. JAMA 293(15):1900–1905
118. Sackner-Bernstein J, Aaronson KD (2005) Nesiritide—not verified. N Engl J Med 353(14):1525–1527
119. Anker SD et al (2009) Ferric carboxymaltose in patients with heart failure and iron deficiency. N Engl J Med 361(25):2436–2448
120. Ponikowski P et al (2007) Effect of darbepoetin alfa on exercise tolerance in anemic patients with symptomatic chronic heart failure: a randomized, double-blind, placebo-controlled trial. J Am Coll Cardiol 49(7):753–762
121. Silverberg DS et al (2000) The use of subcutaneous erythropoietin and intravenous iron for the treatment of the anemia of severe, resistant congestive heart failure improves cardiac and renal function and functional cardiac class, and markedly reduces hospitalizations. J Am Coll Cardiol 35(7):1737–1744
122. Phrommintikul A et al (2007) Mortality and target haemoglobin concentrations in anaemic patients with chronic kidney disease treated with erythropoietin: a meta-analysis. Lancet 369(9559):381–388
123. McMurray JJ et al (2009) Design of the Reduction of Events with Darbepoetin alfa in Heart Failure (RED-HF): a Phase III, anaemia correction, morbidity-mortality trial. Eur J Heart Fail 11(8):795–801
124. Teerlink JR et al (2009) Relaxin for the treatment of patients with acute heart failure (Pre-RELAX-AHF): a multicentre, randomised, placebo-controlled, parallel-group, dose-finding phase IIb study. Lancet 373(9673):1429–1439
125. Krum H et al (2009) Catheter-based renal sympathetic denervation for resistant hypertension: a multicentre safety and proof-of-principle cohort study. Lancet 373(9671):1275–1281
126. Felker GM et al (2011) Diuretic strategies in patients with acute decompensated heart failure. N Engl J Med 364(9):797–805
127. Damman K et al (2011) The cardiorenal syndrome in heart failure. Prog Cardiovasc Dis 54(2):144–153
128. Malbrain ML et al (2006) Results from the International Conference of Experts on Intra-abdominal Hypertension and Abdominal Compartment Syndrome. I. Definitions. Intensive Care Med 32(11):1722–1732

Chapter 4
Echocardiography in the Clinical Evaluation of Heart Failure: What Clinicians Need to know and Echocardiographers Should Report

Ivan Stankovic and Jens-Uwe Voigt

Abstract Echocardiography is widely available, safe, and the most cost-effective imaging technique for the diagnosis and follow-up of structural and functional abnormalities associated with heart failure. In this chapter, we review the use of different echocardiographic modalities for the state-of-the-art evaluation of patients with heart failure. We describe the most important details of the examination technique and review clinically relevant echocardiographic parameters for the assessment of cardiac morphology and function. The role of echocardiography for guiding pharmacological and device-based heart failure therapy and future trends in this field are also discussed.

1 Assessment of Cardiac Morphology

1.1 The Left Heart

Quantification of left cardiac chambers is a fundamental component of an echocardiographic examination. Since many of the quantitative echo parameters have direct diagnostic and prognostic implications, measurements must be obtained and reported in a standardized manner [1]. Reference values for left ventricular and left atrial dimensions and volumes are summarized in (Table 4.1).

I. Stankovic • J.-U. Voigt (✉)
Department of Cardiovascular Diseases, University Hospital Gasthuisberg, Herestraat 49, Leuven 3000, Belgium
e-mail: jens-uwe.voigt@uzleuven.be

J. Bartunek and M. Vanderheyden (eds.), *Translational Approach to Heart Failure*,
DOI 10.1007/978-1-4614-7345-9_4, © Springer Science+Business Media New York 2013

Table 4.1 References ranges for morphology and function parameters of the LV. Modified from Lang RM, Bierig M, Devereux RB, Flachskampf FA et al. (2006) Recommendations for chamber quantification. Eur J Echocardiogr;7(2):79–108

Parameter	Reference range
Morphology	
LV end-diastolic diameter	<59 mm
Septal wall thickness (end-diastole)	<11 mm
Posterior wall thickness (end-diastole)	<11 mm
LV mass	88–224 g
LV volume/BSA (diastole)	35–75 mL/m^2
LA diameter (end-systole)	30–40 mm
LA area	≤20 cm^2
LA volume/BSA	<28 mL/m^2
Function	
LV ejection fraction	≥55 %
LV fractional shortening	25–43 %
Myocardial performance (Tei) index	<0.30
MAPSE	>12 mm
Global longitudinal strain	−18 to 20 %

LV left ventricle, *LA* left atrium, *BSA* body surface area, *MAPSE* mitral annular plane systolic excursion

1.1.1 Left Ventricle

Left ventricular end-diastolic diameter (LVEDD), septal (SWT), and posterior wall thickness (PWT) are key figures of each echo report. They can be measured in parasternal long-axis view (PLAX) using both 2D echo and M-mode imaging. The latter may only be used, however, if the M-mode line can be placed perpendicularly to the long axis of the LV. End-diastolic and -systolic parameters are measured when the ventricle is largest and smallest, respectively.

Left ventricular mass is estimated from linear end-diastolic LV dimensions, using the modified Devereux formula:

$$\text{LVmass(g)} = 0.8 \times [1.04 \times (\text{LVEDD} + \text{PWT} + \text{SWT})^3 \text{-LVEDD}^3] + 0.6$$

Note, that this formula depends on geometrical assumptions of the ventricular shape which may not hold true for ventricles with regional abnormalities.

Relative wall thickness (RWT) is calculated by the formula (2 × PWT)/LVEDD, and is used for categorization of an increase in LV mass as either concentric (RWT ≥ 0.42) or eccentric (RWT ≤ 0.42) hypertrophy.

1.1.2 Left Atrium

The end-systolic antero-posterior diameter of the left atrium (LA) in the parasternal long-axis view is commonly used as a marker for atrial remodeling, but may be insensitive in elongated atria. The measurement of LA volume reflects LA

Table 4.2 References values for morphology and function parameters of the RV. Modified from Rudski LG, Lai WW, Afilalo J, Hua L et al. (2010) Guidelines for the echocardiographic assessment of the right heart in adults. J Am Soc Echocardiogr;23(7):685–713

Parameter	Reference values
Morphology	
RV basal diameter	<42 mm
RV wall thickness (subcostal view)	≤5 mm
RVOT distal diameter	<27 mm
RA major dimension	<53 mm
RA minor dimension	<44 mm
Function	
TAPSE	>18 mm
Myocardial performance (Tei) index	<0.40
Fractional area change	>35 %
Peak systolic tricuspid annular velocity	>10 cm/s

LV left ventricle, *RA* right atrium, *RV* right ventricle, *TAPSE* tricuspid annular plane systolic excursion

remodeling more accurately, particularly if there is a predominant enlargement in the superior–inferior and medial-lateral dimensions. Both the area-length method and the modified Simpson's rule may be used to calculate LA volume from apical four- and two-chamber views.

1.2 The Right Heart

As a qualitative assessment, right ventricular (RV) size may be compared with LV size in a parasternal short-axis and an apical four-chamber views. A quantitative evaluation of RV dimensions is challenging due to its complex anatomy and immediate retrosternal position. Right ventricular (RV) wall thickness can be measured using both 2D and M-mode in subcostal view. In an apical four-chamber view, both the long- and short-axis RV diameters can be measured and the end-systolic and end-diastolic areas can be determined. The diameter of the RVOT can be measured in the parasternal short-axis view, at the aortic valve level. The RA size is usually reported as the minor axis dimension (from the lateral RA border to the interatrial septum). Table 4.2 summarizes reference values of most frequently used parameters for quantitative RV assessment.

Key Point

- Due to the direct clinical implications, the assessment of cardiac dimensions needs particular care and strict standardization. Of note, the majority of quantitative echocardiographic parameters are one-dimensional measurements of moving three-dimensional structures, taken from a single still frame. Therefore, abnormal measurements should be cross-checked in several image planes, and interpreted considering the visual impression and the clinical context.

2 Assessment of Systolic Function

2.1 Assessment of Global Left Ventricular Systolic Function

Gold standard for the definition of the state of myocardial function is the parameter "contractility" which is estimated from complex invasive heamodynamic measurements and which is therefore not feasible for routine clinical use. Instead, surrogate parameters are used in the clinic which usually describe myocardial deformation or ventricular volume changes. Such surrogate parameters reflect contractility only modulated by pre- and afterload of the ventricle as well as by ventricular shape. Despite of that, there is broad evidence that they are powerful predictors of the patient's prognosis and clinically useful to guide therapeutic decisions.

2.1.1 Ejection Fraction

Left ventricular ejection fraction (LVEF) is defined as the stroke volume of the left ventricle relative to its end-diastolic volume.

In daily practice, LVEF is often visually estimated. This approach can provide clinically useful and reliable estimates if performed by a well-trained echocardiographer with sufficient experience [2]. However, insufficient image quality, regional ventricular dysfunction, high or low heart rate and other factors may bias even the well-trained eye. Quantification should therefore be sought whenever possible.

According to the Teichholz method, the (three-dimensional) LV volumes in systole and diastole are estimated from the (one-dimensional) basal internal diameters using extensive geometric assumptions. This method is therefore particularly unreliable in patients with abnormal LV geometry or regional wall motion abnormalities and does not reflect state-of-the-art echocardiography.

The biplane method of discs (modified Simpson's rule) approximates the LV volume with a stack of ellipsoid discs, the diameters of which are derived from manually contouring the LV in the four- and two-chamber view (Fig. 4.1). This method must be regarded as current clinical standard and is recommended by the echocardiographic societies [1] unless 3D data are available. The use of a contrast agent for better endocardial delineation may be considered if less than 80 % of the endocardial contour is visible [1].

Several approaches for the automatic and semiautomatic delineation of the LV endocardial contour have been suggested. Recently, myocardial tracking algorithms are additionally used to track these contours automatically through the cardiac cycle. Although accuracy of the derived LVEF estimates is usually not better than with manual contouring, the limited user-interaction of these algorithms leads to a significant improvement in inter- and intra-observer variability [2].

Three-dimensional (3D) echocardiography allows the reconstruction of LV volumes without geometrical assumptions. Also here, different commercial

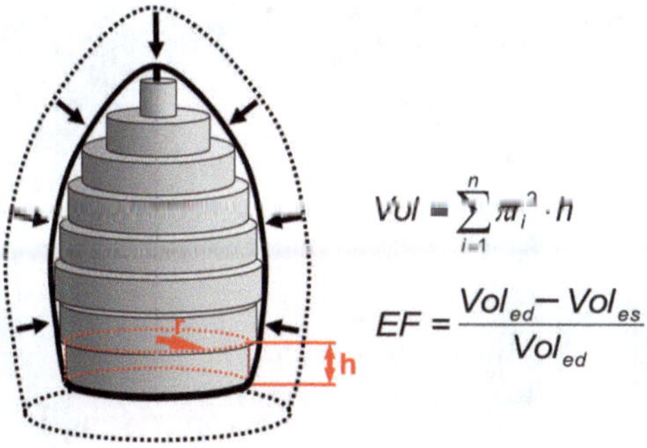

Fig. 4.1 Principle of left ventricular ejection fraction calculation by echocardiography using the Simpson's method (here: mono-plane). After manual (or semi-automated) delineation of the LV endocardial contour, the ventricular volume is calculated as the sum of a stack of cylinders of equal height. Ejection fraction is then calculated as the ratio of LV volume change and LV end-diastolic volume. *EF* ejection fraction, *r* cylinder radius, *h* cylinder height, *Voled* LV end-diastolic volume, *Voles* LV end-systolic volume, *dashed line* end-diastolic contour, *solid line* end-systolic contour

post-processing algorithms support the user in contouring the LV which indicates that endocardial border delineation remains crucial. Under optimal conditions, however, accuracy and reproducibility of 3D echocardiographic EF assessments are fully comparable to MRI [3]. So far, 3D echocardiography has not yet been fully integrated into the clinical routine due to the expensive equipment, the comparably time consuming data acquisition and analysis as well as the limited feasibility in patients with insufficient imaging windows.

2.1.2 Global Strain

Global longitudinal strain (GLS) is defined as the length change of the entire left ventricular circumference in one or all three apical views [4]. It is based on the tracking of myocardial deformation in gray scale images (speckle tracking). The exact methods of estimating global strain differ significantly between vendors so that measurements from different softwares cannot be directly compared.

LVEF and GLS are related parameters. Initial experience shows, however, that GLS has added value in detecting mild changes in LV function (Fig. 4.2). This might be due to the fact that GLS is more susceptible to changes in the longitudinal component of LV function. Further, GLS benefits from the limited user-interaction of all tracking methods so that it shows a somewhat better reproducibility than a regular LVEF estimated by the biplane Simpson's method. Since similar tracking algorithms are used for automated LVEF estimates (see above), this latter advantage may be only true for the comparison to the manual border contouring.

Normal ranges for GLS are yet to be determined, but first experiences indicate that values around –20 % are normal. Further, GLS of ≥–12 % has been shown to define severe LV dysfunction equivalent to an EF ≤35 % [5].

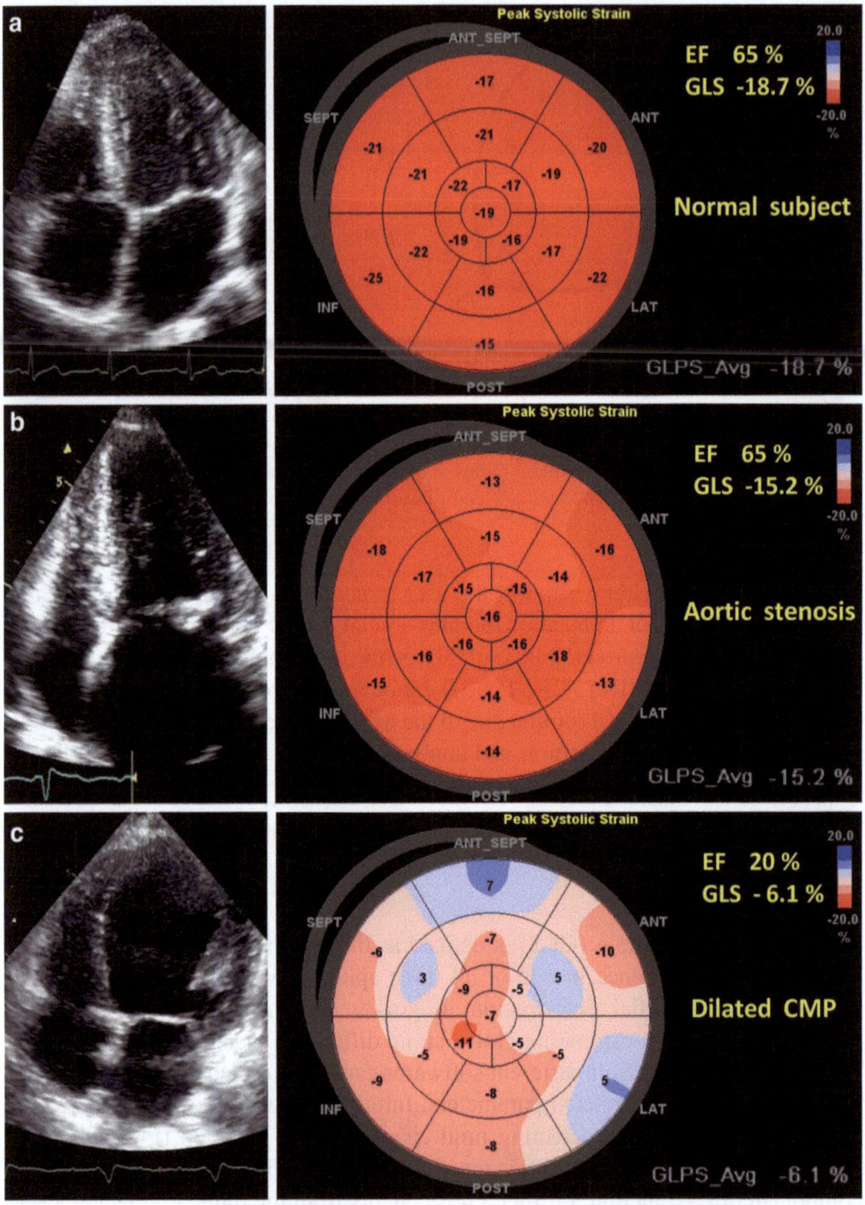

Fig. 4.2 Global left ventricular function assessment using ejection fraction and global longitudinal strain. *Right panels*: Bull's eye display of longitudinal peak systolic strain by speckle tracking echocardiography; segments with normal strain are represented in dark shade of *red*; decreased (less negative) strain is represented in *light red* and different shades of *blue*. (**a**) in a healthy subject, both EF and GLS are normal; (**b**) in a patient with aortic stenosis and concentric LV hypertrophy, EF is preserved whereas GLS is reduced, reflecting subtle left ventricular systolic dysfunction; (**c**) in a patient with dilative cardiomyopathy, both EF and GLS are significantly reduced. *EF* ejection fraction, *GLS* global longitudinal strain, *CMP* cardiomyopathy

2.1.3 Other Indicators of LV Global Function

The mitral annular plane systolic excursion (MAPSE) reflects the deformation of the related myocardial wall and can therefore serve as surrogate for GLS or LVEF. An excursion of >12 mm can be regarded as normal. In patients with regional dysfunction, however, measurements from all six walls need to be averaged.

Tissue Doppler velocities of the mitral ring can similarly be used to asses LV function. Also here, measurements from all walls need to be averaged in patients with regional dysfunction.

The maximum pressure rise in the LV (dP/dt max) is closely related to contractility and can be estimated form the continuous Doppler trace of a mitral regurgitation by measuring the time it takes to rise from 1 to 3 m/s. Values below 1,000 mmHg/s may be regarded as pathologic.

Key Point

- Global LV function is routinely assessed by estimating LV Ejection Fraction. Visual assessment is possible, but should only be performed by well-trained observers. The biplane Simpson's method is the standard. Tracking-based automated EF assessment and the new parameter of Global Longitudinal Strain are emerging alternatives with clinical potential.

2.2 Assessment of Regional Left Ventricular Systolic Function

2.2.1 Visual Assessment

For the assessment of regional function, the left ventricle is divided into 17 segments [1] (Fig. 4.3a). Another common segmentation, using three segments per wall is shown in (Fig. 4.3b). When segmental function is related to perfusion territories of the three coronary arteries, the inherent variability of coronary supply needs to be considered (Fig. 4.3c).

For a semiquantitative description, the function of each segment is graded as "normokinetic" (normal function), "hypokinetic" (reduced wall thickening and/or reduced longitudinal shortening), "akinetic" (no deformation), and "dyskinetic" (regional outward motion of the wall). The grading can be converted into a score ranging from 1 (normokinetic) to 4 (dyskinetic). The average of the scores of all LV segments is called Wall Motion Score Index and has comparable prognostic significance as LVEF.

The limitations of visual wall motion assessment are its subjectivity and the direct impact of image geometry (foreshortening) and image quality (endocardial border detection). While the latter problem can be partially overcomed by the use of contrast agents, the first two reflect the human factor in classic echocardiography, i.e., ability, training, and experience.

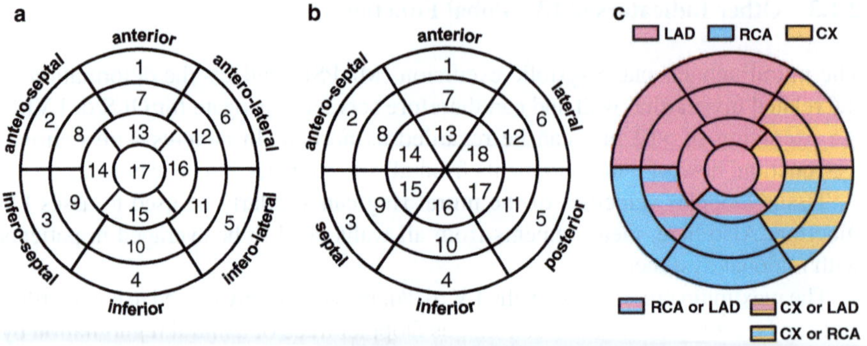

Fig. 4.3 Left ventricular segmentation and assignment of segments to coronary arterial territories. Bulls eye plots showing the left ventricular segments in a 17-segment 0028 (**a**) and an 18-segment (**b**) model; the *outer circle* represents the basal segments, the *middle circle* the mid-ventricular segments and the *inner circle* the apical segments. (**c**) Regional distribution of coronary vascular beds, with variations dependant on coronary artery dominance [1]. *CX* circumflex coronary artery, *LAD* left anterior descending coronary artery, *RCA* right coronary artery

2.2.2 Quantitative Assessment

Regional function can be quantified be measuring deformation (strain) or deformation rate (strain rate) using tissue Doppler or speckle tracking methods. A plethora of post-processing software is offered by all major vendors. Unfortunately, all softwares use different definitions and algorithms so that values cannot be compared between vendors. Further, image data are not interchangeable so that one lab usually has to rely on a proprietary solution from one company.

One added value of quantifying regional deformation is the possibility to assess the time course of deformation during the cardiac cycle in detail. Typical phenomena, such as post-systolic shortening in ischemia cannot be assessed visually [6] (Fig. 4.4). A major limitation of both tissue Doppler and speckle tracking solutions is the necessary effort of post-processing and the relatively high variability of measurement results which limits the feasibility of both techniques for a routine clinical use. In dedicated situations, such as asynchrony assessment or stress echocardiography, this effort appears justified. In the context of clinical research, the possibility to quantify regional myocardial function becomes indispensable and often—particularly if Doppler-based approaches are used—results in a surprising sensitivity to subtle functional changes [4].

Key Point

- In the clinical routine, regional myocardial function is semiquantitatively graded per myocardial segment as normo-, hypo-, a-, and dyskinesia. Regional function can be quantified by tissue Doppler or speckle tracking. Both methods are powerful and valuable research tools but show a relevant variability in individual measurements. Their clinical use is therefore only slowly increasing.

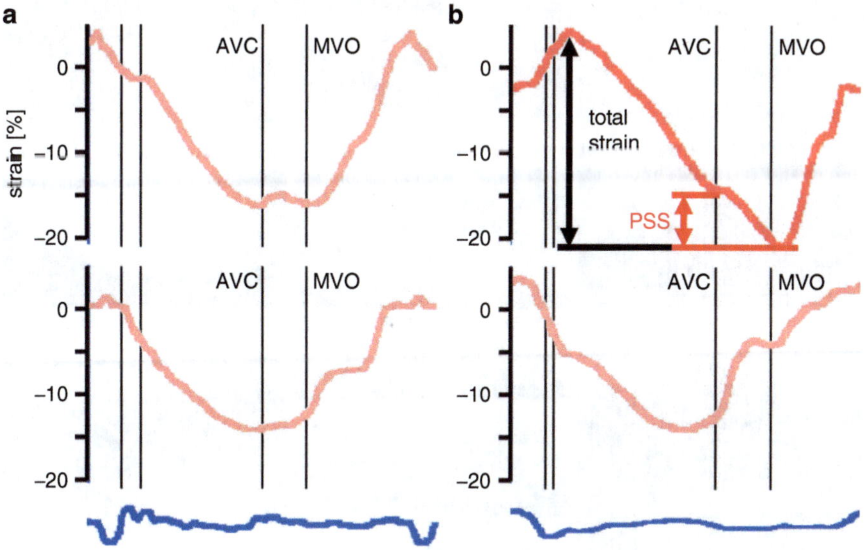

Fig. 4.4 Example of postsystolic shortening during stress-induced ischemia. *Top panels*: segment with ischemic response during stress echocardiography. *Bottom panels*: segment with normal response. (**a**) Normal pattern of baseline strain curves in both segments. (**b**) Ischemic response of the upper segment can be seen as the reduced systolic shortening and the marked postsystolic shortening. The normal segment shows a normal curve pattern under peak dobutamine stress. *AVO* aortic valve opening, *MVC* mitral valve closure, *MVO* mitral valve opening, *PSS* postsystolic shortening (reproduced from Voigt JU, Exner B, Schmiedehausen K, Huchzermeyer C et al. (2003) Strain-rate imaging during dobutamine stress echocardiography provides objective evidence of inducible ischemia. Circulation;107(16):2120-6.)

2.3 *Echocardiographic Assessment of Myocardial Variability*

Echocardiography can identify dysfunctional but viable myocardium by observing the changes in regional function during a low-dose dobutamine challenge. Dobutamine is administered as low as 5, 10, and 20 μg/(kg·min) and regional improvement of function by at least one grade is considered to indicate viability. A biphasic response with a later functional deterioration indicates additionally ischemia and improves predictive accuracy further.

The predictive value of a low-dose dobutamine stress test for functional recovery is comparable to scintigraphy. MRI can accurately distinguish scar and viable myocardium by showing delayed enhancement of scar tissue. Its predictive value for functional recovery, however, is limited due to the lack of a stress test.

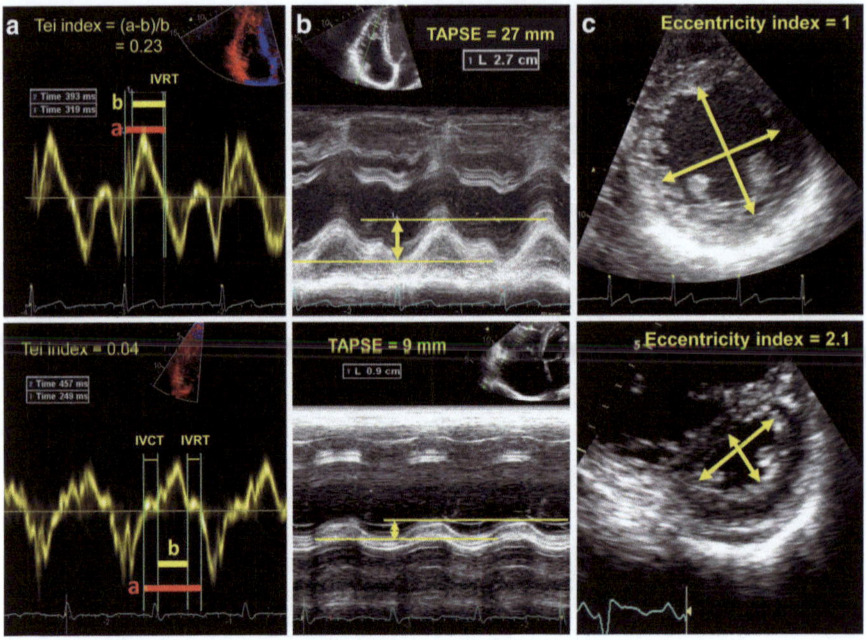

Fig. 4.5 Assessment of right ventricular (RV) function. *Top panels*: a normal subject. *Bottom panels*: a patient with severe pulmonary hypertension. (**a**) Due to prolongation of the isovolumic intervals and a shortening of ejection time, the Tei index is higher in RV dysfunction. Note the increased isovolumic relaxation time, which is almost nonexistent in the normal right ventricle. Also note the reduced peak systolic velocity in pathology. (**b**) Measurements of tricuspid annular plane systolic excursion (TAPSE). Note the reduction in pulmonary hypertension. (**c**) Parasternal short-axis views at the mid-ventricular level illustrating measurements for calculation of the eccentricity index. Normal heart with the eccentricity index of 1 (*upper panel*) and the RV dysfunction with the index of 2.1 (*bottom panel*). *IVCT* isovolumic contraction time, *IVRT* isovolumic relaxation time

2.4 Assessment of Right Ventricular Function

2.4.1 Global Right Ventricular Function

The echocardiographic assessment of right ventricular (RV) function is challenging due to the complex geometry of this chamber, its unfavourable retrosternal position as well as its irregular endocardial border [7].

RV ejection fraction (RVEF) can only be assessed using modern 3D echocardiography. While its reproducibility is comparable to MRI, its feasibility is usually very limited due to the difficult imaging conditions.

Clinically useful parameters to assess RV function are the fractional area change (FAC) and the tricuspid annular plane systolic excursion (TAPSE) [8].

Relative changes in loading conditions due to pathology are much higher in the RV then in the LV. Therefore, the actual pre- and afterload of the RV must be considered when interpreting any functional parameter of the RV (Table 4.2 and Fig. 4.5).

2.4.2 Regional Right Ventricular Function

Regional function may be visually assessed or quantified using tissue Doppler or speckle tracking-based deformation imaging. For the latter, the RV free wall is usually separated into an apical and basal segment only. It has been shown that pathology can have differential effects on both segments. The added clinical value of quantitative regional RV function assessment remains to be determined.

3 Assessment of Diastolic Function

3.1 Guideline-Based Decision Tree

The term "diastolic function" describes the ability of the ventricle to receive a sufficient volume of blood for an optimal ejection. Diastolic function is the result of the complex interaction between relaxation of the muscle fibers, the passive properties of the myocardium and its surrounding tissue, ventricular shape and size, and many other factors. Reduced diastolic function results in an elevated filling pressure of the ventricle. Therefore, the invasive assessment of filling pressures is the gold standard for the evaluation of diastolic function.

With the exception of well-defined restrictive and constrictive diseases, the existence of a pure diastolic dysfunction is subject to debate since in most pathology, diastolic dysfunction of the myocardium may be just one first stage in the continuum towards systolic dysfunction and heart failure. Therefore the term "heart failure with preserved ejection fraction" (HFPEF) has been commonly accepted. The diagnosis of HFPEF is nearly the only clinically relevant application for diastolic function assessment.

Echocardiographic assessment of diastolic function aims at a noninvasive estimate of the LV filling pressure (Fig. 4.6). No single echocardiographic parameter alone can fulfill this task reliably. The assessment of diastolic function remains therefore an integration process considering different echocardiographic measurements and the clinical context [9].

3.1.1 Atrial Size

Elevated filling pressures result in an enlargement of the left atrium. A dilated atrium is a sensitive, but nonspecific indicator of diastolic dysfunction. Conversely, relevant diastolic dysfunction becomes highly unlikely if the atrial size is normal (<34 mL/m^2).

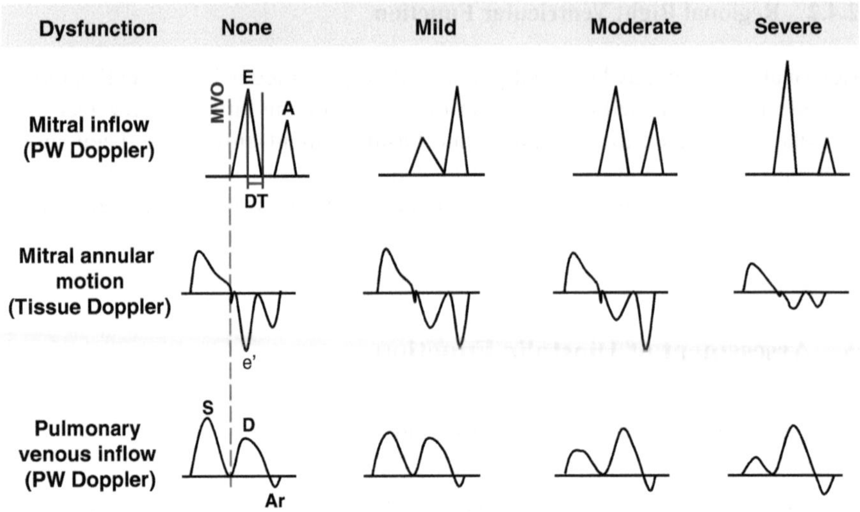

Fig. 4.6 Evaluation and grading of left ventricular diastolic function using different Doppler techniques. *E* peak early filling velocity, *A* velocity at atrial contraction, *DT* mitral E velocity deceleration time, *MV* mitral valve, *e′* velocity of mitral annulus early diastolic motion, *S* systolic forward flow, *D* diastolic forward flow, *AR* pulmonary venous atrial reversal flow

3.1.2 Mitral Inflow Profile

Acceleration and deceleration of the flow over the mitral valve is caused by the pressure difference between the left ventricle and the left atrium. Therefore, the measurement of the inflow profile over the non-stenotic mitral valve allows to a certain extend conclusions about the LV diastolic function.

Under normal conditions, the early diastolic flow over the mitral valve is higher than the late diastolic flow (E:A ratio > 1) in young and middle aged people. As a first sign of mild diastolic dysfunction, the end-diastolic "push" from the atrium increases resulting in an A-wave velocity exceeding the E-wave velocity (E:A ratio < 1). With increasing dysfunction, also the early diastolic filling pressure is rising which leads to a pseudo-normalization of the E:A ratio (>1). Initially, this pseudo-normalization is reversible by unloading the left atrium (Valsalva maneuver) but remains fixed in a more advanced state of the disease.

Similar considerations allow to explain the changes in the LV isovolumic relaxation time (IVRT) and the deceleration time of the mitral inflow E-wave (DT). The biphasic response of all of these echocardiographic indices is the biggest challenge in the correct assessment of diastolic function (Fig. 4.6).

3.1.3 Pulmonary Venous Inflow Profile

The inflow profile from the pulmonary veins is strongly influenced by filling LV pressures. Besides changes in the early and late filling peaks (S and D waves), the duration of backflow during atrial contraction (Ar) has been shown to be a relevant parameter, particularly if compared to the duration of the A-wave of the mitral inflow. A time difference of Ar–A>30 ms indicates elevated LV filling pressure. Unfortunately, the acquisition of sufficient pulmonary vein flow profiles is difficult and usually not successful in half of the patients.

3.1.4 Mitral Ring Velocity and E/e' Ratio

The early diastolic velocity of the mitral ring (e') is modulated by myocardial relaxation in a monophasic way. Consequently, the calculation of the E/e' ratio leads to a parameter which is linearly related to LV filling pressures. Unfortunately, ventricular size, shape, and systolic function are also reflected in the early diastolic velocity of the mitral ring which makes the E/e' ratio fail to predict LV filling pressures in patients with depressed LV function, conduction delays, and several other conditions.

The current guidelines on the assessment of diastolic function [9] recommend therefore a differential approach depending on LV function (Fig. 4.7a–c). In preserved LV function, the e' velocity is the first parameter to look at, while in depressed LV function, the E:A ratio comes first. Different cut-off values for mitral ring velocities are used. Higher values can be expected in the free lateral wall, while the septum has lower values. Ring velocities should be averaged in case of regional wall motion abnormalities.

3.1.5 Assessment of Diastolic Function in Patients with Atrial Fibrillation

Evaluation of diastolic function in patients with atrial fibrillation (AF) is challenging but feasible. Several parameters can also be applied in the absence of a regular atrial contraction. These include the isovolumic relaxation time (IVRT), the deceleration time of the mitral inflow (DT) and the E/e' ratio. Measurements should be averaged over 5–10 consecutive cycles if RR intervals vary more than 20 % [9].

Key Point

- Clinically relevant indications for diastolic function assessment are rare; the diagnosis of heart failure with preserved ejection fraction is one of them. Diastolic function assessment by echocardiography is not straight forward and requires the integration of several measurement parameters with the clinical context. The current guidelines provide a clinically useful and feasible decision tree based on systolic function, E:A ratio, E/e′-ratio and additional parameters if needed.

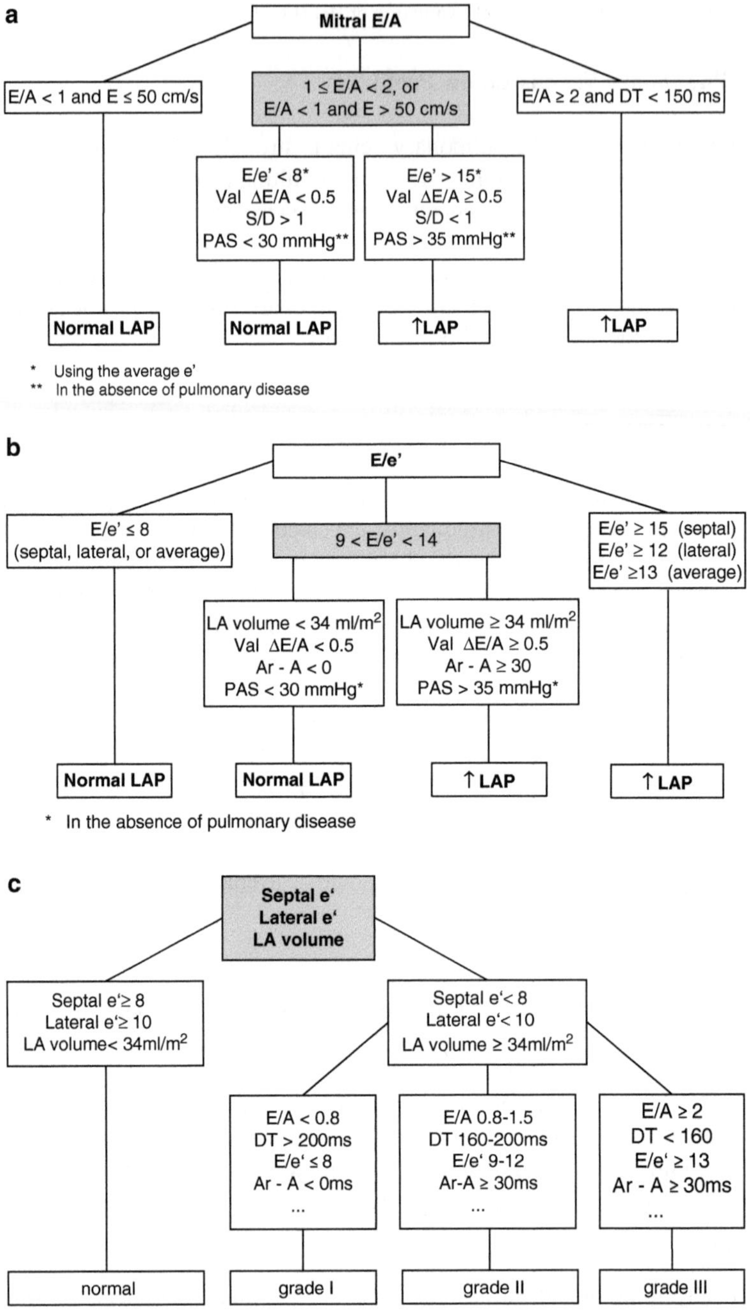

Fig. 4.7 Algorithms for the estimation of LV filling pressures and grading diastolic dysfunction. (**a**) Estimation of filling pressures of LV with reduced ejection fraction (<50 %). (**b**) Estimation of filling pressures of LV with preserved EF (>50 %). (**c**) Practical approach to grade LV diastolic dysfunction. Modified from Nagueh SF, Appleton CP, Gillebert TC, Marino PN, et al. (2009) Recommendations for the evaluation of left ventricular diastolic function by echocardiography. Eur J Echocardiogr;10(2):165–93

3.2 The Myocardial Performance Index (Tei index)

The myocardial performance index (Tei index) is a simple Doppler parameter that provides global assessment of systolic and diastolic function [10]. It is defined as the sum of the isovolumic contraction and isovolumic relaxation times divided by the ejection time of the respective ventricle. All time intervals necessary for its calculation can be obtained either from Doppler interrogation of the valves or from tissue Doppler traces (Fig. 4.5).

The Tei index can be calculated for both, the LV and the RV, but different cut-off values have to be used (RV Tei < 0.30 and LV Tei < 0.40 are considered "normal"). The index rises with increasing dysfunction of the ventricle. The major drawback of the index is its nonspecific nature as it does not allow to distinguish systolic from diastolic components. Further, pseudonormalization of the Tei index can be observed in severe dysfunction since increasing atrial pressures lead to a shortening of the IVRT and with this to a normalization of the index.

Key Point

- The Tei index is an unspecific marker of both systolic and diastolic ventricular dysfunction and is usually not part of the standard echocardiographic report. Its use might be considered if other approaches to assess ventricular function fail, e.g., due to poor echogenicity of the patient.

4 Glossary on the Noninvasive Assessment of Hemodynamics

Cardiac catheterization allows the direct and reliable measurement of cardiac pressures. Echocardiography allows to estimate most of the clinically relevant pressures parameters fast, noninvasively and without risk for the patient (Fig. 4.8). The reliability of the different estimates differs substantially and will be discussed below. Besides that, echocardiography is one of the few noninvasive imaging modalities that can directly measure hemodynamics, i.e., the motion of the blood.

4.1 Stroke Volume and Cardiac Output

The left ventricular stroke volume (SV) can be estimated from the difference of the diastolic and systolic volume of the LV as described in Sect. 1.2. A second "hemodynamic" approach integrates the velocity curve of the LV outflow tract during systole, derived from pulsed wave (PW) Doppler, and multiplies this "stroke length" with the cross-sectional area of the LV outflow tract (LVOT), which is estimated from the LVOT diameter under the assumption of its circular shape (Fig. 4.9). Both measurements are critical. If the PW Doppler sample volume is placed too far in the

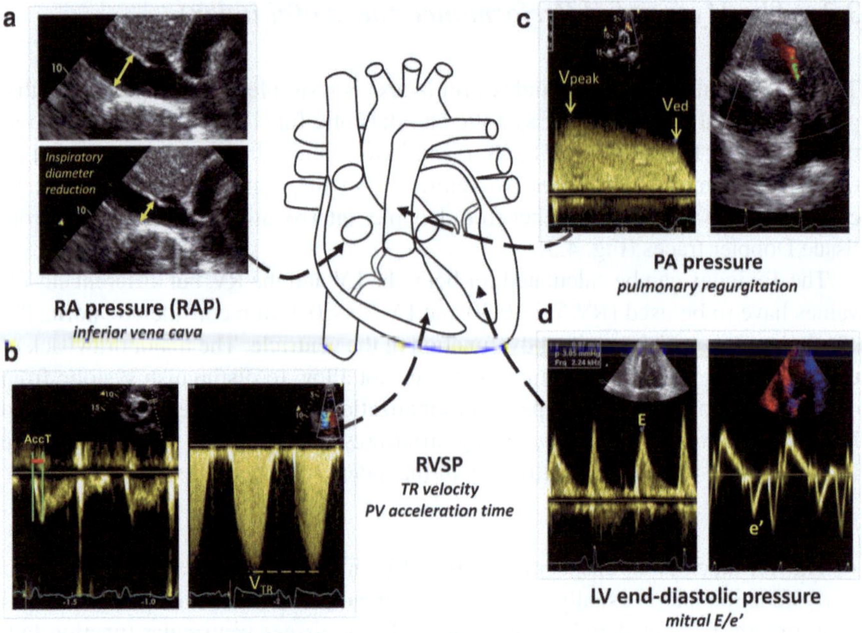

Fig. 4.8 Noninvasive hemodynamic assessment of the heart. *RA* right atrium, *RAP* right atrial pressure, *RVSP* right ventricular systolic pressure, *PA* pulmonary artery, *PV* pulmonary valve, *LV* left ventricle, *TR* tricuspid regurgitation

ventricle, the stroke volume will be underestimated, if it is placed too close to the aortic valve, potential flow acceleration towards an aortic stenosis will result in an overestimation of the SV. Further, due to the assumption of a circular shape, LVOT diameter measurement errors affect SV estimates to the power of 2.

Right ventricular stroke volumes can be assessed similarly. Since the RV outflow tract is often not well aligned with the Doppler beam, measurements may also be taken from the main pulmonary artery.

Cardiac output (CO) is calculated by multiplying the SV with the heart rate.

4.2 Left Ventricular and Left Atrial Pressures

In the absence of any aortic stenosis, the LV systolic pressure is in a first approximation equal to the cuff pressure measurements on the arm and need no echocardiographic assessment.

The end-diastolic pressure of the LV (and with this, of the LA) can be assessed as described in the chapter on diastolic function assessment (Fig. 4.7). Echocardiography allows usually to distinguish "normal" from "elevated" (Fig. 4.8d).

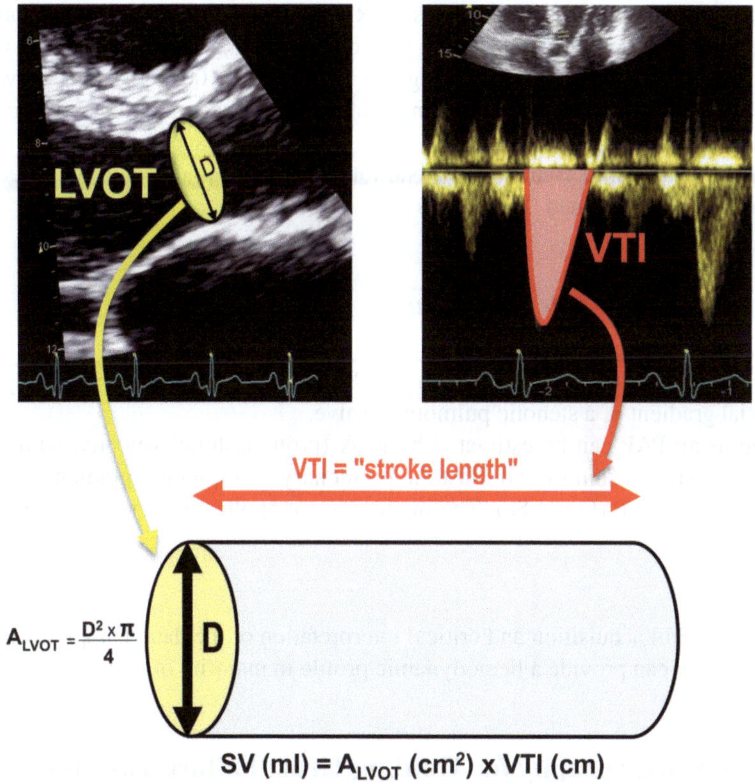

Fig. 4.9 The stroke volume can be interpreted as a cylindrical column of blood, the base of which is similar to the LVOT cross-sectional area. The length of the blood column is derived from the time integral of the blood flow velocities during ejection ("stroke length"). The cross-sectional area of the LVOT is assumed to be circular and approximated by measuring the LVOT diameter in the parasternal long axis. A_{LVOT} cross-sectional area of the LV outflow tract, *SV* stroke volume, *VTI* velocity-time integral

4.3 Right Ventricular and Right Atrial Pressures

The right atrial pressure can be estimated from the subcostal view by assessing the inferior vena cava diameter and its response to breathing maneuvers (Fig. 4.8a). Echocardiography usually allows to distinguish "normal" (inspiratory collapse of the vein) from "elevated" (dilated IVC, no response to breathing). A finer classification has been is proposed but is not reliably possible in the clinical setting.

The right ventricular systolic pressure can be determined from the maximum systolic pressure gradient across the tricuspid valve by adding the estimated right atrial pressure to the measurement. Since the estimate of the RA pressure is unreliable, it has been proven clinically useful to report the tricuspid pressure gradient as such.

If no tricuspid regurgitation is present RV pressures can be estimated from the acceleration time (AT) of the systolic flow over the non-stenotic pulmonary valve. Echocardiography can usually distinguish "normal" (>100 ms) from "elevated" (<100 ms) (Fig. 4.8b). Further, the length of the RV isovolumic relaxation may be measured from Doppler traces of the RV valves or the tissue Doppler trace of the right lateral tricuspid ring. If a measurable RV IVRT is detected, elevated RV pressures can be assumed (Fig. 4.5).

4.4 Pulmonary Artery Pressure

The systolic pulmonary artery pressure (PAP) is equal to the RV pressure plus a potential gradient of a stenotic pulmonary valve.

The mean PAP can be estimated by peak (protodiastolic) velocity, while end-diastolic PAP is a sum of end-diastolic pulmonary regurgitation gradient (PA-RV-gradient) and RAP (Fig. 4.8c). The method is not applicable in severe pulmonary regurgitation.

Key Point

- With careful acquisition and critical interpretation of the data, Doppler echocardiography can provide a hemodynamic profile in majority of patients.

5 Echocardiography for Guiding Heart Failure Therapy

5.1 Guiding Pharmacotherapy

Left ventricular EF is the most frequently used parameter for initiation of a certain drug classes. According to the latest ESC guidelines, unless contraindicated or not tolerated, ACE inhibitors and beta-blockers should be used in all symptomatic patients with a LVEF ≤40 %, whereas a low dose of an aldosterone antagonist should be administered to those with EF of ≤35 % [11].

After initial diagnosis, short term repetition of echocardiography is usually not indicated unless new symptoms require it. Even an acute decompensation of preexisting heart failure will usually lead to elevated pulmonary pressures and an increase of a mitral regurgitation which will resolve after successful re-compensation, but will deliver otherwise no relevant new information.

5.2 Monitoring Cardiotoxic Treatment

Echocardiography is the standard technique for monitoring LV function during the treatment with cardiotoxic drugs (such as anthracycline agents) and radiotherapy

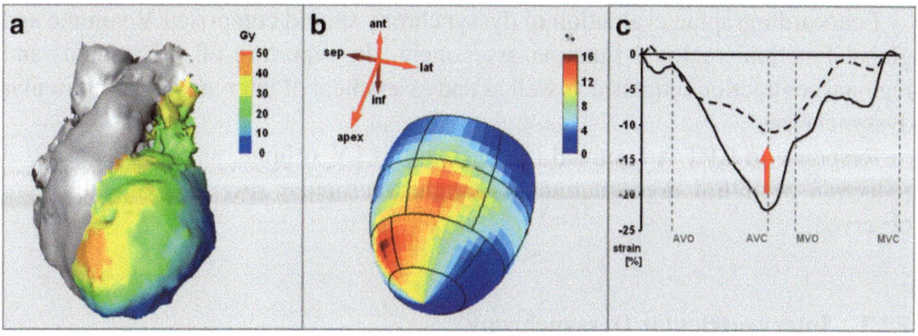

Fig. 4.10 Radiotherapy (RT) effects on systolic myocardial function detected by strain-rate imaging in a left-breast cancer patient [12]. (**a**) Three-dimensional (3D) CT reconstruction of the patient's heart. The surface of the LV was color-coded according to radiation dose distribution. (**b**) 3D model of the LV displaying the color-coded change (relative decrease) in the percentage of regional longitudinal strain post-RT. Note the concordance between radiation dose distribution and regional functional impairment. (**c**) The change in end-systolic longitudinal strain (*red arrow*) in the anteroapical segmental strain (*solid line* before RT; *dashed line* after RT; AVO; AVC; MVO; MVC, aortic and mitral valve opening and closure)

[12, 13]. With increasing long term survival, iatrogenic cardiac dysfunction after cancer treatment becomes a relevant problem. Currently, therapy is stopped or modified in 17 % of patients for cardiac problems, mostly documented as decrease in LVEF.

Serial echocardiographic evaluations using advanced quantitative echocardiographic methods, such as tissue Doppler and speckle tracking-based deformation imaging have been shown to identifying cardiotoxicity by detecting subtle changes in cardiac function earlier than by using conventional LVEF [12, 13] (Fig. 4.10).

5.3 Cardiac Resynchronization Therapy

Cardiac resynchronization therapy (CRT) is recommended for symptomatic heart failure patients (NYHA II-IV) with prolonged QRS duration (QRS width > 120 ms), who are resistant to optimal medical treatment [14]. However, one-third of the patients selected by current criteria do not respond to therapy while an unknown number of patients who may have benefitted is rejected.

Echocardiography has been suggested as selection technique since CRT aims at re-synchronizing the dyssynchronous contraction of the heart walls and echocardiography is able to measure myocardial motion and deformation with high temporal resolution [14]. A plethora of echocardiographic parameters, mostly based on timing of regional myocardial velocity peaks, has been proposed. Currently, there is conflicting evidence on the value of these parameters and the development goes towards the use of parameters which are based on the direct assessment of myocardial deformation.

Echocardiographic evaluation of dyssynchrony should comprise LV volume and global function, regional function assessment, the reporting of scar regions and regional contraction sequence as well as and assessment of inter- and intraventricular dyssynchrony.

Response to CRT is assumed if a decrease in LV volume, an increase in EF, a reduction of mitral regurgitation or a right ventricular reverse remodeling are observed.

5.3.1 Interventricular Dyssynchrony

Interventricular dyssynchrony is assumed if the difference between LV and RV pre-ejection time exceeds 40 ms. Alternatively, the onset of systolic motion in the basal right ventricular free wall versus the most delayed basal LV segment can be measured by Tissue Doppler. A delay of >56 ms is considered to indicate interventricular dyssynchrony [15]. Interventricular dyssynchrony has a limited value for predicting CRT response.

5.3.2 Intraventricular Dyssynchrony

Intraventricular dyssynchrony can be evaluated by conventional echocardiography, tissue velocity measurements, and deformation imaging.

Conventional Echocardiography

Conventional echo markers of dyssynchrony involve LV pre-ejection time (cut-off>140 ms) and septal-posterior wall motion delay (cut-off>130 ms). Feasibility and predictive value of these methods are disputed [16].

Tissue Velocity Imaging

Regional myocardial velocities are measured either directly with PW tissue Doppler or retrospectively from high frame rate (>90 frames/s) color tissue Doppler, usually acquired from the apical window. Parameters can be broadly divided into (1) time delays between opposing walls and (2) standard deviations of time-to-peak systolic velocities. The reproducibility and predictive value of these parameters is subject to debate.

One example of a time delay parameter is the maximum delay between any systolic velocity peak in four basal LV segments. A delay >65 ms is considered predictive for CRT success [16].

Similarly, the calculation of the standard deviation of the time-to-peak systolic velocity in 6 basal or 12 basal and mid-wall segments of the LV can be used.

A cut-off value of >36.5 ms (6 segments) and >32.3 ms (12 segments) has been suggested to predict response to CRT [16].

Deformation Imaging

In contrast to the timing of myocardial velocity peaks, myocardial deformation parameters (strain, strain rate) depend less on tethering between segments and offer true regional information on myocardial function. Doppler-based deformation data are noisier and more angle dependent compared to velocities, while 2D speckle tracking-derived data have limited temporal resolution.

Currently, the time difference of peak systolic radial strain between the basal anterior-septal and basal posterior segments of more than 130 ms appears as one of the most promising simple parameters to predict CRT success [16].

More complex approaches try to compare areas of regional lengthening and shortening during ejection in order to determine the "wasted energy." Although conceptually convincing and promising in first studies, these parameters are still subject to further research.

Septal Flash and Apical Rocking

Septal flash and apical rocking describe the direct mechanical consequences of dyssynchronous contraction induced by left bundle branch block. A short initial septal contraction within the isovolumic contraction period results of a short inward motion of the septum (septal flash) and causes the apex to move septally (Fig. 4.11). The delayed activation of the lateral wall pulls then the apex laterally during the ejection time while stretching the septum. This typical motion pattern of the apex is described as "apical rocking." The presence of septal flash and apical rocking can be both visualized and quantified and have been shown to have predictive value for a CRT response which is superior to velocity-based parameters of LV dyssynchrony [17–19].

3D Echocardiography

At present, there is no sufficient evidence to recommend 3D echocardiography for dyssynchrony assessment.

Key Point

- Echocardiography provides several guideline criteria for CRT indication, such as LV volume and LVEF. Echocardiography appears further as the obvious tool to assess the treatment target of CRT, which is the asynchronous contraction of different LV walls. No robust evidence base is available, but asynchrony markers based on myocardial deformation and epiphenomena, such as apical rocking and septal flash, appear favorable.

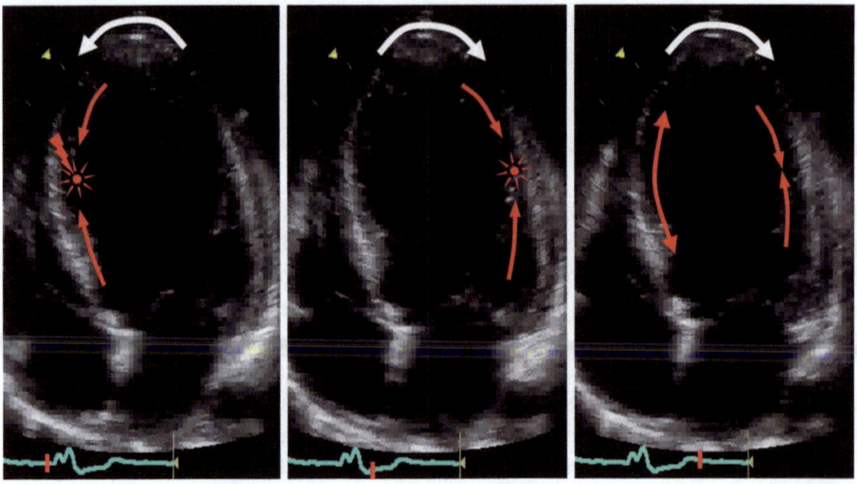

Fig. 4.11 Typical contraction sequence in LBBB: a short initial (apical) septal contraction causes the apex to move septally. The lateral wall is activated with delay, pulling the apex laterally and stretching the septum

5.3.3 CRT Optimization

AV Delay Optimization

Optimization of atrio-ventricular (AV) and interventricular (VV) delays has been suggested to improve the response to CRT. The AV delay may be optimized by evaluating the mitral inflow pattern. If the A-wave is absent or truncated, the AV delay is probably too short. If the E and A waves are merged, the AV delay is most likely too long. Further, the maximization of the VTI of the mitral inflow and the LV filling time is attempted. Optimization is usually done by changing the AV interval iteratively in steps of 20 ms and echocardiographic guidance.

Independent of the echocardiography guided optimization, the AV delay must be so short that a reliable capture of the LV is be guaranteed. It should be noted that optimal settings for varying physical activity or body size are unknown.

Delay Optimization

The VV delay optimum is highly individual. For optimization, VV delay is changed stepwise in a range of −80 ms (RV first) to +80 ms (LV first) and parameters are measured at each step. At least ten beats of stabilization should be allowed before echocardiographic measurements are done. Care has to be taken of the definition of VV delay which may differ depending on the vendor (time delay relative to the first lead, time delay relative to the RV lead, etc.) and which may result in an unwanted

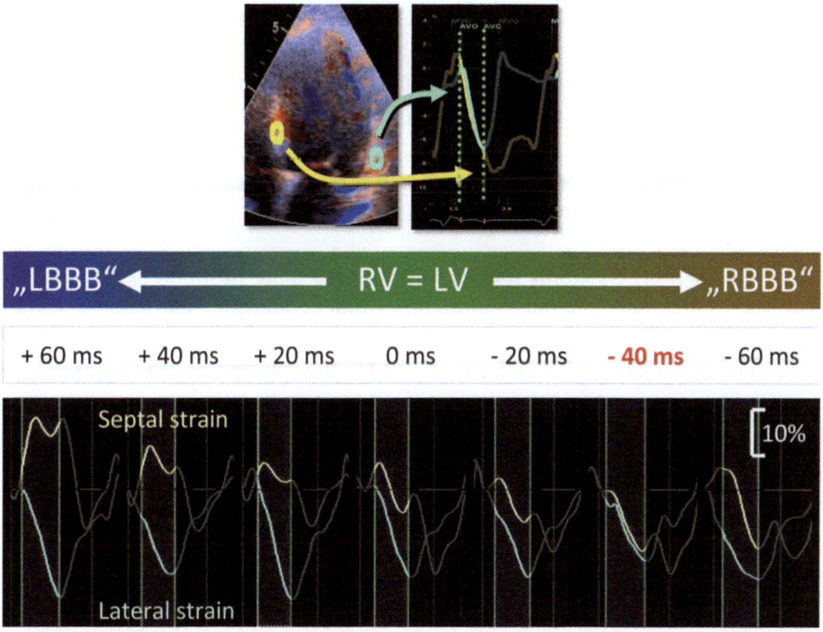

Fig. 4.12 VV delay optimization using Tissue Doppler-derived longitudinal strain curves from the septum and the lateral wall. VV delay intervals were altered in 20 ms steps, and the optimal delay was determined as the value minimizing the temporal differences between the strain peaks of basal septal and lateral segments. Note that VV delay of –40 ms abolished positive strain in the septal segment and resulted in simultaneous LV contraction

change in AV timing. At present, there is no consensus favoring a certain parameter for optimization. Both hemodynamic (LV stroke volume, mitral inflow VTI) and regional function parameters (interventricular dyssynchrony, time to peak velocity in 6 basal segments) have been proposed (Fig. 4.12).

Key Point

- Echocardiography can be used for an iterative attempt to optimize AV and VV setting on CRT patients. While AV settings are usually optimized based on the improvement of the mitral inflow, no clear standards exist for VV delay optimization.

5.4 Implantable Cardioverter-Defibrillators

5.4.1 Dilated and Ischemic Cardiomyopathy

LV systolic dysfunction and heart failure symptoms are among the strongest predictors of risk for sudden cardiac death. In the vast majority of studies, LV systolic function as described by LVEF has been used while the actual modality and method for measuring LVEF has been varying. Currently LVEF of <30–35 % is a cut-off for ICD implantation. Functional recovery after revascularization and optimal treatment has to be excluded since premature ICD implantation has shown no benefit [20].

5.4.2 Other Cardiomyopathy

Echo has a leading role in the diagnosis of hypertrophic cardiomyopathy and contributes to establish the diagnosis of an arrhythmogenic right ventricular cardiomyopathy (ARVC). Usually, multimodality imaging and clinical aspects are considered. For detailed information, the reader is referred to the appropriate guidelines [21, 22].

6 Sources of Further Information

6.1 Textbooks

Galiuto L (ed) (2011) The EAE textbook of echocardiography. Oxford University Press, Oxford, NY

This book covers the core syllabus of echocardiographic knowledge as proposed by the European Association of Echocardiography.

6.2 Position Papers and Guidelines

1. Mor-Avi V et al. Current and evolving echocardiographic techniques for the quantitative evaluation of cardiac mechanics [Ref. # 4].

   Valuable consensus document, outlining the use of echocardiographic methods to evaluate cardiac mechanics. The document discusses a variety of techniques for evaluating mechanics of all cardiac chambers, and summarizes their strengths, limitations, and potential clinical applications.

2. Nagueh SF et al. Recommendations for the evaluation of left ventricular diastolic function by echocardiography [Ref. # 9].

   Well balanced summary of available echocardiographic methods for the assessment of LV diastolic function, comprehensive review of the significance of diastolic parameters, as well as feasible recommendations for nomenclature and reporting of diastolic data in routine clinical practice.

6.3 Recent Journal Articles

7. Jurcut R et al. The echocardiographic assessment of the right ventricle: what to do in 2010? [Ref. # 7].

   State-of-the-art review of the utility of conventional and advanced echocardiographic techniques in the assessment of the right ventricle which may also serve as a practical guide to the RV evaluation in a daily routine.

16. Anderson LJ et al. Patient selection and echocardiographic assessment of dyssynchrony in cardiac resynchronization therapy [Ref. # 16].

   A critical review of the current role of echocardiography in cardiac resynchronization therapy and a detailed overview over many CRT studies from the past years.

17. Voigt JU et al. Apical transverse motion as surrogate parameter to determine regional left ventricular function inhomogeneities: a new, integrative approach to left ventricular asynchrony assessment [Ref. # 17].

   This study sheds new light on the dyssynchrony assessment, introducing apical rocking—a surrogate parameter, reflecting both temporal and functional inhomogeneities in the left ventricle with left branch bundle block.

7 Future Trends in the Field

Wider use of both handheld ultrasound machines and three-dimensional echocardiography, as well the translation of myocardial deformation imaging into a readily available diagnostic tool for the clinical arena will further strengthen the role of echocardiography in the assessment of patients with heart failure.

When used by adequately trained physicians, pocket-sized ultrasound devices allow fast and reliable assessment of cardiac morphology and function, which makes them a suitable tool for screening and initial evaluation of patients with suspected heart failure. With further technical improvements, these "stethoscopes of the future" could become an indispensable gadget for physical examination of cardiovascular system in everyday clinical practice.

If further advances in imaging technology and processing software make three-dimensional echocardiography more feasible for the clinical routine, these systems may become more widely used and routine assessment of cardiac morphology and function will be regularly performed in a quality which is comparable to so called "gold standard" techniques.

Myocardial deformation imaging has already entered the clinical arena. If further improvements in robustness and comparability of measurements and parameters between different vendors are achieved, this diagnostic tool will become indispensable for the diagnosis and follow-up of heart failure patients.

Nevertheless, for both pocket-sized devices and advanced techniques, appropriate training of physicians and sonographers will be critical to avoid serious consequences of misdiagnosing heart disease. Efforts have to be made by the national and European imaging societies and legislation to foster standardized training in echocardiography and to continuously ensure quality control.

References

1. Lang RM, Bierig M, Devereux RB, Flachskampf FA, Foster E, Pellikka PA, Picard MH, Roman MJ, Seward J, Shanewise J, Solomon S, Spencer KT, St John Sutton M, Stewart W, American Society of Echocardiography's Nomenclature and Standards Committee, Task Force on Chamber Quantification, American College of Cardiology Echocardiography Committee, American Heart Association, European Association of Echocardiography, European Society of Cardiology (2006) Recommendations for chamber quantification. Eur J Echocardiogr 7(2):79–108
2. Szulik M, Pappas CJ, Jurcut R, Magro M, Peeters E, Goetschalckx K, Rademakers F, Desmet W, Voigt JU (2011) Clinical validation of a novel speckle-tracking-based ejection fraction assessment method. J Am Soc Echocardiogr 24(10):1092–1100
3. Nikitin NP, Constantin C, Loh PH, Ghosh J, Lukaschuk EI, Bennett A, Hurren S, Alamgir F, Clark AL, Cleland JG (2006) New generation 3-dimensional echocardiography for left ventricular volumetric and functional measurements: comparison with cardiac magnetic resonance. Eur J Echocardiogr 7(5):365–372
4. Mor-Avi V, Lang RM, Badano LP, Belohlavek M, Cardim NM, Derumeaux G, Galderisi M, Marwick T, Nagueh SF, Sengupta PP, Sicari R, Smiseth OA, Smulevitz B, Takeuchi M, Thomas JD, Vannan M, Voigt JU, Zamorano JL (2011) Current and evolving echocardiographic techniques for the quantitative evaluation of cardiac mechanics: ASE/EAE consensus statement on methodology and indications endorsed by the Japanese Society of Echocardiography. Eur J Echocardiogr 12(3):167–205
5. Voigt JU (2011) Quantification of left ventricular function and synchrony using tissue Doppler, strain imaging, and speckle tracking. In: Galiuto L (ed) The EAE textbook of echocardiography. Oxford University Press, New York
6. Voigt JU, Exner B, Schmiedehausen K, Huchzermeyer C, Reulbach U, Nixdorff U, Platsch G, Kuwert T, Daniel WG, Flachskampf FA (2003) Strain-rate imaging during dobutamine stress echocardiography provides objective evidence of inducible ischemia. Circulation 107(16):2120–2126
7. Jurcut R, Giusca S, La Gerche A, Vasile S, Ginghina C, Voigt JU (2010) The echocardiographic assessment of the right ventricle: what to do in 2010? Eur J Echocardiogr 11(2):81–96
8. Rudski LG, Lai WW, Afilalo J, Hua L, Handschumacher MD, Chandrasekaran K, Solomon SD, Louie EK, Schiller NB (2010) Guidelines for the echocardiographic assessment of the right heart in adults: a report from the American Society of Echocardiography endorsed by the European Association of Echocardiography, a registered branch of the European Society of Cardiology, and the Canadian Society of Echocardiography. J Am Soc Echocardiogr 23(7):685–713
9. Nagueh SF, Appleton CP, Gillebert TC, Marino PN, Oh JK, Smiseth OA, Waggoner AD, Flachskampf FA, Pellikka PA, Evangelisa A (2009) Recommendations for the evaluation of left ventricular diastolic function by echocardiography. Eur J Echocardiogr 10(2):165–193
10. Tei C, Ling LH, Hodge DO, Bailey KR, Oh JK, Rodeheffer RJ, Tajik AJ, Seward JB (1995) New index of combined systolic and diastolic myocardial performance: a simple and reproducible measure of cardiac function–a study in normals and dilated cardiomyopathy. J Cardiol 26(6):357–366

11. Dickstein K, Cohen-Solal A, Filippatos G, McMurray JJ, Ponikowski P, Poole-Wilson PA, Strömberg A, van Veldhuisen DJ, Atar D, Hoes AW, Keren A, Mebazaa A, Nieminen M, Priori SG, Swedberg K, ESC Committee for Practice Guidelines (CPG) (2008) ESC Guidelines for the diagnosis and treatment of acute and chronic heart failure 2008: the Task Force for the Diagnosis and Treatment of Acute and Chronic Heart Failure 2008 of the European Society of Cardiology. Developed in collaboration with the Heart Failure Association of the ESC (HFA) and endorsed by the European Society of Intensive Care Medicine (ESICM). Eur Heart J 29(19):2388–2442
12. Erven K, Jurcut R, Weltens C, Giusca S, Ector J, Wildiers H, Van den Bogaert W, Voigt JU (2011) Acute radiation effects on cardiac function detected by strain rate imaging in breast cancer patients. Int J Radiat Oncol Biol Phys 79(5):1444–1451
13. Jurcut R, Wildiers H, Ganame J, D'hooge J, De Backer J, Denys H, Paridaens R, Rademakers F, Voigt JU (2008) Strain rate imaging detects early cardiac effects of pegylated liposomal Doxorubicin as adjuvant therapy in elderly patients with breast cancer. J Am Soc Echocardiogr 21(12):1283–1289
14. Authors/Task Force Members, Dickstein K, Vardas PE, Auricchio A, Daubert JC, Linde C, McMurray J, Ponikowski P, Priori SG, Sutton R, van Veldhuisen DJ; ESC Committee for Practice Guidelines (CPG), Vahanian A, Auricchio A, Bax J, Ceconi C, Dean V, Filippatos G, Funck-Brentano C, Hobbs R, Kearney P, McDonagh T, Popescu BA, Reiner Z, Sechtem U, Sirnes PA, Tendera M, Vardas P, Widimsky P; Document Reviewers, Tendera M, Anker SD, Blanc JJ, Gasparini M, Hoes AW, Israel CW, Kalarus Z, Merkely B, Swedberg K, Camm AJ. 2010 Focused Update of ESC Guidelines on device therapy in heart failure: an update of the 2008 ESC Guidelines for the diagnosis and treatment of acute and chronic heart failure and the 2007 ESC guidelines for cardiac and resynchronization therapy. Developed with the special contribution of the Heart Failure Association and the European Heart Rhythm Association. Eur Heart J. 2010;31(21):2677–2687
15. Penicka M, Bartunek J, De Bruyne B, Vanderheyden M, Goethals M, De Zutter M, Brugada P, Geelen P (2004) Improvement of left ventricular function after cardiac resynchronization therapy is predicted by tissue Doppler imaging echocardiography. Circulation 109(8):978–983
16. Anderson LJ, Miyazaki C, Sutherland GR, Oh JK (2008) Patient selection and echocardiographic assessment of dyssynchrony in cardiac resynchronization therapy. Circulation 117(15):2009–2023
17. Voigt JU, Schneider TM, Korder S, Szulik M, Gürel E, Daniel WG, Rademakers F, Flachskampf FA (2009) Apical transverse motion as surrogate parameter to determine regional left ventricular function inhomogeneities: a new, integrative approach to left ventricular asynchrony assessment. Eur Heart J 30(8):959–968
18. Szulik M, Tillekaerts M, Vangeel V, Ganame J, Willems R, Lenarczyk R, Rademakers F, Kalarus Z, Kukulski T, Voigt JU (2010) Assessment of apical rocking: a new, integrative approach for selection of candidates for cardiac resynchronization therapy. Eur J Echocardiogr 11(10):863–869
19. Parsai C, Bijnens B, Sutherland GR, Baltabaeva A, Claus P, Marciniak M, Paul V, Scheffer M, Donal E, Derumeaux G, Anderson L (2009) Toward understanding response to cardiac resynchronization therapy: left ventricular dyssynchrony is only one of multiple mechanisms. Eur Heart J 30(8):940–949
20. Hohnloser S, Kuck K, Dorian P et al (2004) on behalf of the DINAMIT Investigators. Prophylactic use of an implantable cardioverter-defibrillator after myocardial infarction. N Engl J Med 351:2481–2488
21. Marcus FI, McKenna WJ, Sherrill D, Basso C, Bauce B, Bluemke DA, Calkins H, Corrado D, Cox MG, Daubert JP, Fontaine G, Gear K, Hauer R, Nava A, Picard MH, Protonotarios N, Saffitz JE, Sanborn DM, Steinberg JS, Tandri H, Thiene G, Towbin JA, Tsatsopoulou A, Wichter T, Zareba W (2010) Diagnosis of arrhythmogenic right ventricular cardiomyopathy/dysplasia: proposed modification of the task force criteria. Circulation 121(13):1533–1541
22. Gersh BJ, Maron BJ, Bonow RO, Dearani JA, Fifer MA, Link MS, Naidu SS, Nishimura RA, Ommen SR, Rakowski H, Seidman CE, Towbin JA, Udelson JE, Yancy CW, American College

of Cardiology Foundation/American Heart Association Task Force on Practice Guidelines, American Association for Thoracic Surgery; American Society of Echocardiography, American Society of Nuclear Cardiology; Heart Failure Society of America, Heart Rhythm Society, Society for Cardiovascular Angiography and Interventions, Society of Thoracic Surgeons (2011) 2011 ACCF/AHA guideline for the diagnosis and treatment of hypertrophic cardiomyopathy: a report of the American College of Cardiology Foundation/American Heart Association Task Force on Practice Guidelines. Circulation 124(24):e783–831

Chapter 5
Back to Earth: "Common Sense" in the Management of Heart Failure

Marc Goethals

Never before has the diagnosis and treatment of heart failure been as challenging as it is today. This may sound paradoxical because there is a wealth of evidence-based medicine and guidelines for diagnosis and treatment. However, the ageing population and ever increasing standards of health care make medicine a lot more complicated than it was before. In addition the narrowing scope of super specialized physicians is ill adapted to the complex multi-organ pathology of a geriatric population. Blind confidence in guidelines, in numerical computer-generated patient data and a startling lack of "common sense" pose even a threat to the care of the cardiac patient. Within the scope of this chapter, it is not useful to reiterate once more on the published and widely distributed guidelines. Instead, I will try to hand over some practical thoughts and challenges that I meet every day in the care of my heart failure patients.

1 Three Basic Questions

Being confronted with a patient (often within the geriatric age) who is suspected of having "heart failure" I ask myself three basic questions.

1. Has the patient cardiac disease and/or heart failure and if so what is the pathophysiology of it?
2. Is heart failure his/her main problem?
3. How can I find a way out?

To sort out whether the patient has heart failure not only his/her present complaints and symptoms should be looked at but his/her complete medical history should be scrutinized, including not only numerical data but as much as possible

M. Goethals (✉)
Cardiovascular Centre, OLV Hospital, Moorselbaan 164, Aalst 9300, Belgium
e-mail: marc.goethals@olvz-aalst.be

J. Bartunek and M. Vanderheyden (eds.), *Translational Approach to Heart Failure*,
DOI 10.1007/978-1-4614-7345-9_5, © Springer Science+Business Media New York 2013

also the original tracings, images, and a detailed history of his/her medical treatments and the effects thereof on the clinical course, laboratory, and technical data. With the help of echocardiography, invasive hemodynamic and laboratory data (natriuretic peptides have revolutionized the management of heart failure!) it is most of the time possible to precisely establish a cardiac diagnosis.

However, once a diagnosis of cardiac disease/heart failure has been made the (superspecialized) cardiologist often becomes blinded for the pathology of other organ systems that may be more life threatening to the patient and/or more limiting his/her physical capacity than the eye catching cardiac pathology. Therefore the second question is often overlooked and it may be more relevant and more difficult to answer than the first question: Is this cardiac pathology really the main problem of the patient? Is this pathology really responsible for his/her symptoms and/or loss of quality of life? Can it be justified to aggressively treat this cardiac pathology if it is not causing symptoms, just for prognostic reasons in an 80-year-old person? Therefore, a multidisciplinary approach is of utmost importance to avoid to manage an innocent cardiac bystander at the cost of the accompanying complications.

Once it is established that the cardiac diagnosis of heart failure is the main problem it is obvious that a way out to solve or at least stabilize/improve the situation should be searched for. It is obvious that a thorough search should be undertaken for precipitating events on the one hand and correctable causes on the other hand besides the well-known basic treatment of heart failure.

2 Precipitating Events

Often in the relatively recent past history of the patient presenting with new onset or worsening heart failure something happened that may be of key importance to understand the physiopathology and to find a solution for his/her problem. In addition, if such a "precipitating event" can be found the patient and/or referring physician can be instructed to correct and/or avoid this in the future. Common "precipitating events" are listed in Table 5.1.

3 Correctable Causes of Heart Failure

The next step should be the search for correctable elements in the physiopathology of the patient. Common and sometimes overlooked correctable factors in the management of heart failure are briefly discussed (Table 5.2).

1. Atrial fibrillation and/or flutter

   (a). When the patient with heart failure and low ejection fraction has spiraled down the vicious cycle of heart failure and atrial fibrillation (AF), it is almost

Table 5.1 Precipitating events leading to heart failure

1. Volume overload due to non compliance of the patient (holidays, restaurant visits, etc.)
2. Medical interventions (i.e., surgery with perioperative intravenous infusions)
3. Intercurrent consultations of other physicians and/or hospitalizations with inadvertent changes in the dosages of active cardiac medication (mainly beta-blocking agents, diuretics, digitalis, etc.)
4. Use of non steroidal anti inflammatory drugs
5. Anemia (dual or triple anti thrombotic therapy!)
6. Inadequate or inadvertent use of other drugs
(a) Antiarrhythmic drugs (with the exception of amiodaron): especially when it was failed to appreciate that atrial fibrillation/flutter was accompanied by heart failure (even more often the case in heart failure with normal ejection fraction)
(b) Calcium antagonists
(c) Long acting beta-2 mimetics (inhalation) with or without atrial arrhythmias
(d) Anti tussive sirups with ephedrin (analogs)
(e) Anti depressant drugs (noradrenaline re-uptake blokkers)
(f) Thiazolidinediones (oral antidiabetic drugs: e.g., rosiglitazone)
(g) Monoclonal antibodies: e.g., Imatinib (Glivec), anti TNF etc.
7. Arrhythmias, often atrial fibrillation sometimes due to alcohol (ab)use, hyperthyroidism, long acting beta-2-mimetics, theophylline, …
8. Unjustified withdrawal of active medication because of (pseudo)—intolerance
(a) Amiodaron: hypothyroidism is not sufficient justification for discontinuation whereas hyperthyroidism duly is
(b) ACE-Inhibitors are often unjustly withdrawn because of:
(i) Asymptomatic hypotension
(ii) Coughing which sometimes is due to pulmonary congestion
(iii) Pseudo hyperkalemia due to hemolysis
(iv) Severe deterioration of renal function which in itself may be a hint that the patient has significant bilateral renal artery stenosis or stenosis in a single kidney
(c) Spironolacton is even more often unjustly withdrawn because of:
(i) Gynecomastia
(ii) (Pseudo) hyperkalemia due to incorrect sampling/handling of blood with hemolysis
(d) Beta-blocking agents:
(e) Digitalis is well known for its withdrawal effects
9. Metabolic diseases: hyperthyroidism (often due to amiodaron)
10. Pacemaker/ICD implantation/changes in pacemaker programming:
(a) Common pacemaker implant: if not enough care is taken to avoid RV apical pacing as much as possible or if it cannot be avoided at all (importance of pre implant assessment of LVEF for pure bradycardia indications for pacemaker implantation)
(b) CRT: "non responders" actually may be worse after implant due to non viable tissue in the posterolateral wall, LV electrode mal positioning/dislodgment, to high lower rate or to sensitive rate responsive programming

impossible to sort out this chicken-egg dilemma (i.e., which of both comes first). In addition, the extent of the "tachycardiomyopathy" component in the diminished systolic function is unpredictable. Therefore, when the atrial fibrillation/flutter is of relatively recent onset (<1 year) restoration of sinus rhythm should be attempted by electrical cardioversion (or if recurrent

Table 5.2 Correctable causes of heart failure

1. Atrial fibrillation/flutter
2. Conduction disease
3. Pacemaker tachycardia and/or various inadequate pacemaker programming modalities
4. Aortic stenosis eventually low flow aortic stenosis
5. Constrictive pericarditis

by interventional techniques) but *after* meticulous titration of diuretics and aldosterone antagonists). Class 1 and class 3 antiarrhythmic drugs with the exception of amiodaron are contraindicated. Moreover, in young patients the toxicity of amiodaron is such that it cannot be a long-term option.

(b). In the patient with heart failure and normal ejection fraction strangely enough atrial fibrillation is often the only presenting symptom and due to limited mobility/level of activity the symptoms of congestion are often less pronounced. In those patients return to a euvolemic state and restoration of sinus rhythm should also be attempted without antiarrhythmic drugs.

2. Conduction disease

(a). Resynchronization therapy by means of biventricular pacing is an established treatment modality in patients with (wide QRS) left bundle branch block and/or high likelihood of constant ventricular pacing and low ejection fraction.

(b). In patients with low ejection fraction that are paced from the right ventricular apex, especially when it can be demonstrated that ejection fraction was still normal at the time of pacemaker implant, the most straightforward treatment modality is to try to restore native conduction by reprogramming the pacemaker and/or alterations in the drug regimen. This means that I advise to decrease the dosage or to stop the treatment with various bradycardia provoking agents like digitalis and/or even beta-blocking agents—which at first sight seems counterintuitive and against guidelines in heart failure with low ejection fraction.

3. Pacemaker tachycardia and/or various "inappropriate" pacemaker programming modalities. Various inappropriate pacemaker programming modalities (pacemaker circus movement tachycardia, mode switching failure due to undersensing of weak atrial fibrillation waves, or atrial flutter waves (atrial lock-in), too short AV delay or excessively rate adaptive AV delay programming, aggressive rate response programming,…) that result in excessive pacing from the right ventricular apex and/or inappropriate high ventricular rates can provoke heart failure and should be searched for and if possible corrected.
4. Valvular aortic stenosis, especially in the elderly, often with only faint or barely audible ejection murmur may be overlooked as a cause of heart failure. If not recognized as such and if inappropriately treated with beta-blocking agents, the

patient with critical aortic stenosis may deteriorate dramatically. On the other hand, if the gradient is low (suspicion of "low flow significant aortic stenosis") the decision to replace the aortic valve may be a difficult one. It is important to remind the clinician that low ejection fraction is not synonymous with low flow over the aortic valve. Indeed, the gradient over de aortic valve correlates with stroke volume and not with ejection fraction! An easy way to exclude significant aortic stenosis in a patient with low ejection fraction and a low gradient is the mixed venous saturation on right heart catheterization. If the mixed venous saturation is normal or high, a critical aortic stenosis can be excluded.

5. Constrictive pericarditis may still be a difficult diagnosis. It is an extreme model of heart failure with impaired diastolic function and beta-blocking agents are relatively contraindicated and ill-supported.

4 Pitfalls and Uncertainties in Medical Management of Heart Failure

1. Angiotensin-converting enzyme inhibitors (ACEI)/Angiotensin receptor blockers (ARB)
   Heart failure guidelines emphasize that the patient should be treated with the "target dose" of ACEI of ARB such as in the trials. However, the evidence behind this recommendation is very weak. ACEI trials were among the first in the long series of trials that built up the present treatment guidelines for heart failure and the only trial addressing explicitly this subject was the ATLAS trial comparing low and high doses of lisinopril in heart failure with low ejection fraction [1]. No mortality benefit could be demonstrated in favor of the high dose of lisinopril. And indeed, in real life increasing the dose of ACEI (or ARB) in severe heart failure patients up to the target dose often severely limits the addition of beta-blocking agents due to hypotension. In practice, therefore I recommend to start with the lowest possible dose of ACEI (or ARB) and instead of increasing the dose to the "target dose" to give priority to the addition of and progressively increasing dose of the beta-blocking agent because beta-blocking agents have a much stronger effect on mortality and reverse remodeling than ACEI (or ARB).
2. Beta-blocking agents
   It is very rare that it is really impossible to add and progressively increase the dose of beta-blocking agents in chronic heart failure. If it is deemed impossible, it is often due to inadequate assessment of the patient and/or inadequate timing as, e.g., when the patient is still volume overloaded, if the blood pressure is too low due to inadequate ("target") dosing of ACEI/ARB.
3. Aldosteron antagonists
   Aldosteron antagonists are of utmost importance in the treatment of heart failure with low ejection fraction [2, 3] and are often inappropriately withdrawn due to relatively minor side effects such as gynecomastia or potentially life-threatening electrolyte disturbances such as hyperkalemia. Strict dosing of the aldosterone

antagonist according to clinical evolution, renal function, and electrolytes with correct sampling and processing of blood analysis in order to avoid hemolysis is important. The difference between the high rate of hyperkalemia in the pilot RALES trial [2] and the almost negligible rate of hyperkalemia in the RALES trial [3] was due to the flexible dosing and strict follow up of renal function and electrolytes in the main trial. We feel that even after return to NYHA class 1 or 2 and after reverse remodeling the aldosterone antagonist should be continued if possible. This has been confirmed in the EMPHASIS HF trial [4].

4. Revascularization
   It is common practice to evaluate the patient with recent onset heart failure for ischemic heart disease, even in the absence of a history of myocardial infarction or symptoms of angina and if reversible ischemia can be demonstrated to proceed with revascularization, either by CABG or by PCI. However, the evidence in favor of this strategy is very weak and often patients with severe heart failure undergo risky procedures without ever been demonstrated that such a strategy prolongs their life. To the contrary, there was no mortality benefit for the patients treated with CABG versus the patients treated with medical therapy alone in the STICH trial [5]. This is not surprising at all-in view of the fact that in the beta-blocker trials recent coronary revascularization was an exclusion. And indeed, many patients with coronary artery disease, even if "significant" have non ischemic cardiomyopathy with low ejection fraction that has no causal relation to the coronary artery disease.
5. Functional mitral regurgitation
   Functional mitral regurgitation remains essentially a disease of the left ventricle. Although it is well known that in patients with heart failure with low ejection fraction functional mitral regurgitation adversely impacts outcome, it has never been proven that surgical correction of *functional* mitral regurgitation will improve life expectancy. Moreover, medical treatment (correction of volume overload and beta-blocking agents) and cardiac resynchronization therapy improve mitral regurgitation and life expectancy. It is less well known that functional mitral regurgitation occurs also frequently in the setting of heart failure with normal ejection fraction in the elderly and can be corrected by appropriate medical treatment.
6. Cardioversion in AF/Aflutter
   In order to successfully and sustainably convert atrial fibrillation to sinus rhythm in the patient with heart failure it is of extreme importance that the patient is in a normovolemic state with adequate dosing of loop diuretics and aldosteron antagonist. In addition, we still prefer a rhythm control strategy in the patient with heart failure if after correction of volume overload sinus rhythm does not spontaneously recur. Return to sinus rhythm may be accomplished by electrical cardioversion (but without antiarrhythmic drugs) or by interventional techniques.

7. Medical "overtreatment"
   After the sometimes aggressive treatment of acute heart failure or once medical treatment or cardiac resynchronization therapy has induced significant "reverse remodeling" with increase in left ventricular ejection fraction, decrease in left ventricular and left atrial volumes, it is sometimes forgotten to downsize dosage of loop diuretics, causing symptoms of weak exercise tolerance or "shortness of breath" very similar to the symptomatology of low output and congestion with heart failure.

References

1. Packer M, Poole-Wilson PA, Armstrong PW, Cleland JG, Horowitz JD, Massie BM, Rydén L, Thygesen K, Uretsky BF (1999) Comparative effects of low and high doses of the angiotensin-converting enzyme inhibitor, lisinopril, on morbidity and mortality in chronic heart failure. ATLAS Study Group. Circulation 100:2312–2318
2. Rales investigators (1996) Effectiveness of spironolactone added to an angiotensin-converting enzyme inhibitor and a loop diuretic for severe chronic congestive heart failure (the Randomized Aldactone Evaluation Study [RALES]). Am J Cardiol 78:902–907
3. Pitt B, Zannad F, Remme WJ et al (1999) The effect of spironolactone on morbidity and mortality in patients with severe heart failure. Randomized Aldactone Evaluation Study Investigators. N Engl J Med 341:709–717
4. Zannad F, McMurray JJ, Krum H, van Veldhuisen DJ, Swedberg K, Shi H, Vincent J, Pocock SJ, Pitt B, EMPHASIS-HF Study Group (2011) Eplerenone in patients with systolic heart failure and mild symptoms. N Engl J Med 364:11–21
5. Velazquez EJ, Lee KL, Deja MA, Jain A, Sopko G, Marchenko A, Ali IS, Pohost G, Gradinac S, Abraham WT, Yii M, Prabhakaran D, Szwed H, Ferrazzi P, Petrie MC, O'Connor CM, Panchavinnin P, She L, Bonow RO, Rankin GR, Jones RH, Rouleau JL, STICH Investigators (2011) Coronary-artery bypass surgery in patients with left ventricular dysfunction. N Engl J Med 364:1607–1616

Part II
Conduction Abnormalities and Rhythm Disturbances in Heart Failure

Chapter 6
Atrial Fibrillation and Heart Failure: Rate Versus Rhythm Control

Mackram F. Eleid, Yong-Mei Cha, and Win-Kuang Shen

Abstract Atrial fibrillation and heart failure are commonly coexisting conditions with important pathophysiologic interactions impacting patient management. Treatment of atrial fibrillation with impaired ventricular function is focused towards preventing adverse hemodynamic effects that may result in more symptoms and decreased exercise tolerance. While rate control using medications or atrioventricular nodal ablation combined with pacing is the primary emphasis of management, rhythm control using pharmacologic or pulmonary vein isolation remains a feasible alternative strategy for some patients. The prevalence, mechanisms, and management strategies of atrial fibrillation and heart failure are reviewed in this chapter.

1 Introduction

Atrial fibrillation (AF) and heart failure (HF), two increasingly common and coexisting conditions encountered in the aging population, interact in ways that are distinct from the general population of AF patients without heart failure. In AF, the primary treatment goals focus on control of symptoms and reducing risk of stroke. Additionally, in the patient with AF and impaired ventricular function, treatment is focused towards preventing adverse hemodynamic effects that may result in more symptoms and decreased exercise tolerance.

Patients with heart failure have a higher risk of developing AF compared to the normal population. The prevalence of AF increases with worsening New York Heart

M.F. Eleid, M.D. • Y.-M. Cha, M.D.
Division of Cardiovascular Diseases, Department of Internal Medicine, Mayo Clinic College of Medicine, 200 First Street SW, Rochester, MN 55905, USA

W.-K. Shen, M.D. (✉)
Division of Cardiovascular Diseases, Department of Internal Medicine, Mayo Clinic College of Medicine, 5777 East Mayo Boulevard, Phoenix, AZ 85054, USA
e-mail: wshen@mayo.edu

J. Bartunek and M. Vanderheyden (eds.), *Translational Approach to Heart Failure*, DOI 10.1007/978-1-4614-7345-9_6, © Springer Science+Business Media New York 2013

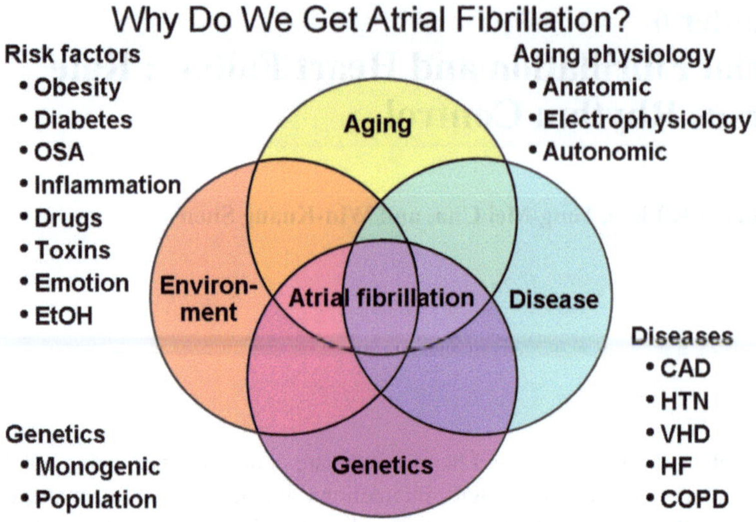

Fig. 6.1 Atrial fibrillation is a multifactorial condition resulting from an interaction between cardiovascular disease effects, aging, genetics, and environmental factors. *CAD* coronary artery disease, *COPD* chronic obstructive pulmonary disease, *EtOH* alcohol use, *HF* heart failure, *HTN* hypertension, *OSA* obstructive sleep apnea, *VHD* valvular heart disease

Association (NYHA) functional class [1]. Additionally, patients with abnormal diastolic function but no clinical heart failure diagnosis also have an increased risk of developing AF [2].

Atrial fibrillation is a disease of the elderly, with 3 out of 4 AF patients between the ages of 65 and 85 years. Interplay between advancing age, comorbidities, and environmental and genetic factors contributes to the development of AF (Fig. 6.1). The prevalence of AF is currently 1–2 %, and is expected to increase with the aging population [3, 4]. Comorbid medical conditions associated with AF including hypertension (HTN), heart failure, valvular heart disease (VHD), cardiomyopathies, coronary artery disease (CAD), obesity, diabetes mellitus, chronic obstructive pulmonary disease (COPD), sleep apnea, and chronic kidney disease are more frequent in the elderly, play a role in propagating AF, and increase morbidity and mortality [5]. Hospitalizations for AF in the United States have increased dramatically (two to threefold) in the last 15 years [6]. The prevalence of heart failure also increases with age, with a lifetime risk of developing heart failure in men and women aged 40 years of 1 in 5 [7].

This chapter reviews the current understanding of the pathophysiology of AF in patients with heart failure, providing an in-depth discussion of evidence-based therapies for rhythm versus rate control therapy. Additionally, this chapter will discuss the rationale for pulmonary vein isolation (PVI) versus atrioventricular (AV) nodal ablation and pacing therapies in patients with AF and heart failure. Evidence for benefit of cardiac resynchronization therapy (CRT) in the setting of AF and heart failure will be highlighted.

2 Pathophysiology of Atrial Fibrillation and Heart Failure

2.1 *Atrial Fibrillation as a Cause of Heart Failure*

2.1.1 Mechanisms

In experimental animal models, it has been observed that chronic tachycardia can result in left ventricular (LV) dilatation with or without systolic dysfunction [8]. Persistent tachycardia depletes cellular high-energy stores in dogs such as creatine, phosphocreatine, and adenosine triphosphate [9]. These changes manifest in a reduced percentage of myocytes and reduced shortening velocity despite a higher LV mass [10]. The depletion of energy stores may be mediated by changes in cellular metabolism with mitochrondrial injury, increased activity of oxidative enzymes, and ischemia [11, 12]. In humans this now well-established entity of reversible congestive heart failure (CHF) in association with chronic tachycardia has been termed tachycardia-mediated cardiomyopathy [13–15].

Atrial fibrillation can also impair myocardial function by its irregular rhythm that produces variable durations of important components of the cardiac cycle, which can impair cardiac output. Furthermore, loss of atrial systole has a negative impact on ventricular filling and cardiac output [16].

The fall in cardiac output associated with AF often results in activation of neurohumoral vasoconstrictors including angiotensin II and norepinephrine, which may further impair ventricular function [17, 18]. Increased sympathetic nerve activity associated with AF is an effect that is partly mediated by the irregular ventricular response [19].

2.2 *Heart Failure as a Cause of Atrial Fibrillation*

2.2.1 Neurohumoral Activation and Mechanoelectrical Feedback

In CHF, neurohumoral activation of substances including angiotensin II and norepinephrine may promote atrial fibrosis [20, 21] with resultant changes in conduction properties that may predispose to AF. Acute atrial wall stretch is associated with increased dispersion of refractoriness and alterations in anisotropic and conduction properties facilitating AF [22]. Elevated filling pressures that occur in ventricular dysfunction lead to left atrial dilatation, which may stimulate stretch-activated channels and increase vulnerability to AF. Blockade of stretch-activated channels reduces the propensity for AF despite elevated atrial pressure and/or volume [23]. Additionally, left atrial enlargement may facilitate the stability and persistence of atrial fibrillation [24].

Key Points

- Atrial fibrillation can cause heart failure via tachycardia-mediated cardiomyopathy, impairment of cardiac output due to irregular cycle length and loss of atrial systole, and increased neurohumoral activation.
- Heart failure contributes to AF by neurohumoral and hemodynamic effects on atrial tissue including fibrosis, acute wall stretch, and chamber dilatation.

3 Prognosis of Atrial Fibrillation and Heart Failure

Several studies have suggested the development of AF is associated with a worse prognosis in patients with preexisting left ventricular (LV) dysfunction. In the Studies of Left Ventricular Dysfunction (SOLVD) prevention and treatment trial [25], AF at baseline was an independent predictor of mortality and morbidity, primarily related to heart failure, death, or rehospitalization for heart failure. In a substudy of the Danish Investigators of Arrhythmia and Mortality ON Dofetilide (DIAMOND) trial [26] of patients with an ejection fraction of 35 % or less, maintenance of sinus rhythm at 1 year was strongly and independently associated with survival, either with placebo or dofetilide. Further evidence that AF causes hemodynamic deterioration in patients with underlying LV dysfunction was provided by an observational study of 344 patients with compensated heart failure who were followed for 19 months [27]. The development of AF in 8 % of these patients was associated with worsening of NYHA functional class, an increase in left atrial size, an increase in both mitral and tricuspid regurgitation, and a reduction in cardiac index and peak oxygen consumption.

4 Current Management

Historically, rate control was considered a "fallback" therapy for AF after failed rhythm control. However, in recent years the practice has shifted from rhythm control to rate control, with rate control being a very feasible alternative therapy for management of AF.

4.1 Rate Control Strategy

The concept of rate control for AF centers on the idea that the primary mechanism for symptoms in AF is tachycardia and the resultant shortening of the diastolic filling period. In addition to symptomatic improvement, many patients with LV dysfunction and AF experience an improvement in ejection fraction following control of the ventricular rate [28, 29], likely reflecting an improvement in tachycardia-mediated ventricular dysfunction.

4.1.1 Medications

Beta-blockers are the preferred agent for rate control in atrial fibrillation, primarily due to their established beneficial effects in heart failure. When a second agent is required, digoxin is often a good choice, with the consideration that patients with impaired renal dysfunction are at higher risk for digoxin toxicity and require closer monitoring. Heart rate should be evaluated both at rest and with activity to determine if control is adequate. In patients with decompensated heart failure and rapid AF, increasing beta-blocker doses is contraindicated and digoxin can be used in this setting. When beta-blockers and digoxin are ineffective, amiodarone can be used alone or in combination with other rate-slowing agents to achieve rate control. Dronedarone slows the heart rate by 10 bpm [30] and should be avoided in any patients with NYHA class III or IV symptoms of heart failure due to its association with increased mortality [31]. Non-dihydropyridine calcium channel blockers carry a risk of exacerbating CHF and thus are generally avoided for this population.

Key Points

- Effective rate control medications for patients with AF and heart failure include beta-blockers, digoxin, and amiodarone.
- Rate control drugs to avoid in AF and symptomatic heart failure include dronedarone and calcium channel blockers.

4.1.2 Trials of Rate Control

Potential benefit of rate control in patients with heart failure was observed in a retrospective analysis of the US Carvedilol Congestive Heart Failure trial where 136 of 1,094 patients with heart failure due to systolic dysfunction had AF [28]. In this study, patients treated with carvedilol had a significant increase in the LV ejection fraction (from 23 to 33 % compared with 24 to 27 % with placebo), demonstrating a beneficial effect of carvedilol in this setting. There was also a trend towards a reduction in the primary endpoint of death or CHF hospitalization ($p=0.06$). An important caveat is that the study did not prove that the benefit seen was due solely to rate control as opposed to the other neurohumoral effects of beta blockade.

The AF-CHF trial randomized patients with heart failure and paroxysmal AF to medical therapy with either rhythm (amiodarone, sotalol, or dofetilide) or rate control (beta-blockers) [32]. After a 3-year follow-up period, there was no difference in cardiovascular mortality between the two groups (Fig. 6.2). This study supports the concept that a rate control strategy is a more reasonable initial approach for the majority of patients with AF and heart failure due to the increased cost, complexity

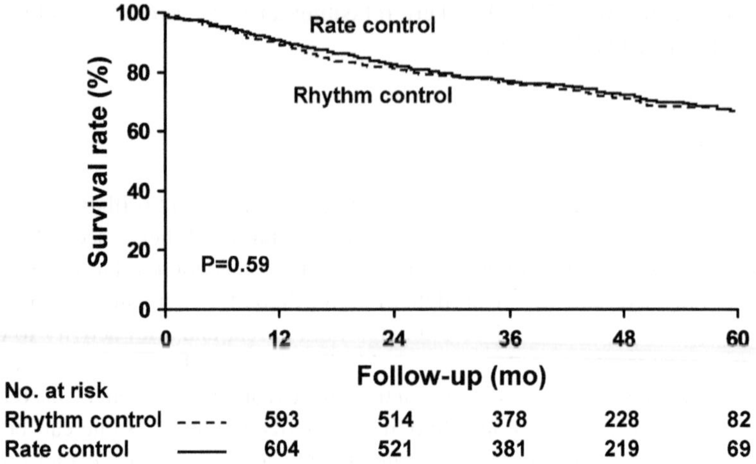

Fig. 6.2 Kaplan Meier estimates for death from cardiovascular causes for patients with atrial fibrillation and heart failure treated with either rate or rhythm control [32]. Permission obtained from The Massachusetts Medical Society

of medical regimen, and potential adverse affects associated with antiarrhythmic therapy.

The RACE II trial compared strict (resting heart rate <80 bpm and heart rate during moderate exercise <110 bpm) versus lenient (resting heart rate <110 bpm) rate control in the AF population [33]. In this study 10 % of patients also had a history of heart failure, and there was no significant difference in the outcome of death from cardiovascular causes, hospitalization for heart failure, stroke, embolism, bleeding, and life-threatening arrhythmic events between the two groups. Based on this trial and other data in the literature (Table 6.1), a goal of average resting heart rate <110 bpm may be a reasonable starting point. However, more data on degree of rate control are needed in the heart failure population.

Key Points

- Rate control of AF in patients with heart failure is associated with improved clinical outcomes.
- Available evidence suggests that rate control has similar benefits as rhythm control in AF and heart failure.

4.1.3 Effect of Pacemaker Therapy on Risk of Atrial Fibrillation and Heart Failure

The choice of dual chamber pacing versus single chamber pacing in patients who require a permanent pacemaker may have an impact on their subsequent risk of AF and heart failure. In 2002, the MOST study randomized 2,010 patients with sinus node dysfunction requiring a pacemaker to either dual chamber or single chamber

Table 6.1 Trials of rate control in atrial fibrillation and heart failure

Author/year	Population	Design	Primary endpoint	Results
Joglar et al. [28]	Symptomatic CHF, EF <35 % with AF (136 patients)	Retrospective analysis of a randomized trial of carvedilol versus placebo	Death or CHF hospitalization	Trend towards reduction in primary endpoint (7 % versus 19 %, $p=0.06$) and improvement in EF (24–33 %, $p=0.001$) w/ carvedilol versus placebo
Roy et al. [32] (AF-CHF)	Symptomatic CHF, EF <35 % with AF (1,376 patients)	Randomized multicenter trial of rate versus rhythm control	Cardiovascular death	No difference in primary endpoint at 3 years (25 % versus 27 %, $p=0.59$)
Van Gelder et al. [33] (RACE II)	Persistant AF (10 % of patients had prior hospitalization for CHF)	Randomized multicenter trial of lenient versus strict rate control	Composite of death from cardiovas-cular causes, hospitalization for CHF, and stroke, systemic embolism, bleeding, and life-threatening arrhythmic events	No difference in primary endpoint at 3 years (12.9 % versus 14.9 %, non-inferiority $p<0.001$)

AF atrial fibrillation, *CHF* congestive heart failure, *EF* ejection fraction, *RACE II* rate control efficacy in permanent atrial fibrillation trial ventricular pacing to determine if there was a difference in the primary endpoint of death or nonfatal stroke [34]. The median age of this population was 74 and comorbidities included prior myocardial infarction in 26 %, prior heart failure in 20 %, diabetes in 22 %, and history of AF in 46 %. There was no difference in the primary endpoint ($p = 0.48$), however a lower incidence of AF and heart failure was observed in the dual chamber pacing group, at almost 3 years of follow-up suggesting a protective effect of dual chamber pacing in this population. This data reinforces that dual chamber pacing is preferred for patients requiring a permanent pacemaker, in order to maintain AV synchrony and reduce the long-term risk of AF and heart failure.

4.1.4 AV Nodal Ablation with Pacing

AV nodal ablation and pacing provides an attractive means to control AF, particularly in patients with drug-refractory AF or in those who cannot tolerate medications due to intolerances or impaired ventricular function. AV nodal ablation is highly effective (>95 % procedural success), but is also a more invasive option that leaves patients pacemaker-dependent. Emerging evidence in the population undergoing AV nodal ablation for AF supports the role of CRT due to the beneficial effects associated with preserved ventricular synchrony (Table 6.2). PVI, although a preferred rhythm-control option for drug-refractory AF patients with normal LV function, has been infrequently used in heart failure population due to a higher prevalence of comorbidities and structural features that are associated with reduced procedural success.

In a prospective, small randomized trial of 81 patients with class II or III heart failure and ejection fraction <40 % who had symptomatic, drug-refractory AF, PVI for rhythm control was compared with AV nodal ablation and biventricular (BiV) pacing for rate control [35]. At 6 months, PVI was associated with statistically significant improvements in left ventricular ejection fraction (35 % versus 28 %), 6-min walk distance (340 versus 297 m), and score on the Minnesota Living with Heart Failure questionnaire. The improvements in ejection fraction and functional capacity were greater for those with nonparoxysmal compared to paroxysmal AF. In addition, approximately 30 % of patients treated with AV node ablation and biventricular pacing had progressive AF (e.g., paroxysmal to persistent AF); such progression was not seen in patients treated with PVI. Although encouraging, this study only provided short-term data, and the long-term efficacy of PVI in the AF and heart failure population is unknown.

The dual-chamber and VVI implantable defibrillator (DAVID) trial randomized over 5,000 patients with ejection fraction <40 % and indication for an implantable cardioverter defibrillator to either ventricular back-up pacing at 40/min or dual-chamber rate-responsive pacing at 70/min [36]. Patients in the dual chamber pacing group had an increased combined endpoint of mortality and hospitalization for CHF. The increased heart failure and mortality was believed to be due to the maladaptive features of RV stimulation, where ventricular electrical activation proceeds

Table 6.2 Trials of CRT in chronic AF

Authors	Year	Number studied	Population	Intervention	Outcome	Results
Leclerq et al.	2002	59	NYHA class III systolic heart failure undergoing pacemaker implant	CRT versus RV pacing	6 min walk distance and oxygen uptake	Favors CRT (mean walk distance increased 9.3 % ($p=0.05$) and peak VO_2 increased by 13 % ($p=0.04$) over RV pacing)
Linde et al.	2002	33	NYHA class III heart failure and pacemaker dependent from either acquired AV block or induced AV nodal ablation	CRT versus RV pacing	6 min walk distance and NYHA class	Favors CRT (mean walk distance improved by 17% ($p=0.004$) and NYHA class improved by 27 % over RV pacing ($p=0.0001$))
Brignole et al.	2005	56	Age 70 ± 8 years with symptomatic persistent AF and either uncontrolled ventricular rate or heart failure	CRT versus RV pacing	Quality of life questionnaires, NYHA class, 6 min walk distance, and ejection fraction	Favors CRT (NYHA class improved by 11 % pacing, 6 min walk distance improved by 4 m, and EF improved by 5 % compared with RV ($p<0.05$ for all))
Doshi et al.	2005	184	Age 69 ± 10 years undergoing AVN ablation	CRT versus RV pacing	6 min walk distance and ejection fraction	Favors CRT (6 min walk 31 % improvement with CRT versus 24 % improvement with RV pacing over baseline, $p=0.04$) EF 46 ± 13 % versus 41 ± 13 % ($p=0.03$)

AF atrial fibrillation, *CRT* cardiac resynchronization therapy, *EF* ejection fraction, *NYHA* New York Heart Association, *RV* right ventricular, *VO_2* oxygen consumption from the right ventricular apex instead of through the existing conduction system, leading to ventricular desynchronization. Although this mechanism was not proven to be the cause of worse outcome, it supported the concept that patients with heart failure requiring frequent ventricular pacing would benefit from CRT.

Observational studies and small randomized trials support the value of CRT for improving symptoms and left ventricular function in patients with poorly controlled AF who have reduced LV systolic function or heart failure [37, 38]. In a small randomized control trial of patients with symptomatic, medically refractory, chronic, rapid AF assigned to AV nodal ablation with either RV pacing or CRT, the group with CRT showed greater improvement in exercise tolerance and greater preservation of ejection fraction [39]. A meta-analysis of three randomized CRT AF trials [37, 40–42] showed a trend towards improved survival among patients randomized to CRT but the difference in survival among patients randomized to CRT versus RV pacing was not statistically significant [43].

A recent observational cohort study of patients with AF and heart failure who received CRT-D showed that AV nodal ablation for definitive biventricular pacing provided a greater improvement in NYHA class and survival benefit compared with drug therapy for rate control [44]. In 154 patients with a median follow-up of 274 days, the median (Q1, Q3) percentage of biventricular pacing after CRT was 99.0 % (95–100 %) in the AV nodal ablation group compared to 96.0 % (85.5–99.0 %) in the drug-treated group ($p=0.05$). After CRT, both groups had significant improvements in NYHA class, LV ejection fraction, and LV end diastolic dimension. Improvement in NYHA class was significantly greater in the AV nodal ablation group compared to the drug-treated group (0.7 ± 0.8 versus 0.4 ± 0.8, $p=0.04$), while improvement in echocardiographic parameters was not significantly different between the two groups.

Key Points

- Dual chamber pacing helps maintain AV synchrony and reduces the long-term risks of AF and heart failure in patients requiring a permanent pacemaker.
- Radiofrequency ablation of the AV node combined with permanent right ventricular endocardial pacing is a highly effective treatment for controlling the ventricular response of AF.
- The elderly population is particularly suited to AV nodal ablation and permanent pacing for treatment of AF due to higher frequency of comorbidities, risks of medication intolerance, and the relative safety and simplicity of the procedure.
- CRT is beneficial for patients with AF and reduced left ventricular systolic function who require frequent pacing.

4.2 Rhythm Control Strategy

Rhythm control may be a reasonable approach in patients with heart failure who are hemodynamically unstable or who are persistently symptomatic despite adequate rate control [45]. Several factors impact the likelihood of successful restoration and long-term maintenance of sinus rhythm, including how long a patient has been in persistent AF, their age, the presence of associated structural heart disease, and left atrial size. Antiarrhythmic drug therapy and radiofrequency catheter ablation are the two primary therapies for rhythm control.

Direct current electrical cardioversion is a useful therapy for patients with new onset AF alone or in combination with antiarrhythmic therapy, and can also be helpful for patients with symptoms that are not clearly attributable to AF. In such patients, when symptoms and functional status improve after cardioversion to sinus rhythm, AF is probably an important factor. In this way cardioversion is helpful in the diagnostic approach to symptoms. Cardioversion is also useful in the management of hemodynamically unstable patients with AF and LV dysfunction. In this group, cardioversion can rapidly improve hemodynamics via restoration of normal cardiac cycle, atrial systole, and decreasing heart rate thus improving diastolic filling time. Cardioversion is more likely to result in sustained maintenance of sinus rhythm in this population when combined with an antiarrhythmic drug.

4.2.1 Antiarrhythmic Therapy

Amiodarone and dofetilide are the first-line therapies for maintenance of sinus rhythm in patients with AF and heart failure recommended by the ACC/AHA/HRS guidelines [46]. Amiodarone has the advantage of being a potassium channel blocker with both beta-blocking and calcium channel-blocking effects. As a result, it has a negative inotropic effect and tends to control the ventricular rate when in atrial fibrillation. Furthermore, amiodarone has been shown to have a low incidence of QT prolongation and less pro-arrhythmia when used in low doses (400 mg per day or less) in patients with heart failure [47]. Compared with dofetilide, additional advantages of amiodarone include its once daily dosing, reduced cost, and ability to start therapy as an outpatient.

4.2.2 Pulmonary Vein Isolation

Although not commonly used as a treatment strategy in the AF population with heart failure, catheter ablation of AF can be successful in patients with concomitant heart failure. In a small observational study of 58 patients undergoing catheter ablation for AF with NYHA class II or greater symptoms and LV ejection fraction <45 %, symptoms, LV function, and exercise capacity were all improved at 12 months [48]. In another observational study 94 patients with impaired LV systolic function (mean ejection fraction 36 %) underwent PVI [49]. After approximately 1 year of follow-up 73 % of the study patients remained AF-free compared to 87 % in a control group of patients with ejection fraction >50 % ($p<0.001$). In this study, there was a nonsignificant trend towards improved ejection fraction following ablation in the study group. These data provide some evidence that PVI can improve clinical outcomes in heart failure patients up to 1 year following ablation. However, the long-term durability of the procedure in this population remains unknown.

Key Points

- Rhythm control in AF and heart failure is useful in patients who are hemodynamically unstable or patients with persistent symptoms from AF despite adequate rate control.
- Electrical cardioversion (usually combined with antiarrhythmic medication) is useful for hemodynamically unstable patients and in patients with symptoms that are not clearly attributable to AF.
- First-line antiarrhythmic medications are amiodarone and dofetilide for AF and heart failure.
- Catheter ablation of AF can be successful in patients with heart failure, but long-term durability remains unknown.

5 Future Trends

The CHALLENGE pilot study is currently recruiting patients to test the hypothesis that AV nodal ablation compared to drug therapy improves outcomes in patients with AF and symptomatic heart failure undergoing CRT. This study is based on the idea that intermittent AV nodal concealed penetrance and ventricular conduction during AF can interrupt CRT pacing and ventricular synchrony, especially in situations of increased myocardial demand (i.e., during exercise). Occurrence of fusion or pseudo-fusion beats may overestimate the amount of "effective" CRT pacing. As a result, optimal clinical benefits may not be achieved even when the device records greater than 80–85 % pacing. It is anticipated that the study will offer valuable insight into whether the ability of AV nodal ablation to achieve 100 % CRT pacing provides a superior clinical effect.

6 Conclusions

Atrial fibrillation and heart failure are two increasingly common conditions in the developed world. In patients with underlying structural heart disease and LV dysfunction, AF can precipitate hemodynamic deterioration and adverse clinical events. AF is also a cause of reversible LV dysfunction in patients without structural heart disease (AF-induced cardiomyopathy) and should be considered when patients present with newly recognized heart failure or AF. When rate control of AF is achieved by either medications or AV nodal ablation with pacing, many hemodynamic consequences of tachycardia may be abated, and ventricular function can improve. In patients with AF and heart failure requiring pacing, increasing data supports the use of CRT to optimize ventricular mechanical synchrony. Ongoing studies will help determine whether AV nodal ablation improves response to CRT in this population. Rhythm control with drug therapy or PVI remains an option, but is generally less successful than rate control.

References

1. Maisel WH, Stevenson LW (2003) Atrial fibrillation in heart failure: epidemiology, pathophysiology, and rationale for therapy. Am J Cardiol 91(6A):2D–8D
2. Tsang TS, Gersh BJ, Appleton CP, Tajik AJ, Barnes ME, Bailey KR, Oh JK, Leibson C, Montgomery SC, Seward JB (2002) Left ventricular diastolic dysfunction as a predictor of the first diagnosed nonvalvular atrial fibrillation in 840 elderly men and women. J Am Coll Cardiol 40(9):1636–1644
3. Go AS, Hylek EM, Phillips KA, Chang Y, Henault LE, Selby JV, Singer DE (2001) Prevalence of diagnosed atrial fibrillation in adults: national implications for rhythm management and stroke prevention: the AnTicoagulation and Risk Factors in Atrial Fibrillation (ATRIA) Study. JAMA 285(18):2370–2375
4. Stewart S, Hart CL, Hole DJ, McMurray JJ (2001) Population prevalence, incidence, and predictors of atrial fibrillation in the Renfrew/Paisley study. Heart 86(5):516–521
5. Camm AJ, Kirchhof P, Lip GY, Schotten U, Savelieva I, Ernst S, Van Gelder IC, Al-Attar N, Hindricks G, Prendergast B, Heidbuchel H, Alfieri O, Angelini A, Atar D, Colonna P, De Caterina R, De Sutter J, Goette A, Gorenek B, Heldal M, Hohloser SH, Kolh P, Le Heuzey JY, Ponikowski P, Rutten FH, Vahanian A, Auricchio A, Bax J, Ceconi C, Dean V, Filippatos G, Funck-Brentano C, Hobbs R, Kearney P, McDonagh T, Popescu BA, Reiner Z, Sechtem U, Sirnes PA, Tendera M, Vardas PE, Widimsky P, Agladze V, Aliot E, Balabanski T, Blomstrom-Lundqvist C, Capucci A, Crijns H, Dahlof B, Folliguet T, Glikson M, Goethals M, Gulba DC, Ho SY, Klautz RJ, Kose S, McMurray J, Perrone Filardi P, Raatikainen P, Salvador MJ, Schalij MJ, Shpektor A, Sousa J, Stepinska J, Uuetoa H, Zamorano JL, Zupan I (2010) Guidelines for the management of atrial fibrillation: the Task Force for the Management of Atrial Fibrillation of the European Society of Cardiology (ESC). Europace 12(10):1360–1420
6. Wattigney WA, Mensah GA, Croft JB (2003) Increasing trends in hospitalization for atrial fibrillation in the United States, 1985 through 1999: implications for primary prevention. Circulation 108(6):711–716
7. Roger VL, Go AS, Lloyd-Jones DM, Adams RJ, Berry JD, Brown TM, Carnethon MR, Dai S, de Simone G, Ford ES, Fox CS, Fullerton HJ, Gillespie C, Greenlund KJ, Hailpern SM, Heit JA, Ho PM, Howard VJ, Kissela BM, Kittner SJ, Lackland DT, Lichtman JH, Lisabeth LD, Makuc DM, Marcus GM, Marelli A, Matchar DB, McDermott MM, Meigs JB, Moy CS, Mozaffarian D, Mussolino ME, Nichol G, Paynter NP, Rosamond WD, Sorlie PD, Stafford RS, Turan TN, Turner MB, Wong ND, Wylie-Rosett J (2011) Heart disease and stroke statistics–2011 update: a report from the American Heart Association. Circulation 123(4):e18–e209
8. Shinbane JS, Wood MA, Jensen DN, Ellenbogen KA, Fitzpatrick AP, Scheinman MM (1997) Tachycardia-induced cardiomyopathy: a review of animal models and clinical studies. J Am Coll Cardiol 29(4):709–715
9. Moe GW, Montgomery C, Howard RJ, Grima EA, Armstrong PW (1993) Left ventricular myocardial blood flow, metabolism, and effects of treatment with enalapril: further insights into the mechanisms of canine experimental pacing-induced heart failure. J Lab Clin Med 121(2):294–301
10. Spinale FG, Holzgrefe HH, Mukherjee R, Arthur SR, Child MJ, Powell JR, Koster WH (1995) LV and myocyte structure and function after early recovery from tachycardia-induced cardiomyopathy. Am J Physiol 268(2 Pt 2):H836–H847
11. Spinale FG, Hendrick DA, Crawford FA, Smith AC, Hamada Y, Carabello BA (1990) Chronic supraventricular tachycardia causes ventricular dysfunction and subendocardial injury in swine. Am J Physiol 259(1 Pt 2):H218–H229

12. O'Brien PJ, Ianuzzo CD, Moe GW, Stopps TP, Armstrong PW (1990) Rapid ventricular pacing of dogs to heart failure: biochemical and physiological studies. Can J Physiol Pharmacol 68(1):34–39
13. Gaasch WH, Zile MR (1984) Evaluation of myocardial function in cardiomyopathic states. Prog Cardiovasc Dis 27(2):115–132
14. Gillette PC, Smith RT, Garson A Jr, Mullins CE, Gutgesell HP, Goh TH, Cooley DA, McNamara DG (1985) Chronic supraventricular tachycardia. A curable cause of congestive cardiomyopathy. JAMA 253(3):391–392
15. Packer DL, Bardy GH, Worley SJ, Smith MS, Cobb FR, Coleman RE, Gallagher JJ, German LD (1986) Tachycardia-induced cardiomyopathy: a reversible form of left ventricular dysfunction. Am J Cardiol 57(8):563–570
16. Linderer T, Chatterjee K, Parmley WW, Sievers RE, Glantz SA, Tyberg JV (1983) Influence of atrial systole on the Frank-Starling relation and the end-diastolic pressure-diameter relation of the left ventricle. Circulation 67(5):1045–1053
17. Cardin S, Li D, Thorin-Trescases N, Leung TK, Thorin E, Nattel S (2003) Evolution of the atrial fibrillation substrate in experimental congestive heart failure: angiotensin-dependent and -independent pathways. Cardiovasc Res 60(2):315–325
18. Tisdale JE, Borzak S, Sabbah HN, Shimoyama H, Goldstein S (2006) Hemodynamic and neurohormonal predictors and consequences of the development of atrial fibrillation in dogs with chronic heart failure. J Card Fail 12(9):747–751. doi:S1071-9164(06)00859-1
19. Wasmund SL, Li JM, Page RL, Joglar JA, Kowal RC, Smith ML, Hamdan MH (2003) Effect of atrial fibrillation and an irregular ventricular response on sympathetic nerve activity in human subjects. Circulation 107(15):2011–2015
20. Cha YM, Dzeja PP, Shen WK, Jahangir A, Hart CY, Terzic A, Redfield MM (2003) Failing atrial myocardium: energetic deficits accompany structural remodeling and electrical instability. Am J Physiol Heart Circ Physiol 284(4):H1313–H1320
21. Li D, Fareh S, Leung TK, Nattel S (1999) Promotion of atrial fibrillation by heart failure in dogs: atrial remodeling of a different sort. Circulation 100(1):87–95
22. Solti F, Vecsey T, Kekesi V, Juhasz-Nagy A (1989) The effect of atrial dilatation on the genesis of atrial arrhythmias. Cardiovasc Res 23(10):882–886
23. Bode F, Katchman A, Woosley RL, Franz MR (2000) Gadolinium decreases stretch-induced vulnerability to atrial fibrillation. Circulation 101(18):2200–2205
24. Shinagawa K, Shi YF, Tardif JC, Leung TK, Nattel S (2002) Dynamic nature of atrial fibrillation substrate during development and reversal of heart failure in dogs. Circulation 105(22):2672–2678
25. Dries DL, Exner DV, Gersh BJ, Domanski MJ, Waclawiw MA, Stevenson LW (1998) Atrial fibrillation is associated with an increased risk for mortality and heart failure progression in patients with asymptomatic and symptomatic left ventricular systolic dysfunction: a retrospective analysis of the SOLVD trials. Studies of Left Ventricular Dysfunction. J Am Coll Cardiol 32(3):695–703
26. Pedersen OD, Bagger H, Keller N, Marchant B, Kober L, Torp-Pedersen C (2001) Efficacy of dofetilide in the treatment of atrial fibrillation-flutter in patients with reduced left ventricular function: a Danish investigations of arrhythmia and mortality on dofetilide (diamond) substudy. Circulation 104(3):292–296
27. Pozzoli M, Cioffi G, Traversi E, Pinna GD, Cobelli F, Tavazzi L (1998) Predictors of primary atrial fibrillation and concomitant clinical and hemodynamic changes in patients with chronic heart failure: a prospective study in 344 patients with baseline sinus rhythm. J Am Coll Cardiol 32(1):197–204
28. Joglar JA, Acusta AP, Shusterman NH, Ramaswamy K, Kowal RC, Barbera SJ, Hamdan MH, Page RL (2001) Effect of carvedilol on survival and hemodynamics in patients with atrial fibrillation and left ventricular dysfunction: retrospective analysis of the US Carvedilol Heart Failure Trials Program. Am Heart J 142(3):498–501

29. Redfield MM, Kay GN, Jenkins LS, Mianulli M, Jensen DN, Ellenbogen KA (2000) Tachycardia-related cardiomyopathy: a common cause of ventricular dysfunction in patients with atrial fibrillation referred for atrioventricular ablation. Mayo Clin Proc 75(8):790–795
30. Davy JM, Herold M, Hoglund C, Timmermans A, Alings A, Radzik D, Van Kempen L (2008) Dronedarone for the control of ventricular rate in permanent atrial fibrillation: the Efficacy and safety of dRonedArone for the cOntrol of ventricular rate during atrial fibrillation (ERATO) study. Am Heart J 156(3):e521–e529
31. Kober L, Torp-Pedersen C, McMurray JJ, Gotzsche O, Levy S, Crijns H, Amlie J, Carlsen J (2008) Increased mortality after dronedarone therapy for severe heart failure. N Engl J Med 358(25):2678–2687
32. Roy D, Talajic M, Nattel S, Wyse DG, Dorian P, Lee KL, Bourassa MG, Arnold JM, Buxton AE, Camm AJ, Connolly SJ, Dubuc M, Ducharme A, Guerra PG, Hohnloser SH, Lambert J, Le Heuzey JY, O'Hara G, Pedersen OD, Rouleau JL, Singh BN, Stevenson LW, Stevenson WG, Thibault B, Waldo AL (2008) Rhythm control versus rate control for atrial fibrillation and heart failure. N Engl J Med 358(25):2667–2677
33. Van Gelder IC, Groenveld HF, Crijns HJ, Tuininga YS, Tijssen JG, Alings AM, Hillege HL, Bergsma-Kadijk JA, Cornel JH, Kamp O, Tukkie R, Bosker HA, Van Veldhuisen DJ, Van den Berg MP (2010) Lenient versus strict rate control in patients with atrial fibrillation. N Engl J Med 362(15):1363–1373
34. Lamas GA, Lee KL, Sweeney MO, Silverman R, Leon A, Yee R, Marinchak RA, Flaker G, Schron E, Orav EJ, Hellkamp AS, Greer S, McAnulty J, Ellenbogen K, Ehlert F, Freedman RA, Estes NA III, Greenspon A, Goldman L (2002) Ventricular pacing or dual-chamber pacing for sinus-node dysfunction. N Engl J Med 346(24):1854–1862
35. Khan MN, Jais P, Cummings J, Di Biase L, Sanders P, Martin DO, Kautzner J, Hao S, Themistoclakis S, Fanelli R, Potenza D, Massaro R, Wazni O, Schweikert R, Saliba W, Wang P, Al-Ahmad A, Beheiry S, Santarelli P, Starling RC, Dello Russo A, Pelargonio G, Brachmann J, Schibgilla V, Bonso A, Casella M, Raviele A, Haissaguerre M, Natale A (2008) Pulmonary-vein isolation for atrial fibrillation in patients with heart failure. N Engl J Med 359(17):1778–1785
36. Wilkoff BL, Cook JR, Epstein AE, Greene HL, Hallstrom AP, Hsia H, Kutalek SP, Sharma A (2002) Dual-chamber pacing or ventricular backup pacing in patients with an implantable defibrillator: the Dual Chamber and VVI Implantable Defibrillator (DAVID) trial. JAMA 288(24):3115–3123
37. Brignole M, Gammage M, Puggioni E, Alboni P, Raviele A, Sutton R, Vardas P, Bongiorni MG, Bergfeldt L, Menozzi C, Musso G (2005) Comparative assessment of right, left, and biventricular pacing in patients with permanent atrial fibrillation. Eur Heart J 26(7):712–722
38. Leon AR, Greenberg JM, Kanuru N, Baker CM, Mera FV, Smith AL, Langberg JJ, DeLurgio DB (2002) Cardiac resynchronization in patients with congestive heart failure and chronic atrial fibrillation: effect of upgrading to biventricular pacing after chronic right ventricular pacing. J Am Coll Cardiol 39(8):1258–1263
39. Doshi RN, Daoud EG, Fellows C, Turk K, Duran A, Hamdan MH, Pires LA (2005) Left ventricular-based cardiac stimulation post AV nodal ablation evaluation (the PAVE study). J Cardiovasc Electrophysiol 16(11):1160–1165
40. Leclercq C, Walker S, Linde C, Clementy J, Marshall AJ, Ritter P, Djiane P, Mabo P, Levy T, Gadler F, Bailleul C, Daubert JC (2002) Comparative effects of permanent biventricular and right-univentricular pacing in heart failure patients with chronic atrial fibrillation. Eur Heart J 23(22):1780–1787
41. Linde C, Braunschweig F, Gadler F, Bailleul C, Daubert JC (2003) Long-term improvements in quality of life by biventricular pacing in patients with chronic heart failure: results from the Multisite Stimulation in Cardiomyopathy study (MUSTIC). Am J Cardiol 91(9):1090–1095
42. Linde C, Leclercq C, Rex S, Garrigue S, Lavergne T, Cazeau S, McKenna W, Fitzgerald M, Deharo JC, Alonso C, Walker S, Braunschweig F, Bailleul C, Daubert JC (2002) Long-term

benefits of biventricular pacing in congestive heart failure: results from the MUltisite STimulation in cardiomyopathy (MUSTIC) study. J Am Coll Cardiol 40(1):111–118
43. Bradley DJ, Shen WK (2007) Atrioventricular junction ablation combined with either right ventricular pacing or cardiac resynchronization therapy for atrial fibrillation: the need for large-scale randomized trials. Heart Rhythm 4(2):224–232
44. Dong K, Shen WK, Powell BD, Dong YX, Rea RF, Friedman PA, Hodge DO, Wiste HJ, Webster T, Hayes DL, Cha YM (2010) Atrioventricular nodal ablation predicts survival benefit in patients with atrial fibrillation receiving cardiac resynchronization therapy. Heart Rhythm 7(9):1240–1245
45. Cha YM, Redfield MM, Shen WK, Gersh BJ (2004) Atrial fibrillation and ventricular dysfunction: a vicious electromechanical cycle. Circulation 109(23):2839–2843
46. Wann LS, Curtis AB, January CT, Ellenbogen KA, Lowe JE, Estes NA III, Page RL, Ezekowitz MD, Slotwiner DJ, Jackman WM, Stevenson WG, Tracy CM, Fuster V, Ryden LE, Cannom DS, Le Heuzey JY, Crijns HJ, Olsson SB, Prystowsky EN, Halperin JL, Tamargo JL, Kay GN, Jacobs AK, Anderson JL, Albert N, Hochman JS, Buller CE, Kushner FG, Creager MA, Ohman EM, Ettinger SM, Guyton RA, Tarkington LG, Yancy CW (2011) 2011 ACCF/AHA/HRS focused update on the management of patients with atrial fibrillation (updating the 2006 guideline): a report of the American College of Cardiology Foundation/American Heart Association Task Force on Practice Guidelines. Circulation 123(1):104–123
47. Vorperian VR, Havighurst TC, Miller S, January CT (1997) Adverse effects of low dose amiodarone: a meta-analysis. J Am Coll Cardiol 30(3):791–798
48. Hsu LF, Jais P, Sanders P, Garrigue S, Hocini M, Sacher F, Takahashi Y, Rotter M, Pasquie JL, Scavee C, Bordachar P, Clementy J, Haissaguerre M (2004) Catheter ablation for atrial fibrillation in congestive heart failure. N Engl J Med 351(23):2373–2383
49. Chen MS, Marrouche NF, Khaykin Y, Gillinov AM, Wazni O, Martin DO, Rossillo A, Verma A, Cummings J, Erciyes D, Saad E, Bhargava M, Bash D, Schweikert R, Burkhardt D, Williams-Andrews M, Perez-Lugones A, Abdul-Karim A, Saliba W, Natale A (2004) Pulmonary vein isolation for the treatment of atrial fibrillation in patients with impaired systolic function. J Am Coll Cardiol 43(6):1004–1009

Chapter 7
Repetitive ICD Shocks and Incessant VTs in Heart Failure: What to Do?

Martin Eisenberger, Tom De Potter, and Peter Geelen

Abstract Repetitive implantable cardiac defibrillator (ICD) shocks and incessant ventricular tachycardias are not uncommon in patients with heart failure. Data on the prognostic significance of both appropriate and inappropriate ICD shocks and ventricular tachyarrhythmias suggest a poor outcome. Management of these patients is challenging and depends on the number of shocks, their appropriateness and the patients clinical condition. Initial management involves 12-lead ECG, assessment of patients history and identifying and correcting the transient causes. Antiarrhythmic medication is often administered to reduce the tendency for ICD shocks and incessant ventricular tachycardias. ICD interrogation helps to discriminate appropriate and inappropriate shocks and recognize possible device malfunction. Catheter ablation has developed into a successful treatment strategy for patients with recurrent ventricular tachycardias resistant to antiarrhythmic drugs. Recently, concepts of prophylactic and emergency catheter ablations have been studied. Other non-pharmacologic therapy options, such as LV assist devices and intra-aortic balloon pump placement, might be an acceptable indication to suppress incessant ventricular tachyarrhythmias.

M. Eisenberger, M.D., Ph.D.
Cardiovascular Centre, OLV Hospital,
Moorselbaan 164, 9300 Aalst, Belgium

University of South Bohemia, Ceske Budejovice, Czech Republic

T. De Potter, M.D. • P. Geelen, M.D., Ph.D. (✉)
Cardiovascular Centre, OLV Hospital,
Moorselbaan 164, 9300 Aalst, Belgium
e-mail: peter.geelen@olvz-aalst.be

J. Bartunek and M. Vanderheyden (eds.), *Translational Approach to Heart Failure*,
DOI 10.1007/978-1-4614-7345-9_7, © Springer Science+Business Media New York 2013

1 Background and Definitions

Repetitive shocks in implantable cardiac defibrillator (ICD) patients and incessant ventricular tachycardias are often described as electrical storms. Electrical storm is defined as a state of electrical instability manifested by three or more separate episodes of ventricular tachycardia (VT) or ventricular fibrillation (VF) within 24 h [1]. Monomorphic ventricular tachycardia accounts for 90 % of electrical storm episodes but it can also occur due to polymorphic VT or VF, mainly in the context of myocardial ischemia [2]. Incessant ventricular tachycardia is defined as tachycardia that does not terminate spontaneously or recurs immediately after termination.

ICD therapy has become an established treatment in patients at risk of developing life-threatening ventricular arrhythmias [3]. It is estimated that 120,000 patients received an ICD worldwide in 2008 and the number of implants is increasing [4]. This is mainly due to the expansion of ICD indications for primary prevention of sudden cardiac death in patients with impaired left ventricular function, the continuous rise of heart failure prevalence and due to the better availability of devices. When electrical storm happens in an individual with an ICD, the patient presents with ICD therapies such as repetitive shocks or antitachycardia pacing (ATP) from the device. Electrical storm occurs in 10–20 % of ICD recipients within 3 years of implant [5] and is more common when the ICD is placed for secondary versus primary prevention and in patients with heart failure [6].

Appropriate shocks are delivered to terminate life-threatening ventricular arrhythmias whereas inappropriate shocks are most often caused by supraventricular tachyarrhythmias or signal misinterpretation due to lead fracture, myopotentials or T-wave oversensing. Unnecessary shocks are due to hemodynamically stable non-sustained arrhythmias or due to inadequate device programming. Phantom shocks, defined as a sensation of ICD therapies that cannot be confirmed by device interrogation, are occasionally reported, often in patients who have experienced multiple shocks in the past.

Most cases of electrical storm occur without any apparent trigger [7]. However, it is important to exclude any causes that might have led to electrical instability, such as modification of medical therapy (especially administration of antiarrhythmic drugs), new or worsened heart failure, myocardial ischemia, infection with high fever, and electrolyte abnormalities. Correction of a precipitating factor is usually the first step in electrical storm treatment.

Key Points

- Repetitive shocks in ICD patients and incessant ventricular tachycardias are described as electrical storms.
- Monomorphic ventricular tachycardia accounts for majority of electrical storm episodes.

2 Clinical and Prognostic Significance

Data on the prognostic significance of electrical storm suggest a poor outcome. In the Antiarrhythmics Versus Implantable Defibrillators (AVID) trial, electrical storm occurred in 90 out of 457 recruited patients. The relative risk of subsequent death was 2.4 and the risk of death was greatest 3 months after the storm [8]. In MADIT II patients experiencing electrical storm, the relative risk for death in the first 3 months after the storm was 17.8 in comparison with those with no ventricular arrhythmias [6]. Incessant ventricular tachycardias invariably lead to heart failure in a population with depressed LV function.

It might follow that patients with more severe cardiovascular disease show a greater risk of potentially fatal ventricular arrhythmias and that ICD shocks are particularly life saving in such a population. However, recently published data showed that in a primary prevention population, both appropriate and inappropriate shocks are associated with increased mortality compared to patients who receive no shocks [9], the so-called paradox of ICD shocks. Explanation for this might be the fact that frequent ventricular and supraventricular arrhythmias are markers for worsening heart failure. It is also believed that ICD shocks can negatively transform the natural history of the disease, cause myocardial injury and exert proarrhythmic and negative inotropic effects [10]. In other words, even though the device probably saved patients lives at the time of therapy, it may have postponed death for a short period of time and possibly promote it further. A recent analysis of 2,135 ICD patients from four trials showed that shocked episodes increased the risk of death by 20 %, whereas ATP did not increase mortality risk, confirming the detrimental effects of ICD shocks [11] but not ATP. In the DINAMIT trial, which randomized patients with impaired left ventricular function who were within 40 days after myocardial infarction to ICD vs. no ICD, the greatest mortality was in patients who received any kind of shock, whether appropriate or inappropriate [12].

Key Point

- Electrical storm is associated with a poor prognosis. Not only appropriate but also inappropriate shocks increase mortality in ICD patients—"paradox of ICD shocks."

3 Management of Repetitive ICD Shocks and Incessant VTs in Heart Failure Patients

3.1 General Measures

Management of repetitive ICD shocks and incessant VTs in a heart failure population is challenging and depends on the number of shocks, their appropriateness and the patients clinical condition. Effective treatment requires knowledge of arrhythmia mechanism, ICD programming, use of antiarrhythmic drugs and also emerging technologies such as catheter ablation. Several review articles have addressed these issues [13, 14].

After experiencing a device shock, the patient should contact the ICD facility. In case of a single or two shocks without clinical instability, the healthcare provider responsible for device follow-up should be contacted within the next working day to interrogate the device. Recently, home monitoring systems have become more available to check the device-related information remotely as described later in this chapter.

In the presence of persisting severe symptoms, such as chest pain, palpitations and shortness of breath, or in case of multiple shocks, there is a need for immediate medical evaluation through hospital emergency units. In the emergency unit, all patients should have a 12-lead ECG recorded and a continuous rhythm monitoring should be established as soon as possible. Telemetry observed at the time of an ICD-delivered therapy generally can help determine the appropriateness of the shocks even before the ICD has been interrogated. Management of incessant ventricular arrhythmias based on initial 12-lead ECG classification is depicted in Fig. 7.1. The ECG differentiation of VT from supraventricular tachycardia with aberrant conduction can be challenging without an intracardiac recording but several algorithms have been published [15]. An ambiguous wide-complex tachycardia should be considered VT, especially in patients with structural heart disease.

The 12-lead ECG during tachycardia gives important clues for the presumed arrhythmia mechanism. Monomorphic VT is usually due to re-entry around an anatomic barrier, mostly scar tissue after remote myocardial infarction. The critical zone of slow conduction, essential for maintaining re-entry, lies within the heterogeneously scarred myocardium where surviving myofibrils can provide a pathway for stable re-entry. This is usually found at the border of the scar between dense fibrotic tissue and healthy myocardium. Polymorphic VT is often associated with acute ischemia, but is also seen in the setting of a prolonged QT interval, requiring serious consideration of acquired causes. The common mechanism of ventricular fibrillation is ischemia, but spatially stable (i.e., monomorphic) triggering premature ventricular beats (often originating in the Purkinje system) must be searched for as they are amenable to catheter ablation with excellent results.

Last but not least, the 12-lead ECG will be helpful in localizing ventricular tachycardia origin in case the patient will undergo catheter ablation. It will help the electrophysiologist to determine whether the tachycardia induced in the electrophysiology laboratory was a clinical one and whether it has been abolished by the subsequent ablation.

Assessment of patients history, recent changes in medication, hemodynamics, electrolyte levels including potassium and magnesium and cardiac function should be performed in all cases. Multiple separate shocks at rest occurring hours apart usually signify recurrent appropriately treated ventricular arrhythmias. On the other hand, multiple repetitive shocks occurring within seconds or minutes during physical activity are usually inappropriate, for example for sinus tachycardia.

An important step is to identify and correct any reversible causes, such as electrolyte disturbances, tricyclic overdose and acute myocardial ischemia. Acute

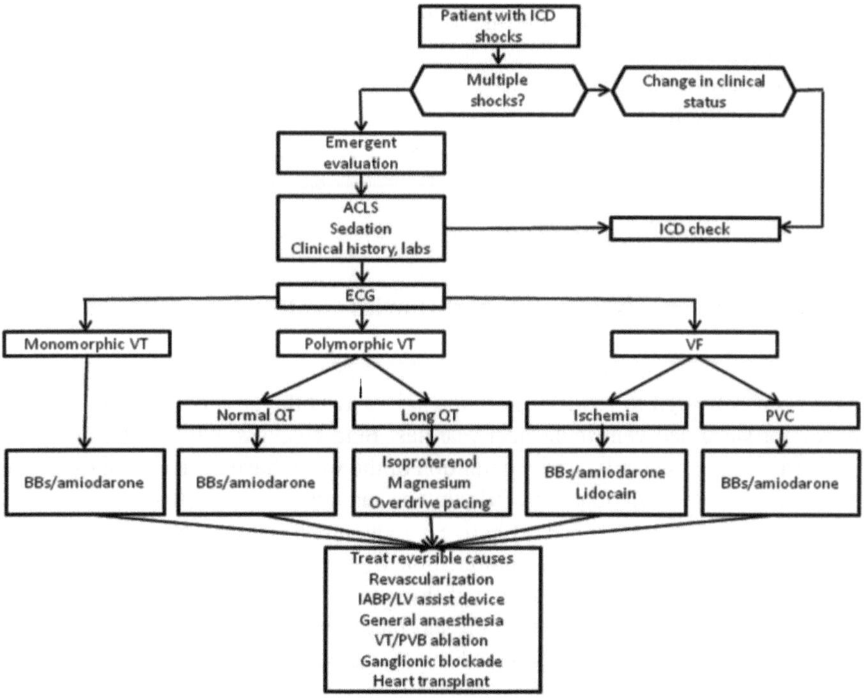

Fig. 7.1 Emergency management of a patient with ICD shocks based on initial evaluation and ECG morphology. *BBs* betablockers, *ACLS* advanced cardiac life support, *PVC* premature ventricular contractions, *IABP* intra-aortic balloon pump

coronary syndrome needs to be excluded by means of cardiac enzymes and in selected patients, a coronary angiogram should be undertaken. It needs to be emphasized that transient ST-segment changes and mildly elevated cardiac troponin levels are common after multiple shocks. As the majority of ICD patients suffer from heart failure, optimization of medical therapy with regards to beta-blockers and ACE inhibitors is important as a general measure. All aspects of critical care, such as management of compromised airways, hypotension and bradycardia, need to be incorporated into the treatment plan. Contact with the ICD clinic should be established as soon as possible to check the device function and interrogate intracardiac ECGs.

In case of ongoing arrhythmia with hemodynamic compromise, urgent treatment is needed, preferably by external direct current cardioversion as IV antiarrhythmic drugs carry the risk of further deterioration of cardiac function. In case of repetitive ICD shocks in the absence of ventricular arrhythmia, e.g. in the presence of fast atrial fibrillation, or due to tachyarrhythmias that are hemodynamically well tolerated, a magnet should be placed over the device to inhibit further ICD therapies. Magnet placement temporarily disables shock deliveries, so it is mandatory to maintain continuous ECG monitoring to detect and treat potentially life-threatening arrhythmias. Inhibition of detection and therapy delivery lasts as long as the magnet is positioned over the ICD. Of note is that applying a magnet does not alter the pacing ability of the ICD.

3.2 Pharmacological Treatment

3.2.1 Prevention of Ventricular Arrhythmias and Repetitive ICD Shocks

Antiarrhythmic medication is often initiated in patients with ICDs before any shocks have been delivered to reduce the frequency of ICD therapy by reducing the tendency for sustained ventricular tachycardias. Beta-blockers, while not considered antiarrhythmic drugs in the strict definition of the word, have been shown to reduce the incidence of ventricular tachyarrhythmias and are usually the first choice unless contraindicated. Amiodarone is effective in reducing the number of ICD shocks and the OPTIC trial showed that a combination with a beta-blocker is more effective than beta-blocker alone [16]. Although long-term amiodarone therapy is usually successful, it may be associated with substantial side effects such as pulmonary fibrosis, hypo- or hyperthyroidism and liver toxicity. Amiodarone may increase the ventricular defibrillation threshold thus possibly requiring re-evaluation. Recent data, however, suggest that this may not be necessary. Sotalol can reduce shocks more than beta-blockers but is significantly inferior to amiodarone, so it may play its role when amiodarone is contraindicated [16]. Also, in contrast to amiodarone and beta-blockers, there is a definite risk of proarrhythmia (mainly due to QTc prolongation) with sotalol. Azimilide, a novel class III antiarrhythmic, reduced the incidence of appropriate ICD discharges but failed to improve mortality and is not approved in many countries [17]. Class IC antiarrhythmic drugs may be justified to prevent inappropriate shocks due to supraventricular arrhythmias such as fast atrial fibrillation, but they are contraindicated in patients with ischemic heart disease and heart failure, so of no use in a heart failure population. Apart from antiarrhythmic drugs, statins and ACE inhibitors may reduce the ventricular arrhythmia burden as shown in retrospective trial analyses [18, 19].

3.2.2 Treatment of Ventricular Arrhythmias and Repetitive ICD Shocks

Sympathetic activity plays a key role in the genesis of electrical storm and a reduction in sympathetic tone by beta-blockers and sedation is essential. Beta-blockers increase the fibrillation threshold and the improvement is greater with propranolol than metoprolol [20]. Because propranolol can exacerbate heart failure in patients with poor systolic function, its use in these patients should be carefully monitored. Intravenous amiodarone is widely used in the treatment of electrical storm due to its high efficacy and few negative electrophysiological and inotropic effects, making it the first choice treatment in patients with failing hearts. In the ARREST trial, IV amiodarone improved survival to admission in the hospital in patients who had had an out-of-hospital cardiac arrest with VF or pulseless VT [21]. Lidocaine may have some beneficial effect, especially if electrical storm is associated with acute ischemia. However, outside the setting of ischemia, its antiarrhythmic properties are relatively weak and inferior to amiodarone [22]. Importantly, most antiarrhythmic drugs may slow the rate of the arrhythmia to a point where it can drop below the device tachycardia detection rate, resulting in no ICD therapy. All patients with electrical storm should be sedated with propofol or benzodiazepines as the physical and emotional stress associated with the storm and multiple shocks often perpetuates the arrhythmia. Bailout options for refractory cases include intra-aortic balloon pump insertion, intubation and general anaesthesia. Beyond drug therapy, sympathetic blockade by left stellate ganglionic blockade exerts beneficial effect in patients with electric storm [23]. Unfortunately, few surgeons maintain the volume of procedures needed to build and keep enough experience.

In polymorphic VT, intravenous administration of magnesium sulphate, potassium and overdrive pacing may be effective in suppressing the arrhythmia. This is particularly true for patients with triggering ventricular extrasystoles that occur in long-short-long cycles due to delayed afterdepolarizations, such as seen in torsade de pointes. In patients with polymorphic VT and QT prolongation, isoproterenol may terminate incessant arrhythmias and prevent recurrent episodes [24].

3.3 *ICD Interrogation and Programming*

ICD interrogation after delivery of an electrical shock helps to discriminate appropriate and inappropriate shocks and recognize possible device malfunction (Fig.7.2). Most frequent causes of appropriate and inappropriate shocks are depicted in Table 7.1. Strategic ICD programming is important to reduce inappropriate shocks without compromising the ICD efficacy. Evaluation of the stored electrograms has to be done using a programmer made by the ICD manufacturer.

3.3.1 ICD Programming to Reduce Shocks

All efforts should be made to avoid inappropriate shock therapies because they decrease battery life and are associated with poor quality of life and unfavourable outcomes, and decrease battery life. ATP is either a burst of pacing impulses at a rate slightly faster than the VT rate or a rapidly decelerating train of beats that may terminate the ongoing ventricular tachycardia. Large studies have shown that ATP can effectively terminate up to 94 % of episodes of spontaneous VT [25]. In the PainFree Rx II study, one sequence of eight ATP pulses at 88 % of the tachycardia cycle length successfully terminated three out of four fast ventricular tachycardia episodes that were initially considered as not suitable for overdrive pacing [26].

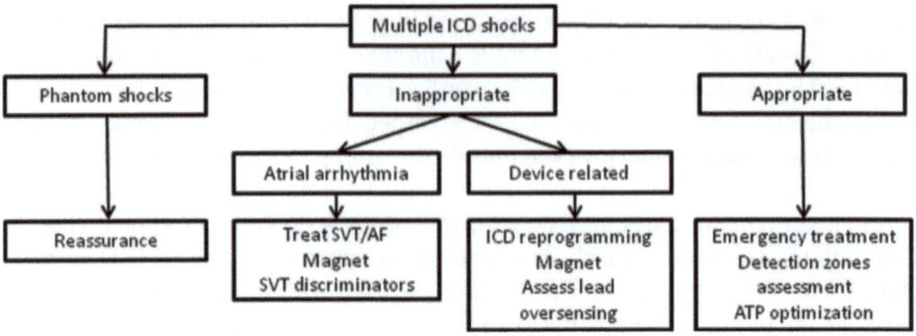

Fig. 7.2 ICD check of a patient with multiple shocks

Table 7.1 Causes of appropriate and inappropriate ICD shocks

Causes of appropriate shocks	Causes of inappropriate shocks
Monomorphic VT	*Arrhythmia different from VT or VF*
Polymorphic VT	Atrial fibrillation/flutter/tachycardia
Ventricular fibrillation	Supraventricular tachycardia (AVNRT, AVNRT, etc.)
Torsade de pointes	Sinus tachycardia
	Multiple premature ventricular beats
	Device related
	T-wave oversensing
	Double counting of QRS complexes
	Oversensing due to lead failure or insulation break
	Oversensing of diaphragmatic myopotentials
	Electromagnetic interference

The PREPARE investigators have shown that in primary prevention it is useful to set detection threshold for VT at 182 bpm and VF for rates above 250 bpm that were maintained for at least 30 of 40 beats [27]. From the same dataset, programming a slow VT monitor zone was shown to be helpful in detecting slower arrhythmias, without giving ICD treatment. Time to detection and time to therapy (to allow spontaneous termination of non-sustained arrhythmias) may be extended without compromising safety. Strategic programming can be performed empirically with preset parameters and such approach is not inferior to tailored programming (Fig. 7.3) [28]. Most modern ICDs now have the possibility to use ATP during charging for a shock and this should be programmed on.

3.3.2 Appropriate Shocks

ICD shocks are appropriately delivered for monomorphic and polymorphic VT, ventricular fibrillation and torsade de pointes VT (Table 7.1). Twenty-two to thirty-five percentage of patients will receive appropriate ICD therapy within 3 years of

Detection zone	Therapy 1	Therapy 2	Therapy 3
Slow VT (182-200 bpm)	ATP x3	ATP x3	35J x5
Fast VT (200-250 bpm)	ATP x1	35J	35J x5
VF (>200 bpm)	35J (ATP during charging)	35J	35J x4

Fig. 7.3 Empirical ICD programming

implant with an annual ICD shock rate of 5 % [29]. In case of repetitive ICD shocks, the appropriateness of the therapy needs to determined by evaluation of the stored electrograms. Tachyarrhythmia settings, such as detection zones or programmed therapies must be evaluated. When no obvious cause for a single or a couple of ICD shocks is evident after a thorough clinical assessment, simply reassuring the patient may be all that is required. In patients who present with frequent albeit isolated appropriate ICD shocks, clinicians may consider optimizing the programming of ATP or adjustment of detection zones together with pharmacologic therapy as outlined above. Also, the possibility of ablation therapy should be considered.

In ICD patients without CRT, it is important to avoid unnecessary RV pacing, and in those with CRT-D, the percentage of biventricular stimulation should be as high as possible. If poor rate control during atrial fibrillation causes insufficient resynchronisation therapy, ablation of the AV node is considered appropriate.

3.3.3 Inappropriate Shocks

Inappropriate shocks can be a relatively frequent occurrence. In a review of 449 patients randomly assigned to receive ICD therapy in the AVID trial, 22 % of patients received inappropriate therapy [30]. The main cause of inappropriate therapy is atrial arrhythmia, usually atrial fibrillation with rapid ventricular conduction (Fig. 7.4a). Large heart failure databases suggest that the overall incidence of AF in heart failure patients is 10–50 %, making the potential of inappropriate detection a significant problem. Pharmacologic therapy can be used to reduce inappropriate shocks caused by atrial fibrillation and are often also effective for other supraventricular tachycardias (e.g. atrial flutter), but catheter ablation must certainly be considered. Appropriate programming of algorithms for the discrimination between supraventricular and ventricular tachycardias may help to reduce the number of inappropriate therapies. To distinguish sinus tachycardia from VT, nearly all ICDs can implement an algorithm to detect a sudden increase in the ventricular rate at the onset of the tachycardia. Stability criterion comparing variability of heart rate is effective for excluding atrial fibrillation that generally has a more unstable heart rate than VT. Morphology discriminators take advantage of the difference in appearance of the local electrograms sensed by the ventricular lead during VT when compared with a stored electrogram obtained during sinus rhythm. The downside of all these features is that they might withhold therapy if the algorithm fails. A dual chamber ICD can be programmed to look for the AV relationship and properly distinguish the large majority of ventricular from supraventricular tachycardias. One should realize, however, that although a dual chamber ICD theoretically should help to reduce the occurrence of inappropriate shocks, randomized studies have shown no clear benefit [31].

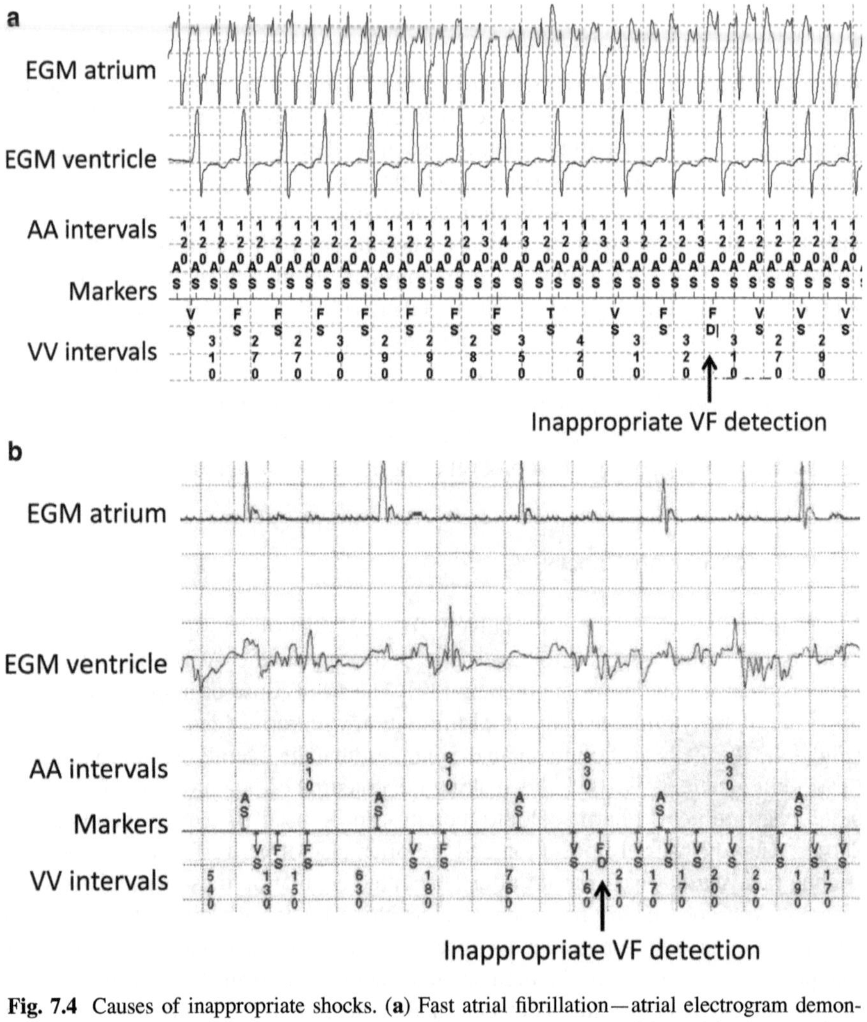

Fig. 7.4 Causes of inappropriate shocks. (**a**) Fast atrial fibrillation—atrial electrogram demonstrates atrial fibrillation, whereas the ventricular electrogram reveals fast and irregular activity falling in the ventricular fibrillation zone. (**b**) Lead failure—noise in the ventricular lead misinterpreted as ventricular fibrillation. (**c**) T-wave oversensing—high voltage T-wave detected as an R-wave. (**d**) Double sensing of wide ventricular complexes

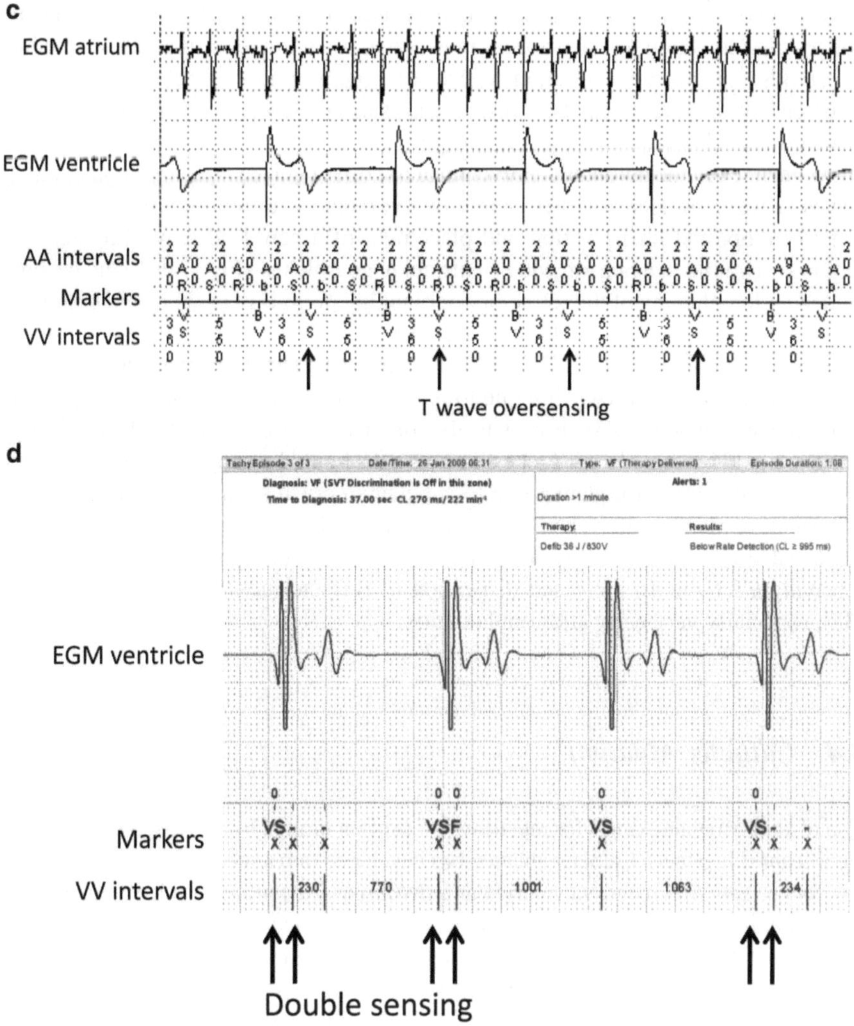

Fig. 7.4 (continued)

The second cause of inappropriate shocks is related to device dysfunction. Mechanical lead problems, such as lead fracture, dislodgment and insulation failure can be diagnosed by abnormal lead impedance or by analysis of intracardiac electrograms and a failure to sense or capture appropriately (Fig. 7.4b). Inappropriate shocks due to lead dysfunction are rarely avoidable by device programming, due to the high frequency of noise signals leading to detection in the VF zone (where SVT algorithms do not apply). Lead fracture or insulation failure therefore almost always requires close monitoring until the lead is revised or replaced. T-wave oversensing due to false detection of a T-wave as an R-wave, often in the setting of low sensing thresholds, is another common cause of inappropriate shocks (Fig. 7.4c). Oversensing of T-waves can be transient and is usually corrected with changing the sensitivity level or adjusting the refractory period. In some devices, specific features allow changes in the automatic gain control to correct chronic sensing of late, tall T waves. T-wave oversensing that cannot be overcome with reprogramming may be due to suboptimal lead position and placement of a new lead may ultimately be required. Double sensing of wide ventricular complexes (Fig. 7.4d) can be prevented by lengthening of the refractory or blanking periods or again by changing the sensing decay algorithm. Pectoral myopotentials as well as electromagnetic interference are uncommon and rarely cause inappropriate shocks because ICD sensing is always bipolar. If oversensing due to myopotentials or lead failure is suspected, provocative manoeuvres such as Valsalva or manipulation with the device in the pocket should be considered. A chest radiograph should be obtained to look for lead dislodgement, insulation defect due to subclavian crush syndrome or altered connection of the lead to the generator. Even though CRT may reduce the incidence of electrical storm, several cases of pacing related ventricular arrhythmias in patients receiving CRT due to increased dispersion of refractoriness have been described [32], especially very early after implantation.

3.4 Catheter Ablation

Use of antiarrhythmic drugs for repetitive VT is often limited by decreased efficacy and significant side effects. Catheter ablation has developed into a successful treatment strategy for patients with recurrent ventricular arrhythmias. According to current guidelines, catheter ablation of ventricular tachycardia is recommended for symptomatic sustained VT necessitating frequent ICD therapies despite antiarrhythmic drug treatment or when antiarrhythmic drugs are not tolerated or not desired. There is a general trend to consider catheter ablation early in the treatment of patients with recurrent VT. However, current recommendations are based largely on uncontrolled trials and single-centre reports. Several ablation strategies have been described depending on the hemodynamic tolerance and VT morphology.

3.4.1 Catheter Ablation of Stable Monomorphic VT

Monomorphic ventricular tachycardias that do not lead to hemodynamic compromise can be mapped using conventional mapping strategies, such as activation mapping, pacemapping or entrainment mapping. Activation mapping is used to localize the origin of tachycardia by identifying the site of the earliest activation, or in case of re-entrant arrhythmias, to delineate the circuit and find an area of slow conduction. Pacemapping, i.e. pacing near the origin of tachyarrhythmia during sinus rhythm, may reproduce the same QRS morphology as the clinical tachycardia. Entrainment mapping involves pacing from the ablation catheter during tachycardia at a slightly faster rate and evaluating the response of the tachycardia to confirm catheter location is within the re-entry circuit. The ablation target can also be identified by isolated diastolic electrograms during ongoing re-entrant tachycardias. However, the tachycardia needs to be inducible during the electrophysiological study and ideally a 12-lead ECG of the clinical VT should be available to confirm the morphology. Moreover, the arrhythmia needs to be hemodynamically tolerated to allow for mapping. A stored intracardiac electrogram downloaded using the ICD programmer may be used to confirm the cycle length of induced tachycardia if the surface ECG is not available.

To treat stable monomorphic VT not suppressible by antiarrhythmic drugs, knowing the mechanism of VT is of key importance to select the appropriate ablation strategy. In rare cases of a focal origin, the critical portion is contained in a small area so a discrete lesion can abolish VT. In the majority of patients with scar-related re-entrant tachycardias, ablation is aimed at transecting the critical tachycardia isthmus. The isthmus may be narrow, allowing a discrete lesion to abolish VT, or broad, requiring larger ablation areas. Most re-entry circuit isthmuses can be transected using an endocardial approach. However, critical re-entry circuit sites can be intramural or subepicardial in some patients.

3.4.2 Substrate Mapping and Ablation

Substrate mapping using voltage criteria has been introduced to allow substrate modification in cases where ventricular tachycardia is not inducible or is unstable, or multiple VTs are present. Electroanatomic mapping systems such as CARTO or EnSite NavX are beneficial to guide mapping and ablation. They allow a 3D reconstruction of the chamber of interest and colour-coded display of various electrophysiological parameters for endocardial or epicardial mapping. In post-myocardial infarction patients, the infarcted area is usually defined during sinus rhythm by electrograms with an amplitude ≤1.5 mV, dense scars are defined by electrograms with an amplitude ≤0.5 mV (Fig. 7.5). Conducting channels within the scar area might be identified by setting the value for scar at ≤0.2 mV and finding continuous electrograms differentiated from the surrounding scar tissue by a higher amplitude. In patients with unstable arrhythmias, pace mapping can support the involvement of the conducting channel on the basis of the long stimulus-to-QRS interval and on the 12-lead ECG match. Sequential lesions are created to transect any isthmuses and to connect the lowest-amplitude signals areas to healthy endocardium across the borders of abnormal endocardium, the so-called substrate pacification. Linear lesions might be created to connect scar areas to a valve continuity [33, 34]. Another strategy is to encircle the infarct area, but a continuous line may be difficult to

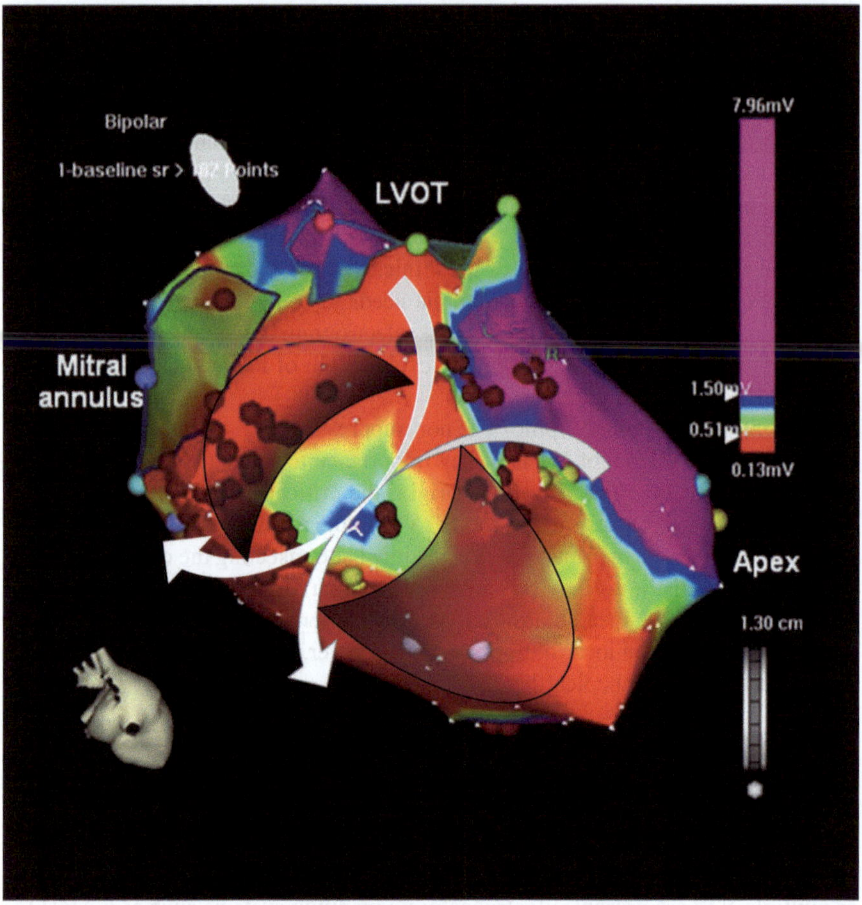

Fig. 7.5 Substrate mapping in a patient with a history of inferior myocardial infarction and recurrent ventricular tachycardias. Scar region is identified by electrogram amplitude below 0.5 mV (*red colour*, shown by the *oval shape*). Potential channels within the low-voltage scar have been found and late and split potentials were recorded in this region during sinus rhythm. *White arrows* show anticipated direction of the tachycardia waveform across the scar region within the channel. Targeting the isthmus together with the exit and entry point made ventricular tachycardia non-inducible

achieve around large scars. The endpoint is to abolish all inducible sustained VT but if this is not feasible, ablation of the clinical VT with persistent non-inducibility should be achieved as a minimal requirement.

3.4.3 Early Catheter Ablation

Recently, the concept of catheter ablation in post-myocardial infarction patients with an ICD indication has been studied in a randomized fashion. In a group of patients with either documented cardiac arrest and planned ICD in secondary prevention, or ICD in primary prevention with later appropriate therapy, patients who underwent VT ablation on top of ICD received fewer shocks than did those who underwent ICD implantation alone [35]. In a similar multicenter trial, patients with stable VT, a history of MI and low LV ejection fraction undergoing RF ablation plus ICD implantation had longer times to recurrence of VT than patients who received an ICD without ablation [36]. These findings support the early use of ablation in patients who receive an ICD and remain at high risk of recurrent VT.

3.4.4 Emergency Catheter Ablation

Emergency catheter ablation can be used to treat electrical storm and repetitive ICD shocks. In the largest consecutive series of 95 ICD patients undergoing ablation for drug-refractory electrical storm, arrhythmia was acutely suppressed in all patients. Many of them were critically ill and required hemodynamic support. At a median follow-up of 22 months, 92 % of patients were free of electrical storm and 66 % were free of VT recurrence. Interestingly, of the ten patients who continued to have inducible VT, eight had recurrent electrical storm and four died despite appropriate ICD therapy [37].

In some cases, repetitive polymorphic VT and VF seem to be triggered by monomorphic premature ventricular beats (Fig. 7.6) [38]. Ventricular ectopy after myocardial infarction has been associated nearly exclusively with surviving Purkinje system fibbers after myocardial infarction. Moreover, the majority of premature ventricular beats originate from the conduction system in the border zone of infarcted area as pioneered by Haissaguerre et al. [39]. Ablation of polymorphic VT and VF aims at eliminating the ectopic focus triggering VF (Fig. 7.7). Acute success rate of electrical storm ablation is high, very likely due to the very superficial endocardial location of the targeted tissue. Recent EHRA expert consensus recommends catheter ablation for recurrent polymorphic VT and VF refractory to antiarrhythmic therapy when there is a suspected trigger that can be targeted by ablation [3].

3.4.5 Epicardial and Surgical Ablation

Some ventricular tachycardias originate from an epicardial scar and might be resistant to endocardial ablation. These arrhythmias mostly occur in patients with non-ischaemic cardiomyopathy and especially is patients with right ventricular arrhythmogenic dysplasia or Chagas disease. Compared with endocardial ventricular tachycardias, they typically have a wider QRS interval with the so-called pseudo-delta wave [40]. Epicardial ablation requires the insertion of a sheath into the pericardial space using a needle and a guidewire under fluoroscopic control [41]. A recent study has shown that combined endo- and epicardial ablation significantly increases freedom from ventricular tachycardia in patients with electrical storms [42].

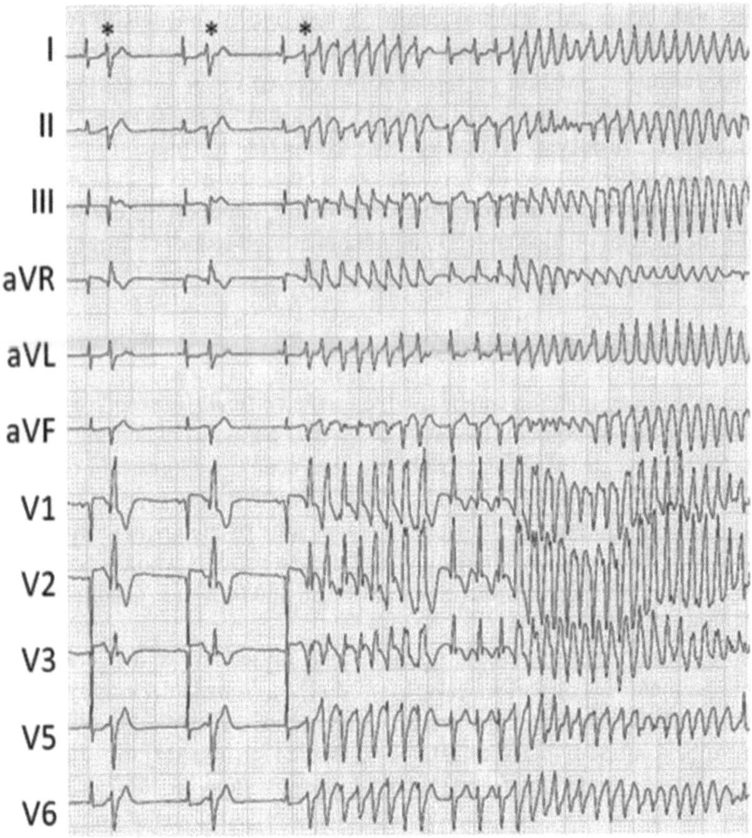

Fig. 7.6 Repetitive episodes of ventricular fibrillation triggered by monomorphic premature ventricular beats originating in the distal posterior fascicle

The surgical approach for the treatment of ventricular tachycardia has been largely replaced by percutaneous techniques. However, it might be an alternative in patients with ventricular aneurysms, especially when coronary artery disease requiring revascularization is present [43]. Surgery is also an option for selected patients with tachycardias late after repair of Tetralogy of Fallot and in some cases of failed catheter ablation.

3.4.6 Aalst Experience with Catheter Ablation for Ventricular Tachyarrhythmias

Between January 2009 and July 2012, 107 patients (female 23, mean age 64 ± 14 years) with structural heart disease underwent mapping and ablation for ventricular tachyarrhythmias in the OLV Hospital, Aalst, Belgium. Mean LV ejection fraction

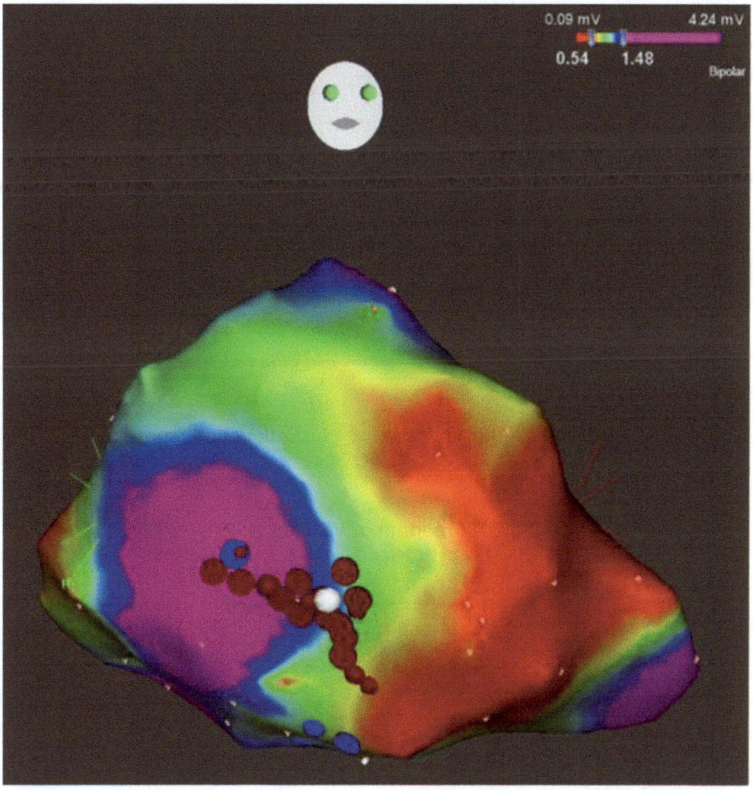

Fig. 7.7 Mapping and ablation of a trigger in a distal Purkinje system. Electro-anatomical voltage map of the left ventricle (*red*—low voltage, *violet*—normal voltage). *Blue tags*—sites with Purkinje potentials during sinus rhythm, *red tags*—ablation points, *white tag*—site with the earliest ventricular activation during the premature ventricular contraction (ectopic focus)

was 35 ± 14 %. Ten patients required epicardial puncture after failed endocardial ablation. Acute procedural success defined as non-inducibility of previously inducible ventricular tachyarrhythmia was 84 %. No patient died during the procedure or as its consequence. During a mean follow-up of 12 months (range 0–39 months) survival rate was 85 % (Fig. 7.8), whereas ventricular arrhythmia-free survival rate at 11 months was 83 % (Fig. 7.9).

4 Other Non-pharmacological Treatment Options

Placing an intra-aortic balloon pump or percutaneous LV assist device is an accepted indication to suppress malignant arrhythmias. These devices increase coronary perfusion pressure and can dramatically relieve the ischemic substrate. The mechanical effects might be directly antiarrhythmic, because this therapy has been effective even

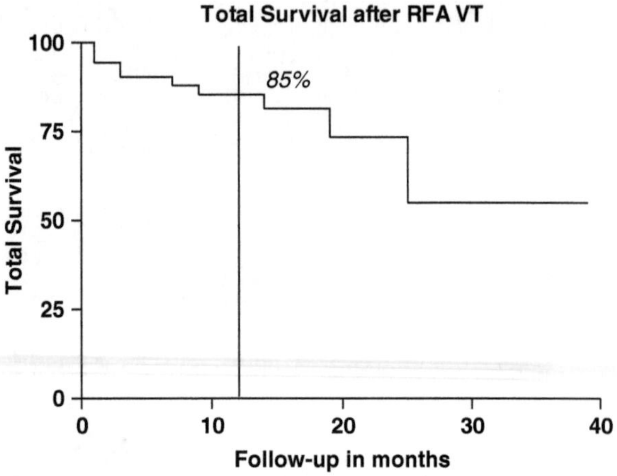

Fig. 7.8 Total survival after catheter ablation for ventricular tachyarrhythmias

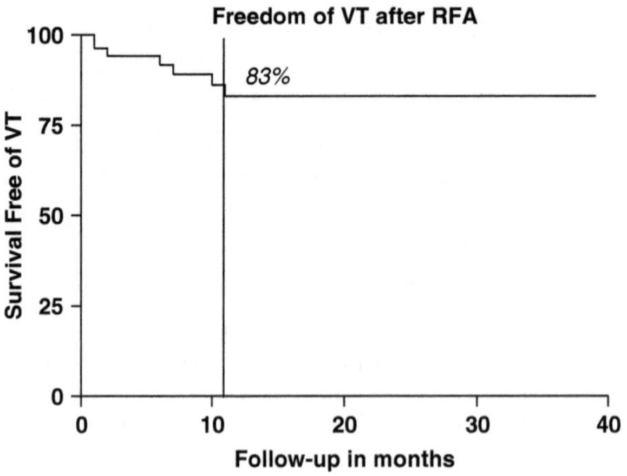

Fig. 7.9 Ventricular tachyarrhythmia-free survival after catheter ablation. *Key Points:* Management of repetitive ICD shocks and incessant ventricular tachycardias in heart failure patients include emergency measures, pharmacological and non-pharmacological therapy. Catheter ablation has emerged as a successful treatment strategy in patients with drug-refractory ventricular tachycardias

outside the presence of ischaemia. The mechanism may involve reduction in afterload, LV size and wall tension. Cardiac transplantation might be the only option in some patients if all measures fail to suppress incessant tachycardias or ICD shocks.

Key Point

- Other non-pharmacological treatment options include an intra-aortic balloon pump, percutaneous LV assist device and heart transplantation.

5 Remote Monitoring

Remote monitoring offers continuous surveillance of the ICD performance and information stored by the device. It is now offered by most ICD manufactures and all systems allow notifications to be sent to a service centre via the internet or GSM network. This allows a prompt evaluation of the appropriateness of detection and effectiveness of delivered therapy. If device function is considered appropriate and the clinical status is stable, the patient can be reassured. However, if there is a device malfunction suspected or there is an issue associated with an increased risk for shock delivery, such as fast atrial fibrillation or recurrent self-limited VT, early intervention may prevent clinical deterioration or unnecessary shock therapies. In a study of 54 patients undergoing an ICD lead revision due to malfunction of the ICD lead, inappropriate shocks due to oversensing occurred in 53.4 % patients without remote monitoring system and only in 27.3 % in the remote monitoring group [44]. Home monitoring has been shown to save hospital and travel costs and it also reduces overall patient visits. Several studies are ongoing and some of them may answer whether monitoring of fluid status in heart failure patients can reduce the risk for hospitalization, repetitive ICD shocks and incessant ventricular arrhythmias. Remote monitoring has been recommended as a standard clinical practice in the expert consensus [45] but the post-implant in-office follow up after 1 month and at least once a year should be maintained.

Key Point

- Remote monitoring allows continuous ICD performance surveillance and early intervention.

6 Future Trends

It is believed that deep re-entry circuits contribute to a relatively high number of recurrences and that new ablation technologies including intramural needle ablation catheters may help to overcome some limitations. Intraprocedural contact-force measurement may improve transmural lesion formation. First-in-man experience with renal sympathetic denervation for the treatment of electrical storm has been described [46]. There is no evidence so far that ventricular tachycardia ablation reduces mortality. A future prospective study using standardized ablation protocols will need to answer this important question

Key Point

- Some future trends include new ablation technologies including intramural needle ablation and renal denervation.

7 Conclusion

Patients with repetitive ICD shocks and incessant ventricular arrhythmias have a poor outcome. ECG morphology during arrhythmia and sinus rhythm and the presence or absence of structural heart disease provide important diagnostic clues about the mechanism of electrical storm. Initial management involves identifying and correcting the transient causes of arrhythmia and interrogating the ICD. Pharmacological treatment, especially beta-blockers and amiodarone, are the cornerstone of therapy in patients with appropriate shocks due to ventricular arrhythmias. Device programming and identification of possible device malfunctions are important steps in diagnosis and the treatment of ICD patients. Catheter ablation has emerged as a promising tool in recurrent VT and in drug-refractory electrical storms. Other non-pharmacological therapy options, such as LV assist devices and intra-aortic balloon pump placement, may be successful to suppress malignant arrhythmias.

8 Sources of Further Information

Sources of further information on the topic of repetitive ICD shocks and incessant ventricular tachycardias in heart failure are provided in the reference list. More information can be obtained from the conference papers and webcasts, book series and medical company websites and presentations.

References

1. Israel CW, Barold SS (2007) Electrical storm in patients with an implanted defibrillator: a matter of definition. Ann Noninvasive Electrocardiol 12:375–382
2. Hohnloser SH, Al-Khalidi HR, Pratt CM, Brum JM, Tatla DS, Tchou P, Dorian P (2006) Electrical storm in patients with an implantable defibrillator: incidence, features, and preventive therapy: insights from a randomized trial. Eur Heart J 27(24):3027–3032
3. Zipes DP, Camm AJ, Borggrefe M, Buxton AE, Chaitman B, Fromer M, Gregoratos G, Klein G, Moss AJ, Myerburg RJ, Priori SG, Quinones MA, Roden DM, Silka MJ, Tracy C, Blanc JJ, Budaj A et al (2006) ACC/AHA/ESC 2006 guidelines for management of patients with ventricular arrhythmias and the prevention of sudden cardiac death. Europace 8(9):746–837
4. Braunschweig F, Boriani G, Bauer A, Hatala R, Herrmann-Lingen C, Kautzner J, Pedersen SS, Pehrson S, Ricci R, Schalij MJ (2010) Management of patients receiving implantable cardiac defibrillator shocks: recommendations for acute and long-term patient management. Europace 12:1673–1690
5. Arya A, Haghjoo M, Dehghani MR, Fazelifar AF, Nikoo MH, Bagherzadeh A, Sadr-Ameli MA (2006) Prevalence and predictors of electrical storm in patients with implantable cardioverter-defibrillator. Am J Cardiol 97(3):389–392
6. Sesselbergh HW, Moss AJ, Mc Nitt S, Zareba W, Daubert JP, Andrews ML et al (2007) Ventricular arrhythmia storms in post-infarction patients with implantable defibrillators for primary prevention indications: a MADIT-II substudy. Heart Rhythm 4(11):1395–1402

7. Credner SC, Klingenheben T, Mauss O, Sticherling C, Hohnloser SH (1998) Electrical storm in patients with transvenous implantable cardioverter-defibrillators: incidence, management and prognostic implications. J Am Coll Cardiol 32:1909–1915
8. Exner DV, Pinski SL, Wyse DG, Renfroe EG, Follmann D, Gold M et al (2001) Electrical storm presages nonsudden death: the antiarrhythmics versus implantable defibrillators (AVID) trial. Circulation 108(16):2066–2071
9. Poole JE, Johnson GW, Hellkamp AS, Anderson J, Callans DJ, Raitt MH et al (2008) Prognostic importance of defibrillator shocks in patients with heart failure. N Engl J Med 359:1009–1017
10. Xie J, Weil MH, Sun S, Tang W, Sato Y, Jin X et al (1997) High-energy defibrillation increases the severity of postresuscitation myocardial dysfunction. Circulation 96:683–688
11. Sweeney MO, Sherfesee L, DeGroot P, Wathen M, Wilkoff BL (2010) Differences in effects of electrical therapy type for ventricular arrhythmias on mortality in ICD patients. Heart Rhythm 7:353–360
12. Dorian P, Hohnloser SH, Thorpe KE et al (2010) Mechanisms underlying the lack of effect of implantable cardioverter-defibrillator therapy on mortality in high-risk patients with recent myocardial infarction: insights from the Defibrillation in Acute Myocardial Infarction Trial (DINAMIT). Circulation 122(25):2645–2652
13. Gehi AK, Mehta D, Gomes JA (2006) Evaluation and management of patients after implantable cardioverter-defibrillator shock. JAMA 296:2839–2847
14. Eifling M, Razavi M, Massumi A (2011) The evaluation and management of electrical storm. Tex Heart Inst J 38(2):111–121
15. Brugada P, Brugada J, Mont L, Smeets J, Andres EW (1991) A new approach to the differential diagnosis of a regular tachycardia with a wide QRS complex. Circulation 83(5):1649–1659
16. Connolly SJ, Dorian P, Roberts RS, Gent M, Bailin S, Fain ES et al (2006) Comparison of beta-blockers, amiodarone plus betablockers, or sotalol for prevention of shocks from implantable cardioverter defibrillators: the OPTIC Study: a randomized trial. JAMA 295(2):165–171
17. Dorian P, Borggrefe M, Al-Khalidi HR, Hohnloser SH, Brum JM, Tafia DS (2004) Schock inhibition evaluation with azimilide (SHIELD) investigators: placebo-controlled, randomized clinical trial of azimilidie for prevention of ventricular tachyarrhythmias in patients with an implantable cardioverter defibrillator. Circulation 110:3646–3654
18. Domanski MJ, Exner DV, Borkowf CB, Geller NL, Rosenberg Y, Pfeffer MA (1999) Effect of angiotension converting enzyme inhibition on sudden cardiac death in patients following acute myocardial infarction. A meta-analysis of randomized clinical trials. J Am Coll Cardiol 33:598–604
19. Vyas AK, Guo H, Moss AJ, Olshansky B, McNitt SA, Hall WJ et al (2006) Reduction in ventricular tachyarrhythmias with statins in the Multicenter Automatic Defibrillator Implantation Trial (MADIT)-II. J Am Coll Cardiol 47:769–773
20. Anderson JL, Rodier HE, Green LS (1983) Comparative effects of beta-adrenergic blocking drugs on experimental ventricular fibrillation threshold. Am J Cardiol 51(7):1196–1202
21. Kudenchuk PJ, Cobb LA, Copass MK, Cummins RO, Doherty AM, Fahrenbruch CE, Hallstrom AP, Murray WA, Olsufka M, Walsh T (1999) Amiodarone for resuscitation after out-of-hospital cardiac arrest due to ventricular fibrillation. N Engl J Med 341(12):871–878
22. Dorian P, Cass D, Schwartz B, Cooper R, Gelaznikas R, Barr A (2002) Amiodarone as compared with lidocaine for shock-resistant ventricular fibrillation. N Engl J Med 346(12):884–890
23. Nademanee K, Taylor R, Bailey WE, Rieders DE, Kosar EM (2000) Treating electrical storm. Sympathetic blockade versus advanced cardiac life support—guided therapy. Circulation 102:742–747
24. Belhassen B, Glick A, Aiskin S (2004) Efficacy of quinidine in high-risk patients with Brugada syndrome. Circulation 110(13):1731–1737
25. Nasir N Jr, Pacifico A, Doyle TK, Earle NR, Hardage ML, Henry PD (1997) Cadence Investigators. Spontaneous ventricular tachycardia treated by antitachycardia pacing. Am J Cardiol 79:820–822

26. Wathen MS, DeGroot PJ, Sweeney MO, Stark AJ, Otterness MF, Adkisson WO et al (2004) Prospective randomized multicenter trial of empirical antitachycardia pacing versus shocks for spontaneous rapid ventricular tachycardia in patients with implantable cardioverter-defibrillators: Pacing Fast Ventricular Tachycardia Reduces Shock Therapies (PainFree Rx II) trial results. Circulation 110:2591–2596
27. Wilkoff BL, Williamson BD, Stern RS, Moore SL, Lu F, Lee SW et al (2008) Strategic programming of detection and therapy parameters in implantable cardioverter-defibrillators reduces shocks in primary prevention patients: results from the PREPARE (Primary Prevention Parameters Evaluation) Study. J Am Coll Cardiol 52:541–550
28. Wilkoff BL, Ousidigian KT, Sterns LD, Wang ZJ, Wilson RD, Morgan JM (2006) A comparison of empiric to physician-tailored programming of implantable cardioverter-defibrillators: results from the prospective randomized multicenter EMPIRIC trial. J Am Coll Cardiol 48:330–339
29. Moss AJ, Greenberg H, Case RB et al (2004) Long-term clinical course of patients after termination of ventricular tachyarrhythmia by an implanted defibrillator. Circulation 110:3760–3765
30. Klein RC, Raitt MH, Wilkoff BL et al (2003) Analysis of implantable cardioverter defibrillator therapy in the Antiarrhythmics Versus Implantable Defibrillators (AVID) trial. J Cardiovasc Electrophysiol 14:940–948
31. Swerdlow CD, Chen PS, Kass RM, Allard JR, Peter CT (1994) Discrimination of ventricular tachycardia from sinus tachycardia and atrial fibrillation in a tiered-therapy cardioverter-defibrillator. J Am Coll Cardiol 23:1342–1355
32. Nayak HM, Verdino RJ, Russo AM, Gerstenfeld EP, Hsia HH, Lin D, Dixit S, Cooper JM, Callans DJ, Marchlinski FE (2008) Ventricular tachycardia storm after initiation of biventricular pacing: incidence, clinical characteristics, management, and outcome. J Cardiovasc Electrophysiol 19(7):708–715
33. Marchlinski FE, Callans DJ, Gottlieb CD, Zado E (2000) Lienar ablation lesions for control of unmappable ventricular tacycardia in patients with ischemic and nonischemic cardiomyopathy. Circulation 101:1288–1296
34. Soejima K, Suzuki M, Maisel WH, Brunckhorst CB, Delacretaz E, Blier L, Tung S, Khan H, Stevenson WG (2001) Catheter ablation in patients with multiple and unstable ventricular tachycardias after myocardial infarction: short ablation lines guided by reentry circuit isthmuses and sinus rhythm mapping. Circulation 104:664–669
35. Reddy VY, Reynolds MR, Neuzil P, Richardson AW, Taborsky M, Jongnarangsin K et al (2007) Prophylactic catheter ablation for the prevention of defibrillator therapy. N Engl J Med 357(26):2657–2665
36. Kuck KH, Schaumann A, Eckardt L, Willems S, Ventura R, Delacretaz E et al (2010) Catheter ablation of stable ventricular tachycardia before defibrillator implantation in patients with coronary heart disease (VTACH): a multicentre randomised controlled trial. Lancet 375(9708):31–40
37. Carbucichio C, Santamaria M, Trevisi N, Maccabelli G, Giraldi F, Fassini G, Riva S, Moltrasio M, Cireddu M, Veglia F, Della BP (2008) Catheter ablation for the treatment of electrical storm in patients with implantable cardioverter-defibrillators. Circulation 117:462–469
38. Kohsaka S, Razavi M, Massumi A (2007) Idiopathic ventricular fibrillation successfully terminated by radiofrequency ablation of the distal Purkinje fibers. Pacing Clin Electrophysiol 30(5):701–704
39. Haissaguerre M, Shoda M, Jais P, Nogami A, Shah DC, Kautzner J et al (2002) Mapping and ablation of idiopathic ventricular fibrillation. Circulation 106(8):962–967
40. Berruezo A, Mont L, Nava S et al (2004) Electrocardiographic recognition of the epicardial origin of ventricular tachycardias. Circulation 109:1842–1847
41. Sosa E, Scanavacca M, d'Avila A, Oliveira F, Ramires JA (2000) Nonsurgical transthoracic epicardial catheter ablation to treat recurrent ventricular tachycardia occurring late after myocardial infarction. J Am Coll Cardiol 35(6):1442–1449

42. Di Biase L, Santangeli P, Burkhardt DJ, Bai R et al (2012) Endo-epicardial homogenization of the scar versus limited substrate ablation for the treatment of electrical storms in patients with ischemic cardiomyopathy. J Am Coll Cardiol 60(2):132–141
43. Krishnan SC, Josephson ME (2000) Surgery for postinfarction ventricular tachycardia: is it obsolete? Pacing Clin Electrophysiol 23:1295–1301
44. Spencker S, Coban N, Koch L, Schirdewan A, Muller D (2009) Potential role of home monitoring to reduce inappropriate shocks in implantable cardioverter defibrillator patients due to lead failure. Europace 11(4):483–488
45. Wilkoff BL, Auricchio A, Brugada J, Cowie M et al (2008) HRS/EHRA expert consensus on the monitoring of cardiovascular implantable electronic devices (CIED): description of techniques, indications, personnel, frequency and ethical considerations. Heart Rhythm 5(6):907–925. doi:10.1016/j.hrthm.2008.04.013
46. Ukena C, Bauer A, Mahfoud F, Schreieck J et al (2012) Renal sympathetic denervation for treatment of electrical storm: first-in-man experience. Clin Res Cardiol 101(1):63–67

Chapter 8
Dyssynchronous Heart Failure: From Bench to Bedside

Caroline J.M. van Deursen, Lars B. van Middendorp, and Frits W. Prinzen

Abstract Dyssynchronous heart failure (HF) has only recently been recognized as a specific entity of heart failure. It entails abnormal timing of electrical activation, which has a major impact on ventricular contraction, resulting in acute and chronic adaptations.

In this chapter, we first describe the pathophysiology of dyssynchrony in combination with the acute effects on heart function. Subsequently, the adaptive responses will be discussed, including structural, electrical, and contractile remodeling. Throughout the chapter we will link the results obtained in bench research to clinical practice.

Abbreviations

^{18}F-FDG	Fluorodeoxyglucose
AAI	Atrial pacing
AF	Atrial fibrillation
APD	Action potential duration
AV	Atrioventricular
BBB	Bundle branch block
Ca^{2+}	Calcium
CM	Cardiac memory
CREB	cAMP response element binding
CRT	Cardiac resynchronization therapy
CV	Conduction velocity
Cx43	Connexin43
DDD_R	Dual-chamber rate responsive pacing

C.J.M. van Deursen, M.D. • L.B. van Middendorp, M.D. • F.W. Prinzen, Ph.D. (✉)
Department of Physiology, Cardiovascular Research Institute Maastricht, University of Maastricht, P.O. Box 616, 6200 MD, Maastricht, The Netherlands
e-mail: frits.prinzen@maastrichtuniversity.nl

J. Bartunek and M. Vanderheyden (eds.), *Translational Approach to Heart Failure*,
DOI 10.1007/978-1-4614-7345-9_8, © Springer Science+Business Media New York 2013

ECG	Electrocardiogram
ECM	Extracellular matrix
HF	Heart failure
I_{CaL}	L-type calcium current
ICD	Implantable cardioverter defibrillator
ICTP	Carboxyterminal telopeptide of type I collagen
I^{k1}	Inward rectifier current
I^{kr}	Rapid rectifier current
I^{ks}	Slow rectifier current
I_{to}	Transient outward current
IVCD	Intraventricular conduction delay
K^+	Potassium
LBBB	Left bundle branch block
LV	Left ventricular
MBF	Myocardial blood flow
MMP	Matrix metallo proteinases
MRI	Magnetic resonance imaging
mRNA	Messenger RNA
MVO_2	Myocardial oxygen consumption
Na^+	Sodium
NCX	Sodium calcium exchanger
P/V	Pressure/volume
PET	Positron emmission tomograhy
PICP	Carboxyterminal propeptide collagen type I
PIIICP	Carboxyterminal propeptide collagen type III
PIIINP	Aminoterminal propeptide collagen type III
PINP	Aminoterminal propeptide collagen type I
PLN	Phospholamban
POH	Pressure overloaded hyperthrophy
RBBB	Right bundle branch block
RV	Right ventricular
SERCA2a	Sarcoplasmic reticulum CA^{2+} ATPase
SR	Sarcoplasmatic reticulum
TAVI	Transcathteter aortic valve implantation
TIMP	Tissue inhibitor metalloproteinases
VVI	Ventricular demand pacing
β_1-AR	β_1-Adrenergic receptor

1 Introduction

Dyssynchronous HF is a recently introduced term and relates to the condition that HF is accompanied with timing differences in electrical activation and/or contraction. The term dyssynchrony is not clearly defined. In many publications "asynchrony" refers to timing differences in electrical activation, whereas "dyssynchrony" often refers to mechanical timing differences. However, this difference is not used consistently throughout literature. Therefore, we use "dyssynchrony" in this chapter for both electrical and mechanical timing differences.

It is still not known whether dyssynchrony is caused by HF or the other way around. This lack of understanding is mainly due to the fact that most types of dyssynchrony, such as left bundle branch block (LBBB), develop silently and are accompanied by much comorbidity.

However, since cardiac resynchronization therapy (CRT) was introduced in 2000, it became clear that resynchronization reduces the burden of HF, thus supporting the idea that dyssynchrony may at least contribute to the development of HF. Moreover, during the last decade animal models have been developed were dyssynchrony is induced. The results from these models shed interesting light on the pathogenesis of dyssynchronous HF.

Hence, while CRT was applied in patients almost without any animal experiments, subsequent bench research has contributed significantly to the understanding of the underlying pathophysiology and helped to improve current treatment. Below we will discuss both clinical and experimental studies on dyssynchronous HF and CRT.

2 Prevalence and Prognosis

2.1 Prevalence

The interest in individuals with a bundle branch block (BBB) has primarily focused on its role as a predictor of mortality in patients with cardiovascular diseases. Most epidemiological data is therefore derived from hospitalized patients [1–5]. The prevalence of BBB depends on the population studied, ranging from approximately 1 % in a general hospital population to as high as 24 % in patients with symptomatic HF.

Only a few large epidemiological studies for the prevalence of BBB have been conducted in a general healthy, nonhospitalized population. The results varied a little between these studies, mainly because of differences in age and health status of the subjects. However, they all show that the prevalence of isolated BBB is relatively low and affects approximately 1 in every 1,000 subjects [6–11]. In healthy subjects right bundle branch block (RBBB) is more common than LBBB. The prevalence of a BBB markedly increases with age, from 0.1 % under the age of 45 to more than 1.0 % in the age group above 65 years [9]. This is further emphasized in a cohort of healthy airline personnel, both pilots and ground personnel, of the US Air Force where no case of isolated LBBB was found under the age of 25, but where prevalence increased to 3 per 10,000 subjects over the age of 35. The apparent rarity of LBBB in a group of medically healthy declared subjects indicates that LBBB is not an asymptomatic congenital abnormality but probably an acquired abnormality indicative of an underlying structural disease [10].

Besides intrinsic conduction abnormalities, also conventional right ventricular (RV) pacing causes disruptions in the normal electrical activation pattern and its adverse effects gained broad interest in the 1990s. However, a large amount of pacemakers are implanted each year for anti-bradycardia therapy, yet symptomatic HF in these patients is rare. The best estimate of the number of pacemakers implanted, comes from a worldwide cardiac pacing survey involving 61 countries and conducted in 2009 [12]. This review revealed that 737,840 new pacemakers were implanted, which was approximately 80 % of the worldwide implantation rate for 2009, thus leading to the conclusion that per year almost a million new pacemaker are implanted worldwide of which less than 5 % are CRT pacemakers.

2.2 Prognosis

In recent decades, there was some speculation concerning the importance of the electrocardiogram (ECG) as a prognostic marker in patients with HF. One of the first studies showed a fairly high mortality rate in HF patients with an increase in QRS duration [13], while later studies could not corroborate these findings [9, 11]. These conflicting results can, at least partly, be explained by differences in age, etiology of the underlying heart disease and criteria used for QRS prolongation/BBB. Nonetheless, overall it seems that QRS prolongation is an independent predictor of mortality in HF patients [2, 8, 14–21].

Subsequent research has shown that the ECG and the parameters derived therefrom such as QRS duration and morphology are important prognostic markers in heart disease. Even in patients without apparent structural heart disease the ECG contains prognostic value. For example, subjects with isolated LBBB without any underlying structural heart disease have a higher risk of sudden cardiac death compared to matched controls [22]. Likewise, patients with isolated LBBB are more susceptible to develop a total atrioventricular conduction block necessitating the implantation of a pacemaker [8].

Studies that additionally subdivided patients with a QRS prolongation into patients with LBBB, RBBB, and intraventricular conduction delay (IVCD) showed that the patients with LBBB have a strikingly higher mortality rate and have a higher risk of HF compared to patients with RBBB or IVCD [8, 14, 19]. Surprisingly, the risk of death is approximately the same for HF patients with RBBB and IVCD as compared to HF patients with a normal QRS duration [14]. These observations lead to the conclusion that LBBB has a more deleterious effect on the heart than RBBB and/or IVCD. The importance of LBBB is further accentuated by the effect of CRT on patients with LBBB. CRT partially restores the normal conduction in the left ventricle, antagonizing the effect of LBBB. In the MADIT-CRT study patients with LBBB that received an implantable cardioverter defibrillator (ICD), which does not restore normal conduction, had a worse prognosis than patients with RBBB or IVCD. However this difference was completely reversed in the groups treated by CRT (Fig. 8.1) [23].

The effect of conventional RV pacing on prognosis is clearly shown in a retrospective treatment comparison study of patients with sick sinus syndrome. A significantly higher incidence of permanent atrial fibrillation (AF) was found in patients

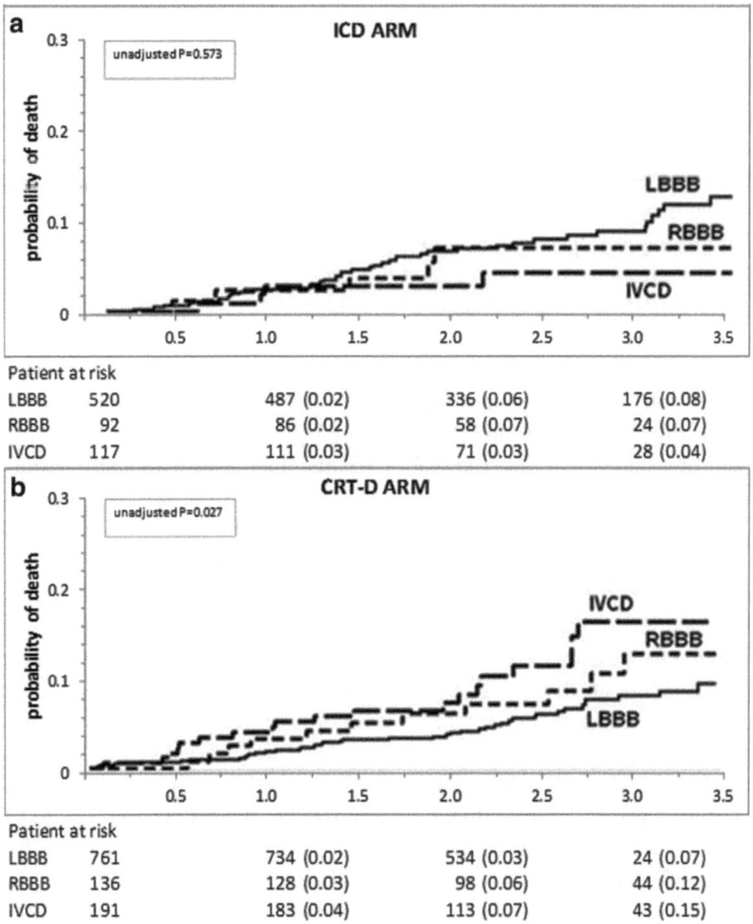

Fig. 8.1 Cumulative probability of death according to QRS morphology in the ICD arm (**a**) and CRT-D arm (**b**) of the multicenter automatic defibrillator implantation trial–cardiac resynchronization therapy (MADIT-CRT) [23]

treated with ventricular (VVI) pacing compared to atrial (AAI) pacing (47 % vs. 6.7 %) [24, 25]. Moreover, congestive HF occurred significantly more often in the VVI group than in the AAI group (37 % vs. 15 %). Even more important, overall mortality was significantly increased in the ventricular pacing group (23 % vs. 8 %) after an average follow-up period of 4 years.

Likewise, in a prospective study with sick sinus syndrome patients randomized to either atrial or ventricular pacing, overall survival was significantly higher in atrial pacing (relative risk 0.66 (95 % CI 0.44–0.99)) after a follow-up period of 8 years [26]. Survival from cardiovascular death was also significantly higher in atrial pacing (0.47 (0.27–0.82)). Furthermore, atrial pacing was associated with less AF, lower NYHA functional class with less increase during follow-up, less use of diuretics, and fewer thromboembolic complications than ventricular pacing [26, 27].

Initially it was considered that single-chamber ventricular pacing can interfere with AV synchrony. Dual-chamber (DDDR) pacing was developed 3 decades ago to restore AV synchronization. This led to an emphasis of AV synchronization in cardiac pacing, and DDDR was quickly adopted as the "physiologic" pacing mode. However, large randomized clinical trials in sinus or AV-nodal disease have reached a consensus that despite maintenance of AV synchrony, DDDR pacing does not reduce death compared with single-chamber ventricular pacing (VVIR) and has surprisingly modest or even negligible benefits for progression of HF and AF that emerge only after many years of follow-up [28–30].

Clearly, the benefit of preserving AV synchrony is outweighed by the detrimental effects of ventricular dyssynchronization during single site RV pacing. This was demonstrated in the MOST trial that studied a large population of sick sinus syndrome patients. A strong association between the percentage of ventricular pacing and the development of HF and AF was found [31]. With regard to this "dose" of dyssynchrony-dependent risk, the risk of HF also increases with augmenting paced QRS duration [32].

In perspective of the adverse effects of RV pacing, the DAVID trial showed even more detrimental effects on mortality and hospitalization for congestive HF. This was a randomized clinical trial where patients with an indication for ICD therapy and compromised left ventricular (LV) systolic function were assigned to have the ICDs programmed to ventricular backup pacing at 40/min (VVI-40) or dual-chamber rate responsive pacing at 70/min (DDDR-70). Dual-chamber pacing revealed a higher incidence of the combined endpoint of death or hospitalization for HF compared to ventricular backup pacing (26.7 % vs. 16.1 %) within 12 months [33]. Moreover, the adverse effects of dual-chamber pacing were larger in this study performed in patients with compromised LV systolic function compared to the MOST trial where LV systolic function was not compromised in patients, indicating that poor cardiac function as a substrate intensifies the adverse effects of RV pacing.

In conclusion, both morbidity and mortality are increased in patients with LBBB and long-term conventional RV apical pacing and the adverse effects seem to be larger when cardiac function is already compromised. Detrimental effects of LBBB and RV apical pacing are comparable, because the altered ventricular activation sequence that causes unidirectional wavefront propagation throughout the LV is similar in both conditions.

3 Pathophysiology of Dyssynchrony

3.1 Normal Electrical Impulse Conduction and Activation of the Ventricles

Ventricular contraction normally occurs in a highly coordinated fashion, caused by the rapid spread of electrical signals via the His–Purkinje fibers. The His bundle divides into right and left bundle branches that lie underneath the endocardium on the two respective sides of the ventricular septum. Each branch spreads downward to the apex of the ventricle, subdividing and becoming Purkinje fibers. From the ventricular apex, the Purkinje fibers course around the ventricular chamber and back towards the base of the heart. The Purkinje fibers penetrate about one third into the ventricular muscle mass towards the epicardial surface where they end in Purkinje-myocardial junctions [34]. The ventricles are thus activated from the apical region to the basal regions (ensuring efficient pump function) and from the endocardium to the epicardium [35, 36].

The Purkinje fibers have a particularly important quality; they transmit action potentials at high velocity (1.5–4.0 m/s, approximately 4 times faster than the ventricular muscle fibers). This enables an almost immediate transmission of the cardiac impulse throughout the entire remainder of the ventricular muscle. The rapid transmission of action potentials by Purkinje fibers is presumably the result of a high level of permeability in the gap junctions at the intercalated discs between the successive cardiac cells that make up the Purkinje fibers. Within just 30 ms after entering of the cardiac impulse into the bundle branches in the ventricular septum, the cardiac impulse reaches the terminations of the Purkinje fibers and excites the slower conducting ventricular muscle fibers [36].

The action potential triggers calcium (Ca^{2+}) influx through L-type calcium channels into the cardiac myocytes, initiating Ca^{2+}-induced Ca^{2+} release by the sarcoplasmatic reticulum (SR) [37]. The now abundant Ca^{2+} binds to troponine, causing tropomyosine to dislocate, by which it enables the myosine/actine cross-bridging of the sarcomere (contraction). The time needed for transport and binding of Ca^{2+} released from the SR, results in a time delay between the depolarization and onset of force development of approximately 30 ms [38].

Thus, it is because of the specialized rapid ventricular conduction system, that the ventricles are synchronously depolarizing and because of the excitation-contraction coupling, subsequently synchronously contracting. All portions of the ventricular muscle in both ventricles begin contracting at approximately the same time, by which effective ventricular pumping is achieved.

3.2 *Left Bundle Branch Block*

In case of LBBB, transmission of the cardiac impulse through the left bundle branch is blocked or at least significantly slowed down, resulting in slow cell-to-cell conduction via the ventricular muscle fibers (velocity of 0.3–0.5 m/s). The anatomically fixed or functional conduction block can be located at any segment of the left-sided intraventricular conduction system, from the fibers of the distal (or even proximal) His bundle to the main left bundle branch or both its subdivisions (it remains the question if the latter can be defined as complete LBBB). The result is that the RV is activated through the intact right sided Purkinje system, whereas the LV is not. The activation wavefront then spreads slowly through muscular conduction from the RV to the LV side of the septum and enters the LV endocardium at a septal or anterior

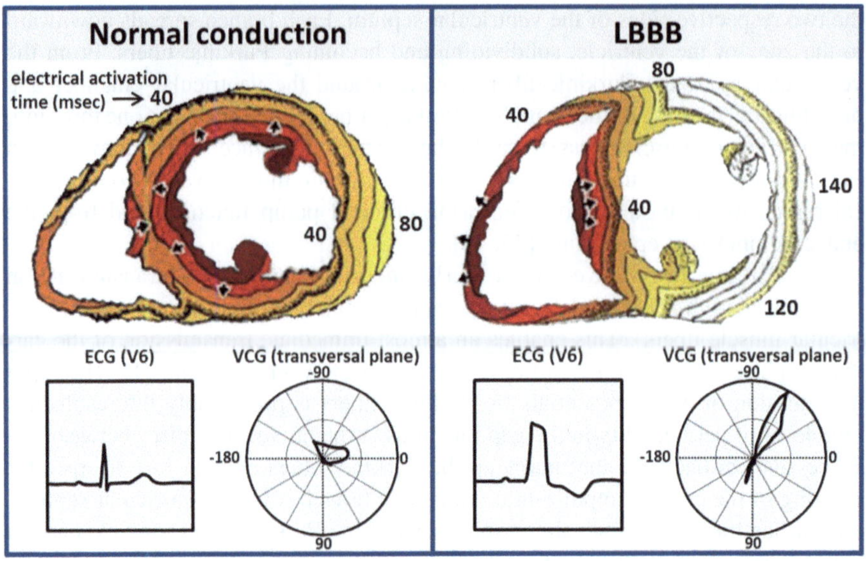

Fig. 8.2 Cross-section of ventricular electrical activation maps of a patient with normal conduction (*left*) and a patient with LBBB (*right*) [40]. Electrical activation starts at the *small arrows* and spreads in a wavefront, with each *colored line* representing successive 10 ms. Underneath, ECGs (lead V6) with corresponding VCGs (transversal plane) of a patient with normal ventricular conduction (*left*) and a patient with LBBB (*right*)

region, usually 40–70 ms later than the earliest RV activation (Fig. 8.2) [39]. Actually, one single LV endocardial breakthrough site with a right-to-left transseptal conduction time of 40 ms or more is a required condition for genuine complete LBBB [40]. Similarly, when pacing the RV, endocardial mapping revealed that virtually all patients have one single LV breakthrough site [41]. From the anteroseptal breakthrough site, the activation wavefront slowly proceeds to the lateral and posterolateral region of the LV endocardium (which takes approximately 50 ms because the electrical depolarization is not conducted in the rapid Purkinje system when it reaches the LV endocardium), ending at the basal region of the posterolateral wall near the mitral valve annulus [39, 42]. Finally, the LV posterolateral wall including the epicardial surface is activated within another 50 ms. In patients with HF, conduction capacities can be further depressed by variable degrees of injury and disarray in different layers and regions, caused by fibrosis, hypertrophy and cellular uncoupling or pathologic ion channel functioning.

The consequence of LBBB is that the RV and the septal part of the LV wall are activated, and thus contract, before the LV posterolateral wall, thereby causing a significant depression in the overall pumping effect [43]. The significance of the LBBB initiated depression in pump function is particularly apparent in patients with already compromised ventricular systolic function.

Interestingly, little is known about causal factors of LBBB, partly because it often has a silent onset and it is associated with widespread comorbidity. Myocardial infarction and LBBB as a complication of a surgical procedure are obvious causes, but these causes comprise only a minority of all LBBB cases. In most cases LBBB develops as a degenerative process, of which the cause is incompletely understood and its onset not known.

In an upcoming interventional technique for high-risk patients with aortic valve stenosis, transcatheter aortic valve implantation (TAVI), the proximal left bundle branch is damaged more frequently than with traditional surgical valve replacement, thereby inducing LBBB. While the incidence of permanent postoperative LBBB is 6 % for surgical aortic valve replacement, it ranges between 15 and 30 % for TAVI [44, 45]. Occurrence of TAVI-induced LBBB is influenced by prosthesis type, prosthesis implantation depth, and balloon/aortic annulus size ratio [45, 46]. Clearly, TAVI-induced LBBB cannot be regarded as a beneficial side effect, but it may be a very useful model to further unravel the consequences of LBBB in human hearts.

LBBB can be recognized by a prolonged QRS duration (slowness of impulse conduction) with a specific LBBB morphology on the surface ECG (Fig. 8.2). Recently, Strauss et al. proposed a minimum threshold of QRS duration for complete LBBB of ≥140 ms in men and ≥130 ms in women instead of the conventional threshold of 120 ms [40]. The need to prolong the threshold is because of the evidence that in human at least 140 ms is required to depolarize the heart in case of LBBB (40 ms for right-to-left transseptal activation + 50 ms for LV endocardial activation + 50 ms for activation of the posterolateral wall), while the threshold of 120 ms was based on observations in dogs. The sex-specific difference in threshold is postulated, because in general men have larger hearts that take longer to depolarize. Following this idea, QRS duration might also be normalized to LV mass, thereby possibly also accounting for the problem of prolonged QRS duration caused by LV hypertrophy mistaken for LBBB [40]. LBBB morphology is characterized by a negative QRS complex in V1 and a broad positive QRS complex in the lateral leads, because the depolarization potentials generated by the two ventricles appear sequentially and do not neutralize each other. Also, mid-QRS notching or slurring in the lateral leads (V5, V6, I, and avL) seems to be an important indicator of LBBB on the ECG [40]. The first peak of the notch represents the right-to-left transseptal activation, the gap represents the slow activation around the LV cavity and the second peak represents the endo- to epicardial posterolateral wall activation. Dyssynchronous contraction as with LBBB can also be recognized by echocardiographic imaging, by which a typical septal-to-lateral apical motion or "shuffle" pattern of the LV can be visually observed or abnormal measurements of contraction timing and paradoxal septal stretch can be revealed (see further in Sect. 3.4) [47–52].

3.3 Pacing-Induced Dyssynchrony

Almost any ventricular pacing disturbs the normal physiological sequence of electrical activation. Pacing at the conventional pacing site, the RV apex, causes an LV electrical activation pattern similar to that of LBBB [53]. Ectopically generated impulses rarely penetrate the rapid specialized conduction system, causing the activation sequence to spread slowly through the working myocardium and prolonging the time required for activation of the entire ventricular muscle [54]. Moreover, conduction velocity is slower because of its perpendicular direction to muscle fiber length (anisotropic conduction), instead of isotropic conduction (direction parallel to muscle fiber length) [55]. Besides, fibers close to the endocardial surface, even though not part of the Purkinje system, conduct impulses faster than the intramyocardial and epicardial fibers [56]. The difference with LBBB is, however, that during LBBB RV activation is normal whereas it is abnormal during RV pacing.

3.4 Regional Contraction Patterns and Myocardial Work

Dyssynchronous electrical activation of the ventricles, as during LBBB and ventricular pacing, is associated with dyssynchronous timing of contraction [38, 57]. In case of LBBB or RV apical pacing, LV septal regions are contracting early during systole, whereas LV posterolateral regions are contracting late. Quantification of the dyssynchrony as the timing differences in onset or peak of shortening was initially measured using M-mode (septum to posterior wall motion delay) or Tissue Doppler Imaging (peak velocity differences between two or more regions), later also using speckle tracking analysis [48–51]. However, such "mechanical dyssynchrony" proved not uniformly useful in selecting patients for CRT [58]. The explanation might be that there is an even more important effect of LBBB and RV apical pacing than just the shift in onset of contraction between various regions. Due to the mechanical interaction between the various regions in the ventricular wall, the shape of the contraction pattern also differs between regions. The early activated and contracting regions stretch the later activated ones, whereupon the latter show amplified and prolonged contraction [59, 60]. As a consequence, dyssynchronous activation leads to discoordination of contraction.

Initially, contraction patterns in dyssynchronous hearts have been explored using magnetic resonance imaging (MRI) tagging, by which deformation patterns and myocardial fiber strains can be measured. More recently, assessment of regional myocardial deformation is also possible by speckle tracking analysis on echocardiographic images. This technique tracks natural acoustic reflections or unique "speckle" patterns frame to frame and angle independent, producing 2D- and 3D-based images. Comparing circumferential strain patterns of septal to posterolateral LV wall regions, differences in time course and extent of shortening are relatively small during right atrial pacing [60]. During RV apical pacing on the other hand, septal regions show a rapid onset of shortening (negative strain) during the early systolic phase, which is followed by a rebound stretch and a second phase of shortening (Fig. 8.3). In posterolateral regions, considerable early systolic stretch is followed by pronounced shortening during the ejection phase. These different strain patterns during RV apical pacing change gradually when moving from the early (septal) to the late (posterolateral) activated regions [60].

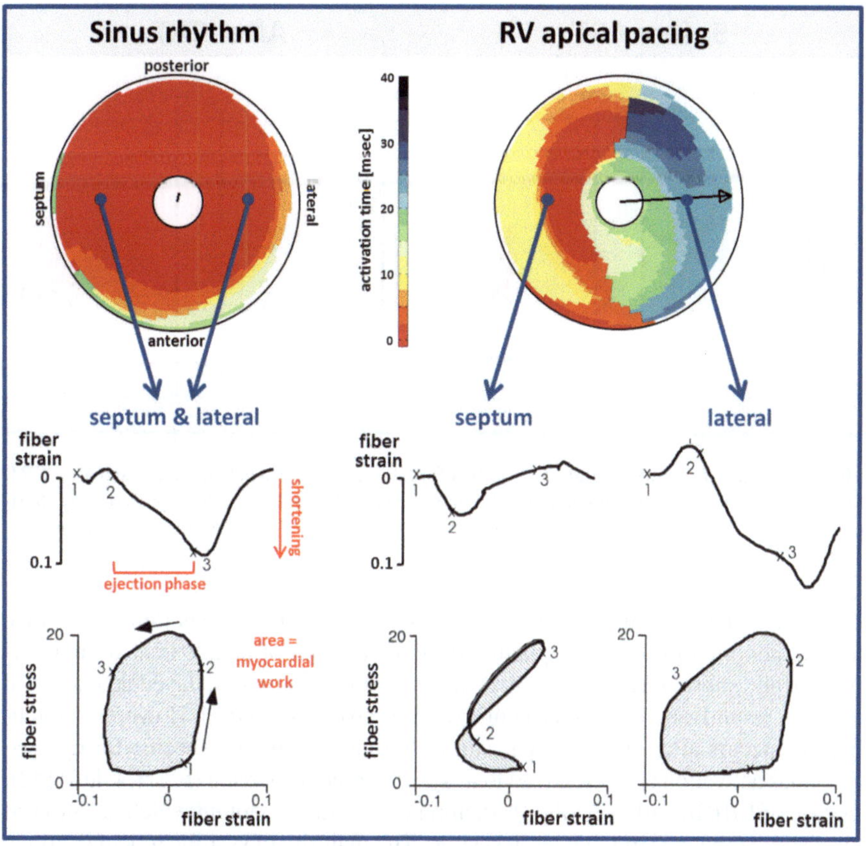

Fig. 8.3 LV endocardial activation maps acquired by noncontact mapping and septal and lateral strain patterns with corresponding fiber stress–strain loops of a healthy canine heart during intrinsic sinus rhythm (*left*) and RV apical pacing (*right*) [145]. Numbers 1, 2, and 3 indicate end-diastole, begin of ejection, and end of ejection respectively

The regionally different contraction patterns are presumably caused by regional differences in fiber (and sarcomere) length, induced by the dyssynchronous activation [61]. As with LBBB and RV apical pacing, the septum starts to shorten early and vigorously because the cavity pressure is still low and all other muscle fibers are passive. The opposing lateral LV free wall is being pre-stretched, because it is not yet activated and the force generated by the contracting septum pushes it outwards. The passive stretch in this area causes a lengthening of the myocardial fibers and as a consequence of the Frank–Starling mechanism, contraction (fiber length shortening) is stronger here. Therefore, the regional differences in contraction pattern during dyssynchronous activation are most likely caused by regional differences in effective local preload [61].

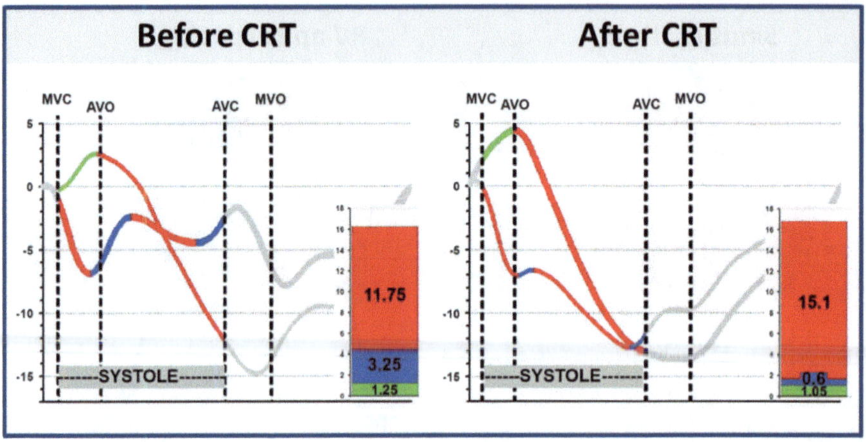

Fig. 8.4 Septal (*thick*) and lateral (*thin*) wall deformation curves in a patient before and after CRT. Systolic total shortening is depicted in *red*, systolic rebound stretch (stretching preceded by shortening) in *blue*, and systolic pre-stretch (early stretching not preceded by shortening) in *green* [52]

Instead of assessing timing differences of onset or peak shortening, cardiac motion abnormalities can be quantified by the amount of paradoxical stretch during systolic shortening. Systolic stretch is not only a cause of delayed activation, it can also result from regional ischemia or excessive loading [62]. However, stretching that occurs after initial early systolic shortening is highly specific for dyssynchronous activation and is referred to as systolic rebound stretch (Fig. 8.4; left) [52]. In case of LBBB, early systolic shortening occurs in the septum which is followed by systolic rebound stretch later in systole. The majority of systolic rebound stretch can thus be found in the septum in LBBB. Recently, it became clear that the measurement of septal systolic rebound stretch provides a better prediction of CRT response in terms of improvement in LV end-systolic volume than mechanical dyssynchrony [52]. This emphasizes the importance of abnormal wall motion patterns ("discoordination") in the pathophysiology of dyssynchronous HF.

Do these abnormal locally different contraction patterns also result in regional differences in myocardial work within the LV wall? The answer came from a study that explored regional myocardial work by constructing fiber stress–strain loops by which the loop area represented myocardial work [60]. Fiber stress was estimated using data on LV midwall deformation in combination with additional hemodynamic and structural data (LV cavity pressure and LV cavity to wall volume ratio). Myocardial strain was measured using MRI tagging. During RV apical pacing in a canine heart, the pattern of the stress–strain loop differed between early and late activated myocardial segments (Fig. 8.3). In early activated regions, contraction (fiber strain shortening) initially occurred at low fiber stress levels (the late activated region is not contracting yet), and subsequently, when the late activated regions are contracting, the fiber stress increases while fibers are being stretched, resulting in a figure-of-eight shaped loop. The net area of the stress–strain loop in early activated regions is almost zero, indicating low external work. In late activated regions, passive stretch in early systole (contraction of the early activated regions) generated increased stress before contraction, resulting in a wide loop with a large stress–strain loop area. Therefore, besides a different pattern in stress–strain loop between early and late activated regions, myocardial work is reduced in early activated regions, whereas it is augmented to values twice as high as normal in late activated regions [60, 63].

In HF patients, LV dilatation could increase regional mechanical nonuniformity that results from discoordinated activation with the potential consequence of further impairment in cardiac function. In a computational model of ventricular electromechanics it was shown that LBBB combined with LV dilatation synergistically increased nonuniformity in regional work and decreased regional cardiac function [64]. A possible explanation is that in the dilated heart, stress levels are increased and a larger variability of strain is needed to maintain force equilibrium when electrical dyssynchrony is included [64].

Regional differences in contraction patterns and mechanical load heterogeneity as a result of dyssynchronous activation can be corrected by ventricular resynchronization as obtained by biventricular pacing [52, 65–67]. The paradoxical systolic rebound stretch of the LV septum in LBBB is almost completely normalized after induction of CRT (Fig. 8.4; right), with a subsequent gain in septal shortening during systole.

3.5 *Effect of Dyssynchronous Activation on Blood Flow and Metabolism*

In patients with LBBB, other cardiovascular problems are common. Coronary artery disease can cause perfusion defects which can be detected by noninvasive myocardial imaging. However, in patients with LBBB, septal perfusion defects are frequently found even in the absence of any significant coronary artery disease [68–72]. The question is whether these differences are due to coronary artery disease or due to the abnormal contraction patterns.

To investigate regional myocardial blood flow (MBF) the microsphere deposition method can be used. After injection of radioactive or fluorescent-labeled microspheres, local deposition can be measured, thereby providing information on regional flow. During sinus rhythm in healthy canine hearts blood flow is homogenous and equally distributed. In contrast, MBF in dyssynchronous HF is heterogeneous with 20 % decrease in local MBF in the early activated regions and 20 % increased flow in late activated regions [43, 59, 73–75].

Closely related to MBF is myocardial oxygen consumption (MVO_2). Not surprisingly, MVO_2 shows a similar distribution as MBF in a dyssynchronous heart, where early activated regions show a reduction in MVO_2, whereas a near normal oxygen consumption is observed in the latest activated regions [73, 75]. Therefore, one theory is that the reduced perfusion in the septum of LBBB patients is due to redistribution of mechanical work, and so reduced demands in

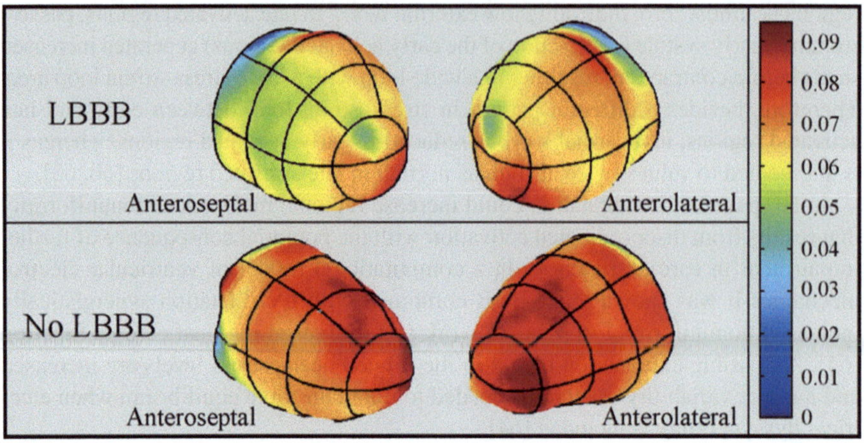

Fig. 8.5 Anteroseptal and anterolateral view of parametric 3-D myocardial oxygen consumption (MVO2) map in dilated cardiomyopathy with LBBB and without LBBB. MVO2 is more homogeneously distributed over the myocardial walls (septal-to-lateral ratio 0.96) in the non-LBBB than in the LBBB patient who exhibits a higher MVO2 in the lateral wall than in the septum (septal-to-lateral ratio 0.83). MVO2 (k2) is given in 1/min [76]

the septum. This hypothesis is confirmed in a quantitative study of MBF and MVO_2 in a group of HF patients with LBBB. Both MBF and MVO_2 are globally reduced in patients with HF. Moreover, in patients with HF and LBBB, MVO_2 is significantly higher in the lateral wall compared to the septum (Fig. 8.5) [76]. Another hypothesis says that the abnormal contraction may hamper blood flow by prolonging the systolic phase. Such an effect may be exaggerated when heart rate is higher, thereby becoming a possible explanation for exercise-induced angina in these patients.

The aforementioned changes in MBF and workload are paralleled by changes in metabolism. In dyssynchrony induced by RV pacing, glucose uptake in the septum is markedly reduced in a similar fashion as the redistribution of MBF [74]. In patients with LBBB, comparable defects are observed in glucose metabolism assessed by fluorodeoxyglucose (^{18}F-FDG) positron emission tomography (PET) imaging. PET images of metabolism in LBBB hearts display a relative reduction of glucose uptake in the septum. There are several hypotheses to explain the mechanism of reduced glucose uptake, but the underlying cause is still not well understood. In fact the hypotheses that are postulated for hampered glucose uptake in LBBB are probably also applicable to explain changes in MBF. It is speculated that glucose uptake is hampered by the abnormal depolarization or by a decrease in systolic function and augmented intramyocardial pressure during dyssynchrony [74, 77–79]. A caveat here is that glucose uptake is often displayed in relative terms, so it is not clear whether glucose uptake deficit in the septum is due to increased glucose uptake in the lateral wall or reduced uptake in the septum.

In line with a reduced metabolism in early activated regions, the genes that regulate metabolism are also downregulated, implying a reduction in local metabolic demand [80]. Besides regional changes in metabolism, a recent study indicates that long-term dyssynchrony in canine hearts leads to changes in the mitochondrial proteome, globally across the LV. Eventually, this leads to a decreased function of mitochondria [81]. Mitochondria are the major source of chemical energy in cells, but also play a role in apoptosis and cell differentiation.

Like abnormal systolic strains and work load normalize upon resynchronization, myocardial glucose metabolism, oxygen consumption, and perfusion homogenize as well by CRT [65, 82]. The improvement in oxygen supply/demand ratio may improve contraction and the lower oxygen consumption may also lead to less formation of oxygen radicals. CRT also restores alterations in gene expression to a near normal homogeneous expression profile [74, 80]. Besides, CRT partially restores the mitochondrial proteome by altering posttranslational enzymes involved in the Krebs cycle, thereby increasing ATP production and fuel efficiency [81]. This improvement in mitochondrial performance may be important in improving hemodynamics and cardiac function in dyssynchronous HF.

Thus redistribution of local work in dyssynchronous hearts leads to alterations in metabolism. This is reflected by changes in local oxygen demand, glucose uptake, and gene expression profile. All of which can be partially restored by resynchronization via CRT.

3.6 Hemodynamic Consequences

One can imagine that the wall motion abnormalities as observed in dyssynchronously activated hearts by LBBB or RV apical pacing can result in mechanical inefficiency (Fig. 8.6). Contraction of the anteroseptal regions of the LV wall in early systole results in pre-stretch of the still inactive posterolateral wall, rather than causing intracavitary pressure to rise and the mitral valve to close [83]. The abnormal septal motion not only results in a diminished contribution of the interventricular septum to LV ejection, it also jeopardizes the contractile efficiency of the opposing wall. After all, when the LV posterolateral wall finally contracts in late systole, it leads to a corresponding stretch of the anteroseptal region, instead of building up powerful aortic ejection and cardiac output. Contraction is not only discoordinated, but also prolonged, causing isovolumic phases to last longer, thereby diminishing effective ejection time and decreasing cardiac output [84].

Dyssynchrony also impairs the uniformity of the relaxation process, resulting in a delayed and prolonged relaxation process, which in turn decreases diastolic filling time [85]. The result is a decrease in preload- and length-dependent activation, which reduces contractile force and cardiac output. Also, the shorter effective diastole along with the prolonged systolic phase may hamper coronary perfusion, which may be especially relevant at higher heart rates. A further decline in cardiac pump function is generated by functional mitral regurgitation, caused by the delay in LV intracavitary pressure rise and discoordinated papillary muscle contraction [86, 87].

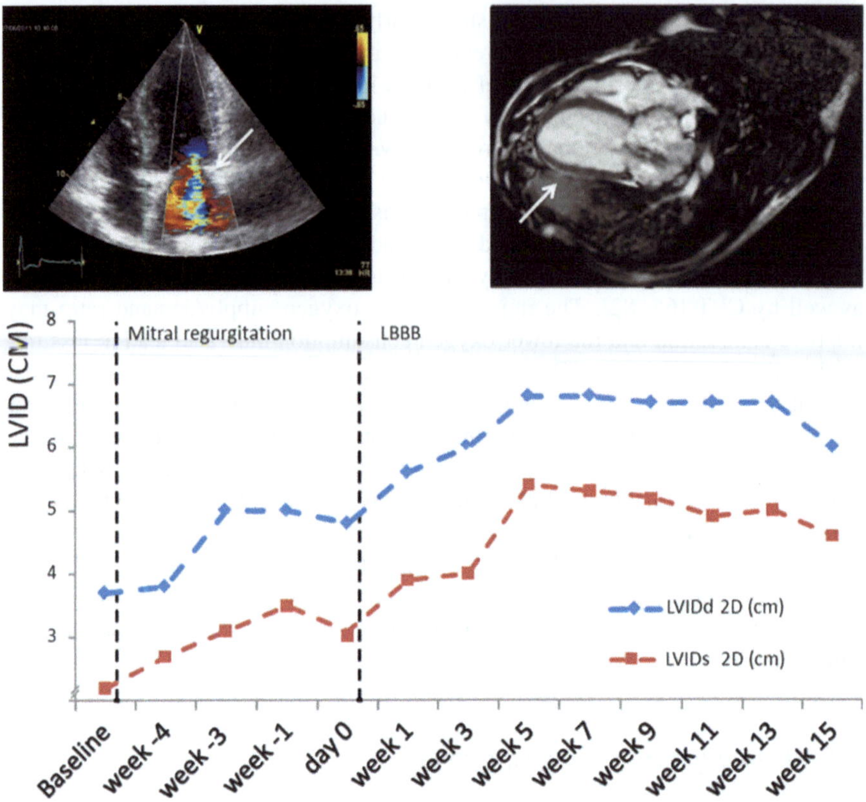

Fig. 8.6 *Top left*: echocardiographic image just after creation of mitral regurgitation, *arrow* is indicative of the site of mitral valve damage. *Top right*: MRI image after 15 weeks of mitral regurgitation and left bundle branch block, *arrow* clearly points out a mitral regurgitation jet. Note the enlarged atrium and signs of heart failure (pulmonary edema, pericardial effusion). *Bottom*: Biweekly echocardiographic follow-up of a canine with HF. HF is induced by creating mitral regurgitation. Four weeks later the left bundle branch is ablated. Note the steep increase in end-diastolic (LVIDd) and end-systolic internal diameter (LVIDs) of the left ventricle after superimposing LBBB upon mitral regurgitation

The effect of LV dyssynchrony on global systolic LV function can be perceived from LV pressure/volume (*P*/*V*) loop registrations. In dyssynchronous contracting ventricles induced by RV pacing, stroke volume is decreased as can be observed by the decreased width of the *P*/*V* loop in Fig. 8.7 [88–91]. In addition, the end-systolic *P*/*V* relationship is shifted to the right with an increase in end-systolic volume, causing an increase in the LV end-systolic wall stress.

When inducing LBBB in canine hearts, an immediate decrease in cardiac output without changes in LV end-diastolic pressure can be observed (Fig. 8.7) [43, 65]. LV dP/dt_{max}, the maximal rate of LV pressure rise and a sensitive marker of systolic function in stable cardiac loading conditions, declines as well. In addition, LV dP/dt_{min},

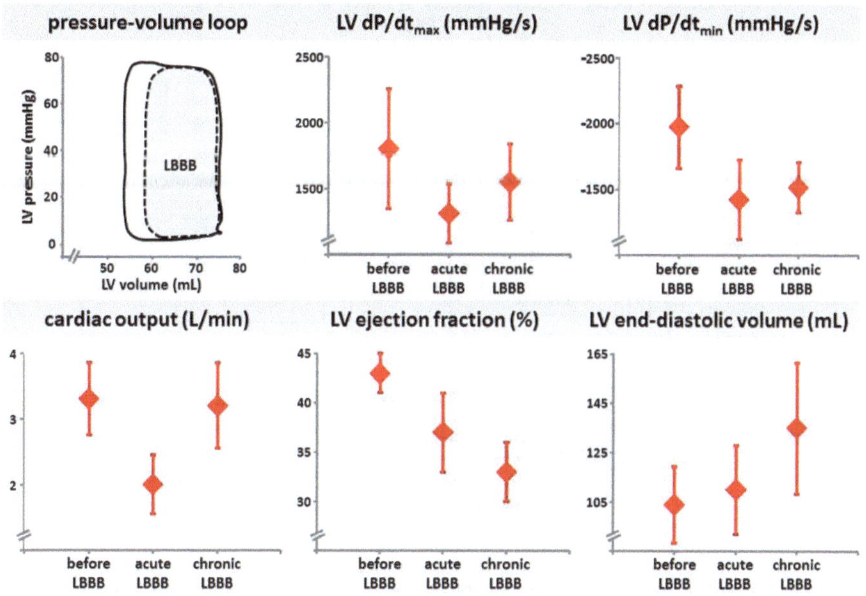

Fig. 8.7 *Left upper*: pressure/volume loop of a canine heart before (*solid line*) and after (*dashed line*) induction of LBBB. *Upper*: mean values of left ventricular (LV) dP/dt_{max} (the maximal rate of LV pressure rise) and LV dP/dt_{min} (the maximal rate of LV pressure decline), and *lower*: cardiac output, LV ejection fraction and LV end-diastolic volume of eight dogs before, acute (for LV ejection fraction and LV end-diastolic volume acute is within 2 weeks) and 16 weeks after induction of LBBB. Data derived from reference [43]

the maximal rate of LV pressure decline and a marker for diastolic function, decreases after induction of LBBB. Echocardiographic measurement of LV ejection fraction shows a significant decrease after 2 weeks of LBBB compared to baseline, with a further decline after 16 weeks of LBBB of 23 %. LV end-diastolic volume tends to increase after 2 weeks of LBBB, and shows a significant increase of 25 % after 16 weeks of LBBB. Cardiac output has normalized in chronic LBBB, while LV dP/dt_{min} and LV dP/dt_{max} are still decreased, although less than observed with acute LBBB. While cardiac output normalizes in chronic LBBB, the increase in LV end-diastolic volume indicates that this compensation is not effortless and without consequences [43]. Reduction in contractility and relaxation is also observed after initiation of RV apical pacing in humans [85, 92]. Hence, both systolic and diastolic LV function are compromised after induction of dyssynchronous activation as with LBBB and RV apical pacing.

From the above, it can be appreciated that dyssynchronous LV activation may at least contribute to the development of HF. This is further emphasized in a canine model where LBBB is superimposed on mitral regurgitation. These canine hearts show clear signs of HF on echocardiographic follow-up (Fig. 8.6). Also, the beneficial effects of resynchronization therapy supports the hypothesis that dyssynchrony

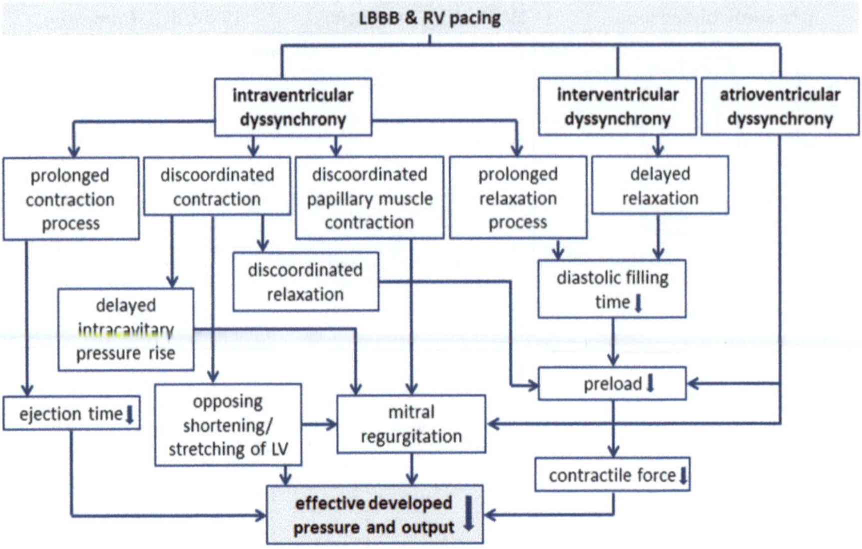

Fig. 8.8 Schematic overview of the pathophysiology of dyssynchronous activation on cardiac function. For details see text

contributes to the development of HF, because CRT immediately improves LV pump function and efficiency and it reverses the remodeling process in the long run in patients with HF in combination with LBBB [93–95]. However, LBBB might also be a consequence of poor cardiac function and ventricular dilatation, for example due to fibrosis and/or reduction in number of gapjunction proteins (connexins). Therefore, LBBB could either be the cause or the consequence of HF, this chicken-or-egg riddle remains unsolved, but in both cases a vicious circle is recognizable.

In patients with HF and LBBB, CRT can accomplish a more coordinated contraction by pacing the LV, thereby restoring inter- and intraventricular coupling. Besides this correction of CRT on dyssynchronous contraction in LBBB, biventricular pacing also reduce the amount of dyssynchrony in hearts without conduction abnormalities when compared to RV apical pacing. As can be appreciated from the schematic overview of how dyssynchronous activation leads to reduced contractile force and cardiac output (Fig. 8.8), one can understand the potential of CRT to reverse all the processes by restoring inter- and intraventricular coupling. The result is an improvement in systolic as well as diastolic function and a reduction of functional mitral regurgitation [93, 95–97]. The improvement in systolic LV function by CRT is achieved at unchanged or even decreased filling pressures, denoting a true improvement of ventricular contractility through improved coordination of contraction [67]. This is also indicated by a leftward shift of the end-systolic P/V relationship during CRT [97]. Furthermore, unlike the oxygen demanding inotropic effect of dobutamine, systolic augmentation with ventricular resynchronization increases LV dP/dt_{max} without increasing myocardial oxygen consumption (mechanical efficiency) [94]. A reduction in left-sided AV uncoupling can also be achieved by CRT, which may further improve diastolic performance and reduce functional mitral regurgitation. These acute beneficial hemodynamic effects of CRT may lead to even more beneficial long-term effects, because structural, electrical, and contractile remodeling consequences of dyssynchronous activation appear to be reversible, as will be discussed in the next sections.

4 Structural Remodeling

Dyssynchrony has been shown to decrease global heart function and to exacerbate HF in a variety of ways. Beside the abovementioned hemodynamic effects, there are a large number of relevant changes at tissue, cellular, and molecular levels that are induced by dyssynchrony. These "remodeling processes" can be divided into structural (muscle mass, fibrosis), electrical (ion channels), and contractile remodeling. As will be discussed below, some of the changes found in dyssynchronous heart can be observed as global up- or downregulation at the mRNA or protein level across the ventricles, whereas other substances show clear differences between early and late activated regions. This implies a very complex regulatory mechanism of remodeling under the influence of both local and global regulatory pathways. Recent studies showed that, in animals driven into HF by rapid RV pacing, rapid biventricular pacing improved EF only to a limited extent. However, biventricular pacing restores uniformity in gene expression and is actually capable of restoring some of the downregulated genes. These genes are involved in important processes such as metabolism, extracellular matrix remodeling, and stress responses. This indicates that strain distribution is a powerful initiator of absolute amount and distribution of gene expression [80, 98].

4.1 Regional Hypertrophy

The ventricular wall is capable of adapting to changes in work load by changing the extracellular matrix composition and hypertrophy of cardiomyoctes. It is not entirely clear which mechanisms are responsible to initiate these changes, but neurohumoral changes and cardiac load have been ascribed to play an important role.

In a canine model of chronic dyssynchrony, induced by pacing the LV free wall for 6 months, the LV showed asymmetrical hypertrophy. In this case, the late activated septum showed an increase in wall thickness after 6 months of pacing. The thickness of the wall segment closest to the pacing location on the other hand, did not change significantly [99]. Similar (opposite) regional hypertrophy was found in dogs where LBBB was induced by ablating the left bundle branch. LBBB induces asymmetric hypertrophy with an increase in wall thickness in the latest activated regions, the LV free wall [43]. The effect of dyssynchrony is further elucidated by inducing dyssynchrony in canine hearts with pressure overloaded hypertrophy (POH) due to constriction of the aorta for 6 months. RV pacing suppresses the POH-induced hypertrophy in the early activated septum, while no additional hypertrophy is observed in the latest activated regions [100].

The observations made in these experimental models are readily translational to the human situation. In patients with LBBB the effect of dyssynchronous activation on regional hypertrophy was qualitatively comparable to that observed in canine models although less pronounced, possibly due to the large heterogeneity and confounding factors such as pre-existing hypertrophy [72, 101].

The local changes in hypertrophy are probably related to the differences in contraction patterns. The more pronounced hypertrophy in the pre-stretched regions indicates that the local mechanical load is an important stimulus in the remodeling process. The potential of local mechanical load to induce hypertrophy is further supported by the fact that stretching of isolated myocytes induces a hypertrophic response [102].

Such hypertrophic response may be opposed by increased apoptosis of cardiac myocytes, as associated with the development of HF. Increased apoptosis is found in patients with dyssynchronous HF and is considered to play an important role in structural remodeling. Apoptosis leads to a lower wall thickness to volume ratio and thereby increases local mechanical stress. Treatment of dyssynchrony by CRT reduces apoptosis and thereby may reduce wall stress [103, 104].

Summarized, a change in local work load will lead to an adaptation of the ventricular wall to cope with the increased or decreased stress. This results in local changes in hypertrophy probably induced by difference in strain patterns.

4.2 *Extracellular Matrix Remodeling*

Cardiac fibrosis plays a major role in the progression of HF. In pathophysiological conditions decompensatory remodeling takes place, mainly by changes in collagen turnover, which ultimately leads to fibrosis [105]. Several biomarkers reflecting collagen synthesis seem useful for risk stratification in HF patients. Collagen type I and III are secreted as procollagens and mature collagen fibrils are formed by splitting off pro-peptides, releasing the aminoterminal (PINP and PIIINP) and carboxyterminal propeptides (PICP and PIIICP). Degradation of collagen type I forms the carboxyterminal telopeptide of type I collagen (ICTP). Breakdown of the extracellular matrix (ECM) is controlled by proteases of which matrix metalloproteases (MMP) and its tissue inhibitors (TIMP) are the most extensively studied [105–108].

In chronic dyssynchronous animal models no fibrosis has been observed [99]. In patients very few data on tissue content of fibrosis is present, although studies with small populations show an increase in collagen content in patients with dyssynchronous HF. Resynchronization by CRT reduces the collagen volume fraction in HF patients [104]. Furthermore, in patients with dyssynchronous HF treated by CRT the PICP/ICTP ratio in serum normalizes, thereby restoring the balance between collagen synthesis and degradation. Especially patients with high PICP levels at baseline, reflecting manifest fibrosis, respond to CRT [106]. MMP and TIMP levels did not change significantly to CRT [106, 107]. However, MMPs are one of the main determinants of ECM degradation and are important to identify HF patients who are at risk for adverse remodeling.

Nonetheless, the scarce observations of cardiac fibrosis in dyssynchronous heart failure must be interpreted with care since these are small observational studies. There is still a lot that is unknown and quite a few questions have to be resolved to translate these promising results from bench to bedside.

5 Electrical Remodeling

5.1 Conduction Velocity and Action Potential Duration

Chronic dyssynchrony has been shown to change conduction velocity (CV) and action potential duration (APD), two hallmarks of myocardial electrophysiology. These changes have been observed using in vitro analysis of wedges from canine hearts (Fig. 8.9). In these preparations conduction velocity (CV) was unchanged in wedges taken from the early activated regions of hearts with chronic LBBB. In contrast, the latest activated regions display a significant reduction in endocardial CV without apparent epicardial changes. At the same time connexin43 (Cx43), the main gap junction protein, is redistributed from the intercalated disks to the longitudinal membrane. In that way, Cx43 provides an etiological mechanism for the differences in conduction velocity. Interestingly, Cx43 redistribution is equal in endo- and epicardial tissue. Therefore, these alternations in cell-coupling cannot entirely explain the different changes in CV between endo- and epicardium [109]. In vivo studies could not corroborate the findings on CV, because in chronic dyssynchronous hearts neither regional differences nor reduction of endocardial CV was observed (Strik et al. Circ AE in press). A possible explanation could be alterations in myocyte connectivity, sodium current density, or cellular architecture due to tissue preparation for in vitro assessment of CV. On the other hand, distances along the endocardium are hard to measure precisely in vivo, making the estimations of CV less accurate.

Changes in APD are not consistent in dyssynchronous hearts [109, 110]. In wedge preparations from canine hearts with chronic LBBB, APD is shorter in the latest than in the earliest activated regions at both endo- and epicardium. Precisely opposite effects are found in myocytes isolated from canine hearts with HF caused by rapid LV pacing. In this model APD is markedly increased in the latest activated regions, whereas no changes are observed in early activated regions compared to control [111, 112]. Because prolongation of APD in the latest activated regions leads to pronounced dispersion of repolarization, the latter changes require further investigation. Of course repolarization is different in isolated cells compared to in vivo measurements because electrotonic potentials are different in isolated vs. coupled cells.

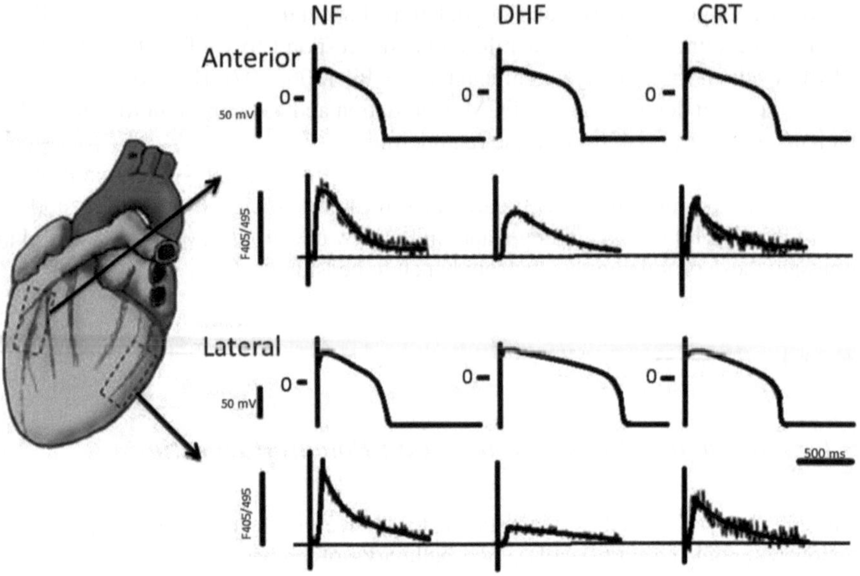

Fig. 8.9 Regional heterogeneity of action potential and Ca^{2+} transient (CaT) in dyssynchronous HF (DHF) and its restoration by CRT in early (anterior) and late (lateral) activated regions. CRT abbreviates DHF-induced prolongation of APD and restores amplitude and decay of CaT in the lateral cells, thus reduced regional heterogeneity of repolarization and Ca^{2+} handling [128]

In conclusion, in vitro observations clearly show changes in local conduction velocity and action potential duration. However these results still have to be validated in in vivo studies.

5.2 *Cardiac Memory*

In hindsight the first evidence of electrical remodeling due to dyssynchrony are the T-wave changes, observed when returning to normal sinus rhythm after a period of altered electrical activation sequence (cardiac memory (CM)) In general, the direction of the T-wave remains in the direction of the paced R-wave. This capability of the heart to "remember" the previous sequence of activation was first observed in a patient with rate-dependent LBBB, who was paced for 96 h at a rate where LBBB was continuously present. After cessation of pacing an inversion of T-wave was observed in all ECG leads [113].

T-wave changes on ECG can give varying results concerning the extent of cardiac remodeling, since different leads have distinct amplitudes and T-wave angles.

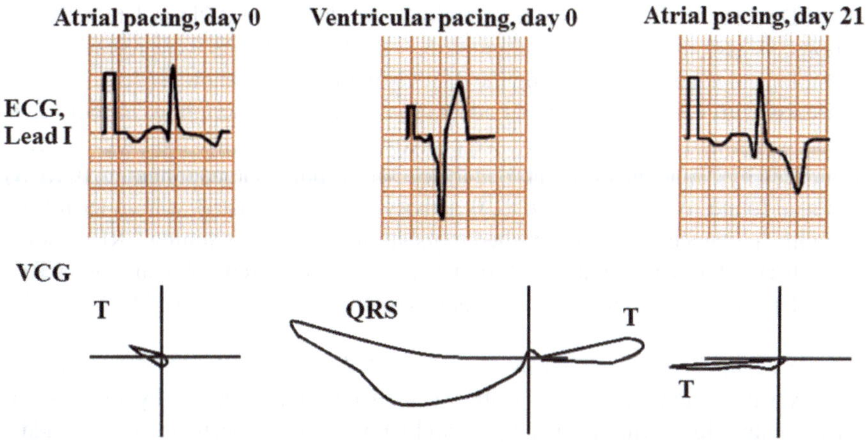

Fig. 8.10 Lead I of ECG and frontal plane VCG during atrial (*left*) and ventricular pacing (*middle*) at 130 beats/min of a dog at day 0 and during atrial pacing after 21 days of ventricular pacing (*right*). Note that on day 21 there are (1) rotation of the average T-wave vector in the direction of the paced QRS, (2) an increase in the average T vector amplitude, and (3) displacement of the average T vector from its control position [115]

This limits any form of quantification in a single lead. Vectorcardiography avoids these problems, since its combines the information of all ECG leads, and therefore gives accurate information on CM. The vector of "learned" T-waves tracks the vector of the altered QRS complex. In addition to the change in vector angle, the amplitude increases when CM evolves (Fig. 8.10) [114, 115].

In vivo canine studies have provided experimental information on CM for short-term (minutes to hours) and long-term (2–5 weeks) CM. Most experimental data is obtained by pacing the LV epicardium. Pacing for 2–3 weeks showed marked T-wave changes, which returned to normal within 1 month after cessation of pacing. Normalization of the T-wave took at least twice as long when the heart was paced for 4–5 weeks. This suggests a cumulative learning effect and a continuous adaptation process.

Patients who receive RV pacing for the treatment of sick sinus syndrome show a comparable evolution of CM, although the development of CM in humans is more rapid and more homogeneous between patients. This difference is possibly explained by a higher percentage of full capture in patient studies compared to canine studies [116]. Interestingly, in patients who receive CRT, signs of CM are already present within the first 24 h. Repolarization continues to adapt in the first 2 weeks following CRT treatment. CRT and RV pacing both show CM although T vector changes are less pronounced in CRT. Indeed both pacing modalities clearly show that the T-wave tracks the paced QRS vector. Therefore CM seems to be a consistent cardiac response even when heart failure is present.

The abnormal T-wave may be explained at least in part by changes in APD. Costard-Jäckle et al. showed in rabbit hearts that development of CM is accompanied by APD increases in early activated regions and decreased APD in late activated regions, as also mentioned in paragraph 5.1. Such adaptations were regarded as a physiological adaptation, reducing the dispersion in repolarization [117].

Hearts with CM display several adaptations in gene transcription. Initially, evidence was found that I_{CaL} and I_{to} were involved. Interestingly, the latter appears influenced by Angiotensin II. Later on the cAMP response element binding (CREB) was also found to be involved. CREB activity is downregulated in long-term CM, providing evidence for the diminished translation of genes containing CRE regions. The observed downregulation of transient outward current (I_{to}) and its CRE-dependent genes (see below) provide confirmation of this hypothesis. More recently, several studies provided evidence that CM is initiated by mechanical stimuli. CM can, for example, be prevented by venting the LV cavity during LV pacing in rabbits, by which ventricular load is almost abolished. Furthermore, by suppressing active contraction during LV pacing using blebbistatin also decreases CM. In addition, applying differences in pressure by in- or deflating a balloon in the LV cavity alters CM [118]. Besides the effects of load, pressure, and contractility, stretch is known to influence CM. This was proven by streptomycin, a stretch/activated channel blocker, which prevents the occurrence of CM.

Recapitulated, such an involvement of mechanics in CM is highly interesting, because, as described earlier, different activation patterns are known to alter local stress–strain relationships in the myocardium. Therefore, it has been suggested that dyssynchrony may not only lead to abnormal electro-mechanics, but that this is accompanied by a mechano-electrical coupling, leading to repolarization changes. This has been observed as reduction in T-wave amplitudes during longer lasting RV pacing and LBBB.

5.3 Potassium Handling

Ion channels and currents are important to create an action potential and are thereby key regulators of cardiac electrical activity. Ion channel remodeling underlies many of the cellular electrophysiological changes in HF. Many changes are initially adaptive, for example increase in APD during bradycardia increases contractility. However, long-term effect of these adaptations may be detrimental for heart function and make the heart more susceptible for arrhythmias [110, 111, 119]. Ca^{2+}channels play a key role in contraction and are therefore described below, together with changes in contractile remodeling. Sodium channels are hardly affected by dyssynchrony and are therefore not included in this chapter.

Potassium (K^+) plays a key role in repolarization. Downregulation of K^+ currents is the most consistent finding in human HF as well as in animal models of HF. The most consistent finding is a decrease in transient outward current and a decrease in its related CRE-dependent genes; Kv4.3 and KChIP2. I_{to} is downregulated homogeneously across the ventricles in HF [110, 111, 119, 120]. Although I_{to} only transiently opens during the action potential, it is a major contributor to the ventricular

APD and action potential shape [121]. In HF less robust alterations of the inward rectifier current (I_{k1}) are found. I_{k1} is important in maintaining the membrane resting potential and during phase 3 (late repolarization) of the action potential. In rabbits with HF induced by rapid pacing of the LV apex, no changes were found in I_{k1} densities [122, 123]. In contrast, canines with HF induced by rapid pacing of the RV apex, a small but significant difference can be found in I_{k1} density [111, 120, 121]. This difference is likely due to variability in duration and severity of the induced HF.

The delayed rapid and slow rectifier currents (I_{kr} and I_{ks}) are relevant for the repolarization phase. I_{kr} is not significantly altered due to HF. I_{ks} is consistently downregulated in HF and possibly plays a role in the increased APD seen in HF [111, 119, 120, 124, 125].

In the animal model of rapid pacing dyssynchronous HF all potassium channels are uniformly affected across the LV. The distribution of I is not altered by treatment with CRT, whereas I_{k1} and I_{ks} adaptations are partially restored by CRT. This suggests that remodeling of potassium channels is not only related with mechanical stress caused by dyssynchronous activation, but also under the influence of neurohumoral and autonomic control [111].

To conclude, changes in potassium channels observed in dyssynchronous heart failure are likely not only the result of dyssynchronous activation but attributable to heart failure in itself. Resynchronization only partly restores potassium handling implying that neurohumoral and autonomic adaptational processes activated by heart failure are responsible for the alterations observed and not local work.

6 Contractile Remodeling

6.1 Calcium Handling

Ca^{2+} plays an important role in excitation-contraction coupling, as can be appreciated from Sect. 3. Ca^{2+} is removed from to the extracellular space through the sodium (Na^+)–Ca^{2+} exchanger (NCX) and simultaneously pumped back into the sarcoplasmic reticulum primarily via the sarcoplasmic reticulum Ca^{2+} ATPase (SERCA2a) [119]. The changes in Ca^{2+} handling caused by HF have important consequences for contractility and arrhythmogenity.

Contractility is generally reduced in HF, but remarkably, L-type calcium current (I_{CaL}) density is not altered [126]. Nevertheless, in failing canine hearts the number of I_{CaL} channels is markedly reduced. To compensate for the loss of I_{CaL} channels, channel opening times are considerably increased, so total I_{CaL} density can be maintained [126, 127]. Dyssynchrony causes regional changes in I_{CaL} with a reduced density and slowed current decay in the late activated regions. In contrast, peak I_{CaL} density is increased in the early activated regions. CRT partially restores these differences, eliminating the anterior to lateral density gradient (Fig. 8.11) [128].

The molecular bases of the changes in Ca^{2+} handling are incompletely understood and often conflicting results are found. The complexity is emphasized by

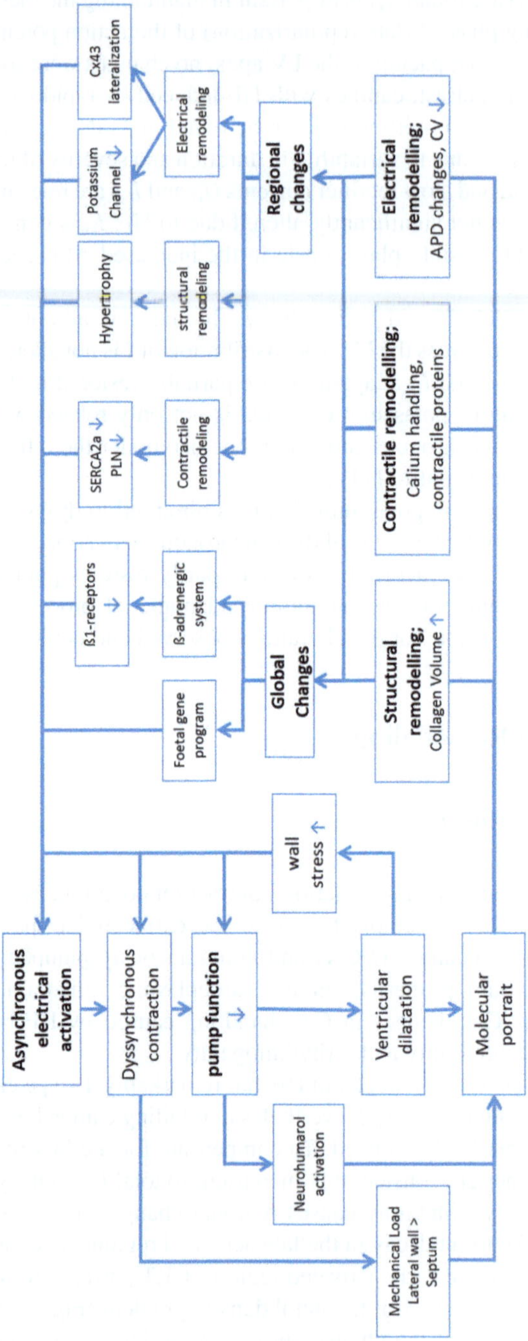

Fig. 8.11 Schematic overview of the remodeling processes addressed in this chapter

studies reporting isoform switching of the I_{CaL} subunits, α1C and β. In the end these alterations probably contribute to a decrease in contractility but further research is needed [129, 130].

NCX is found to be upregulated in HF, which may be explained by the fact that increased NCX activity compensates for depressed SERCA activity. The loss of SERCA function is further exacerbated by reduced phosphorylation of phospholamban (PLN), a small regulatory molecule of SERCA2a. This further impairs SERCA2a function, decreasing the exchange of Ca^{2+} from the cytoplasm to the SR. The changes in NCX, SERCA2a, and PLN ultimately lead to a lower and slower Ca^{2+} transient, and thus weaker contraction accompanied by a prolonged action potential [111, 119, 131, 132]. At the same time, during diastole, Ca^{2+} removal from the cytosol is impaired leading to a slower relaxation. This may ultimately lead to diastolic HF. SERCA2a messengerRNA (mRNA) is upregulated after treatment of HF by LV assist devices or beta-blocker therapy and is associated with improved contractility. In humans treated with CRT, SERCA2a/PLN and, SERCA2a/NCX ratios are increased as compared to before CRT, suggesting that resynchronization may restore calcium handling and thereby improve contractility [133, 134].

Thus calcium handling plays an important role in contractility and APD. Dyssynchrony leads to local adaptations of the Ca^{2+} channels but with a remarkable reserve capacity. However, contractility and relaxation are markedly altered, which ultimately results in diastolic heart failure.

6.2 *β-Adrenergic Receptors*

Almost 5 decades ago it was believed that the β_1-adrenergic receptor (β_1-AR) was specific for cardiac tissue and that the β_2-AR was only present in vascular and bronchial structures. Since then more and more of the cardiac β-adrenergic system was discovered, revealing a complex organization of not only β_1 and β_2-ARs in the heart but also β_3 and possibly β_4-ARs [135, 136].

Stimulation of β_1-AR activates the effector enzyme adenylyl cyclase, which in turn increases the cAMP levels augmenting the phosphorylation via cAMP-dependent protein kinases of several Ca^{2+} regulating proteins, which has positive inotropic, chronotropic, and lusitropic (relaxation) effects [137]. β_2-AR stimulation has many similarities with β_1-AR stimulation, such as its inotropic and lusitropic function, but also has some unique features. Selective stimulation of β_1-ARs with a β-agonist isoprenaline in knockout mice for β_2-AR causes higher mortality and increases apoptosis of myocytes compared to wild-type mice. This suggests a cardiac protective anti-apoptotic effect of β_2-AR stimulation, whereas β_1-AR promotes apoptosis [136, 138, 139].

In HF the sympathetic system is activated strongly and this stimulation is inversely correlated with survival. High catecholamine levels downregulate β-ARs, in particular the β_1-AR [137, 140]. The mechanism behind this specific downregulation of β_1-AR remains elusive. Current therapies, such as β-blockade, angiotensin converting enzyme inhibition and assist devices, decrease the sympathetic drive.

At first instance CRT for dyssynchronous HF does not seem to have a direct effect on neurohormones, as β-blockers do, or loading conditions of the heart, like an assist device does. Surprisingly, CRT improves the β-adrenergic reserve. This improvement is attributable to the effect of CRT on local contraction and indirectly local load. The changes in contraction could lead to activation of signaling pathways of β-AR and the upregulation of β-AR density to near normal levels, thereby increasing contractility and decreasing apoptosis. In addition, CRT reduces sympathetic drive [141–143].

Summarized, heart failure increases the sympathetic drive which acutely may have a beneficial effect but in the end leads to a higher mortality rate. Current medical therapy aims at decreasing the sympathetic drive. Remarkably, CRT also influences the sympathetic drive by decreasing local load and remodeling of β-AR.

7 Future Perspectives

The deleterious effects of dyssynchrony only became acknowledged since the treatment of HF patients with CRT. Interestingly, treatment was started without fully understanding the pathophysiological background of dyssynchrony. Later bench research, especially in animal models of dyssynchrony, began to uncover the complex pathology of this disease. Molecular and genetic pathways are currently being revealed. Uncovering these pathways will hopefully lead to a better understanding of the disease and a better selection of patients who benefit from treatment. Therefore, dyssynchronous HF is quite unique in the sense that it has first become recognized and treated at the bedside, while mechanistic insight was improved by bench research, data from which are in the process of again being translated to the bedside.

Up till now it is often unknown if dyssynchrony is a cause or a consequence of HF in patients. This is because dyssynchrony has a silent onset and often is only first diagnosed when patients present themselves with other comorbidities. TAVI, a new and upcoming technique for treating aortic valve stenosis, can help to solve this chicken-or-egg riddle in humans, since the onset of dyssynchrony is exactly known in case of the (unintended and unwanted) development of LBBB. Again this bedside research will aid in subsequent bench research.

8 Sources of Further Information

In this chapter the highlights of the pathophysiology of dyssynchrony are addressed. For more detailed information on specific subjects, some interesting articles are mentioned below. The authors of these articles are well known for their work in the dyssynchrony field.

- Strauss et al. [40] for better understanding true ECG markers for left ventricular dyssynchrony.
- Prinzen et al. [60] describes the correlation between local strain patterns and MBF.

- Aiba et al. [111] give a very detailed overview of electrophysiological consequences of heart failure and dyssynchrony.
- Vanderheyden et al. [134] and Spragg et al. [144] are one of the first to shed some light on the molecular and genetic portrait of dyssynchrony and its normalization after treatment with CRT.

References

1. Boyle DM, Fenton SS (1966) Left bundle branch block. Ulster Med J 35(1):93–99
2. Hawkins NM et al (2007) Prevalence and prognostic impact of bundle branch block in patients with heart failure: evidence from the CHARM programme. Eur J Heart Fail 9(5):510–517
3. Johnson RP et al (1951) Prognosis in bundle branch block. II. Factors influencing the survival period in left bundle branch block. Am Heart J 41(2):225–238
4. Smith S, Hayes WL (1965) The prognosis of complete left bundle branch block. Am Heart J 70:157–159
5. Sumner G et al (2009) The prognostic significance of bundle branch block in high-risk chronic stable vascular disease patients: a report from the HOPE trial. J Cardiovasc Electrophysiol 20(7):781–787
6. Dhingra R et al (2006) Electrocardiographic QRS duration and the risk of congestive heart failure: the Framingham Heart Study. Hypertension 47(5):861–867
7. Eriksson P et al (1998) Bundle-branch block in a general male population: the study of men born 1913. Circulation 98(22):2494–2500
8. Eriksson P, Wilhelmsen L, Rosengren A (2005) Bundle-branch block in middle-aged men: risk of complications and death over 28 years. The Primary Prevention Study in Goteborg, Sweden. Eur Heart J 26(21):2300–2306
9. Fahy GJ et al (1996) Natural history of isolated bundle branch block. Am J Cardiol 77(14):1185–1190
10. Hiss RG, Lamb LE (1962) Electrocardiographic findings in 122,043 individuals. Circulation 25:947–961
11. Rotman M, Triebwasser JH (1975) A clinical and follow-up study of right and left bundle branch block. Circulation 51(3):477–484
12. Mond HG, Proclemer A (2011) The 11th world survey of cardiac pacing and implantable cardioverter-defibrillators: calendar year 2009—a world Society of Arrhythmia's project. Pacing Clin Electrophysiol 34(8):1013–1027
13. Unverferth DV et al (1984) Factors influencing the one-year mortality of dilated cardiomyopathy. Am J Cardiol 54(1):147–152
14. Baldasseroni S et al (2002) Left bundle-branch block is associated with increased 1-year sudden and total mortality rate in 5517 outpatients with congestive heart failure: a report from the Italian network on congestive heart failure. Am Heart J 143(3):398–405
15. Brenyo A, Zareba W (2011) Prognostic significance of QRS duration and morphology. Cardiol J 18(1):8–17
16. Iuliano S et al (2002) QRS duration and mortality in patients with congestive heart failure. Am Heart J 143(6):1085–1091
17. Kashani A, Barold SS (2005) Significance of QRS complex duration in patients with heart failure. J Am Coll Cardiol 46(12):2183–2192
18. Kearney MT et al (2003) Cardiac size, autonomic function, and 5-year follow-up of chronic heart failure patients with severe prolongation of ventricular activation. J Card Fail 9(2):93–99
19. Schinkel AF et al (2009) Prognostic significance of QRS duration in patients with suspected coronary artery disease referred for noninvasive evaluation of myocardial ischemia. Am J Cardiol 104(11):1490–1493

20. Shamim W et al (1999) Intraventricular conduction delay: a prognostic marker in chronic heart failure. Int J Cardiol 70(2):171–178
21. Silvet H et al (2001) Prognostic implications of increased QRS duration in patients with moderate and severe left ventricular systolic dysfunction. Am J Cardiol 88(2):182–185, A6
22. Rabkin SW, Mathewson FL, Tate RB (1982) The electrocardiogram in apparently healthy men and the risk of sudden death. Br Heart J 47(6):546–552
23. Zareba W et al (2011) Effectiveness of cardiac resynchronization therapy by QRS morphology in the multicenter automatic defibrillator implantation trial-cardiac resynchronization therapy (MADIT-CRT). Circulation 123(10):1061–1072
24. Rosenqvist M, Brandt J, Schuller H (1986) Atrial versus ventricular pacing in sinus node disease: a treatment comparison study. Am Heart J 111(2):292–297
25. Rosenqvist M, Brandt J, Schuller H (1988) Long-term pacing in sinus node disease: effects of stimulation mode on cardiovascular morbidity and mortality. Am Heart J 116(1 Pt 1):16–22
26. Andersen HR et al (1997) Long-term follow-up of patients from a randomised trial of atrial versus ventricular pacing for sick-sinus syndrome. Lancet 350(9086):1210–1216
27. Nielsen JC et al (1998) Heart failure and echocardiographic changes during long-term follow-up of patients with sick sinus syndrome randomized to single-chamber atrial or ventricular pacing. Circulation 97(10):987–995
28. Connolly SJ et al (2000) Effects of physiologic pacing versus ventricular pacing on the risk of stroke and death due to cardiovascular causes. Canadian Trial of Physiologic Pacing Investigators. N Engl J Med 342(19):1385–1391
29. Lamas GA et al (2002) Ventricular pacing or dual-chamber pacing for sinus-node dysfunction. N Engl J Med 346(24):1854–1862
30. Toff WD, Camm AJ, Skehan JD (2005) Single-chamber versus dual-chamber pacing for high-grade atrioventricular block. N Engl J Med 353(2):145–155
31. Sweeney MO et al (2003) Adverse effect of ventricular pacing on heart failure and atrial fibrillation among patients with normal baseline QRS duration in a clinical trial of pacemaker therapy for sinus node dysfunction. Circulation 107(23):2932–2937
32. Sweeney MO, Hellkamp AS (2006) Heart failure during cardiac pacing. Circulation 113(17):2082–2088
33. Wilkoff BL et al (2002) Dual-chamber pacing or ventricular backup pacing in patients with an implantable defibrillator: the Dual Chamber and VVI Implantable Defibrillator (DAVID) Trial. JAMA 288(24):3115–3123
34. Massing GK, James TN (1976) Anatomical configuration of the His bundle and bundle branches in the human heart. Circulation 53(4):609–621
35. Spach MS, Barr RC (1975) Ventricular intramural and epicardial potential distributions during ventricular activation and repolarization in the intact dog. Circ Res 37(2):243–257
36. Durrer D et al (1970) Total excitation of the isolated human heart. Circulation 41(6):899–912
37. Johnson RG Jr, Kranias EG (1998) Cardiac sarcoplasmic reticulum function and regulation of contractility. Introduction. Ann N Y Acad Sci 853:xi–xvi
38. Prinzen FW et al (1992) The time sequence of electrical and mechanical activation during spontaneous beating and ectopic stimulation. Eur Heart J 13(4):535–543
39. Auricchio A et al (2004) Characterization of left ventricular activation in patients with heart failure and left bundle-branch block. Circulation 109(9):1133–1139
40. Strauss DG et al (2008) ECG quantification of myocardial scar in cardiomyopathy patients with or without conduction defects: correlation with cardiac magnetic resonance and arrhythmogenesis. Circ Arrhythm Electrophysiol 1(5):327–336
41. Vassallo JA et al (1986) Left ventricular endocardial activation during right ventricular pacing: effect of underlying heart disease. J Am Coll Cardiol 7(6):1228–1233
42. Vassallo JA et al (1984) Endocardial activation of left bundle branch block. Circulation 69(5):914–923
43. Vernooy K et al (2005) Left bundle branch block induces ventricular remodelling and functional septal hypoperfusion. Eur Heart J 26(1):91–98

44. Piazza N et al (2010) Persistent conduction abnormalities and requirements for pacemaking six months after transcatheter aortic valve implantation. EuroIntervention 6(4):475–484
45. Aktug O et al (2012) Incidence and predictors of left bundle branch block after transcatheter aortic valve implantation. Int J Cardiol 160(1):26–30
46. Nuis RJ et al (2011) Timing and potential mechanisms of new conduction abnormalities during the implantation of the Medtronic CoreValve System in patients with aortic stenosis. Eur Heart J 32(16):2067–2074
47. Jansen AH et al (2007) Qualitative observation of left ventricular multiphasic septal motion and septal-to-lateral apical shuffle predicts left ventricular reverse remodeling after cardiac resynchronization therapy. Am J Cardiol 99(7):966–969
48. Pitzalis MV et al (2002) Cardiac resynchronization therapy tailored by echocardiographic evaluation of ventricular asynchrony. J Am Coll Cardiol 40(9):1615–1622
49. Bax JJ et al (2004) Left ventricular dyssynchrony predicts response and prognosis after cardiac resynchronization therapy. J Am Coll Cardiol 44(9):1834–1840
50. Yu CM et al (2004) Tissue Doppler imaging is superior to strain rate imaging and postsystolic shortening on the prediction of reverse remodeling in both ischemic and nonischemic heart failure after cardiac resynchronization therapy. Circulation 110(1):66–73
51. Gorcsan J III et al (2007) Combined longitudinal and radial dyssynchrony predicts ventricular response after resynchronization therapy. J Am Coll Cardiol 50(15):1476–1483
52. De Boeck BW et al (2009) Septal rebound stretch reflects the functional substrate to cardiac resynchronization therapy and predicts volumetric and neurohormonal response. Eur J Heart Fail 11(9):863–871
53. Lister JW et al (1964) Effect of pacemaker site on cardiac output and ventricular activation in dogs with complete heart block. Am J Cardiol 14:494–503
54. Spach MS, Barr RC (1975) Anaylsis of ventricular activation and repolarization from intramural and epicardial potential distributions for ectopic beats in the intact dog. Circ Res 37(6):830–843
55. Spach MS et al (1981) The discontinuous nature of propagation in normal canine cardiac muscle. Evidence for recurrent discontinuities of intracellular resistance that affect the membrane currents. Circ Res 48(1):39–54
56. Myerburg RJ et al (1978) The role of canine superficial ventricular muscle fibers in endocardial impulse distribution. Circ Res 42(1):27–35
57. Wyman BT et al (1999) Mapping propagation of mechanical activation in the paced heart with MRI tagging. Am J Physiol 276(3 Pt 2):H881–H891
58. Chung ES et al (2008) Results of the Predictors of Response to CRT (PROSPECT) trial. Circulation 117(20):2608–2616
59. Prinzen FW et al (1990) Redistribution of myocardial fiber strain and blood flow by asynchronous activation. Am J Physiol 259(2 Pt 2):H300–H308
60. Prinzen FW et al (1999) Mapping of regional myocardial strain and work during ventricular pacing: experimental study using magnetic resonance imaging tagging. J Am Coll Cardiol 33(6):1735–1742
61. Prinzen FW et al (2011) Mechano-energetics of the asynchronous and resynchronized heart. Heart Fail Rev 16(3):215–224
62. Leenders GE et al (2011) Echocardiographic prediction of outcome after cardiac resynchronization therapy: conventional methods and recent developments. Heart Fail Rev 16(3):235–250
63. Mills RW et al (2009) Left ventricular septal and left ventricular apical pacing chronically maintain cardiac contractile coordination, pump function and efficiency. Circ Arrhythm Electrophysiol 2(5):571–579
64. Kerckhoffs RC et al (2010) Ventricular dilation and electrical dyssynchrony synergistically increase regional mechanical nonuniformity but not mechanical dyssynchrony: a computational model. Circ Heart Fail 3(4):528–536
65. Vernooy K et al (2007) Cardiac resynchronization therapy cures dyssynchronopathy in canine left bundle-branch block hearts. Eur Heart J 28(17):2148–2155

66. Breithardt OA et al (2003) Cardiac resynchronization therapy can reverse abnormal myocardial strain distribution in patients with heart failure and left bundle branch block. J Am Coll Cardiol 42(3):486–494
67. Klimusina J et al (2011) Redistribution of left ventricular strain by cardiac resynchronization therapy in heart failure patients. Eur J Heart Fail 13(2):186–194
68. Hirzel HO et al (1984) Thallium-201 scintigraphy in complete left bundle branch block. Am J Cardiol 53(6):764–769
69. Matzer L et al (1991) A new approach to the assessment of tomographic thallium-201 scintigraphy in patients with left bundle branch block. J Am Coll Cardiol 17(6):1309–1317
70. Hayat SA et al (2008) Effects of left bundle-branch block on cardiac structure, function, perfusion, and perfusion reserve: implications for myocardial contrast echocardiography versus radionuclide perfusion imaging for the detection of coronary artery disease. Circulation 117(14):1832–1841
71. Inanir S et al (2001) Tc-99m sestamibi gated SPECT in patients with left bundle branch block. Clin Nucl Med 26(10):840–846
72. Masci PG et al (2010) Myocardial structural, perfusion, and metabolic correlates of left bundle branch block mechanical derangement in patients with dilated cardiomyopathy: a tagged cardiac magnetic resonance and positron emission tomography study. Circ Cardiovasc Imaging 3(4):482–490
73. Delhaas T et al (1994) Regional fibre stress-fibre strain area as an estimate of regional blood flow and oxygen demand in the canine heart. J Physiol 477(Pt 3):481–496
74. Ono S et al (1992) Regional myocardial perfusion and glucose metabolism in experimental left bundle branch block. Circulation 85(3):1125–1131
75. van Oosterhout MF et al (2002) Relation between local myocardial growth and blood flow during chronic ventricular pacing. Cardiovasc Res 53(4):831–840
76. Lindner O et al (2005) Global and regional myocardial oxygen consumption and blood flow in severe cardiomyopathy with left bundle branch block. Eur J Heart Fail 7(2):225–230
77. Altehoefer C et al (1995) Metabolic mismatch of septal beta-oxidation and glucose utilization in left bundle branch block assessed with PET. J Nucl Med 36(11):2056–2059
78. Neri G et al (2003) Effect of biventricular pacing on metabolism and perfusion in patients affected by dilated cardiomyopathy and left bundle branch block: evaluation by positron emission tomography. Europace 5(1):111–115
79. Zanco P et al (2000) Effects of left bundle branch block on myocardial FDG PET in patients without significant coronary artery stenoses. J Nucl Med 41(6):973–977
80. Barth AS et al (2009) Cardiac resynchronization therapy corrects dyssynchrony-induced regional gene expression changes on a genomic level. Circ Cardiovasc Genet 2(4):371–378
81. Agnetti G et al (2010) Modulation of mitochondrial proteome and improved mitochondrial function by biventricular pacing of dyssynchronous failing hearts. Circ Cardiovasc Genet 3(1):78–87
82. Nowak B et al (2003) Cardiac resynchronization therapy homogenizes myocardial glucose metabolism and perfusion in dilated cardiomyopathy and left bundle branch block. J Am Coll Cardiol 41(9):1523–1528
83. Spragg DD, Kass DA (2006) Pathobiology of left ventricular dyssynchrony and resynchronization. Prog Cardiovasc Dis 49(1):26–41
84. Zhou Q et al (2000) Different effects of abnormal activation and myocardial disease on left ventricular ejection and filling times. Heart 84(3):272–276
85. Zile MR et al (1987) Right ventricular pacing reduces the rate of left ventricular relaxation and filling. J Am Coll Cardiol 10(3):702–709
86. Maurer G et al (1984) Two-dimensional echocardiographic contrast assessment of pacing-induced mitral regurgitation: relation to altered regional left ventricular function. J Am Coll Cardiol 3(4):986–991
87. Mark JB, Chetham PM (1991) Ventricular pacing can induce hemodynamically significant mitral valve regurgitation. Anesthesiology 74(2):375–377

88. Park RC, Little WC, O'Rourke RA (1985) Effect of alteration of left ventricular activation sequence on the left ventricular end-systolic pressure-volume relation in closed-chest dogs. Circ Res 57(5):706–717
89. Burkhoff D, Oikawa RY, Sagawa K (1986) Influence of pacing site on canine left ventricular contraction. Am J Physiol 251(2 Pt 2):H428–H435
90. Rosenqvist M et al (1996) The effect of ventricular activation sequence on cardiac performance during pacing. Pacing Clin Electrophysiol 19(9):1279–1286
91. Boerth RC, Covell JW (1971) Mechanical performance and efficiency of the left ventricle during ventricular stimulation. Am J Physiol 221(6):1686–1691
92. Nahlawi M et al (2004) Left ventricular function during and after right ventricular pacing. J Am Coll Cardiol 44(9):1883–1888
93. Auricchio A et al (1999) Effect of pacing chamber and atrioventricular delay on acute systolic function of paced patients with congestive heart failure. The Pacing Therapies for Congestive Heart Failure Study Group. The Guidant Congestive Heart Failure Research Group. Circulation 99(23):2993–3001
94. Nelson GS et al (2000) Left ventricular or biventricular pacing improves cardiac function at diminished energy cost in patients with dilated cardiomyopathy and left bundle-branch block. Circulation 102(25):3053–3059
95. St John Sutton MG et al (2003) Effect of cardiac resynchronization therapy on left ventricular size and function in chronic heart failure. Circulation 107(15):1985–1990
96. Breithardt OA et al (2003) Acute effects of cardiac resynchronization therapy on functional mitral regurgitation in advanced systolic heart failure. J Am Coll Cardiol 41(5):765–770
97. Kass DA et al (1999) Improved left ventricular mechanics from acute VDD pacing in patients with dilated cardiomyopathy and ventricular conduction delay. Circulation 99(12):1567–1573
98. Kass DA (2009) Pathobiology of cardiac dyssynchrony and resynchronization. Heart Rhythm 6(11):1660–1665
99. van Oosterhout MF et al (1998) Asynchronous electrical activation induces asymmetrical hypertrophy of the left ventricular wall. Circulation 98(6):588–595
100. van Oosterhout MF et al (2001) Remodeling by ventricular pacing in hypertrophying dog hearts. Cardiovasc Res 49(4):771–778
101. Prinzen FW et al (1995) Asymmetric thickness of the left ventricular wall resulting from asynchronous electric activation: a study in dogs with ventricular pacing and in patients with left bundle branch block. Am Heart J 130(5):1045–1053
102. Blaauw E et al (2010) Stretch-induced hypertrophy of isolated adult rabbit cardiomyocytes. Am J Physiol Heart Circ Physiol 299(3):H780–H787
103. Chakir K et al (2008) Reversal of global apoptosis and regional stress kinase activation by cardiac resynchronization. Circulation 117(11):1369–1377
104. D'Ascia C et al (2006) Effects of biventricular pacing on interstitial remodelling, tumor necrosis factor-alpha expression, and apoptotic death in failing human myocardium. Eur Heart J 27(2):201–206
105. de Jong S et al (2011) Biomarkers of myocardial fibrosis. J Cardiovasc Pharmacol 57(5):522–535
106. Garcia-Bolao I et al (2008) Impact of collagen type I turnover on the long-term response to cardiac resynchronization therapy. Eur Heart J 29(7):898–906
107. Umar S et al (2008) Myocardial collagen metabolism in failing hearts before and during cardiac resynchronization therapy. Eur J Heart Fail 10(9):878–883
108. Zile MR et al (2011) Plasma biomarkers that reflect determinants of matrix composition identify the presence of left ventricular hypertrophy and diastolic heart failure. Circ Heart Fail 4(3):246–256
109. Spragg DD et al (2005) Abnormal conduction and repolarization in late-activated myocardium of dyssynchronously contracting hearts. Cardiovasc Res 67(1):77–86
110. Tomaselli GF, Zipes DP (2004) What causes sudden death in heart failure? Circ Res 95(8):754–763

111. Aiba T et al (2009) Electrophysiological consequences of dyssynchronous heart failure and its restoration by resynchronization therapy. Circulation 119(9):1220–1230
112. Jeyaraj D et al (2007) Mechanoelectrical feedback as novel mechanism of cardiac electrical remodeling. Circulation 115(25):3145–3155
113. Rosenbaum MB et al (1982) Electrotonic modulation of the T wave and cardiac memory. Am J Cardiol 50(2):213–222
114. Shvilkin A et al (1998) Evolution and resolution of long-term cardiac memory. Circulation 97(18):1810–1817
115. Coronel R et al (2007) Long-term cardiac memory in canine heart is associated with the evolution of a transmural repolarization gradient. Cardiovasc Res 74(3):416–425
116. Wecke L et al (2005) Temporal characteristics of cardiac memory in humans: vectorcardiographic quantification in a model of cardiac pacing. Heart Rhythm 2(1):28–34
117. Costard-Jackle A et al (1989) Slow and long-lasting modulation of myocardial repolarization produced by ectopic activation in isolated rabbit hearts. Evidence for cardiac "memory". Circulation 80(5):1412–1420
118. Sosunov EA, Anyukhovsy EP, Rosen MR (2008) Altered ventricular stretch contributes to initiation of cardiac memory. Heart Rhythm 5(1):106–113
119. Nattel S et al (2007) Arrhythmogenic ion-channel remodeling in the heart: heart failure, myocardial infarction, and atrial fibrillation. Physiol Rev 87(2):425–456
120. Li GR et al (2002) Transmural action potential and ionic current remodeling in ventricles of failing canine hearts. Am J Physiol Heart Circ Physiol 283(3):H1031–H1041
121. Kaab S et al (1996) Ionic mechanism of action potential prolongation in ventricular myocytes from dogs with pacing-induced heart failure. Circ Res 78(2):262–273
122. Rozanski GJ et al (1997) Electrophysiology of rabbit ventricular myocytes following sustained rapid ventricular pacing. J Mol Cell Cardiol 29(2):721–732
123. Tsuji Y et al (2000) Pacing-induced heart failure causes a reduction of delayed rectifier potassium currents along with decreases in calcium and transient outward currents in rabbit ventricle. Cardiovasc Res 48(2):300–309
124. Rose J et al (2005) Molecular correlates of altered expression of potassium currents in failing rabbit myocardium. Am J Physiol Heart Circ Physiol 288(5):H2077–H2087
125. Tsuji Y et al (2006) Potassium channel subunit remodeling in rabbits exposed to long-term bradycardia or tachycardia: discrete arrhythmogenic consequences related to differential delayed-rectifier changes. Circulation 113(3):345–355
126. Chen X et al (2002) L-type Ca^{2+} channel density and regulation are altered in failing human ventricular myocytes and recover after support with mechanical assist devices. Circ Res 91(6):517–524
127. He J et al (2001) Reduction in density of transverse tubules and L-type Ca(2+) channels in canine tachycardia-induced heart failure. Cardiovasc Res 49(2):298–307
128. Aiba T, Tomaselli GF (2010) Electrical remodeling in the failing heart. Curr Opin Cardiol 25(1):29–36
129. Hullin R et al (2003) Cardiac L-type calcium channel beta-subunits expressed in human heart have differential effects on single channel characteristics. J Biol Chem 278(24): 21623–21630
130. Yang Y et al (2000) L-type Ca^{2+} channel alpha 1c subunit isoform switching in failing human ventricular myocardium. J Mol Cell Cardiol 32(6):973–984
131. Armoundas AA et al (2007) Cellular and molecular determinants of altered Ca^{2+} handling in the failing rabbit heart: primary defects in SR Ca^{2+} uptake and release mechanisms. Am J Physiol Heart Circ Physiol 292(3):H1607–H1618
132. Hobai IA, O'Rourke B (2000) Enhanced Ca(2+)-activated Na(+)-Ca(2+) exchange activity in canine pacing-induced heart failure. Circ Res 87(8):690–698
133. Mullens W et al (2008) Early and late effects of cardiac resynchronization therapy on force-frequency relation and contractility regulating gene expression in heart failure patients. Heart Rhythm 5(1):52–59

134. Vanderheyden M et al (2008) Myocardial gene expression in heart failure patients treated with cardiac resynchronization therapy responders versus nonresponders. J Am Coll Cardiol 51(2):129–136
135. Gauthier C et al (1996) Functional beta3-adrenoceptor in the human heart. J Clin Invest 98(2):556–562
136. Zhu W et al (2005) The enigma of beta2-adrenergic receptor Gi signaling in the heart: the good, the bad, and the ugly. Circ Res 97(6):507–509
137. Post SR, Hammond HK, Insel PA (1999) Beta-adrenergic receptors and receptor signaling in heart failure. Annu Rev Pharmacol Toxicol 39:343–360
138. Patterson AJ et al (2004) Protecting the myocardium: a role for the beta2 adrenergic receptor in the heart. Crit Care Med 32(4):1041–1048
139. Xiao RP et al (2004) Subtype-specific beta-adrenoceptor signaling pathways in the heart and their potential clinical implications. Trends Pharmacol Sci 25(7):358–365
140. Lohse MJ, Engelhardt S, Eschenhagen T (2003) What is the role of beta-adrenergic signaling in heart failure? Circ Res 93(10):896–906
141. Chakir K et al (2009) Mechanisms of enhanced beta-adrenergic reserve from cardiac resynchronization therapy. Circulation 119(9):1231–1240
142. Najem B et al (2006) Sympathetic control after cardiac resynchronization therapy: responders versus nonresponders. Am J Physiol Heart Circ Physiol 291(6):H2647–H2652
143. Vanderheyden M et al (2008) Endomyocardial upregulation of beta1 adrenoreceptor gene expression and myocardial contractile reserve following cardiac resynchronization therapy. J Card Fail 14(2):172–178
144. Spragg DD et al (2003) Regional alterations in protein expression in the dyssynchronous failing heart. Circulation 108(8):929–932
145. Vernooy K et al (2003) Relation between abnormal ventricular impulse conduction and heart failure. J Interv Cardiol 16(6):557–562

Chapter 9
Telemonitoring and Sensor Technologies in Chronic Heart Failure

Matthias Dupont, Wilfried Mullens, and W.H. Wilson Tang

Abstract The high readmission rate and accompanying cost in patients with heart failure are considered unacceptable. It is believed that a good part of hospital admissions can be avoided with closer monitoring of signs, symptoms, and certain physiologic variables of these patients, allowing timely intervention. Modern technologies make this possible without the need for face-to-face contact with the patient. This chapter describes the methodology and evidence for such strategies, going from "simple" disease management over "structured telephone support," to the use of implantable device monitoring. The pathophysiology of acute decompensated heart failure is explained in order to identify opportunities for early detection. The concepts and methods to measure heart rate variability, impedance, and invasive pressures are explained before examining the evidence from observational studies and randomized trials. We conclude that disease management is an essential component of good heart failure care, but that the incremental benefit of more intensive follow-up, even of variables obtained by implantable devices, remains to be determined.

1 Introduction

Despite major advances in the treatment and management of heart failure (HF), it remains one of the major contributors to mortality, morbidity, and societal costs [1]. Approximately 5.7 million Americans ≥20 years of age have HF and it is the most important reason for hospitalization over the age of 65. Sixty to seventy percent of the total cost of HF ($39.2 billion in 2010) which stems from hospitalizations and rehospitalization rates after HF admission is the highest among all medical conditions,

M. Dupont, M.D. • W. Mullens, M.D., Ph.D. • W.H.W. Tang, M.D. (✉)
Department of Cardiovascular Medicine, Heart and Vascular Institute, Cleveland Clinic, 9500 Euclid Avenue, J3-4, Cleveland, OH 44195, USA
e-mail: tangw@ccf.org

J. Bartunek and M. Vanderheyden (eds.), *Translational Approach to Heart Failure*,
DOI 10.1007/978-1-4614-7345-9_9, © Springer Science+Business Media New York 2013

reaching 50 % after 6 months [2–4]. These numbers illustrate the economic need for reduction of recurrent HF hospitalizations. In addition there is evidence that decompensated HF and the accompanying neurohormonal activation accelerate disease progression [5], and reduction of morbidity and mortality (including rehospitalizations) has been demonstrated with aggressive use of neurohormonal blockade.

It was projected that by close follow-up and careful evaluation of several physiologic parameters, early signs of congestion could be recognized and acted upon in order to avoid HF hospitalizations, shifting the clinician's role from a reactive to a more proactive one. However, it is practically impossible to achieve this goal by just flooding already busy outpatient clinics with even more patient visits or patient information with limited infrastructure or management algorithms. This is where modern (communication) technology comes into play. Patients' information can be transferred over the analog or mobile telephone network or the internet and similarly patients can be instructed via this way—hence the terms "telemonitoring" and "structured telephone support." Moreover, a large majority of patients with advanced chronic systolic HF may have implantable cardioverter defibrillators (ICDs) or cardiac resynchronization therapy (CRT) devices implanted. These devices are capable of capturing certain physiologic data that can subsequently be used to evaluate the patients' condition and predict adverse events such as hospitalization for acute decompensated heart failure (ADHF). Frequent transmission of physiologic data obtained by devices can potentially transform evaluation of outpatients from a snapshot approach to an almost continuous one without the confinement of the location of care.

In this chapter we will review the methodology and the evidence of the different remote strategies, starting from its most simple form ("multidisciplinary disease management programs" and "structured telephone support") to more complex forms using invasive technologies. We will start with reviewing some insights in the pathophysiology of ADHF and end with a glimpse at the future.

2 Pathophysiologic Insights Derived from Sensor Technology

Clinical studies performed with implantable devices during the last decade have produced new insights in the pathophysiology about the transition from stable to destabilized states of HF leading to ADHF. It is clear that HF exacerbations do not start at the moment the patient's weight changes or symptoms develop, but long before. In that way, the term "acute" in ADHF is somewhat misleading. Figure 9.1 depicts a timeline of physiologic alterations occurring before hospital admission and potential targets for advanced sensor technologies. The earliest detectable change seems to be a small but consistent increase in filling pressures which can be detected 24–30 days before the event [6–8]. This rise in filling pressures is similar in magnitude but perhaps somewhat more rapid in HF patients with preserved as compared to reduced systolic function [7, 8]. It is hypothesized that the increase in filling pressures results from very small (too small to detect) increases

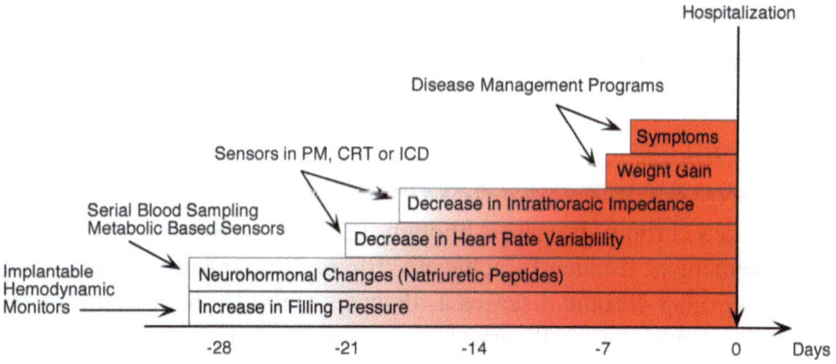

Fig. 9.1 Transition from chronic to acute decompensated heart failure (ADHF) and opportunities for early detection

in intravascular volume (through either gradual accumulation or redistribution) although alterations in vascular tone might also contribute [9, 10]. The increase in filling pressures can then lead to more substantial fluid accumulation (detectable by thoracic impedance measurements on average 18 days before admission), weight gain, and ultimately symptoms (detectable by the patient approximately 1 week before admission) [11, 12]. The extravascular pulmonary fluid accumulation occurs at much higher pressures in chronic HF patients as compared to normals [8]. Before this happens, the body strives to maintain homeostasis by accommodating to the higher filling pressures via sympathetic activation and vagal withdrawal (detected by decreased heart rate variability as early as 21 days before admission), presumably in an attempt to increase cardiac output [9, 13]. Because regular monitoring of neurohormones (e.g., natriuretic peptides or other neurohormones) is more difficult to achieve, less is known about their time course in ADHF. However, animal models suggest that changes occur early, in concert with changes in pressure [14].

The trials with implantable hemodynamic monitors also revealed wide pressure changes during regular daily activities, exercise, and changes in body position [15, 16]. These pressure changes are likely expected "normal biological variations" in chronic HF patients and may not necessarily lead to ADHF episodes. Other electrophysiologic signals also exhibit such fluctuations of physiologic signals, making the design of a treatment algorithm based on changes in these signals somewhat challenging.

Key Points

- Implantable devices, that are able to continuously monitor physiologic variables, helped to improve our understanding of the transition from chronic to ADHF.
- Changes in pressures, heart rate variability, and impedance occur much earlier before admission than originally thought.
- An elevation in filling pressures is the first alteration in the development of ADHF whereas an increase in weight is a late and insensitive symptom.

3 Disease Management, Structured Telephone Support, and Noninvasive Telemonitoring

3.1 The Principle

Heart failure is a chronic disease. Although delay in progression, stabilization, or even improvement is frequently achieved, lifelong treatment is often necessary. Like managing other chronic diseases as diabetes mellitus, the idea originated that HF treatment would be well-served by a more structured, multidisciplinary approach. This also resulted from the observation that one-half to two-thirds of rehospitalizations appeared to be triggered by potentially remediable factors such as poor discharge planning, noncompliance to diet and medication, inadequate follow-up and social support, and delay in seeking medical help [17]. The multidisciplinary initiatives that address this self-care need are labeled as "disease management programs" and involve [18]:

- Identification of target patient population.
- Patient education.
- Caregiver education.
- Optimizing treatment prescriptions.
- Importance of adherence to medication.
- Dietary recommendations.
- Structured telephone support.
- Self-monitoring (weight and symptoms).
- Self-management (self-adjustment of the treatment regimen).
- Personnel: nurses, case managers, physicians, pharmacists, social workers, dietitians, physical therapists, psychologists.

When "disease management" incorporates some form of systematic structured evaluation of physiologic variables in the outpatient setting, this is often labeled as "home monitoring." The concept also implies that, when abnormalities are detected, appropriate action (treatment) will be applied [19, 20].

3.2 The Evidence

Table 9.1 gives an overview of the most important trials regarding disease management and noninvasive telemonitoring in HF. Rich et al. published the landmark trial in 1995, demonstrating simultaneous improvements in readmission rates and quality of life while saving costs, after the implementation of a nurse-led multidisciplinary intervention for the management of HF [21]. Many randomized trials have been published since then with mixed results [22–35]. The earlier trials were mainly positive whereas more recent trials are predominantly negative. A meta-analysis performed by Clark et al. showed a 20 % reduction in all-cause mortality and a 21 % reduction in hospitalization for HF [36]. Another meta-analysis by Inglis et al.

Table 9.1 Overview of randomized disease management trials using telephone support and noninvasive telemonitoring

Study acronym, first author	Year of publication	Number and type of patients	Study design	Intervention	Control-group	Duration (months)	Endpoints	Results
	1995	$N=282$	Single-center	Patient education	Standard of care (no disease management)	3	Survival without admission	Less readmissions ($p=0.02$)
Rich et al.		≥70 years	Prospective	Diet prescription			Heart failure admission	↓56 % readmissions for HF
		Admission for HF		Social service consultation			All-cause admission	↓28 % readmissions for other causes
				Medication review			Quality of life	Improvement in QOL ($p=0.001$)
				Intense follow-up (telephone contact)			Costs	Cost-saving (–460$ per patient)
WHARF	2003	$N=280$	Multicenter	Electronic weight and symptom monitoring by AlereNet system (telemonitoring)	Disease management program with advice for weight and symptom monitoring	6	Rehospitalization	Rehospitalization similar
Goldberg et al.		Admission for HF	Prospective				Mortality	56 % mortality reduction ($p<0.003$)
		NYHA III or IV						
		EF ≤35 %						

(continued)

Table 9.1 (continued)

Study acronym, first author	Year of publication	Number and type of patients	Study design	Intervention	Control-group	Duration (months)	Endpoints	Results
SPAN-CHF	2004	$N=200$	Multicenter	Home visit	Standard of care (no disease management)	3 (short-term)	HF hospitalization	Less readmission for HF ($p=0.027$)
Kimmelstiel et al.		Admission for HF	Prospective	Medication and diet education		9 (long-term)	Cardiac hospitalization	Less days in hospital ($p<0.001$)
				Self-monitoring			All-cause hospitalization	Effects largely disappear at 9 months
				Teaching booklet			Number of days in hospital	
				Telephone contact				
TEN-HMS	2005	$N=426$	Multicenter	Two intervention groups	Standard of care (no disease management)	8	Days death or hospitalized	No difference between 3 groups
Cleland et al.		Admission for HF	Prospective	(1) Monthly nurse telephone support				Lower mortality in both intervention groups ($p=0.032$)
		EF <40 %		(2) Home monitoring (= twice daily measurement of HR, rhythm, BP, weight, and automatic transmission)				No additional benefit of home monitoring

	2006	N=406	Multicenter	Initial one-time appointment	Standard of care (no disease management)	12	Hospitalization	Less hospitalizations in intervention group at 12 months
Sisk et al.		Ambulatory	Prospective	Structured telephone support			Functional level	No difference in hospitalizations thereafter
		Systolic dysfunction		Coordination with clinician				Better quality of life
COACH	2008	N=1023	Multicenter	Two intervention groups	Standard of care by cardiologist (follow-up after 2 months)	18	Time to death or HF rehospitalization	No reduction in hospitalization or death in both intervention groups
Jaarsma et al.		Admission for HF	Prospective	(1) Basic nurse support			Days lost to death or rehospitalization	
		NYHA II–IV		(2) Intensive multidisciplinary support				

(continued)

Table 9.1 (continued)

Study acronym, first author	Year of publication	Number and type of patients	Study design	Intervention	Control-group	Duration (months)	Endpoints	Results
HFHC	2008	$N=315$	Multicenter	Computer-based home disease management program with daily evaluation and transmission of symptoms and weight (telemonitoring)	Disease management with education, medication optimization, and digital home scale	6	Cardiovascular death or HF rehospitalization	No differences in death, rehospitalization, or length of stay
Soran et al.		Medicare	Prospective				Length of hospital stay when rehospitalized	
		Older women, nonwhite men						
	2009	$N=460$	Multicenter	Weekly or 2-weekly structured telephone support (telemonitoring) or when symptoms (teleassistance)	Disease management with education, medication optimization, and dietary advice	12	Cardiovascular readmission	Lower readmission and less costs in intervention group ($p<0.01$)
Giordano et al.		Admission for HF EF <40 %	Prospective	Transmission of ECG strip				

HOME-HF	2009	$N=182$	Multicenter	Honeywell HomeMed telemonitoring equipment for HR, BP, saturation, weight, and questionnaire (daily transmission)	Disease management with education, medication optimization, and dietary advice	6	Days alive out of hospital	No difference
Dar et al.		Admission for HF NYHA II–IV	Prospective				Number and duration of HF hospitalization QOL	Less "unplanned" admissions in intervention group
HHH	2009	$N=461$	Multicenter	Three layers of intervention	Standard of care by cardiologist	12	Cardiac death and HF hospitalization	No difference
Mortara et al.		Admission for HF NYHA II–IV EF <40 %	Prospective	(1) Monthly structured telephone support (2) ↑ weekly transmission of vital signs, weight, symptoms (3) ↑ monthly 24 h cardiorespiratory recordings			Bed day occupancy for HF	

(continued)

Table 9.1 (continued)

Study acronym, first author	Year of publication	Number and type of patients	Study design	Intervention	Control-group	Duration (months)	Endpoints	Results
HART	2010	$N=902$	Single-center	Self-management counseling	HF education including medication optimization and dietary advice	30	Death or HF hospitalization	No difference
Powell et al.			Prospective					
DIAL	2010	$N=1518$	Multicenter	Structured telephone support	Standard of care by cardiologist	12 and 36 months	Death or HF hospitalization	Lower rate of death or HF hospitalization at 1 ($p=0.13$) and 3 years ($p=0.05$)
Ferrante et al.		Ambulatory	Prospective	Education				Driven by less HF hospitalizations ($p=0.0004$)
				Nurses could adjust diuretic dose				
TELE-HF	2010	$N=1653$	Multicenter	Telemonitoring of weight, symptoms via daily telephone interrogation with daily review by nurses	Disease management with education, medication optimization, and dietary advice	6	All-cause death or rehospitalization	No difference
Chaudhry et al.		Admission for HF	Prospective				HF hospitalization	
							Number of days in hospital	

TIM-HF	2010	*N*=710	Multicenter	Telemonitoring of weight, HR, BP, ECG (daily)	Disease management with education, medication optimization, and dietary advice	26	Death from any cause	No difference
Koehler et al.		Ambulatory	Prospective				Death and HF rehospitalization	
		NYHA II–III EF <35 %						
	2012	*N*=605	Multicenter	Multisession self-care counseling including structured telephone support	Single, 40 min session education	12	All-cause death or hospitalization	No difference
DeWalt et al.		Ambulatory	Prospective					People with low literacy benefit more from multiple sessions
		NYHA II–IV						

HF heart failure, *QOL* quality of life, *BP* blood pressure, *HR* heart rate, *NYHA* New York Heart Association, *EF* ejection fraction demonstrated reduction in HF hospitalizations by both structured telephone support (23 %) and telemonitoring (21 %), while a reduction in mortality could only be demonstrated with telemonitoring (34 %) [37]. However, these meta-analyses were followed by two large randomized trials (The Telemedical Interventional Monitoring in Heart Failure [TIM-HF] and Telemonitoring to Improve Heart Failure Outcome [TELE-HF]) that did not show any benefit [33, 34]. The general belief is that disease management works and this is incorporated in the guidelines in both the USA and Europe [38, 39]. However, the largest effect seems to stem from initial education and counseling of patients. It is less clear whether there is a dose–response relationship and whether there is much gain of more intensive follow-up or telemonitoring [20].

3.3 Potential Reasons for Inconsistent Results of the Strategy

Because disease-comprehension and adherence with medication and diet go hand in hand, it may come as no surprise that patients included in disease management programs experience fewer hospitalizations and lower mortality. This explains the success of the earlier trials. Once patients understand these concepts, further benefit from structured telephone support or telemonitoring should derive from early detection and treatment of (imminent) HF decompensation. However, as explained earlier, the signs (edema, weight gain, shortness of breath, tachycardia) and symptoms, typically screened for by telemonitoring, occur fairly late in the development of ADHF (Fig. 9.1). In addition the signs and symptoms are not very sensitive. Substantial weight gain (i.e., 2 lb), the most frequently used screening symptom, occurs in less than 50 % of patients admitted with ADHF. Therefore, there is an evolving concept suggesting that there is often volume redistribution instead of volume gain which is not easily detectable by weight changes [12, 40]. Other clinical signs (elevated jugular venous pressure, edema, rales) are notoriously imprecise in detecting elevated left-sided filling pressures [41]. Furthermore, it remains unsure how to best handle the obtained information to prevent hospitalization.

Many clinicians believe that success could be achieved when more sensitive methods, that predict ADHF earlier in its course, could be developed. The resulting technology either stands alone or is incorporated in existing devices such as pacemakers (PMs), ICDs, or CRTs that are implanted in many of the contemporary advanced HF patients. The next section describes these variables and the technologic principles to measure them.

Key Points

- Disease management programs involve patient education, dietary advice, and optimizing drug prescriptions and compliance. They have proven effects in many chronic diseases including HF.
- Active efforts to follow certain physiologic variables, when the patient is ambulatory, are called telemonitoring, remote monitoring, or home monitoring.
- The incremental benefit of these more intensified methods of follow-up remains uncertain.

4 Variables Measurable with Sensor Technology in Implantable Devices

4.1 *Common Device-Based Electrophysiologic Parameters*

Pacemakers, CRTs, and ICDs are in the first place developed to measure cardiac electrical activity, used for timing purposes. Changes in several of these variables can be incorporated in algorithms to predict ADHF. Examples of these variables are:

- Heart rate (HR)
- Heart rate at night
- Heart rate variability (HRV)
- Heart rhythm (% atrial fibrillation)
- % biventricular pacing
- Anti-tachypacing events or shocks

These parameters have been developed and utilized to ensure the integrity and functionality of the device operations, and were not originally intended as a monitoring tool for HF longitudinal care. Nevertheless, information about these variables can be continuously collected by the device and either analyzed by the clinician during office visits or sent from the patient's home to a central server (see below). This strategy that is already in place for checking the status of the device (battery, lead performance, etc.) is called remote follow-up.

The Home CARE pilot study (Home monitoring in cardiac resynchronization therapy) showed that 70 % of hospitalizations were preceded by an increase in mean heart rate at rest and during 24 h and that 43 % of patients experienced a decrease in biventricular pacing before admission [42]. A parameter of particular interest is HRV. The atrial-to-atrial depolarization interval is not a constant in humans but has certain variability. The degree of variability is directly correlated to the amount of vagal influence at the sinoatrial node [43]. Vagal withdrawal and an autonomic imbalance favoring the sympathetic nervous system will thus result in reduced HRV. HRV can be measured as the standard deviation of 5-min median atrial–atrial intervals (SDAAM) over a 24 h period. It was demonstrated that reduced HRV predicts sudden cardiac death and HF rehospitalization with a sensitivity of 70 % and 2.4 false-positives per patient year of follow-up in one study [13, 44]. HRV started to decrease as early as 21 days before admission. In addition early HRV improvement does predict CRT response [45]. However, a recent trial (Decompensation detection study [DECODE]) showed a much lower sensitivity of an algorithm incorporating HRV to detect HF hospitalization [46].

4.2 *Patient Activity, Saturation, and Ventilation*

Implantable devices are also capable of detecting the activity level of patients by interpreting data from accelerometers, which are already incorporated in the device for rate adaptive pacing. It sounds indeed reasonable that activity decreases before hospitalization. One way of measuring this is by integrating activity counts from accelerometers each minute. A minute then counts as active if the counts exceed a certain threshold that corresponds to a walking rate of 70 steps per minute [13, 47]. A low activity day can then be defined as less than 1 h of activity per day. Information about activity was, for example, incorporated in the algorithm (together with nightly HR, HRV, impedance, atrial fibrillation, and device therapy) of the PARTNERS-HF (Program to access and review trending information and evaluate correlation to symptoms in heart failure patients) trial demonstrating a 5.5 times higher risk of hospitalization after device diagnostics became positive [48]. Similarly, minute ventilation can reveal whether the patient is becoming short of breath. Minute ventilation can be measured by devices through changes in impedance (see below) [49]. Finally, mixed venous saturation can be measured continuously by oxygen saturation sensors constructed on a lead and connected with a can [50]. This type of sensor is however not commonly used.

4.3 Intrathoracic Impedance

Impedance (Z, expressed in ohms Ω) is a measure of the degree a medium resists the flow of electrical current at a given (alternate) voltage. It thus depends on the specific conducting characteristics of that medium. Applied to the human thorax, this translates to lower impedance when the tissue characteristics change as a result of changes in extracellular or intracellular fluid content (water is a good conductor compared to other substances). It has to be said that the exact source of the ultimate impedance signal is not completely understood and definitely dependent on more than just fluid accumulation [51]. Nevertheless, it is extrapolated that intrathoracic impedance measurements may serve as a physiologic marker of lung water based on the hypothesis that pulmonary circulatory engorgement or interstitial fluid increases as HF congestion progresses.

Aside from measurements by implantable devices, impedance can also be measured externally by a band electrode method, the classic impedance cardiography [52, 53]. The first derivative of impedance over time can then be used to calculate stroke volume, cardiac output, and systemic vascular resistance. However, the correlation with pulmonary artery catheter-obtained values is rather low and this technique will not be discussed further [54].

Implantable devices (PM, CRT, ICD) classically measure impedance between the right ventricular (RV) lead tip and the can (Fig. 9.2) although alternative configurations are possible. In fact, in a comparative study, the vector between the left ventricular lead and the can had the fastest and largest change in impedance when patients developed ADHF [55]. There is ample evidence that impedance values correlate well with fluid status and also with invasively obtained wedge pressure [8, 11, 56, 57]. To decide whether a certain drop in impedance is relevant, specific algorithms have been developed. A clinically available one (®OptiVol fluid index,

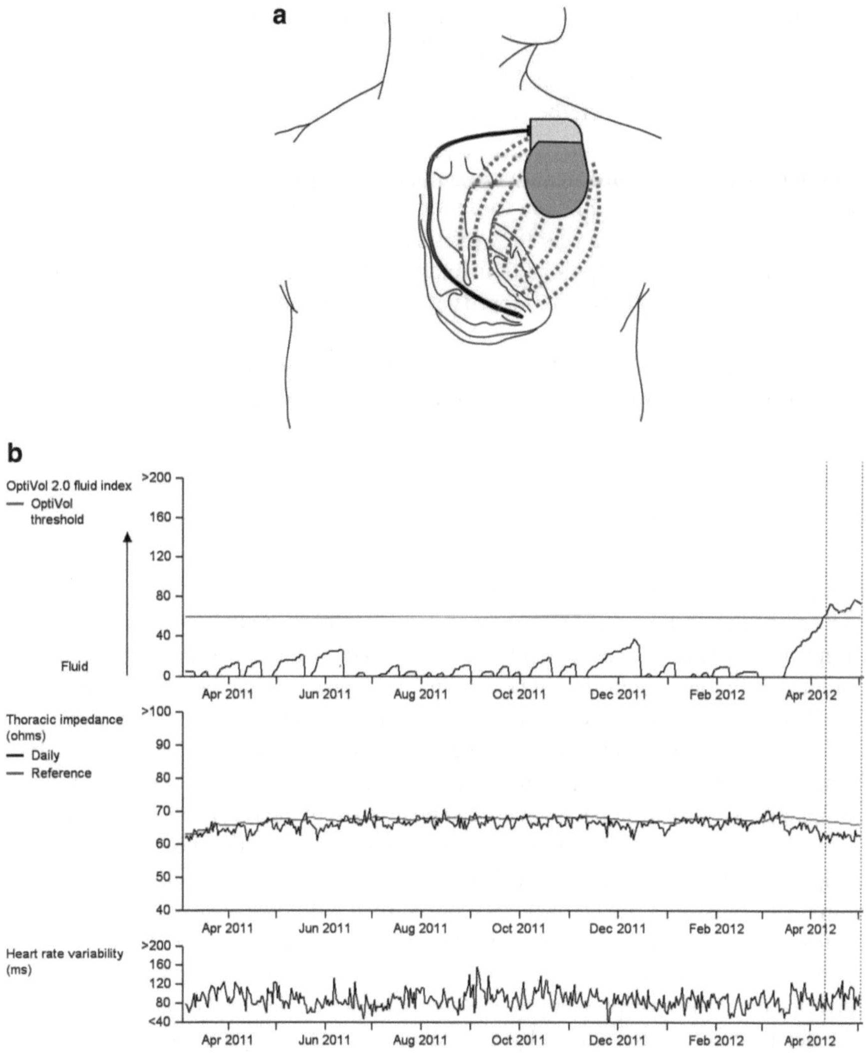

Fig. 9.2 Impedance measurement. (**a**) Schematic drawing of a device measuring impedance in the classic configuration (vector between RV tip and can). (**b**) Example of a threshold crossing event (*right side* of the strip). Telephone contact with the patient revealed that he increased fluid intake after an episode of nephrolithiasis. There were no symptoms of worsening heart failure (yet). Heart rate variability (HRV) is also shown on this strip without a clear change

Medtronic Inc, Minneapolis, MN) compares average daily impedance measurements with a 30-day running average, supposed to reflect the patient's own baseline. Differences in daily impedance values that are persistently below the running average accumulate, using a cumulative sum algorithm, until an arbitrary threshold (e.g., 60 Ω-days) is crossed suggesting a significant increase in lung-water volume (Fig. 9.2). The predictive ability of impedance drops for ADHF admission has been investigated in several studies with mixed results. Earlier studies demonstrate sensitivity in the order of 60–77 %, with 0.2–1.9 false-positive alerts (events without hospitalization) per patient year. The positive predictive value is therefore around 60 % [11, 58, 59]. However, the recently published SENSE-trial (sensitivity of the Insync sentry optivol feature for the prediction of heart failure study) reported a disappointing 21 % sensitivity (although improving to 42 % with time after implantation) and 5 % positive predictive value for HF hospitalization. The positive predictive value for worsening HF was 38 % [60]. These findings suggest that the predictive accuracy of future HF hospitalizations may not be as desirable even though alterations in impedance signals may identify a sicker population.

A similar algorithm, known as CorVue™, has been incorporated in devices from St. Jude Medical. It displays the impedance trend (every 2 h) and compares with a running average. How it performs regarding prediction of HF events is not yet clear.

4.4 Hemodynamics

Elevation of ventricular filling pressure is essential in the pathophysiology of ADHF, and one of the earliest changes documented [7]. Because clinicians strive to keep filling pressures as low as possible in chronic HF without compromising cardiac output, continuous monitoring of hemodynamics appeals attractive. Several implantable devices have been developed to measure intracardiac pressures (Fig. 9.3).

The Chronicle® intracardiac hemodynamic monitor (Medtronic Inc, Minneapolis, MN) utilizes a variable capacitance pressure sensor integrated into a unipolar passive fixation pacemaker lead positioned in the right ventricular outflow tract. This lead is connected with a stand-alone device or ICD. The device continuously monitors right ventricular (RV) pressure, dP/dt, and estimates end-diastolic pulmonary pressure (ePAD) as the RV pressure at pulmonary valve opening which occurs at maximal dP/dt. In the absence of pulmonary vascular disease, ePAD approximates wedge pressure [61]. The device measures absolute pressures that are corrected for barometric pressure by a reference device carried by the patient at all time. The device can be interrogated by a handheld radiofrequency wand that transmits the data through the home monitor over a telephone line to a secure server. The pressures obtained by the device correlate very well with Swan-Ganz-derived pressures [62, 63]. In an initial feasibility study, RV pressure increased by 25 % on average in 9 out of 12 patients hospitalized for HF [64].

The HeartPOD® device (St. Jude Medical, St. Paul, MN) is a permanent implantable left atrial pressure sensor, inserted after transseptal puncture. The sensor is connected to a subcutaneous antenna which can be interrogated and powered by 125-kHz radiofrequency telemetry after placing an external handheld advisor module over the subcutaneous antenna. The advisor module also alerts patients with reminders to take medications. The initial experience with this device was positive in the sense that implantation was safe and pressure measurements accurate when compared to Swan-Ganz [65]. The small non-randomized HOMEOSTASIS trial

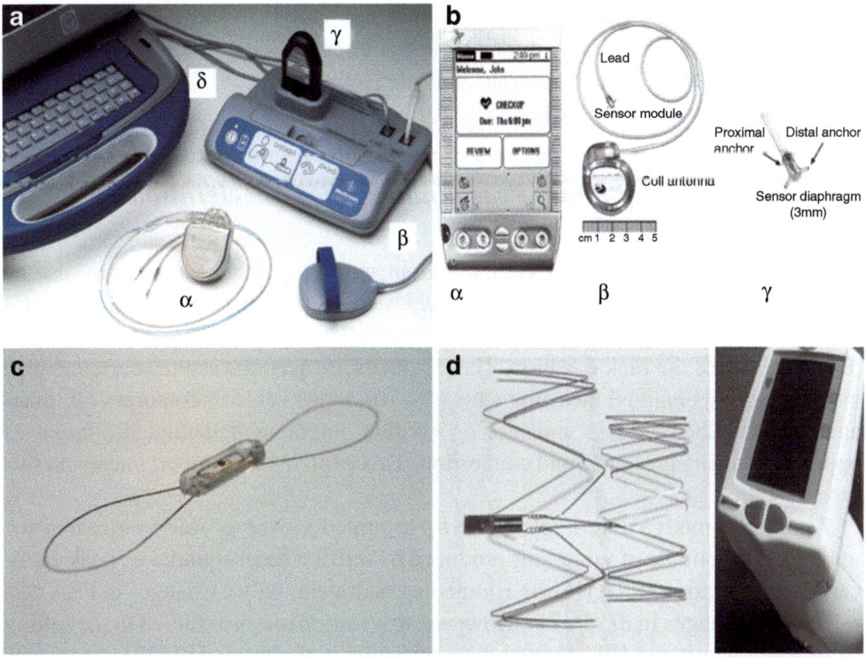

Fig. 9.3 Different implantable hemodynamic monitoring systems. (**a**) *Chronicle*® ICD system composed of α = ICD can with shock lead and pressure sensor, β = home monitor and telemetry wand, γ = reference device for barometric pressure correction, and δ = standard programmer. (**b**) *HeartPOD*® left atrial pressure monitoring device with α = patient advisor module, β = coil antenna and sensor lead, γ = detail of anchor-fixation system and sensing diaphragm. (**c**) *CardioMEMS*® implantable pressure device. (**d**) *Impressure*® pressure monitoring system with pulmonary artery implant (*left*) and handheld unit (*right*) (with permission from Adamson et al., Verdejo et al., Hoppe et al. [68, 69, 92])

(Hemodynamically guided home self-therapy in severe heart failure patients) showed that self-management guided by left atrial pressure resulted in lower pressures, more neurohormonal uptitration, and less diuretic use [66]. A larger trial (Left atrial pressure monitoring to optimize heart failure therapy [LAPTOP-HF]) is currently ongoing [67].

The CardioMEMS® heart sensor (CardioMEMS Inc, Atlanta, GA) is a wireless device deployed in the pulmonary artery via right heart catheterization. It consists of a three-dimensional coil housed in a pressure-sensitive capacitor that is tethered by two nitinol loops to avoid migration. It only measures pressure when it is interrogated by an external antenna using radiofrequency electro-mechanical coupling. The antenna measures the resonant frequency of the device. The shift in resonant frequency is proportional to the intrapulmonary pressure after correcting for atmospheric pressure. The measurements correlate well with invasively obtained Swan-Ganz pressures [68]. The Impressure® pressure-monitoring system (Boston Scientific Inc, Natick, MA, USA) is similar to the CardioMEMS device deployed in the pulmonary artery and responds to ultrasonic signal. In the PAPIRUS II trial (Pulmonary artery pressure by implantable device responding to ultrasonic signal II study) it demonstrated to be accurate and safe [69].

4.5 *Cardiac Output and Peak Endocardial Acceleration*

The continuous monitoring of cardiac output via implantable sensors can also be performed with a high degree of accuracy. Usually this is achieved through photosensitive diodes that measure oxygen saturation allowing calculation of cardiac output by the use of the Fick equation. These sensors are accurate as they correlate well with invasively obtained measurements [50, 70]. However, contemporary HF management has focused less and less on cardiac output as a therapeutic target as opposed to filling pressures and congestion. This explains the limited interest in this type of sensor.

Another hemodynamic implantable tip-mounted sensor is able to measure the maximum amplitude of vibrations produced by the first heart sound, i.e., peak endocardial acceleration (PEA) (Sorin Biomedica, Saluggia, Italy). Changes in PEA correlate with changes in dP/dt [71]. However, this sensor is more studied in the setting of AV-optimization in CRT than in the management of chronic HF [72].

Key Points

- The most commonly used device-based variables to predict worsening HF are heart rate (variability), patient activity, impedance, and intracardiac pressures.
- Impedance is inversely related to pulmonary fluid content.
- The sensitivity of a 60 Ω-days threshold crossing (drop in impedance) for HF admission varies between 21 and 77 % depending on the study.
- Several devices measure filling pressures in either the right ventricle (®Chronicle), pulmonary artery (CardioMEMS® or Impressure®), or left atrium (HeartPOD®).

5 Existing Device-Based Remote Monitoring Platforms

The preceding paragraph makes it clear that contemporary devices are capable of measuring a wide variety of physiologic variables. The next step however is to make the data available for HF nurses and physicians in a secure and save way via remote transmission. Each major device company therefore developed its own platform for remote transmission (Table 9.2) [73]. The general principles are similar: The implanted device is equipped with a micro-antenna that communicates with an external device known as the patient transmitter or patient device. The communication either requires active participation of the patient (via a wand) or occurs automatically (wandless). Data are then transferred via standard analog telephone lines or via cellular phone transmission to a secure central database organized by the company.

Table 9.2 Existing remote monitoring platforms (modified with permission from Samara et al. [74])

	Biotronik	Medtronic	St. Jude	Boston Scientific
Parameter	Home Monitoring®	Carelink® Network	Merlin.net Patient Care Network™	Latitude®
Available in	PM CRT ICD	PM CRT ICD	PM CRT ICD	 CRT ICD
Electrophysiologic variables	Device info (battery, leads, etc.) HR/HRV Afib + ventricular rate VES VT/Vfib + ATP + shocks IEGM % pacing, % biv pacing	Device info (battery, leads, etc.) HR/HRV Afib + ventricular rate VES VT/Vfib + ATP + shocks IEGM % pacing, % biv pacing	Device info (battery, leads, etc.) HR/HRV Afib + ventricular rate VES VT/Vfib + ATP + shocks IEGM % pacing, % biv pacing	Device info (battery, leads, etc.) HR/HRV Afib + ventricular rate VES VT/Vfib + ATP + shocks IEGM % pacing, % biv pacing
Additional variables	Patient activity	Patient activity OptiVol® impedance monitoring	Patient activity CorVue™ impedance monitoring	Patient activity Weight change BP cuff Questionnaire
Name of patient transmitter	CardioMessenger®	CareLink® Home Monitor	HouseCall Plus™ Merlin@home™	Latitude® communicator
Portable or stationary (transmitter)	Portable	Stationary	Stationary	Stationary
Patient participation required	No (wireless)	Yes (wand-operated) or no (wireless)	Yes (wand-operated) or no (wireless)	Yes (wand-operated) or no (wireless)

(continued)

Table 9.2 (continued)

Parameter	Biotronik: Home Monitoring®	Medtronic: Carelink® Network	St. Jude: Merlin.net Patient Care Network™	Boston Scientific: Latitude®
Frequency of data transmission	Daily (fixed time) +	Scheduled (every 21 days at most)	Scheduled	Scheduled (typically every week)
	Patient activated +	Patient activated (after events)	Patient activated (after events)	Patient activated (after events)
	Event activated (immediately)			
Long range transmission	Analog landline or GSM network	Analog landline or M-link cellular accessory	Analog landline	Analog landline
Patient trigger to take action (data transmission)	CardioMessenger call-back light	Audible alert	Vibration alert	Audible alert
Data storage	Home monitoring service center (central database in Europe)	®PaceART	Merlin.net™	®Latitide
Alert notification in case of event	Text messaging	Text messaging		Phone
	Fax		Fax	Fax
	E-mail	E-mail	E-mail	E-mail
Integration with electronic medical record	Software available	Software available	Software available	Software available
Impact of daily monitoring on battery longevity	Low	High	High	High

Last updated on June 15, 2012 (Biotronik: http://www.biotronik-healthservices.com, Medtronic: http://www.medtronic.com, St. Jude Medical: http://www.sjm.com/devices, Boston Scientific: http://www.aboutlatitude.com)

PM pacemaker, *CRT* cardiac resynchronization therapy, *ICD* implantable cardiac defibrillator, *HR* heart rate, *HRV* heart rate variability, *Afib* atrial fibrillation, *VES* ventricular extrasystoly, *VT* ventricular tachycardia, *Vfib* ventricular fibrillation, *ATP* anti-tachypacing, *IEGM* intracardiac electrogram

The overview in Table 9.2 stresses the similarities and differences between the platforms. The most important facts are:

- The Biotronik Home Monitoring system was the first approved system and is the only one that uses daily wireless data transfer via the mobile network without the need for patient involvement and with a portable patient transmitter.
- The Medtronic devices can transfer ®OptiVol impedance information via the CareLink network.
- The St. Jude devices transfer CorVue™ impedance and other electrophysiologic signals via the Merlin.net network.
- The Boston Scientific devices transfer not only device-based information but also scripted questions and body weight/blood pressure information via external devices thru the LATITUDE system.
- Interrogation and transfer of data requires power and can cause a substantial reduction in the longevity of the battery.

This remote technology is becoming more and more common for device follow-up (battery status, lead integrity, etc.). However, although technically feasible, no system allows remote reprogramming of the device due to legal issues.

6 What to Do with the Obtained Information?

The ultimate goal of the collection of the aforementioned variables is not to just monitor them, but to develop a strategy whereby these variables are used to avoid (re) hospitalizations and improve long-term outcomes. The variables from the implanted devices can first of all be used to improve risk stratification [74]. The PARTNERS-HF trial demonstrated how a combination of device-based variables can be used to predict risk of hospitalization [48]. It was also shown that impedance threshold crossings identify HF patients at increased risk for mortality [75]. The unique aspect of these device-acquired variables, as they are continuously monitored, is that they characterize the dynamic nature of the disease.

The more appealing idea is that the information from the implantable devices will be used in an event-directed management strategy, meaning that a treatment response is expected in case a certain event is detected. Although this might seem logic, several conditions have to be fulfilled to make this strategy work (Fig. 9.4) [76, 77]. It first of all requires a parameter that can be accurately measured and is both sensitive and specific for worsening HF. This information should quickly be made available for either the patient (self-management) or his caregivers (physician or HF nurse). The information has to be interpreted and the right treatment plan has to be made and communicated to the patient. The treatment has to be implemented and again monitored to see if the intended effect is accomplished. Potential delays reside in data transmission and in the often required communication between nurses and physicians. To make the loop as short as possible, the ideal scenario might be self-management by the patient in a similar way as a diabetic regulates his insulin. It is also important to realize that the obtained information could be used not only

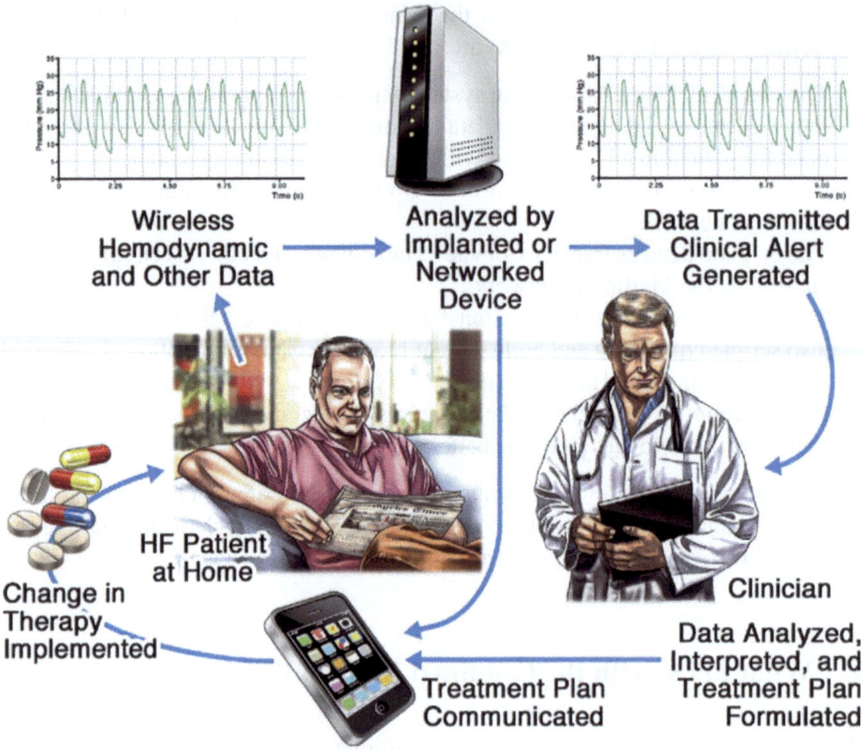

Fig. 9.4 Circle from home to heart failure disease management. Hemodynamic information is taken as an example but the principle is similar for other variables such as impedance, heart rate variability, or patient activity (with permission from Bui et al. [77])

for increasing diuretics in case of increasing congestion but also for increasing or starting vasodilators or decreasing diuretics and uptitrating of neurohormonal blockers in the case of euvolemia.

7 Evidence from Randomized Trials

Table 9.3 summarizes the methods and results from trials specifically designed to test the hypothesis that hospital admissions and/or mortality could be avoided by incorporating information from variables obtained by implantable devices into the daily management of ambulatory HF patients [78–82]. The most important findings are:

- Only one randomized trial (CHAMPIONS: CardioMEMS heart sensor allows monitoring of pressure to improve outcomes in NYHA class III heart failure patients trial) and one non-randomized observational trial (Catanzariti et al.) are positive (less HF hospitalizations) so far [78, 82].

Table 9.3 Overview of trials using (invasive) implantable devices for telemonitoring

Study acronym, first author	Year of publication	Number and type of patients	Study design	Intervention	Control-group	Duration (months)	Endpoints	Results
COMPASS-HF	2008	$N=274$	Multicenter	Right ventricular pressure monitoring by Chronicle® (Medtronic)	Also had the device implanted but information not used	6	HF events (hospitalization or emergency department visits)	Primary endpoint not met
Bourge et al.		NYHA III or IV	Prospective	At least weekly review of data	Received phone calls as well		Freedom from complications	Nonsignificant 21 % reduction in HF events
		HF hospitalization within 6 months	Randomized					Time to first HF event was reduced ($p=0.03$)
		Includes HFpEF						
	2009	$N=532$	Multicenter	Impedance measured by OptiVol® (Medtronic)	Audible alert was programmed OFF	12	HF hospitalization + cardiac death + HTX	AHFS in 7 % ON-group vs. 20 % OFF-group
Catanzariti et al.		NYHA I–IV	Observational	Audible alert when threshold crossing				Lower cardiac death and HF hospitalization in ON-group ($p=0.007$)
		CRT-D	Non-randomized					

(continued)

Table 9.3 (continued)

Study acronym, first author	Year of publication	Number and type of patients	Study design	Intervention	Control-group	Duration (months)	Endpoints	Results
DOT-HF	2011	N=335	Multicenter	Impedance measured by OptiVol® (Medtronic)	Audible alert was programmed OFF	15	All-cause mortality and HF rehospitalization	Trial stopped due to slow enrollment
Van Veldhuisen et al		NYHA II–IV (60 % II, 36 % III)	Prospective	Audible alert when threshold crossing followed by patient–physician contact				29 % in ON-group vs. 20 % in OFF-group (p=0.06)
		LVEF ≤35 %	Randomized	No remote access (no CareLink)				No benefit of impedance monitoring
		ICD or CRT-D						
REDUCE-HF	2011	N=400	Multicenter	Right ventricular pressure monitoring by Chronicle® (Medtronic)	HF disease management and telephone calls by nurses	12	HF events (hospitalization, emergency department visit, urgent clinic visit)	Stopped prematurely because of lead failure
Adamson et al.		NYHA II or III	Prospective	Weekly review of data				Not powered to analyze outcome
		ICD	Randomized					No difference between groups (HR 0.99)
		HF hospitalization within 12 months						

CHAMPION	2011	$N=550$	Multicenter	Pulmonary artery CardioMEMS® (CardioMEMS)	Standard of care	6	HF hospitalization	39 % reduction in heart failure hospitalization ($p<0.0001$)
Abraham et al.		NYHA III	Prospective	Daily transmission of measurements	Only heart failure centers			Freedom from device complications 98.6 %
		HF hospitalization within 12 months	Randomized	At least weekly review of data				Vasodilators were main treatment strategy

HF heart failure, *HTX* heart transplantation, *NYHA* New York Heart Association, *CRT-D* cardiac resynchronization therapy-defibrillator, *LVEF* left ventricular ejection fraction

- The CHAMPIONS-trial observed a 39 % reduction in HF hospitalization through daily transmissions of pulmonary artery pressures by the ®CardioMEMS device.
- The DOT-HF (The diagnostic outcome trial in heart failure) trial nearly showed an increase ($p = 0.06$) in hospitalizations in the group randomized to treatment with available impedance values. There was however no remote monitoring via CareLink in this trial which resulted in mandatory patient–physician contact after audible alerts [80].
- COMPASS-HF (Chronicle offers management to patients with advanced signs and symptoms of heart failure), a randomized trial based on RV pressure monitoring with the ®Chronicle device, demonstrated a trend towards less HF hospitalizations. REDUCE-HF (The reducing decompensation events utilizing intracardiac pressures in patients with chronic heart failure study), planned to be a larger trial with the same sensor, was stopped early due to lead failure in other trials causing an end on the further development of this system [79, 81].
- Several other randomized trials are still ongoing (LAPTOP-HF, OptiLink HF) [67, 83].

Another important finding is that the success of the CHAMPIONS-trial was predominantly achieved by intervention with vasodilators in the group randomized to pulmonary artery pressure-based treatment [84]. This contrasts with earlier observations in disease management programs that pointed towards adjustment of diuretics as the most important adaptation made after hospitalization [85].

To avoid that every audible alert necessarily results in an outpatient visit, remote monitoring seems essential when implantable devices are used to screen for threatening decompensation as recently proven in the evolution of management strategies of heart failure patients with implantable defibrillators study (EVOLVO-trial) [86, 87].

Key Points

- All device companies developed their own platform for the remote transmission and storage (on a secure server) of acquired physiologic data.
- Data obtained by implantable devices can be used for risk stratification or for event-directed management.
- The successful implementation of event-directed management is represented by a loop from the patient to caregiver and back to the patient (Fig. 9.4).
- Only one randomized trial (CHAMPIONS) using the ®Chronicle device demonstrated a reduction in HF admissions.

8 Financial and Medicolegal Aspects

The steep rise in the prevalence of HF, in general and in patients with devices in particular, implies that a great number of patients are potential candidates for telemonitoring with or without implantable devices. Filtering the relevant signals from the noise of physiologic data provided by remote monitoring platforms is challenging and time-consuming. One way to decrease the amount of received information is by being alerted only when there are changes in measured variables above or below certain thresholds. The direct incorporation of the data in the electronic medical record would also be of great value. Even this approach however will demand a larger workforce of midlevel personnel specialized in HF management. In many countries there are no reimbursement strategies for telemedicine. The initial concept was that remote monitoring was going to be cost-saving or at least cost-effective for society. However, the infrastructure and personnel required to perform telemonitoring, in combination with the uncertain effects on rehospitalization, puts this into question.

Another important question relates to who is responsible to act on the received data or alerts and what time delay is acceptable, particularly at night, weekend, or holidays. It has been proposed that the creation of dedicated telemedical centers that operate 24 h a day, 7 days a week, might be a more effective model to guarantee optimal care [88]. However, this might not be appropriate as long as there are no improvements in the approach and interpretation (sensitivity and specificity) of the physiologic data. Another potential threat is that the internet server database, containing patient information, could be hacked or even worse that devices with wireless capability could be accessed and reprogrammed (including commanded shocks). Although it is believed that the latter is theoretically possible, it requires considerable technical expertise and has never happened so far [89].

A third limiting factor particularly related to device-based management strategies has been the comfort level of healthcare providers to broadly utilize such device information, which stems from the lack of knowledge base regarding modern device technology, the lack of reliable algorithms that would guide management, and lack of incentives to better utilize these devices. In many ways, there have not been any consistent results in clinical studies to demonstrate the safety and efficacy despite broad clinical availability. Much work is needed to clarify and refine their clinical utility before any efforts in expanding their implementation. All the aforementioned factors make that telemonitoring for HF, although available, is not yet widely implemented in clinical practice.

9 Future Perspectives

At this point in time, it is somewhat uncertain whether telemonitoring for HF management will live up to its full potential and fulfill its initial promise. Clearly, the whole concept and the use of remote technology fit our modern way of life, but that on itself is not enough to justify its use in the absence of clear benefit. In our view, there are two mean reasons why telemonitoring has not demonstrated the envisioned results so far. First, HF and especially ADHF have a very heterogeneous pathophysiology. This makes it difficult to find one variable which is sensitive and specific enough to predict (in advance) imminent decompensation. A substantial amount ($\approx$40 %) of rehospitalizations in HF patients is even not for HF in the first place [33]. Likely, the solution will come from algorithms that combine several variables. Nevertheless, the search for other important measurable variables (e.g., neurohormones, natriuretic peptides, inflammatory markers, etc.) continues. Metabolite-based sensors that are capable of measuring circulating levels of metabolites could be of value [47, 90]. The second problem is treatment itself. Most often, the loop still involves the physician which means that, after an event, the patient gets in contact with the HF nurse who contacts the physician after which a treatment plan is made. This strategy can cause a substantial time lag. More ideal would be that this evolves into self-management whereby the patient interprets his own data and treats himself in the same way a diabetic regulates his own glycemia. To extend the parallel with diabetic treatment (i.e., insulin pumps) even more, some foresee a coupling of the implantable sensor to an effective and robust effector in the same device. This is already in use for the detection and treatment of arrhythmias [47]. Appropriate patient selection will be essential. It is believed that cardiologists with specific training in HF combined with device-training are best suited for this task [91]. Finally, newer and better drugs to treat ADHF would be welcome as well. After all, the same drugs (diuretics, neurohormonal antagonists, and vasodilators), given to patients admitted with ADHF, are used to treat patients who are telemonitored.

10 Conclusion

The care for patients with HF does not end with scheduling a follow-up appointment 3 months after a hospital admission. It starts during hospitalization with education about drugs, diet, and self-monitoring and includes a thorough explanation of the etiology, signs, and symptoms of HF. The patient should be given directions what to do and who to contact in the case of worsening symptoms. There is little or no doubt that this strategy, labeled "disease management," is effective in improving quality of life, avoiding hospital admissions, and even in reducing mortality. To what amount more intensive strategies, either structured telephone support or telemonitoring with or without information obtained from implantable devices, result in incremental benefit remains uncertain.

11 Sources of Further Information

We can advise the following articles for more detailed explanation and better understanding of telemonitoring and sensor technologies:

- Reviews:

  Samara et al. [74] Clearly explain the current device monitoring strategies.

  Bui et al. [77]. Give a concise overview of the present and future role of home monitoring.

  Jung et al. [73]. Describe the advantages and disadvantages with the different commercial monitoring platforms.

Konstam et al. and Desai et al. [19, 20]. Discuss the role of home monitoring in a "controversies in cardiovascular medicine" (pro-con) series.

Desai and Stevenson [76]. Classic editorial about how the ideal telemonitoring set-up would look like.

- Pathophysiology of ADHF:

Zile et al. [7]. Report the findings from continuous RV pressure monitoring regarding the pathophysiology of ADHF.

Adamson et al. [9]. Bundle our current knowledge about the transition from chronic to ADHF.

- What is impedance?

Tang et al. [51]. Describe in very detail what impedance is, how it can be measured, and what the current applications are.

- Large clinical trials to remember:

Rich et al. [21]. Landmark trial demonstrating the benefit of disease management.

CHAMPIONS (Abraham et al.) [82]. The only randomized controlled trial using an implantable monitoring device that showed reduction in HF hospitalization.

DOT-HF (van Veldhuisen et al.) [80]. Negative trial showing no benefit of impedance monitoring with audible alert.

References

1. Roger VL et al (2012) Heart disease and stroke statistics—2012 update: a report from the American Heart Association. Circulation 125(1):e2–e220
2. Krumholz HM et al (1997) Readmission after hospitalization for congestive heart failure among Medicare beneficiaries. Arch Intern Med 157(1):99–104
3. Lee WC et al (2004) Economic burden of heart failure: a summary of recent literature. Heart Lung 33(6):362–371
4. Jencks SF, Williams MV, Coleman EA (2009) Rehospitalizations among patients in the Medicare fee-for-service program. N Engl J Med 360(14):1418–1428
5. Ahmed A et al (2008) Incident heart failure hospitalization and subsequent mortality in chronic heart failure: a propensity-matched study. J Card Fail 14(3):211–218
6. Zile MR et al (2011) Hemodynamic factors associated with acute decompensated heart failure: part 1—insights into pathophysiology. J Card Fail 17(4):282–291
7. Zile MR et al (2008) Transition from chronic compensated to acute decompensated heart failure: pathophysiological insights obtained from continuous monitoring of intracardiac pressures. Circulation 118(14):1433–1441
8. Vanderheyden M et al (2010) Continuous monitoring of intrathoracic impedance and right ventricular pressures in patients with heart failure. Circ Heart Fail 3(3):370–377
9. Adamson PB (2009) Pathophysiology of the transition from chronic compensated and acute decompensated heart failure: new insights from continuous monitoring devices. Curr Heart Fail Rep 6(4):287–292

10. Fallick C, Sobotka PA, Dunlap ME (2011) Sympathetically mediated changes in capacitance: redistribution of the venous reservoir as a cause of decompensation. Circ Heart Fail 4(5): 669–675
11. Yu CM et al (2005) Intrathoracic impedance monitoring in patients with heart failure: correlation with fluid status and feasibility of early warning preceding hospitalization. Circulation 112(6):841–848
12. Chaudhry SI et al (2007) Patterns of weight change preceding hospitalization for heart failure. Circulation 116(14):1549–1554
13. Adamson PB et al (2004) Continuous autonomic assessment in patients with symptomatic heart failure: prognostic value of heart rate variability measured by an implanted cardiac resynchronization device. Circulation 110(16):2389–2394
14. Rademaker MT et al (2011) Monitoring of heart failure: comparison of left atrial pressure with intrathoracic impedance and natriuretic peptide measurements in an experimental model of ovine heart failure. Clin Sci (Lond) 120(5):207–217
15. Ohlsson A et al (2003) Central hemodynamic responses during serial exercise tests in heart failure patients using implantable hemodynamic monitors. Eur J Heart Fail 5(3):253–259
16. Adamson PB et al (2006) Ambulatory hemodynamic monitoring from an implanted device: components of continuous 24-hour pressures that correlate to supine resting conditions and acute right heart catheterization. Congest Heart Fail 12(1):14–19
17. Michalsen A, Konig G, Thimme W (1998) Preventable causative factors leading to hospital admission with decompensated heart failure. Heart 80(5):437–441
18. Krumholz HM et al (2006) A taxonomy for disease management: a scientific statement from the American Heart Association Disease Management Taxonomy Writing Group. Circulation 114(13):1432–1445
19. Konstam MA (2012) Home monitoring should be the central element in an effective program of heart failure disease management. Circulation 125(6):820–827
20. Desai AS (2012) Home monitoring heart failure care does not improve patient outcomes: looking beyond telephone-based disease management. Circulation 125(6):828–836
21. Rich MW et al (1995) A multidisciplinary intervention to prevent the readmission of elderly patients with congestive heart failure. N Engl J Med 333(18):1190–1195
22. Goldberg LR et al (2003) Randomized trial of a daily electronic home monitoring system in patients with advanced heart failure: the Weight Monitoring in Heart Failure (WHARF) trial. Am Heart J 146(4):705–712
23. Kimmelstiel C et al (2004) Randomized, controlled evaluation of short- and long-term benefits of heart failure disease management within a diverse provider network: the SPAN-CHF trial. Circulation 110(11):1450–1455
24. Cleland JG et al (2005) Noninvasive home telemonitoring for patients with heart failure at high risk of recurrent admission and death: the Trans-European Network-Home-Care Management System (TEN-HMS) study. J Am Coll Cardiol 45(10):1654–1664
25. Sisk JE et al (2006) Effects of nurse management on the quality of heart failure care in minority communities: a randomized trial. Ann Intern Med 145(4):273–283
26. Jaarsma T et al (2008) Effect of moderate or intensive disease management program on outcome in patients with heart failure: Coordinating Study Evaluating Outcomes of Advising and Counseling in Heart Failure (COACH). Arch Intern Med 168(3):316–324
27. Soran OZ et al (2008) A randomized clinical trial of the clinical effects of enhanced heart failure monitoring using a computer-based telephonic monitoring system in older minorities and women. J Card Fail 14(9):711–717
28. Giordano A et al (2009) Multicenter randomised trial on home-based telemanagement to prevent hospital readmission of patients with chronic heart failure. Int J Cardiol 131(2):192–199
29. Dar O et al (2009) A randomized trial of home telemonitoring in a typical elderly heart failure population in North West London: results of the Home-HF study. Eur J Heart Fail 11(3): 319–325
30. Mortara A et al (2009) Home telemonitoring in heart failure patients: the HHH study (Home or Hospital in Heart Failure). Eur J Heart Fail 11(3):312–318

31. Powell LH et al (2010) Self-management counseling in patients with heart failure: the heart failure adherence and retention randomized behavioral trial. JAMA 304(12):1331–1338
32. Ferrante D et al (2010) Long-term results after a telephone intervention in chronic heart failure: DIAL (Randomized Trial of Phone Intervention in Chronic Heart Failure) follow-up. J Am Coll Cardiol 56(5):372–378
33. Chaudhry SI et al (2010) Telemonitoring in patients with heart failure. N Engl J Med 363(24): 2301–2309
34. Koehler F et al (2010) Telemedical Interventional Monitoring in Heart Failure (TIM-HF), a randomized, controlled intervention trial investigating the impact of telemedicine on mortality in ambulatory patients with heart failure: study design. Eur J Heart Fail 12(12):1354–1362
35. Dewalt DA et al (2012) Multisite randomized trial of a single-session versus multisession literacy-sensitive self-care intervention for patients with heart failure. Circulation 125(23): 2854–2862
36. Clark RA et al (2007) Telemonitoring or structured telephone support programmes for patients with chronic heart failure: systematic review and meta-analysis. BMJ 334(7600):942
37. Inglis SC et al (2011) Which components of heart failure programmes are effective? A systematic review and meta-analysis of the outcomes of structured telephone support or telemonitoring as the primary component of chronic heart failure management in 8323 patients: Abridged Cochrane Review. Eur J Heart Fail 13(9):1028–1040
38. Lindenfeld J et al (2010) HFSA 2010 Comprehensive Heart Failure Practice Guideline. J Card Fail 16(6):e1–e194
39. McMurray JJ et al (2012) ESC Guidelines for the diagnosis and treatment of acute and chronic heart failure 2012: The Task Force for the Diagnosis and Treatment of Acute and Chronic Heart Failure 2012 of the European Society of Cardiology. Developed in collaboration with the Heart Failure Association (HFA) of the ESC. Eur Heart J 14(8):803–869
40. Zhang J et al (2009) Predicting hospitalization due to worsening heart failure using daily weight measurement: analysis of the Trans-European Network-Home-Care Management System (TEN-HMS) study. Eur J Heart Fail 11(4):420–427
41. Stevenson LW, Perloff JK (1989) The limited reliability of physical signs for estimating hemodynamics in chronic heart failure. JAMA 261(6):884–888
42. Ellery S et al (2006) Predicting mortality and rehospitalization in heart failure patients with home monitoring—the Home CARE pilot study. Clin Res Cardiol 95(Suppl 3):III29–III35
43. Katona PG, Jih F (1975) Respiratory sinus arrhythmia: noninvasive measure of parasympathetic cardiac control. J Appl Physiol 39(5):801–805
44. La Rovere MT et al (2003) Short-term heart rate variability strongly predicts sudden cardiac death in chronic heart failure patients. Circulation 107(4):565–570
45. Fantoni C et al (2005) Cardiac resynchronization therapy improves heart rate profile and heart rate variability of patients with moderate to severe heart failure. J Am Coll Cardiol 46(10): 1875–1882
46. Gilliam FR 3rd, Ewald GA, Sweeney RJ (2012) Feasibility of automated heart failure decompensation detection using remote patient monitoring: results from the decompensation detection study. J Innov Card Rhythm Manage 3:735–745
47. Merchant FM, Dec GW, Singh JP (2010) Implantable sensors for heart failure. Circ Arrhythm Electrophysiol 3(6):657–667
48. Whellan DJ et al (2010) Combined heart failure device diagnostics identify patients at higher risk of subsequent heart failure hospitalizations: results from PARTNERS HF (Program to Access and Review Trending Information and Evaluate Correlation to Symptoms in Patients With Heart Failure) study. J Am Coll Cardiol 55(17):1803–1810
49. Cole CR et al (2001) Correlation of impedance minute ventilation with measured minute ventilation in a rate responsive pacemaker. Pacing Clin Electrophysiol 24(6):989–993
50. Ohlsson A et al (2001) Continuous ambulatory monitoring of absolute right ventricular pressure and mixed venous oxygen saturation in patients with heart failure using an implantable haemodynamic monitor: results of a 1 year multicentre feasibility study. Eur Heart J 22(11): 942–954

51. Tang WH, Tong W (2009) Measuring impedance in congestive heart failure: current options and clinical applications. Am Heart J 157(3):402–411
52. Patterson RP (1989) Fundamentals of impedance cardiography. IEEE Eng Med Biol Mag 8(1):35–38
53. Luepker RV, Michael JR, Warbasse JR (1973) Transthoracic electrical impedance; quantitative evaluation of a non-invasive measure of thoracic fluid volume. Am Heart J 85(1):83–93
54. Kamath SA et al (2009) Correlation of impedance cardiography with invasive hemodynamic measurements in patients with advanced heart failure: the BioImpedance CardioGraphy (BIG) substudy of the Evaluation Study of Congestive Heart Failure and Pulmonary Artery Catheterization Effectiveness (ESCAPE) Trial. Am Heart J 158(2):217–223
55. Khoury DS et al (2009) Ambulatory monitoring of congestive heart failure by multiple bioelectric impedance vectors. J Am Coll Cardiol 53(12):1075–1081
56. Becher J et al (2010) Device-based impedance measurement is a useful and accurate tool for direct assessment of intrathoracic fluid accumulation in heart failure. Europace 12(5):731–740
57. Luthje L et al (2005) Detection of heart failure decompensation using intrathoracic impedance monitoring by a triple-chamber implantable defibrillator. Heart Rhythm 2(9):997–999
58. Vollmann D et al (2007) Clinical utility of intrathoracic impedance monitoring to alert patients with an implanted device of deteriorating chronic heart failure. Eur Heart J 28(15):1835–1840
59. Abraham WT et al (2011) Intrathoracic impedance vs daily weight monitoring for predicting worsening heart failure events: results of the Fluid Accumulation Status Trial (FAST). Congest Heart Fail 17(2):51–55
60. Conraads VM et al (2011) Sensitivity and positive predictive value of implantable intrathoracic impedance monitoring as a predictor of heart failure hospitalizations: the SENSE-HF trial. Eur Heart J 32(18):2266–2273
61. Reynolds DW et al (1995) Measurement of pulmonary artery diastolic pressure from the right ventricle. J Am Coll Cardiol 25(5):1176–1182
62. Steinhaus DM et al (1996) Initial experience with an implantable hemodynamic monitor. Circulation 93(4):745–752
63. Magalski A et al (2002) Continuous ambulatory right heart pressure measurements with an implantable hemodynamic monitor: a multicenter, 12-month follow-up study of patients with chronic heart failure. J Card Fail 8(2):63–70
64. Adamson PB et al (2003) Ongoing right ventricular hemodynamics in heart failure: clinical value of measurements derived from an implantable monitoring system. J Am Coll Cardiol 41(4):565–571
65. Ritzema J et al (2007) Direct left atrial pressure monitoring in ambulatory heart failure patients: initial experience with a new permanent implantable device. Circulation 116(25):2952–2959
66. Ritzema J et al (2010) Physician-directed patient self-management of left atrial pressure in advanced chronic heart failure. Circulation 121(9):1086–1095
67. ClinicalTrials.gov (2011) Left atrial pressure monitoring to optimize heart failure therapy (LAPTOP-HF). http://clinicaltrials.gov/ct2/show/NCT01121107?term=laptop&rank=2. Cited 19 June 2012.
68. Verdejo HE et al (2007) Comparison of a radiofrequency-based wireless pressure sensor to swan-ganz catheter and echocardiography for ambulatory assessment of pulmonary artery pressure in heart failure. J Am Coll Cardiol 50(25):2375–2382
69. Hoppe UC et al (2009) Chronic monitoring of pulmonary artery pressure in patients with severe heart failure: multicentre experience of the monitoring Pulmonary Artery Pressure by Implantable device Responding to Ultrasonic Signal (PAPIRUS) II study. Heart 95(13):1091–1097
70. Kjellstrom B et al (2004) Six years follow-up of an implanted SvO(2) sensor in the right ventricle. Eur J Heart Fail 6(5):627–634
71. Plicchi G et al (2002) PEA I and PEA II based implantable haemodynamic monitor: pre clinical studies in sheep. Europace 4(1):49–54

72. Dupuis JM et al (2003) Programming optimal atrioventricular delay in dual chamber pacing using peak endocardial acceleration: comparison with a standard echocardiographic procedure. Pacing Clin Electrophysiol 26(1 Pt 2):210–213
73. Jung W et al (2008) Advances in remote monitoring of implantable pacemakers, cardioverter defibrillators and cardiac resynchronization therapy systems. J Interv Card Electrophysiol 23(1):73–85
74. Samara MA, Tang WH (2011) Device monitoring strategies in acute heart failure syndromes. Heart Fail Rev 16(5):491–502
75. Tang WH et al (2012) Threshold crossing of device-based intrathoracic impedance trends identifies relatively increased mortality risk. Eur Heart J 33(17):2189–2196
76. Desai AS, Stevenson LW (2010) Connecting the circle from home to heart-failure disease management. N Engl J Med 363(24):2364–2367
77. Bui AL, Fonarow GC (2012) Home monitoring for heart failure management. J Am Coll Cardiol 59(2):97–104
78. Catanzariti D et al (2009) Monitoring intrathoracic impedance with an implantable defibrillator reduces hospitalizations in patients with heart failure. Pacing Clin Electrophysiol 32(3): 363–370
79. Bourge RC et al (2008) Randomized controlled trial of an implantable continuous hemodynamic monitor in patients with advanced heart failure: the COMPASS-HF study. J Am Coll Cardiol 51(11):1073–1079
80. van Veldhuisen DJ et al (2011) Intrathoracic impedance monitoring, audible patient alerts, and outcome in patients with heart failure. Circulation 124(16):1719–1726
81. Adamson PB et al (2011) Continuous hemodynamic monitoring in patients with mild to moderate heart failure: results of The Reducing Decompensation Events Utilizing Intracardiac Pressures in Patients With Chronic Heart Failure (REDUCEhf) trial. Congest Heart Fail 17(5):248–254
82. Abraham WT et al (2011) Wireless pulmonary artery haemodynamic monitoring in chronic heart failure: a randomised controlled trial. Lancet 377(9766):658–666
83. Brachmann J et al (2011) Fluid status monitoring with a wireless network to reduce cardiovascular-related hospitalizations and mortality in heart failure: rationale and design of the OptiLink HF Study (Optimization of Heart Failure Management using OptiVol Fluid Status Monitoring and CareLink). Eur J Heart Fail 13(7):796–804
84. Costanzo MR et al (2011) Medical management guided by pulmonary artery pressures in NYHA functional class III heart failure patients. J Card Fail 17:S93
85. Shah MR et al (2005) Intensity and focus of heart failure disease management after hospital discharge. Am Heart J 149(4):715–721
86. Landolina M et al (2012) Remote monitoring reduces healthcare utilization and improves quality of care in heart failure patients with implantable defibrillators: the EVOLVO (evolution of management strategies of heart failure patients with implantable defibrillators) study. Circulation 125(24):2985–2992
87. Van Veldhuisen DJ, Maass AH (2012) Telemonitoring of outpatients with heart failure: a search for the holy grail? Circulation 125(24):2965–2967
88. Anker SD, Koehler F, Abraham WT (2011) Telemedicine and remote management of patients with heart failure. Lancet 378(9792):731–739
89. Burri H, Senouf D (2009) Remote monitoring and follow-up of pacemakers and implantable cardioverter defibrillators. Europace 11(6):701–709
90. Porapakkham P et al (2010) B-type natriuretic peptide-guided heart failure therapy: a meta-analysis. Arch Intern Med 170(6):507–514
91. Adamson PB et al (2004) The evolving challenge of chronic heart failure management: a call for a new curriculum for training heart failure specialists. J Am Coll Cardiol 44(7):1354–1357
92. Adamson PB et al (2007) Reducing events in patients with chronic heart failure (REDUCEhf) study design: continuous hemodynamic monitoring with an implantable defibrillator. Clin Cardiol 30(11):567–575

Part III
Functional Mitral Regurgitation in Heart Failure

Chapter 10
Functional Mitral Regurgitation: The Surgeons' Perspective

Jerry Braun and Robert J.M. Klautz

Abstract Physicians who are involved in heart failure treatment are regularly confronted with patients who present with functional mitral regurgitation (MR), occurring in a setting of ischaemic or non-ischaemic cardiomyopathy. For these patients, the current guidelines do not offer clear treatment algorithms, and mitral valve surgery is often not advised. This is however not a proper representation of the currently available literature on this topic, and may lead to patients not being evaluated for an intervention from which they may benefit. This chapter deals with the surgical perspective of functional mitral regurgitation. Topics covered are pathophysiology (with its implications for surgical techniques and annuloplasty ring choice), patient assessment and a critical appraisal of the outcome of different surgical approaches. While the focus lies on the results of undersized restrictive annuloplasty, various additional techniques are discussed in order to provide a tailored medico-surgical approach to this difficult subset of patients.

1 Introduction

Patients with heart failure and functional mitral regurgitation are regularly presented to the heart failure team. Optimal treatment requires an individualized multidisciplinary approach that should also consider surgical options. The cardiac surgeon should therefore always be part of this medico-surgical team to allow a tailor-made solution for each patient. For several reasons the contribution of surgery in the treatment of heart failure patients is still debated. Current guidelines only

J. Braun • R.J.M. Klautz (✉)
Department of Cardiothoracic Surgery, Leids Universitair Medisch Centrum, P.O. Box 9600, 2300 RC, Leiden, The Netherlands
e-mail: R.J.M.Klautz@lumc.nl

J. Bartunek and M. Vanderheyden (eds.), *Translational Approach to Heart Failure*, DOI 10.1007/978-1-4614-7345-9_10, © Springer Science+Business Media New York 2013

recommend a marginal role for mitral valve surgery [1, 2]. This chapter will focus on the existing controversies, analyze their backgrounds and provide a structured approach to patients with heart failure and functional mitral regurgitation (MR). The chapter starts with a brief history of functional MR, presents a clinical perspective in terms of prevalence and outcomes, provides recommendations on assessment of functional MR and discusses the different surgical approaches and their outcomes. We present the structured team approach in our clinic, and end with likely future trends in this area.

2 Defining Functional Mitral Regurgitation

Functional mitral regurgitation is a disease condition in which the macroscopically normal mitral valve becomes insufficient as a consequence of left ventricular wall motion abnormalities. As such, it is also referred to as secondary MR. Depending on its cause, functional MR can be classified as *ischaemic MR* or as *MR in non-ischaemic* or *idiopathic cardiomyopathy*. Regardless of aetiology, functional MR carries a poor prognosis and is an independent risk factor for mortality. There are similarities between ischaemic and non-ischaemic functional MR, but there are also distinct differences. In this chapter we will discuss the disease entities together when possible, but separately when necessary.

Ischaemic MR in heart failure patients is always *chronic* ischaemic MR. Using a proper definition of ischaemic MR is important to differentiate between true chronic ischaemic MR and patients who have organic MR and incidental coronary artery disease (CAD). The latter patient category has a much better prognosis. Basically a definition should appreciate the fact that the mitral insufficiency *is caused by* CAD. This means that a patient should have CAD that has led to left ventricular (LV) wall motion abnormalities (due to ischaemia, infarction or both) that induce mitral insufficiency. In addition, the mitral valve should be free from organic disease. As such, a definition of chronic ischaemic mitral regurgitation would be insufficiency of an anatomically normal mitral valve in a setting of wall motion abnormalities of the left ventricle that are caused by the sequelae of CAD.

3 Historical Notes on Functional Mitral Regurgitation

3.1 Ischaemic Mitral Regurgitation

In 1963 Burch suggested that the sequelae of ischaemia could cause mitral regurgitation as a functional phenomenon—rather than only following papillary muscle rupture caused by myocardial infarction in a report on two patients [3]. He related the occurrence of a new systolic murmur, appearing shortly after myocardial infarction, to a "syndrome of papillary muscle dysfunction", and hypothesized that "failure of the infarcted papillary muscle to contract during systole results in mitral regurgitation", actually suggesting leaflet prolapse. Although experimental studies in dogs showed already in 1971 that damage to the papillary muscle alone does not lead to MR, while MR does occur when this injury also involves the adjacent LV wall [4], papillary muscle dysfunction was considered a major determinant in the development of ischaemic MR for a long time. This gradually changed with the introduction of echocardiography. In the landmark paper by Godley and associates, it was described that most patients who developed MR following myocardial infarction showed that "one or both leaflets were effectively arrested within the cavity of the left ventricle during ventricular systole" [5]. This is a nice description of systolic restrictive motion, which is now considered the echocardiographic signature of functional MR. These patients almost invariably demonstrated dyskinetic wall motion in the region immediately surrounding one of the papillary muscles.

Further insights have gradually replaced the concept of papillary muscle dysfunction. We now realize that all components of the mitral valve complex may play a role in functional MR—regardless of aetiology—which has implications for a therapeutic approach.

3.2 Mitral Regurgitation in Non-ischaemic Dilated Cardiomyopathy

Historically, functional MR in non-ischaemic cardiomyopathy has been less clearly recognized as a distinct disease condition. The presence of MR in idiopathic cardiomyopathy was first quantified by angiography in a series of 36 patients, with MR present in 64 % of patients [6]. The higher LV end-diastolic volume in these patients made the authors conclude that annulus dilatation was involved in causing MR. However, the overlapping range in end-diastolic volumes in patients with and without MR suggested that other factors were also involved, in particular "an altered position of the papillary muscles and their axes of tension", as hypothesized by Perloff and Roberts [7]. The surgical treatment of functional MR was regarded inappropriate for a long time. In their 1982 review article on cardiomyopathies, Johnson and Palacios state: "Severe mitral regurgitation, present in a small number of patients with idiopathic congestive cardiomyopathy, may tempt the physician to advise replacement of the mitral valve. We believe that this temptation should be resisted: the perioperative mortality is high in patients whose LV ejection fraction is as low as it is in idiopathic cardiomyopathy, and long-term survival is probably unimproved by operation" [8].

3.3 Introduction of Undersized or Restrictive Mitral Annuloplasty as a Surgical Treatment for Functional Mitral Regurgitation

For a very long time, the only surgery considered possible in these patients was cardiac transplantation. The poor reputation of mitral valve surgery in end-stage cardiomyopathy was due to the poor outcome of mitral valve replacement in patients with systolic heart failure [9]. A major concern was that by abolishing MR the poorly functioning left ventricle would lose its low-impedance left atrial "pop-off" and deteriorate further. The case series presented by Bach and Bolling from the University of Michigan in 1995 represented a major breakthrough by demonstrating that mitral valve repair using an annuloplasty ring was feasible with low mortality and fairly good early outcome [10, 11]. In the interesting discussion that followed the presentation of Bolling's paper at the meeting of the Western Thoracic Surgical Association, he mentions undersizing the trigone-to-trigone distance "perhaps by one size", and reports a mean ring size of 29. In 1998 the Michigan group reported on 48 patients with end-stage non-ischaemic heart failure with an ejection fraction of 16 %, and severe functional MR with one perioperative death and 2-year survival of 72 % [12]. In the discussion following this manuscript, Bolling mentions that he changed his strategy from undersizing by one ring size to using the "smallest ring possible". These publications introduced the concept of *undersized* or *restrictive mitral annuloplasty*, which is the cornerstone of the surgical treatment of functional MR.

Key Points

- Patients with functional MR and heart failure require an individualized multidisciplinary approach in which surgery plays a role.
- Functional MR can occur in ischaemic and non-ischaemic settings.
- Functional MR is not caused by papillary muscle dysfunction.

4 Pathophysiology of Functional Mitral Regurgitation and Implications for Surgery

The pathophysiology of functional MR has been the subject of many experimental and clinical studies, and the surgeon should appreciate the basic mechanisms underlying functional MR because of their implications for surgical treatment. Functional MR is a *dynamic* phenomenon; this has important consequences for patient assessment, which will be discussed in another paragraph. Mitral valve closure is a result of a *balance of forces*: the closing forces generated by LV contraction and the tethering forces exerted by the (contracting) papillary muscles and chords [13]. In functional MR, the tethering forces are stronger and retain the leaflets in the left ventricular cavity. When LV remodelling sets in, tethering increases and mitral leaflet closure becomes more dependent on closing forces, which are likely to diminish

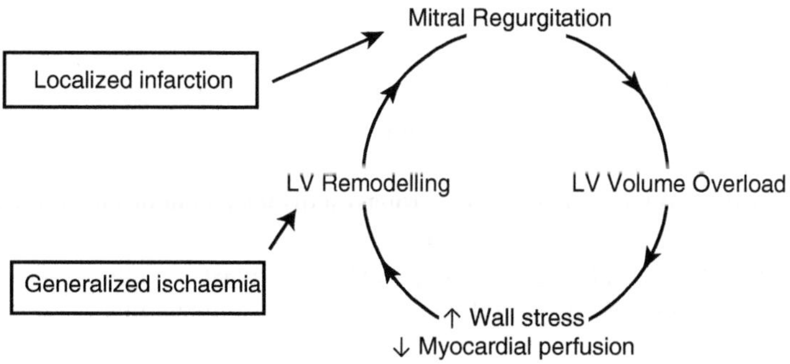

Fig. 10.1 Schematic representation of the vicious cycle involved in ischaemic mitral regurgitation. *LV* left ventricular

further during the continuing remodelling process. A vicious cycle ensues and MR begets MR. This brings us to the next typical feature of functional MR: it is *both a valvular and a ventricular disease*. In functional MR, the left ventricle suffers from both the initial disease (ischaemic or other) and from the volume overload resulting from the insufficiency (Fig. 10.1). It is therefore easy to understand that functional MR will have a more profound effect on cardiac function (and therewith on clinical status and outcome) than organic MR of the same severity.

All components of the mitral valve apparatus may contribute to the development of functional MR. The leaflets may demonstrate insufficient adaptation to an increase in annular area [14]. The mitral annulus shows dilatation, flattening (loss of saddle shape) and lack of systolic area reduction with restricted annular motion [15–17]. However, annulus dilatation by itself does not lead to significant MR because of the twofold surplus of mitral valve tissue available to cover the annular cross-sectional area. In chronic ischaemic animal models, the annulus was found to increase both in the septal-to-lateral dimension and in the commissure-to-commissure dimension. However, only septal-to-lateral dilatation was associated with the development of ischaemic MR [18, 19], and reduction of septal-to-lateral dimension by 15–20 % of baseline diameter abolished MR [20]. Necropsy studies showed that the changes in annular dimensions in cardiomyopathy do not only involve the muscular part of the annulus, but also the fibrous part—including the intercommissural area—to a similar extent [21]. In vivo, the pathological increase in annular area (of approximately 60 % in diastole) and perimeter (of approximately 24 %) was confirmed with 3D transthoracic echocardiography (TTE), together with the finding of restricted annular motion [15, 22].

The role of the papillary muscles has received renewed interest with the advent of resynchronization therapy. Papillary muscle dyssynchrony may contribute to the development or worsening of functional MR. Patients with dilated cardiomyopathy and prolonged QRS (>130 ms) show significant MR twice as often as patients with normal QRS duration [23]. This may be explained by geometrical changes induced by the dyssynchrony itself, as well as by delayed LV pressure generation.

Left ventricular changes associated with functional MR include functional changes (wall motion abnormalities and reduced contractility), dimensional changes (LV dilatation with volume increase) and geometrical changes (globally manifested by increased sphericity and locally by papillary muscle displacement). LV dilatation alone is not sufficient to cause functional MR, but increased sphericity has been related to MR through secondary posterolateral displacement of the papillary muscles [24, 25]. Outward displacement of one or both papillary muscles directly influences mitral valve morphology and mechanics by increasing tenting; this can occur in—but is not limited to—a setting of global LV remodelling with increased sphericity.

5 Functional Mitral Regurgitation and the Left Ventricle

The primary injury and the volume overload caused by MR induce changes in global LV size, mass, shape and function that are collectively referred to as "remodelling". At first, these changes compensate for the loss of pump function resulting from the injury, but over time they become pathological. The heart will maintain stroke volume by increasing its cavity size at the expense of ejection fraction. This causes a right ward shift of the pressure-volume curve with increased end-diastolic volume and end-diastolic pressure. Increased LV wall stress occurs, which can initially be compensated for by secondary hypertrophy. However, the extent of compensatory hypertrophy is limited, and further dilatation will lead to increased wall stress as described by the LaPlace law, which states that wall stress is the product of transmural pressure and radius, divided by wall thickness. These changes increase oxygen demand (which obviously is limited even more in patients with ischaemic disease). Ultimately, myocyte length increases and myofibril content decreases which further leads to contractile dysfunction. In this way a vicious cycle ensues, and dilatation begets dilatation.

A simple mathematical example can demonstrate how a given degree of functional MR influences haemodynamics. Suppose an EF of 50 % and a regurgitant volume of 40 mL. A resting cardiac index of 2 L/min/m^2 for an average man is equivalent to a cardiac output of 4 L/min. At a heart rate of 70 mL, this translates into a forward stroke volume of 57 mL. With a regurgitant volume of 40 mL, this adds up to a total stroke volume of approximately 100 mL. The end-diastolic volume then has to be 200 mL to achieve an EF of 50 %, which is about twice the normal size. This example also demonstrates how EF is only a surrogate marker for LV contractility; it is highly load-dependent and can remain more or less normal in MR while LV contractility decreases, due to the low LV impedance in systole created by the mitral insufficiency. It has been demonstrated that end-systolic volume is the most reliable non-invasive marker for LV contractility since it is not dependent of preload and varies directly and linearly with afterload [26].

The term *reverse remodelling* is applied to a dilated left ventricle that no longer shows progressive dilatation, and instead regresses towards a normal shape and volume. Also in reverse remodelling we can usually only assess global parameters of this process.

There is no consensus on what to consider proof of reverse remodelling [27]. Most studies use cut-off values of 10 or 15 % reduction in LV diameters or volumes.

Key Points

- Functional MR is a dynamic phenomenon, and all components of the mitral valve apparatus may contribute to its development in a patient.
- Functional MR is both a valvular and a ventricular disease.
- Functional MR and left ventricular remodelling occur in a vicious cycle.
- Ejection fraction is not a good marker of LV function in patients with MR.

6 Incidence, Prevalence and Clinical Outcomes of Functional Mitral Regurgitation

Most studies that provide information on incidence and prevalence of functional MR focus on ischaemic MR while some have included both ischaemic and non-ischaemic aetiologies; unfortunately, data are often presented without stratification. While ischaemic MR is relatively common, exact data on its occurrence are hard to provide since studies reporting on this subject are very different. These differences relate to the interval between the ischaemic event and the occurrence of MR (ranging from several hours to months after the infarction); the technique with which MR was diagnosed (angiography vs. echocardiography) and quantified (semi-quantitative vs. quantitative assessment); the severity of MR; and the characteristics of the study population (observational cohorts, patients included in clinical trials, etc.) [28]. Regarding the presence of functional MR in non-ischaemic cardiomyopathy, available studies have similar shortcomings. An important distinction in the development of MR between ischaemic and non-ischaemic MR needs to be pointed out here. In non-ischaemic MR the mitral insufficiency develops rather late in the natural history when considerable remodelling of the left ventricle has taken place. Low EF and the clinical syndrome of heart failure therefore always accompany it. Ischaemic MR can develop in the same way when diffuse ischaemia leads to LV remodelling and thus ischaemic cardiomyopathy. However, more frequently MR results from a local LV wall motion abnormality, following a myocardial infarction or local ischaemia. In this situation the left ventricle (and EF) can be relatively preserved and the syndrome of heart failure may not yet have become manifest (Fig. 10.2).

Table 10.1 provides an overview of the studies that report on this subject [29–39].

It can be seen that the occurrence of post-MR mitral regurgitation of any severity is frequent with a roughly estimated incidence between 20 and 60 % depending on the population studied. Clinically, patients who develop MR following myocardial infarction are often older and more often females, and they show more signs of LV remodelling compared to patients without MR. There is no relationship between infarct size and the occurrence of MR. Several studies indicate a higher prevalence of ischaemic MR following an infarction in the inferior or posterior region, but this is not a consistent finding. Ischaemic MR has a negative effect on prognosis, which is already present in patients with mild MR. This excess

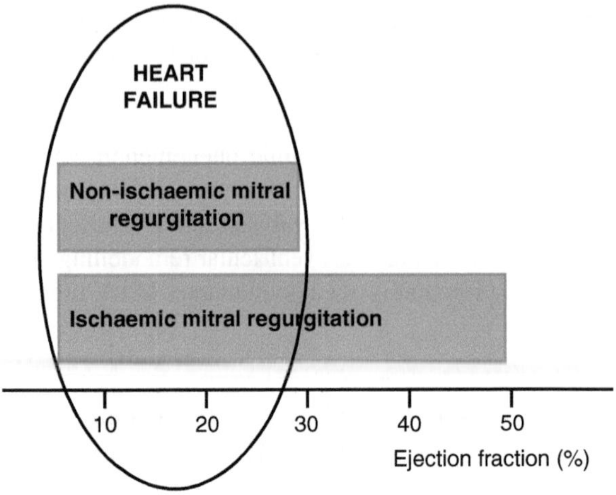

Fig. 10.2 Differences in the range of left ventricular ejection fraction and the presence of heart failure symptoms between ischaemic and non-ischaemic mitral regurgitation

mortality is graded, i.e. related to the degree of MR and independent of LVEF. Finally, ischaemic MR is often clinically silent with the absence of systolic murmur, and has a characteristic dynamic phenomenon.

Functional MR in non-ischaemic patients is also frequently present as summarized in Table 10.1. Mortality is high and related to the severity of MR, although evidence regarding its importance as an independent risk factor is ambiguous. There is an important relationship with tricuspid regurgitation, which may reflect the fact that in non-ischaemic cardiomyopathy both ventricles can be injured. Several studies indicate that prognosis in idiopathic cardiomyopathy is somewhat better than in ischaemic cardiomyopathy.

Key Points

- Functional MR occurs frequently in patients following myocardial infarction, with percentages varying between 20 and 60 %.
- In ischaemic functional MR, left ventricular function may still be relatively preserved and MR may be the result of only local LV wall motion abnormalities.
- Regardless of aetiology, functional MR carries an increased risk of death, which is approximately twofold and is related to the severity of MR.

7 Assessment of Functional Mitral Regurgitation

The dynamic nature of functional MR has important diagnostic implications. While structured intraoperative surgical evaluation of the mitral valve—on the arrested heart—is the cornerstone of mitral valve surgery in organic disease, this analysis has no additional value in functional MR since the valve is structurally normal. Therefore, the diagnosis has to be established prior to surgery by looking at restrictive leaflet motion, LV geometric changes and LV wall motion abnormalities.

Table 10.1 Overview of studies reporting on the presence and severity of functional mitral regurgitation in ischaemic and non-ischaemic aetiologies

Author, year of publication (study interval)	Number of patients	Aetiology	EF (%)	Technique	MR presence and severity	Survival with MR present	Heart failure	Remarks
Lamas 1997 (1987–1990)	727	Ischaemic	32 ± 7	Angiography	19.4 % overall; MR 1+ 75 %, MR 2+ 23 %	71 % at 3.5 years		Survivors ≤16 days following MI, EF ≤ 40 %
Grigioni 2001 (1990–1997)	303 (194 with MR)	Ischaemic	33 ± 14	Quantitative echocardiography		38 % at 5 years		Patients with MI > 16 days
Blondheim 1991 (1986–1988)	91	62 % ischaemic	19 ± 7	Semi-quantitative echocardiography	57 % overall; mild 57 %, moderate 33 %, severe 9 %	22 % at 2.7 years	62 % during follow-up	Patients with dilated cardiomyopathy with EF < 40 % and LVEDD > 60
Koelling 2002 (1986–1990)	1,436	59 % ischaemic	20 ± 5	Semi-quantitative echocardiography	Moderate 30 %, severe 19 %	At 3 years: mild MR 57 %, moderate 50 %, severe 35 %		Patients with EF ≤ 35 %
Trichon 2003 (1986–2000)	2,057	60 % ischaemic	25	Angiography	56 % overall; MR 2+ 70 %, MR 3+/4+ 30 %			Heart failure patients, EF < 40 %
Robbins 2003 (1998)	221 (111 inpatient)	Not specified	28 ± 8	Semi-quantitative echocardiography	59 % moderate or severe; inpatient 74 %, outpatient 45 %	61 % at 5 years		Heart failure patients, EF < 40 %
Patel 2004 (1996–2001)	558	71 % ischaemic	21 ± 7	Quantitative echocardiography	Moderate 22 %, moderate or severe 17 %	At 3 years: ischaemic 40 %, non-ischaemic 70 %		Heart failure patients, EF < 35 %

(continued)

Table 10.1 (continued)

Author, year of publication (study interval)	Number of patients	Aetiology	EF (%)	Technique	MR presence and severity	Survival with MR present	Heart failure	Remarks
Bursi 2005 (1988–1998)	773	Ischaemic	45	Semi-quantitative echocardiography	Mild 38 %, moderate or severe 12 %	At 5 years: mild MR 62 %, moderate or severe MR 40 %, no MR 72 %	RR for heart failure with moderate or severe MR 3.44	Population-based cohort study (Olmsted County) following myocardial infarction
Aronson 2006 (2001–2005)	1,190	Ischaemic	43	Semi-quantitative echocardiography	Mild 40 %, moderate or severe 6 %	At 3.3 years: mild MR 85 %, moderate or severe MR 67 %	Graded relationship with heart failure	Patients with acute MI without previous heart failure
Agricola 2009 (2002–2007)	404	77 % ischaemic	34 ± 11	Quantitative echocardiography	Only patients with MR selected: 41 % mild, 59 % moderate or severe	At 4 years: mild MR 64 %, moderate MR 50 %, severe MR 49 %	Graded relationship with heart failure	Prospective; patients with at least mild MR and EF < 50 %
Rossi 2011	1,256	Both aetiologies included, distribution not provided	32 ± 8	Quantitative echocardiography	Mild to moderate MR 49 %, severe MR 24 %	At 5 years: for ischaemic mild to moderate MR: 60 %, severe MR 23 %; for non-ischaemic mild to moderate MR 50 %, severe MR 27 % at 4 years		Chronic heart failure patients in 4 Italian centres

EF ejection fraction; *MI* myocardial infarction; *MR* mitral regurgitation; *RR* relative risk

7.1 Echocardiographic Assessment of Functional MR

Echocardiography is the most appropriate technique to examine patients with functional MR [40, 41]. Proper assessment of the severity of functional MR is important because of its implications for patient prognosis and treatment. Semi-quantitative techniques using colour flow mapping of regurgitant jet area are easily performed but have limited accuracy, since several technical and physiological factors influence results; for instance, a lower driving pressure will make a jet relatively smaller. Determination of the *vena contracta width* is less sensitive to technical factors. The cross-sectional area of the vena contracta indicates the *effective regurgitant orifice area* (*ERO*), which is the narrowest area of actual flow. Size of the vena contracta is independent of flow rate and driving pressure for a fixed orifice. This means that it can change when the regurgitant orifice is dynamic, as is the case in functional MR. Quantitative techniques are therefore preferred. The *proximal isovelocity surface area* (*PISA*), or *flow convergence* technique is used to calculate ERO and regurgitant volume. Another quantitative flow technique is pulsed wave Doppler. Combining pulsed wave Doppler flow velocities with 2D measurements can provide flow rates and stroke volumes and therewith ERO.

Cut-off values for the echocardiographic assessment of MR severity presented in valve disease guidelines are based on the recommendations by Zoghbi et al. [42]. It should be noted that these values are valid for *organic* MR. Data from the Mayo Clinic suggest, based on patient outcome, that in functional MR lower thresholds should be used for the diagnosis of severe MR: 20 mm^2 for ERO and 30 mL for regurgitant volume [30]. For organic MR these values are 40 mm^2 and 60 mL, respectively. These adapted criteria for functional MR are mentioned in the European guidelines, although without further recommendation, but not in the American guidelines. Furthermore, the ESC guidelines present separate paragraphs on "ischaemic MR" and "functional MR"; the ESC defines functional MR as MR observed in cardiomyopathy and in ischaemic disease with severe LV dysfunction.

New developments in this area include real-time 3D echocardiography (RT3DE). In a head-to-head comparison, RT3DE proved to be better able to quantify ERO and regurgitant volume in functional MR than 2D TTE, compared to the gold standard of 3D velocity encoded MRI [43]. It was shown that 2D echocardiography underestimates the severity of functional MR.

7.2 Exercise Testing in the Diagnosis of Functional MR

The role of echocardiographic exercise testing in functional MR has been extensively evaluated by colleagues from Liège [44]. Exercise-induced ERO changes in ischaemic MR could be related to local rather than global LV remodelling, more specifically to papillary muscle displacement, tethering and increased coaptation height [45]. In patients with an inferior infarction, reduction in ERO was seen following improvement in wall motion. A study by Lancellotti in patients with LV dysfunction (EF < 45 %) and mild ischaemic MR at rest showed that exercise echocardiography could identify patients with a higher risk of cardiac death [46]. Mortality at 19 months follow-up was higher in patients with a resting ERO > 20 mm^2, but also in patients with an ERO that increased during exercise by 13 mm^2 or more (value determined using receiver operating characteristic analysis). No mortality occurred in patients with decreasing MR severity during exercise. These results could not be confirmed by others, however [47]. The Lancellotti study underlines the fact that even mild ischaemic MR may be detrimental and therefore warrants additional examinations in such patients to appreciate the true severity of MR.

7.3 Specific Considerations for the Assessment of Functional MR in the Perioperative Setting

The dynamic nature of functional MR also plays a role in the preoperative and intraoperative setting. Patients with functional MR typically show downgrading of MR severity under general anaesthesia [48–50]. Therefore, severity assessment in functional MR should be performed prior to anaesthesia, and the surgical strategy should be determined at that time. For the surgeon it is also important to consider the influence of heart failure therapy and inotropic support on MR severity. Rosario demonstrated how vasodilator and diuretic treatment resulted in reduction of the severity of functional MR [51]. Therapy led to decreased MR by reduction in ERO without reduction in the transmitral gradient. Inotropes can decrease LV volumes and potentially increase LV pressure and lower left atrial pressure and thus raise transmitral pressure, again resulting in decreased MR severity [52].

The reduction of MR severity during general anaesthesia has led to intraoperative simulation of more physiological hemodynamic conditions in patients with mild to moderate ischaemic MR, or MR that is intermittent, to create a situation in which the true severity of MR can be assessed. These so-called loading tests were introduced by Dion et al. [53]. They include a preload test and, if necessary, an afterload test. The preload test is used to increase the pulmonary capillary wedge pressure by 10–15 mmHg by rapid filling through the aortic cannula. An increase of MR severity is considered a positive test and justifies mitral valve repair. A negative test is followed by an afterload test, using a 5 mg IV bolus of phenylephrine (an alpha-agonist that raises systemic vascular resistance without inotropic effects). If MR severity does not increase, mitral valve repair is not performed. In the series presented by Dion, 58 % of patients with intermittent or grade 2+ ischaemic MR showed a significant increase in MR severity following a loading test. Variations of loading tests have been described by others [54–56].

7.4 Geometry of the Mitral Valve Apparatus in Functional MR

With more advanced echocardiographic imaging, more detailed aspects of mitral valve leaflet geometry and the subvalvular apparatus have been described. They can be used in clinical decision making and provide some indication about the feasibility and success of repair, as will be discussed later. For a more detailed description of these parameters and their assessment, the reader is referred to the original publications [22, 57–61]. The most frequently used parameters to describe mitral valve geometry are:

Coaptation length: the length of leaflet apposition.

Coaptation depth (coaptation distance, tenting height, tenting length): the shortest distance between the point of coaptation on the atrial side and the annular plane.

Tenting area: the area enclosed by the mitral leaflets and the annular plane.

7.5 The Value of Cardiac Magnetic Resonance Imaging (MRI) in Functional MR

Cardiac MRI is increasingly used in the evaluation of heart failure patients with cardiomyopathy. MRI provides high spatial resolution and can combine functional and geometrical assessment of the left ventricle in a single examination. A relative disadvantage is the fact that patients with defibrillator/resynchronization therapy devices (a large proportion of the heart failure population) cannot be examined. MRI is currently considered the reference standard for the assessment of ventricular volume and function and for the visualization of scar [62].

Specific use of cardiac MRI in patients with ischaemic cardiomyopathy is found in the assessment of contractile reserve. Late gadolinium enhancement can visualize irreversible myocardial damage. Scar transmurality can predict the likelihood of functional recovery following revascularization, which is high in the absence of scar (78 %) and low if scar is more than 75 % transmural (2 %) [63]. In the intermediate zone predictive value is limited, with a likelihood of recovery of approximately 40 %. In such patients additional low-dose dobutamine stress is advised which can be performed during the same examination; 42 % of segments with an intermediate scar show contractile reserve during stimulation [64]. Predicting functional recovery after revascularization is important, at least in theory, because of its influence on global improvement of LV function, which is related to increased survival [65]. There are no studies that specifically look at the effect of revascularization alone in the setting of ischaemic MR in relation to regional wall motion abnormalities.

The use of MRI in functional MR in non-ischaemic cardiomyopathy is less well defined. Because of the excellent results in volume assessment, which is much less observer-dependent than in echocardiography, MRI can be used as a perfect follow-up tool to observe volumetric and geometric changes in eligible patients.

MRI has also proven its value in the assessment of mitral valve regurgitation, using 3D velocity encoded techniques [66]. MRI can reliably measure regurgitant flow and as such provides a true estimate of ejection fraction, since it can discriminate between true forward flow through the aortic valve and regurgitant flow through the mitral valve. Finally, MRI has demonstrated its usefulness in guiding cardiac resynchronization therapy (CRT). In a comparison with tissue Doppler imaging, MRI was found to have the same accuracy in establishing LV dyssynchrony and LV filling pressures [67].

Key Points

- The dynamic nature of functional MR has specific implications for MR assessment: it should be preferably performed prior to surgery and induction of anaesthesia and should incorporate different techniques in order to assess severity.
- Exercise echocardiography should be performed in patients with heart failure symptoms and non-significant MR at rest.
- Cardiac MRI may have additional value in the assessment of patients with functional MR.

8 Results of Surgery for Ischaemic Mitral Regurgitation

The optimal treatment for ischaemic MR is a subject of ongoing debate in the surgical and cardiology community. Published reports convey ambiguous messages and are essentially difficult to compare because of different patient populations, different definitions of ischaemic MR, different surgical techniques and different follow-up. This controversy is reflected in the guidelines as well. For ischaemic MR, all recommendations have a "C" level of evidence in the European guidelines since randomized trials are absent [41]. For symptomatic patients with severe MR, EF < 30 % and revascularization options, mitral valve surgery has a class IIa recommendation. The same is true for patients with moderate MR undergoing CABG if repair is feasible. Patients with severe MR, EF > 30 %, no revascularization options and low comorbidity have a class IIb recommendation for mitral valve surgery. The American guidelines state that the indication for mitral valve surgery in CABG patients with mild to moderate MR is still unclear, but that there are data indicating benefit of mitral valve repair in such patients [40]. They also state that CABG alone is usually insufficient and leaves many patients with significant residual MR; such patients "would benefit from concomitant mitral valve repair at the time of the CABG". Finally, it is stated that mitral annuloplasty alone with a downsized annuloplasty ring is often effective at relieving MR.

8.1 Results of Revascularization Only

There has been much discussion whether revascularization alone by improving wall motion abnormalities would suffice to treat ischaemic mitral insufficiency, especially in patients with less than severe MR. This would avoid the supposed increased perioperative morbidity and mortality risk associated with a valvular procedure. In addition, proponents of isolated revascularization claim that valve surgery does not influence long-term outcome and survival.

In Table 10.2, studies reporting on the outcomes of revascularization only in chronic ischaemic MR are summarized [50, 68–78]. Although these studies differ in many aspects, it can be stated that ischaemic MR in patients undergoing revascularization only has a negative influence on survival and functional outcome when compared to results from patients with isolated revascularization for CAD. The effect is graded and can be already observed when only mild MR is present. Furthermore, ischaemic MR treated by revascularization only does not improve in two-thirds of patients and leads to ongoing LV remodelling. There are as yet no predictors that reliably identify patients who will improve with revascularization only. And finally, several studies demonstrate how residual mild MR at rest after revascularization may increase during exercise.

8.2 *Results of Mitral Valve Repair with Revascularization*

The literature overview presented in Table 10.3 reflects and explains the continuing controversy regarding the true benefit of mitral valve repair in addition to coronary revascularization in ischaemic MR [79–94]. These studies are difficult to compare because of different baseline patient characteristics. More importantly, the technique of mitral valve repair varies widely, especially with respect to the annuloplasty device used and the use of downsizing. Other important differences relate to the grafting strategy (completeness of revascularization and the use of arterial conduits), and to the completeness and time interval of echocardiographic follow-up.

Poor results with regard to MR recurrence can be explained by the use of incomplete and/or flexible rings. Best results seem to be obtained with complete rigid or semi-rigid rings that are downsized by two ring sizes and achieving sufficient leaflet coaptation length during surgery; 8 mm seems an appropriate value. This approach results in consistent and durable reduction of MR severity and LV reverse remodelling in a majority of patients. Nevertheless, at long-term follow-up approximately 15 % of patients have recurrent MR ≥ grade 2+, which is likely related to extensive LV remodelling prior to surgery, which may be clinically reflected by LV dilatation (LV end-diastolic dimension >65–70 mm) or by mitral valve tethering geometry, as will be discussed later. Due to the absence of randomized trials and relatively short follow-up, a survival benefit resulting from additional mitral valve repair has not been demonstrated.

8.3 *Studies Comparing Mitral Valve Repair and Mitral Valve Replacement*

Obvious differences in patient characteristics and techniques make historical comparisons between mitral valve replacement vs. repair difficult [95–97]. This is nicely addressed in an editorial comment by Miller [98]. Calafiore has advocated to replace the mitral valve in case of excessive coaptation depth exceeding 10 mm, which in his experience occurs in 7 % of cases [99].

Table 10.2 Overview of studies examining the effects of revascularization only on ischaemic MR

Author, year of publication (study interval)	Number of patients	Population characteristics	Early mortality	MR during follow-up	Survival (by preoperative MR grade if available)	Remarks
Aklog 2001 (1992–1999)	136	CABG indication, MR grade 3+. Mean EF 38 %. CABG only performed (at surgeon's discretion)	2.9 %	At 6 weeks: 8 % trace MR, 52 % mild MR, 40 % moderate/severe MR		Study shows that after CABG alone 92 % of patients have at least grade 2+ MR, and 40 % show no improvement at all. Retrospective
Ellis 2002 (1994–1997)	4,221 total; 53 with MR 3–4+	PCI patients (any indication except acute MI)			At 3 years for EF ≤ 40 %: no MR 76 %, moderate/severe MR 47 %	Study shows the adverse effect of MR on survival following PCI. No FU data on MR provided. Retrospective
Tolis 2002 (1986–1996)	75 pts with TEE, 49 with MR (37 % trace, 53 % mild)	Ischaemic cardiomyopathy, EF ≤ 30 %, isolated CABG and MR 1+ to 3+. Mean EF 22 %	2.0 %	At 14 months: mean MR grade decreased from 1.7 to 0.5	With MR present: 65 % at 3 years, 50 % at 5 years	Limitations: low mean MR grade preoperatively; limited data provided. Retrospective
Trichon 2003 (1986–2001)	2,757 total; 1,385 medical treatment, 537 PCI, 687 CABG, 228 CABG + mitral valve surgery. Strategy determined by physician	Ischaemic MR > grade 2+			At 5 years: medical treatment 41 %, PCI 64 %, surgery 69 %	Median follow-up 3.2 years. No additional survival benefit from mitral valve surgery compared to CABG only (although higher NYHA class and higher MR grade in MV surgery stratum, so groups not comparable)

Mallidi 2004 (1994–2002)	489 total; 163 patients with mild to moderate MR, matched 1:2 to 326 patients without MR	Isolated CABG patients ($n=6,443$), MR severity based on preoperative LV angiography	MR 3.5 %, no MR 2.8 % ($p=0.86$)	FU TTE available for 30 % of patients in MR group at 16 months: 31 % showed progression to moderate or severe MR	At 6 years similar survival (81 % with MR, 85 % without MR)	Matched cohort. Mean FU 3.4 years. Lower event-free survival in MR group at 6 years (37 % vs. 65 %), mainly CHF events
Lam 2005 (1980–2000)	467	Isolated CABG patients with grade 2+ ischaemic MR. Propensity matched to CABG patients without MR for survival analysis (210 matched pairs)	MR 3.3 %, no MR 0 ($p=0.01$)	FU TTE available for 33 % of patients (at discretion) at 2 months median FU time. MR 0/1+ 40 %, MR 2+ 38 %, MR 3/4+ 22 %	At 5 years: no MR 85 %, MR 73 % ($p=0.003$)	Mean FU 3.6 years. Moderate ischaemic MR was a risk factor for early mortality after CABG. Moderate ischaemic MR does not reliably resolve after CABG only and leads to reduced survival. Limitation: non-systematic and short echocardiographic FU
Wong 2005 (1991–2001)	251 total; 219 CABG, 32 CABG+MV annuloplasty (variety of rings)	Patients with grade 3+ ischaemic MR. Surgical strategy at surgeon's discretion. Mean EF 39–42 %	5.2 % (CABG only 4.1 %, MV surgery 13 %; $p=0.06$)	Postoperative echo in 109 patients. In CABG only group, 48 % showed MR 3+ or greater. Mean MR CABG only 2.6 vs. 2.0 in CABG+MV surgery	At 1, 5 and 10 years: 84 %, 68 % and 37 %; similar for CABG only and CABG+MV annuloplasty	Median FU 4.3 years. MV surgery not standardized (intraoperatively mean residual MR grade 1.6). Limited echocardiographic FU
Grossi 2006 (1996–2004)	2,242 total; 38 % no MR, 51 % mild MR, 12 % moderate MR	CABG patients with less than severe MR on intraoperative TEE	1.9 %		At 5 years: no MR 86 %, mild MR 84 %, moderate MR 70 % ($p<0.001$)	No data on postoperative MR severity. Mild and moderate MR were independently associated with late mortality

(continued)

Table 10.2 (continued)

Author, year of publication (study interval)	Number of patients	Population characteristics	Early mortality	MR during follow-up	Survival (by preoperative MR grade if available)	Remarks
Di Mauro 2006 (1988–2002)	140 propensity matched patients; 70 with grade 2+ MR, 70 with MR 0/1+	Isolated CABG patients with ischaemic cardiomyopathy (EF < 30 %) and grade 2+ MR or less. Mean EF 27 %, EDV 118 mL	Total 6.4 %; MR 0/1+ 4.3 %, MR 2+ 8.6 % (NS)	At 5 years (TTE in 88 % of patients): MR 0/1+ showed stable results (mean MR grade 0.7), MR2+ increased (mean MR grade from 2.0 to 2.7)	At 8 years: MR 0/1+ 73 %, MR 2+ 47 % (p=0.029)	MR grade 2+ was an independent risk factor for late mortality. MR grade 2+ patients showed NYHA increase, stable LV diameters and volumes and increased MR. In MR 0/1+ patients, NYHA and MR were stable and LV reverse remodelling occurred
Calafiore 2008 (1994–2002)	4,226 total; no MR 2,805; MR 1+ 1,421; MR 2+ 167	Isolated CABG patients and EF > 30 %, ischaemic MR ≤ grade 2+	Total 2.2 %			Median FU 8.5 years. Presence of MR is independent risk factor for cardiac mortality (not all-cause mortality) in patients with EF between 31 and 40 %, but not in patients with EF > 40 %

Fattouch 2010 (2003–2008)	640 total; 180 patients with moderate MR matched 1:2 to patients without MR	Isolated CABG patients with moderate MR (ERO 10–19 mm^2) or without MR	Total 1.9 %; MR 2.2 %, no MR 1.6 % ($p=0.42$)	At 2.5 years: patients with moderate MR showed decrease (mild MR) in 30 % of cases, stable MR in 35 % and increase (severe MR) in 35 %. Exercise TTE in patients with mild MR showed increase of MR severity in 43 %, and in patients with moderate MR in 76 % of cases	At 5 years: no MR 91 %, moderate MR 74 % ($p<0.001$)	Mean FU 2.5 years. MR is significant risk factor for mortality in patients with EF<40 %. Ischaemic MR led to LV remodelling in all patients. No reliable reduction of MR severity with CABG alone. Often increase of MR severity with exercise
Kang 2011 (1996–2008)	185 total; 66 PCI, 119 surgery (51 CABG, 68 CABG with MV annuloplasty)	Patients with ischaemic MR, ERO≥20 mm^2, treated with PCI or surgery at discretion of physician. All patients had evidence of viability	Surgery 1.7 %, PCI 3 % ($p=0.62$)	At 6 months TTE in 98 % of survivors: improvement of MR after PCI in 54 % and after surgery in 79 % of patients ($p=0.001$)	At 7 years: surgery 60 %, PCI 55 % ($p=0.21$). Event-free survival after surgery 58 %, after PCI 50 % ($p=0.034$)	Registry study. Median FU 4.4 years. In surgery group better functional improvement (by NYHA class) and better EF improvement. Comparing CABG only to CABG+MV surgery, the latter had higher event-free survival, more improvement of MR (95 % vs. 57 %) and lasting reduction of LV volumes

CABG coronary artery bypass grafting; *CHF* congestive heart failure; *EF* ejection fraction; *ERO* effective regurgitant orifice area; *FU* follow-up; *LV* left ventricle/ventricular; *MI* myocardial infarction; *MR* mitral regurgitation; *MV* mitral valve; *NS* not significant; *NYHA* New York Heart Association; *PCI* percutaneous coronary intervention; *RR* relative risk; *TEE* transoesophageal echocardiogram; *TTE* transthoracic echocardiogram

Table 10.3 Overview of studies combining revascularization with mitral valve repair in ischaemic mitral regurgitation

Author, year of publication (study interval)	Number of patients and characteristics	Techniques	Early mortality	MR during follow-up	Actuarial survival and reoperation rate	Remarks
Bax, 2004	51 patients, MR grade 3-4+, mean EF 31 %, LVEDD 64 mm	CABG with 3.3 grafts. Complete semi-rigid rings, downsizing by 2 ring sizes (mean size 28)	5.6 %	Complete echo FU. At 1.5 years mean MR grade 0.8; MR grade 2+ in 2 %, MR 1+ in 22 %	At 2 years: 84 %. Reoperation rate 2.1 %	Significant functional improvement (NYHA from 3.4 to 1.3). Mean LVEDD from 64 to 58 and LVESD from 51 to 43 mm. LVRR (10 % reduction LVEDD) in 58 % of patients. Stringent MV repair protocol and FU
Mc Gee Jr, 2004 (1985–2002)	585 patients, MR 2–4+	No CABG data. MV annuloplasty: 21 % rigid ring (no downsizing), 68 % incomplete flexible band, 11 % bovine pericardium	6.3 %	In 75 % of patients. Median FU 8 days. 75 % of echocardiograms made within 2 months, 17 % after 1 year. At 6 months: MR 3–4+ in 28 %	At 1 year: 82 %, at 5 years 60 %. Freedom from reoperation at 5 years 97 %	Median FU 2.3 years. Use of pericardium risk factor for recurrent MR. Limitations: non-uniform MV repair; no intraoperative echocardiography; very limited echocardiographic FU; no details on bypass grafts
Glower, 2005 (1993–2002)	141 patients, moderate/severe MR, mean EF 40 %	MV annuloplasty: complete (semi-) rigid ring. Undersizing by 1 ring size. Median size 26	6.4 %	Mean FU 1.4 years, in 58 % of patients. Recurrence rate moderate or severe MR 11 %	At 5 years: 56 %. Reoperation rate 2.1 %	Study compares results to patients with non-functional MR; lower survival for ischaemic MR is explained by differences in preoperative risk factors and not by ischaemic MR per se

Braun, 2005 (2000–2004)	87 patients, MR grade 3-4+, mean EF 32 %, LVEDD 64 mm	CABG with 3.3 grafts. Complete semi-rigid rings, downsizing by 2 ring sizes (mean size 26). Intraoperative goal of 8 mm coaptation length	8.0 %	Complete echo FU. At 1.5 years mean MR grade 0.6; MR grade 2+ in 8 %, MR 1+ in 44 %	At 2 years: 86 %. Reoperation rate 2.5 %	Study identifies preoperative LVEDD $\leq$65 mm as predictor for LVRR. LVRR (10 % reduction of LVEDD) in 61 % of patients Mean LVEDD decreased from 64 to 58 and LVESD from 52 to 44 mm. Significant functional improvement (NYHA from 3.0 to 1.3). Stringent MV repair protocol and FU
Geidel, 2005 (2001–2004)	38 patients, MR grade 3–4+, EF $\leq$45 % (mean 31 %), mean LVEDD 60 mm	CABG with 2.3 grafts. Complete flexible ($n=8$) or semi-rigid rings. Dynamic downsizing by 2–4 ring sizes. Intraoperative goal of $\geq$5 mm coaptation length	2.6 %	Complete FU. Mean 13 months; 17 % MR grade 2+, 31 % grade 1+	At 1 year: 85 %. No reoperations	Significant functional improvement. Mean LVEDD from 60 to 57 and LVESD from 47 to 42 mm. LVRR (10 % reduction) for LVEDD in 38 % of patients and for LVEDV in 48 %. Stringent MV repair protocol and FU

(continued)

Table 10.3 (continued)

Author, year of publication (study interval)	Number of patients and characteristics	Techniques	Early mortality	MR during follow-up	Actuarial survival and reoperation rate	Remarks
Mihaljevic, 2007 (1991–2003)	390 patients, MR grade 3–4+, EF<45 %. 100 patients CABG only, 290 patients CABG+MV annuloplasty (at surgeon's discretion). By propensity matching 54 pairs	CABG without mammary artery in 40 % of cases. MV annuloplasty: 22 % rigid ring, 71 % incomplete flexible band, 7 % bovine pericardium. Unclear downsizing	CABG only 7.4 %, CABG+MV surgery 3.7 % ($p=0.7$)	Median TTE FU CABG only 5.5 months, CABG+MV surgery 1.1 month. Postoperative MR grade 3/4+ after 7 weeks in CABG only in 45 % of patients, in CABG+MV surgery 5 %. After 7.4 years: 45 % vs. 20 % (estimate)	Similar survival for matched pairs and total cohort. For matched pairs at 5 years: CABG only 75 %, CABG+MV surgery 75 %. At 10 years: 47 % and 39 %, respectively ($p=0.6$)	Median FU 5 years for CABG, 4 years for CABG+MV surgery. Similar functional improvement in both groups, no survival difference. High percentage of MR recurrence after CABG only. Limitations: non-uniform MV repair; no intraoperative echocardiography; low use of mammary artery grafts; limited echocardiographic FU. Selection bias in treatment groups likely. Exact data on MR recurrence not presented in a clear way

Gelsomino, 2007 (2001–2007)	220 patients with mild to severe ischaemic MR. Patients with MV replacement ($n=3$) and residual MR ≥ grade 2+ ($n=11$) were excluded and only survivors were studied (from the original 251 patients)	CABG with 2.2 grafts (complete as defined per territory). Complete (semi-) rigid rings with downsizing by 2 ring sizes; mean ring size 27. Intraoperative goal of ≥5 mm coaptation length	0.8 %		Prospective TTE FU; after 1 year 85 % of patients, after 3 years 55 %, after 5 years 28 %. Mean MR grade at 1 year 0.3, at 3 years 1.2, at 5 years 2.1. After 5 years, grade 3–4+ in 44 % of patients. LV volumes decreased at 1 year, but re-increased beyond that point	At 5 years: 83 %. Freedom from reoperation at 5 years 78 %	Median FU 2.8 years. Selected patients. High MR recurrence; predictors were sphericity index, myocardial performance index, LV end-systolic volume (≥145 mL) and wall motion score index (≥1.5)
Gelsomino, 2008 (2001–2006)	204 patients with mild to severe ischaemic MR. Patients with MV replacement ($n=4$) and residual MR ≥ grade 2+ ($n=12$) excluded, as well as early deaths ($n=4$)	Same as in 2007 study. Median ring size 28			Prospective TTE FU: early, mid-term (median 6 months) and late (median 2.9 years). Depending on late echocardiogram, 41 % of patients were classified as responders (≥15 % reduction of indexed LV end-systolic volume). Recurrent MR ≥ grade 2+ in 2 % of responders and in 44 % of non-responders	At 5 years: 83 % for whole population, 89 % for responders and 79 % for non-responders ($p=0.036$)	Median FU 2.9 years. Selected patients. Non-responders had more tethering and more LV remodelling signs on preoperative echo. During FU, they also had an MV coaptation length <5 mm

(continued)

Table 10.3 (continued)

Author, year of publication (study interval)	Number of patients and characteristics	Techniques	Early mortality	MR during follow-up	Actuarial survival and reoperation rate	Remarks
Ngaage, 2008 (1978–2002)	179 patients with mostly severe MR and EF ≤ 35 %	30 % MV replacement, 70 % repair (60 % downsized flexible incomplete band, 9 % repair without annuloplasty)	9.5 %	TTE in 109 patients (no data on time interval provided): freedom from moderate or severe MR at 3 years 63 %	At 3 years: 71 %, at 5 years: 51 %. Reoperation rate 5 %	Median FU 2.6 years. Heterogeneous approach to mitral valve, also affected by time era. No differences in survival between MV repair or replacement, but repair patients had significantly better improvement of EF
Crabtree, 2008 (1996–2005)	257 patients; MR grade 3–4+, mean EF 35 %	CABG + MV annuloplasty with complete ring (56 %) or band (44 %); mean ring size 27	10.1 %	TTE in 57 % of patients with mean interval of 1.7 years. Recurrent MR grade 3–4+ in 28 % of patients	At 3 years 68 %, at 5 years 52 %	Mean FU 3.2 years. Observed mortality higher in patients with recurrent MR. Limitations: no data on grafting strategy provided; no data on LV geometry provided; limited echocardiographic FU

Braun, 2008 (2000–2004)	100 patients, MR grade 3–4+, mean EF 27 %, mean LVEDD 61 mm	CABG with 3.3 grafts. Complete semi-rigid rings, downsizing by 2 ring sizes (median size 26). Intraoperative goal of 8 mm coaptation length	8 %	Complete TTE FU, mean 3.8 years. MR ≥ grade 2+ in 16 % of patients (1 patient grade 3+, others grade 2+). In patients with preoperative LVEDD > 65 mm, only 25 % of survivors show LVRR (defined as 10 % decrease of LVEDD)	At 3 years: 80 %, at 5 years: 71 % for the whole population. When stratified by LVEDD ≤ 65 mm, at 3 years: 87 %, at 5 years: 80 %, and for LVEDD > 65 mm at 3 years: 61 %, at 5 years: 49 % (p = 0.002)	Mean FU 4.3 years. Cut-off value of preoperative LVEDD 65 mm identified as independent predictor of mortality, and as a predictor for long-term LVRR
Onorati, 2009 (2004–2007)	64 patients, NYHA III/IV, MR ≥ grade 3+	CABG with 2.3 grafts. Complete semi-rigid rings (including disease-specific rings) used, downsizing by 2 ring sizes; median ring size 26	6.2 %	At discharge, 6 months, and late FU (mean 1.8 years). At 2 years MR ≥ grade 2+ in 27 % of patients	At 2 years: 97 %	Mean FU 1.8 years. More CHF episodes in patients with MR recurrence. Patients with preoperative LVEDD > 70 mm have more heart failure and more often developed recurrent MR
Williams, 2009 (1999–2006)	222 patients, MR severity not provided. Median EF 30 %, mean LVEDD 54 mm, LVESD 43 mm	CABG with 2.8 grafts. Almost exclusively complete nonflexible rings (mean ring size 24.8)	6.3 %	TTE FU available for 68 % of patients, median 10.6 months. Severe recurrent MR in 1.3 % of patients, moderate MR in 9.4 %	At 2 years: 72 %, at 5 years: 55 %	Median FU 2.2 years Limitations: no details on ring sizing provided (small mean size suggests adequate downsizing); limited echocardiographic FU

(continued)

Table 10.3 (continued)

Author, year of publication (study interval)	Number of patients and characteristics	Techniques	Early mortality	MR during follow-up	Actuarial survival and reoperation rate	Remarks
Fattouch, 2009 (2003–2007)	100 patients with MR grade 2+, randomized to CABG only ($n=52$) or CABG+MV repair ($n=48$). Mean EF 43 %, mean LVEDD 58 mm, LVESD 44 mm	CABG with 2.9 grafts, 98 % left ITA use. Complete semi-rigid rings, downsizing 8–10 mm based on echocardiographic anterior mitral leaflet length; no data on ring size. Intraoperative goal of 8 mm coaptation length	2.9 % for whole group; CABG only 1.8 %, CABG+MV surgery 4 % ($p=0.12$)	Complete TTE FU. Mean FU 2.7 years. In CABG+MV surgery group only trivial MR (mean grade 0.08); in CABG only group, 40 % improved, 25 % had moderate MR and 35 % moderate to severe MR	At 3 years CABG only: 93 %, CABG+MV surgery: 96 %; at 5 years CABG only: 89 %, CABG+MV surgery: 94 % (p=NS)	Single centre randomized trial. Mean FU 2.7 years. Better clinical improvement in CABG+MV surgery group (by NYHA class) Significant regression of LV dimensions and PA pressures in CABG+MV surgery group and improvement of EF, all of which were absent in CABG only group. CABG only group showed substantial increase in MR severity on exercise echocardiography. No survival difference (with short FU)

Pocar, 2010 (2000–2007)	57 patients, MR grade 2–3+	CABG with 2.5 grafts, ITA use in all patients. MV annuloplasty with downsizing by 2 ring sizes; complete rigid ring in 18 %, complete flexible ring in 41 %, and posterior pericardial band calibrated on sizer in 40 %; mean ring size 26.8	5.3 %		Recurrent MR grade 2+ in 37 % of patients, grade 3+ in 10 %	At 3 years: 87 %, at 5 years: 66 %	Mean FU 3.6 years Limitations: non-structured approach to annuloplasty type; mean ring size hard to interpret
Grossi, 2011 (2003–2008)	73 patients with severe or moderate symptomatic MR, EF≥25 %, LVEDD<70 mm. Control arm of multicenter randomized controlled trail (RESTOR-MV). Mean MR grade 2.54. Mean EF 38 %	CABG with 2.8 grafts. Variety of MV annuloplasty devices, 21 % non-rigid, mean size 27	4.1 %		At 2 years, moderate or worse recurrent MR in 16 % of patients. Mean MR grade at 1 and 2 years 0.52 and 0.35, respectively. EF increased from 38 to 47 % at 2 years	Crude mortality 24.7 % at 2 years, no actuarial data provided	Control arm of randomized controlled trial. Mean FU 2.1 years Significant improvement of NYHA functional class Limitations: several annuloplasty devices used

CABG coronary artery bypass grafting; *CHF* congestive heart failure; *EF* ejection fraction; *FU* follow-up; *ITA* internal thoracic artery; *LV* left ventricle/ventricular; *LVEDD* left ventricular end-diastolic diameter; *LVESD* left ventricular end-systolic diameter; *LVRR* left ventricular reverse remodelling; *MR* mitral regurgitation; *MV* mitral valve; *NS* not significant; *NYHA* New York Heart Association; *PCI* percutaneous coronary intervention; *TTE* transthoracic echocardiogram

9 Results of Surgery for Functional MR in Non-ischaemic Cardiomyopathy

As stated above, the earliest publications from the Michigan group laid the foundation for successful mitral valve repair using downsized annuloplasty rings in patients with functional MR secondary to idiopathic or non-ischaemic cardiomyopathy [10, 11]. It is important to realize that in ischaemic MR the "ventricular component" of the disease can be addressed through coronary revascularization, while this option is absent in non-ischaemic dilating cardiomyopathy. Compared to ischaemic cardiomyopathy, the number of studies that focus on this pathology are less numerous; an overview is presented in Table 10.4 [12, 100–105]. It can be appreciated that 2-year survival is approximately 70–80 %, and 5-year survival 50–70 %. MR recurrence ≥ grade 2+ is approximately 15–20 % at longer follow-up and—similarly to ischaemic MR—seems dependent on the extent of preoperative LV remodelling. More recent studies have focused on external cardiac restraint to address the ventricular component by decreasing transventricular pressure, with promising results.

Key Points

- Ischaemic MR treated by revascularization only does not improve in two-thirds of patients and leads to ongoing LV remodelling.
- There are no criteria to identify patients with ischaemic MR who may benefit from revascularization only.
- Series reporting on the results of mitral valve repair in functional MR are difficult to compare because of different patient populations and different surgical techniques.
- For ischaemic MR, good and durable results with regard to absence of recurrent MR and reverse LV remodelling are described for complete revascularization and mitral valve annuloplasty with stringent downsizing by two ring sizes, using a semi-rigid or rigid ring and verifying the absence of residual MR with sufficient coaptation length (8 mm).
- This technique seems insufficient in patients with too advanced LV remodelling, which can be assumed in severe LV dilatation (more than 65 mm end-diastolic dimension and/or severe mitral valve tethering).
- Although there are less studies available on patients with non-ischaemic cardiomyopathy, similar guidelines seem to apply although the ventricular component of the disease cannot be addressed in a straightforward manner.

10 Choosing an Annuloplasty Ring in Functional Mitral Regurgitation

The available studies on functional MR reflect different views on ring choice: complete or incomplete, flexible or nonflexible, saddle shaped or flat, and even several so-called disease-specific rings have been introduced for functional MR. The concept

Table 10.4 Overview of studies on mitral valve repair in non-ischaemic functional mitral regurgitation

Author, year of publication (study interval)	Number of patients and characteristics	Techniques	Early mortality	MR during follow-up	Actuarial survival and reoperations	Remarks
Bolling, 1998 (1993–1997)	48 patients, 24 non-ischaemic, 24 ischaemic without ongoing ischaemia. Mean NYHA 3.9. Mean EF 16 %	Undersized flexible ring	2.1 %	Decreased LVEDV from 281 to 206 mL. Increased EF from 17 to 26 %	At 1 year: 82 %, at 2 years: 72 %. One patient underwent HTX	Mean FU 1.8 years. Functional improvement: NYHA from 3.9 to 1.8 Limitations: no exact data on ring size; no data on postoperative MR
Gummert, 2003 (1996–2002)	66 patients, 53 non-ischaemic, 13 ischaemic. Mean EF 25 %, LVEDD 69 mm	Complete downsized semi-rigid ring (mean size 28)	6.1 %	Postoperative mean MR grade 0.7 at early FU and 1.0 at late FU. Stable LVEDD (67 mm, $p=0.093$), increased EF from 25 to 34 % ($p=0.028$)	At 1 year: 86 %, at 5 years: 66 %. Seven patients underwent HTX, 3 underwent reoperation for recurrent MR	Mean FU 2.3 years. Significant functional improvement
Romano, 2004 (1994–2003)	200 patients, mean EF 16 %	Undersized flexible annuloplasty ring	5 %		At 1 year: 82 %, at 3 years: 71 %, at 5 years: 52 %	Mean FU 4.1 years. Limitations: very limited data provided: no data on ring size, no echocardiographic data (MR, LVRR)

(continued)

Table 10.4 (continued)

Author, year of publication (study interval)	Number of patients and characteristics	Techniques	Early mortality	MR during follow-up	Actuarial survival and reoperations	Remarks
Horii, 2006 (1998–2005)	55 patients, 9 underwent emergency surgery. Mean EF 25 %, LVEDD 71 mm, indexed LVEDV 194 mL/m^2, indexed LVESV 148 mL/m^2	MV repair in 67 % of patients: complete downsized (1–2 sizes) semi-rigid ring; mean size 26. Remainder had MV replacement	15 % for total population; 4.3 % for non-emergent cases	Elective patients divided into "small" ($n=21$) and "large" ($n=25$) groups based on preoperative mean indexed LVESV (150 mL/m^2)	For elective patients, at 1 year: 73 %, at 3 years: 58 %, at 5 years: 52 %. For "small LV" group: 84 %, 67 % and 67 %, respectively; for "large LV" group: at 1 year 60 %, at 3 years 42 % ($p=0.03$)	Mean FU 2.4 years. In "small LV" group significant functional improvement and reduction of LVEDD (66–61) and indexed LVESV from 25 to 34 mL/m^2. Significant increase in EF (25–34 %). No beneficial effects in the "large LV" group
Acker, 2006	193 patients, mean EF 24 %, mean LVEDD 70 mm, mean LVESV 270 mL. Part of the Acorn multicenter randomized controlled trial; 102 patients MV surgery only, 91 patients MV surgery + CSD. 6 % ischaemic aetiology	16 % MV replacement, remainder MV annuloplasty: 65 % complete rings, median ring size 26	1.6 %	Between 6 and 18 months >80 % of patients MR 0/1+. Whole group: significant and progressive decrease of LV volumes, and increase of EF. Mean MR grade reduced at 1.5 years (from 2.7 to 0.6). MR 2+ in MV surgery only in 15 % of patients, with CSD in 3 % (p=NS)	At 1 year: 87 %, at 2 years: 35 %	Very low mortality. Patients have highly dilated LV, but relatively low MR severity. Patients with EF up to 45 % included. Significant functional improvement (by NYHA class but also on questionnaires and 6-min walking test). CSD had additional effect on reduction of LV volumes compared to MV surgery alone

Acker, 2011	Same as 2006 study. Aetiology 61 % idiopathic cardiomyopathy, 17 % valvular disease	Same as 2006 study. Ring size <28 in 82 % of patients	1.6 %	At 5 years, freedom from MR grade 3–4+ or redo MV surgery 81 % (5 patients underwent redo MV surgery)	At 1 year: 87 %, at 2 years: 85 %, at 5 years: 70 %. Annual mortality rate 6 % per year	CSD did not influence survival or MR recurrence, but had sustained additive effect on LV volumes and sphericity index
Braun, 2011 (2000–2008)	69 patients, mean EF 26 %, mean LVEDD 67 mm, mean LVEDV 227 mL. 28 patients MV surgery only, 41 patients also CSD implantation (when LVEDD>65 mm, from 2002 onwards)	Complete semi-rigid ring. Median ring size 26. Tricuspid annuloplasty 71 %	5.8 % for whole group; 3.6 % for MV surgery only, 7.3 % for MV surgery+CSD ($p=0.64$)	Median TTE FU 2.3 years, 95 % complete. MR≥grade 2+ in 16 % of patients for whole group; 23 % for MV surgery only, 8.3 % for MV surgery+CSD ($p=0.067$)	For whole group at 1 year: 87 %, at 2 years: 79 %, at 5 years: 63 %. For MV surgery only: 86 %, 75 % and 55 %, respectively; for MV surgery+CSD: 85 %, 82 % and 74 %, respectively ($p=0.27$)	Mean FU 3.1 years

CSD cardiac support device; *EF* ejection fraction; *FU* follow-up; *HTX* heart transplantation; *LV* left ventricle/ventricular; *LVEDD* left ventricular end-diastolic diameter; *LVEDV* left ventricular end-diastolic volume; *LVESV* left ventricular end-systolic volume; *MR* mitral regurgitation; *MV* mitral valve; *NS* not significant; *NYHA* New York Heart Association; *TTE* transthoracic echocardiogram of the (rigid) remodelling annuloplasty ring was introduced by Carpentier, and proved a major factor in long-term durability of mitral valve repair [106]. Duran introduced a flexible ring to preserve the physiologic annular motion [107]. Theoretical advantages of the flexible ring over (semi-)rigid rings have not been proven clinically, however. The current notion is that after implantation and neo-endothelialization of the ring the benefits of flexibility are greatly diminished as the ring becomes more rigid. Another annular remodelling device is the incomplete flexible band designed by Cosgrove et al. [108]. This device would maintain annular motion because of its flexibility while only providing posterior annulus plication. This was considered sufficient based on the assumption that the intertrigonal distance does not dilate. However, several studies have demonstrated that the anterior part of the annulus shows similar dilatation as the posterior part, at least in dilated cardiomyopathy [15, 21]. Based on these considerations, the use of an incomplete ring in functional MR seems inappropriate, since it will not reduce the anterior annular dimension and, more importantly, it will not sufficiently reduce septal-to-lateral dimension, which is the most important factor on an annular level that contributes to MR. The latter consideration also supports the use of a complete nonflexible ring rather than a complete flexible ring, especially when we consider that we have to undersize. Additional reduction or overcorrection of the septal–lateral dimension of the mitral annulus was found to effectively abolish MR studied in a chronic ischaemic ovine model [20]. Since flexible rings have a variable septal-to-lateral dimension throughout the cardiac cycle, their ability to abolish MR completely in functional MR, at least during the first months after implantation, may be insufficient. In addition, undersizing by two ring sizes will put considerable tension on the annular sutures which might be better compensated for by a (semi-) rigid ring. Finally, a nonflexible ring might be better able to achieve the reduction in circumferential radii of curvature of the left ventricle (remodelling of the LV base, as suggested by Bolling et al. [12]) and therewith reduce wall stress, as described in an acute ischaemic MR model [109].

The Michigan group reviewed their experience in functional MR with regard to ring type [110]. From the year 2000 onwards they used only nonflexible rings. The number of reoperations for recurrent MR as a consequence of ongoing remodelling was significantly higher in the flexible ring group. Although several methodological remarks can be made with regard to the study set-up (confounding effect of different time eras in which both rings were used; reoperation was not examined as a time-related event and is a surrogate endpoint for repair failure), the findings suggest that flexible rings might not be the best option for this pathology. Others have made similar observations [111].

In functional MR, the mitral annulus has become flat. The rationale for saddle shaped rings, reduction of leaflet stress to possibly provide a more durable repair, still has to be proven [112]. Theoretically, these rings could be used in functional MR, although exact data regarding the dimensions of these rings, especially with regard to the ratio of the commissure-to-commissure and the septal-to-lateral dimension, and how this ratio varies per ring size, should be carefully taken into consideration.

The fear of creating a relative mitral stenosis by undersizing with the typically used small ring sizes 24 and 26 prompted the introduction of the so-called disease-specific annuloplasty rings. They are designed to provide further reduction in septal-to-lateral dimension while providing a relatively larger orifice area by maintaining or even increasing the commissure-to-commissure dimension. Evaluating and comparing these rings is highly complex, and actually makes a proper ring choice even harder for the surgeon. A paper by Bothe provides measured dimensions of four disease-specific rings and compares them to those of the Physio ring [113]. Disease-specific rings provide a varying amount of additional septal-to-lateral dimension reduction compared to the Physio ring of the same size (10–25 %), but when compared to a Physio ring that is two sizes smaller (so truly undersized) the septal-to-lateral dimension is actually larger in three out of four rings.

The single intermediate term clinical follow-up study in the English literature performed with a disease-specific ring (Edwards GeoForm) does not reveal better freedom from recurrent MR or more extensive LV remodelling after almost 2 years, but does also not show significant mitral stenosis on exercise [114]. In our opinion, disease-specific rings introduce more ambiguity into the discussion on downsizing while their potential benefit is still unproven.

Based on these considerations, we have always adhered to a complete nonflexible annuloplasty ring (Physio ring) in order to provide a reliable downsizing of the septal-to-lateral dimension of the mitral annulus. Sizing is based on the length of the unfurled anterior leaflet, with the ring then chosen two ring sizes smaller (i.e. size 26 when measuring size 30). The ring is inserted using 14–16 U-shaped stitches. At the end of surgery, repair is considered successful when on intraoperative transoesophageal echocardiography MR is absent and coaptation length is 8 mm or more.

Key Point

- There is no proven benefit from the so-called disease-specific rings annuloplasty.

11 Recurrence of Mitral Regurgitation After Restrictive Mitral Annuloplasty

Recurrence of mitral regurgitation following mitral annuloplasty negatively influences the results of surgery. Since functional MR is more than a valvular problem, MR recurrence is also related to the course of the underlying ventricular disease which makes it different from recurrence in organic pathologies. Follow-up studies discussed in this chapter present a wide range of MR recurrence. When interpreting these studies, a distinction should be made between residual MR and true recurrent MR. The first is the result of an inappropriate application of a surgical technique, while the latter might be the consequence of disease progression but may also result from inappropriate surgical repair.

Hung examined MR recurrence following annuloplasty for ischaemic MR and concluded that this was related to continued LV remodelling [115]. Thirty patients underwent CABG and mitral annuloplasty with a variety of rings (47 % flexible, mean ring size 30, without marked downsizing). Early results (4 months) showed that 70 % of patients had mild MR and 30 % severe MR; at late follow-up (4 years), 72 % of patients had moderate to severe recurrent MR. Initially patients showed a reduction in LV volumes followed by a late increase, with a similar pattern for LV sphericity. However, one could argue that the simultaneous occurrence of recurrent MR and ongoing LV remodelling does not necessarily imply a causal relationship.

A Japanese study identified increased posterior leaflet tethering after annuloplasty, leading to reduced coaptation length, as an important determinant of persistent MR in ischaemic MR patients [116]. Similar observations were made by the same group in a study involving patients with longer follow-up: late recurrent MR was seen together with augmented posterior leaflet tethering which was not yet present at early follow-up. These patients had an early decrease of end-systolic volume, but showed an increase at late follow-up. Again it should be appreciated that these phenomena are observed simultaneously without proof of a causal relationship.

Results from the Cleveland Clinic are often cited when it comes to MR recurrence following mitral valve annuloplasty in ischaemic MR [80, 84]. Again, we would emphasize that 80 % of patients in these series had an incomplete annuloplasty (20 % with pericardium), and that echo follow-up was performed at a median of only 8 days. The fact that at 6 months follow-up even with a complete semi-rigid ring 25 % of patients had grade 3 or 4 recurrent MR in our opinion does not suggest disease progression with ongoing LV remodelling but rather an imperfect surgical strategy. The median ring size (size 30) suggests insufficient downsizing, and no strategy is provided with respect to the desired intraoperative result in terms of residual MR and minimum coaptation length. More recently this group focused on late MR recurrence, defined as MR $\geq$ grade 2+ developing at least 6 months after surgery, which occurred in 33 % of patients [117]. Patients with MR recurrence had echocardiographic signs of ongoing LV remodelling, although—again—no temporal relationship between the occurrences of these phenomena is provided.

A properly repaired sufficient mitral valve takes away an important impetus for LV remodelling. MR could then recur secondary to ongoing intrinsic remodelling of the left ventricle. This mechanism is likely present in cases where LV remodelling actually precedes MR recurrence, and can be demonstrated by serial echocardiographic follow-up. De Bonis presented 79 patients who underwent restrictive mitral annuloplasty for end-stage cardiomyopathy with EF $\leq$ 35 % without residual MR at least 6 months after surgery [118]. In patients with early LV reverse remodelling (15 % decrease of indexed end-systolic volume, present in 52 % of patients) 10 % had grade 2+ MR at late follow-up. Patients without reverse remodelling showed a gradual further increase of end-systolic volume that eventually exceeded preoperative values. MR at late follow-up in this group was 2+ in 42 % of patients and 3+ in 19 %.

11.1 Predictors for MR Recurrence Following Restrictive Mitral Annuloplasty

Several studies have tried to identify preoperative echocardiographic predictors for residual or recurrent MR following undersized annuloplasty. In theory, the extent of remodelling of the left ventricle through its effect on the mitral valve apparatus will determine the extent to which undersizing of the annulus will provide sufficient leaflet coaptation in the acute setting, i.e. intraoperatively and in the short-term. Here, remodelling is expressed as a simple geometric phenomenon. The same extent of remodelling will also determine the potential of recovery of the left ventricle necessary to provide durable reverse remodelling after successful abolishment of mitral regurgitation. Here, remodelling is an epiphenomenon, an expression of changes that occur at a cellular or even molecular level, which remain invisible to our observation.

A rough indicator of the extent of LV remodelling can be found in LV diameters or volumes. Cut-off values for LV end-diastolic diameter (LVEDD) have been related to chances of reverse remodelling [82, 89] and MR recurrence [59, 119]; typically, the upper limit for successful recovery has been identified at 65–70 mm. Others have identified detailed aspects of mitral valve geometry that essentially reflect the degree of leaflet tethering [59–61, 120, 121]. Although these studies provide specific cut-off values for several component of mitral valve geometry, their assessment requires advanced echocardiographic skills and an optimal ultrasound window, and as such they have limited value in everyday practice. Nevertheless, these parameters are important because they provide an indication for which cases adjunctive surgical measures—which will be discussed next—may be indicated or, in less experienced hands, when a mitral valve replacement might be better.

Key Points

- MR recurrence should be distinguished from residual MR; recurrence within 6 months after surgery should be considered to result from insufficient repair and not be regarded as recurrence secondary to progress of the underlying ventricular disease.
- MR recurrence may occur in patients without LV reverse remodelling but also in patients with reverse remodelling.
- Specific indicators to predict MR recurrence are not available, but the extent of preoperative LV remodelling might indicate patients in whom adjunctive measures are necessary to prevent recurrence.

12 Alternative and Adjunct Therapies for Functional Mitral Regurgitation

Several alternative or adjunctive therapies have been described for functional MR. These can either address the mitral valve apparatus, or the left ventricle.

12.1 Addressing the Mitral Valve Leaflets

Valvular adjunctive procedures address loss of coaptation due to excessive tethering. Borger presented results of secondary chord cutting as an adjunctive procedure to reduce tethering in ischaemic MR [122]. MR recurrence ≥ grade 2+ was 15 % at 2 years. Theoretically, this approach may further compromise an already diminished LV function because it disrupts the continuity between the mitral valve and the left ventricle. Long-term results are unknown, and we feel that this technique may only be used, if at all, as a bailout procedure in cases where valve replacement should be avoided at all cost.

The edge-to-edge technique has also been applied successfully in functional MR as an adjunct to undersized annuloplasty in patients with excessive tethering (coaptation depth ≥1 cm) [118, 123].

Another valvular approach is posterior leaflet augmentation. The largest clinical series reports on 44 ischaemic MR patients who underwent posterior leaflet augmentation using bovine pericardium followed by insertion of true-sized annuloplasty rings [124]. Freedom from significant MR is high, and this approach might also be used as an adjunct to restrictive annuloplasty in cases of severe tethering, especially when a small posterior leaflet is present, although this might be technically challenging. A single report on anterior leaflet extension was also published, with very limited follow-up, however [125].

12.2 Addressing the Subvalvular Apparatus

Several techniques applied from inside the ventricle have been described to address tethering by direct action on papillary muscle displacement. Hvass combined the papillary muscle sling technique with mitral annuloplasty [126]. This technique involves positioning of a 4 mm polytetrafluoroethylene (PTFE) tube around the base of both papillary muscles which is then tightened and fixed to approximate the muscles. Mitral annuloplasty with moderately undersized or normally sized rings resulted in good clinical outcomes, low MR recurrence and significant LV reverse remodelling at 1-year follow-up. Theoretically, this approach addresses the ventricular problem by influencing subvalvular anatomy, but also by direct volume reduction of the left ventricle, which makes it an interesting approach for functional MR patients with advanced LV dilatation. Unfortunately, no data on coaptation length are provided, and echocardiographic follow-up is limited to 1 year.

Langer introduced the RING + STRING technique, which adds repositioning of the posterior papillary muscle using a 3-0 PTFE suture that is exteriorized through the aortomitral continuity and then tied in the loaded beating heart under echocardiographic guidance, "achieving the most physiological shape of the anterior mitral leaflet along its entire body and locating the coaptation point as close to the annular plane as possible" [127]. This suture is applied through the aortic valve after the ring (a partial flexible ring with 1–2 sizes downsizing) has been inserted. At 2 years, freedom from recurrent MR ≥ grade 2+ was 94 % in a group of 30 ischaemic MR patients.

Upon addressing the mitral leaflet or subvalvular apparatus one should realize that only the problem of MR recurrence is addressed and not that of LV remodelling. This makes these techniques of limited value. Indeed, when the left ventricle is only moderately dilated, a nonflexible undersized annuloplasty ring will provide adequate results, with low recurrence rates and predictable reverse remodelling [89]. If the left ventricle is grossly dilated and consequently the mitral valve shows severe tethering, these additional techniques may lead to better results regarding MR recurrence but presumably not with respect to LV reverse remodelling.

12.3 External Ventricular Restraint or Reshaping

In cases of advanced LV dilatation, external ventricular restraint or reshaping can provide additional support of the mitral valve repair. The CorCap cardiac support device (CSD) provides circumferential diastolic support, passively reduces LV wall stress and thus counteracts the deleterious changes that occur during the remodelling process. Long-term follow-up has demonstrated that the CSD provides a significantly greater decrease in LV end-diastolic volume compared to controls [128]. In primary ischaemic cardiomyopathy, CABG can be combined with CSD implantation, but the grafts should have their course outside the mesh.

Another externally applied device that addresses LV shape is the Coapsys device. This device reshapes the ventricle and reduces wall stress by compressing the mitral annulus and subvalvular apparatus and as such does not require mitral valve repair. Results in the RESTOR-MV trial were promising [129], showing survival benefit for the first time, but the device is currently not on the market.

12.4 Surgical Ventricular Reconstruction

Patients with functional MR with akinesia or dyskinesia of the LV anterior wall should be considered for additional surgical ventricular reconstruction since this will help to promote reverse remodelling of these often highly enlarged left ventricles. We have described our strategy towards functional MR in this patient category [130]. Basically, we recommend performing restrictive mitral annuloplasty in patients with MR ≥ grade 2+, which may also appear after having performed the surgical LV reconstruction; this technique directly affects papillary muscle displacement and has an unpredictable effect on MR severity.

For idiopathic and ischaemic cardiomyopathy with LV end-diastolic dimension >75 mm and akinesia of the septum with preserved lateral wall function, the septal anterior ventricular exclusion procedure has been successfully used as an adjunct to restrictive mitral annuloplasty [131, 132].

12.5 The Tricuspid Valve

Tricuspid regurgitation should always be evaluated in patients with functional MR, especially in idiopathic cardiomyopathy, which may affect both ventricles [133]. We perform a tricuspid ring annuloplasty in patients with regurgitation $\geq$ grade 3+, but also in patients without significant tricuspid regurgitation with annular dilatation, which means a tricuspid annulus >40 mm (or 21 mm/m^2, indexed to body surface area) on TTE. This approach prevents right ventricular dilatation and tricuspid regurgitation [134], which is commonly seen in heart failure patients.

12.6 Cardiac Resynchronization Therapy

CRT is beneficial in moderate to severe heart failure patients with intraventricular conduction delay with regard to improvements in functional class, exercise capacity and quality of life [135], and leads to a significant mortality reduction [136]. Effects of CRT on functional MR severity and LV reverse remodelling have been demonstrated in both short-term [137] and long-term [138, 139], although approximately 30 % of patients are non-responders. In clinical practice, CRT in heart failure patients is often combined with implantable cardiac defibrillation (ICD) to reduce mortality related to cardiac arrhythmias [140]. Guideline indications overlap to a large extent. CRT-ICD therapy has become an important therapeutic alternative or adjunct therapy in the treatment of heart failure patients with functional MR.

12.7 Other Therapies

The role of pharmacological therapy in functional improvement and mortality reduction in heart failure is beyond the scope of this chapter, but should be evident that it has brought major advances in the treatment of heart failure patients and is the cornerstone of medical therapy, also after surgery has been performed.

Since many patients with heart failure and dilated cardiomyopathy die from ventricular arrhythmias, intraoperative therapies directed at their substrate could improve late outcome. Current knowledge in this field is limited, however, especially for patients with idiopathic cardiomyopathy.

Other surgical alternatives include cardiac transplantation and implantation of ventricular assist devices. Transplantation now has a predictable long-term outcome, but is limited by shortage of donor organs which is not expected to change in the future. A more promising evolution is seen with newer assist devices that show lower thromboembolic and infection rates. Experience with these devices as the so-called destination therapy is increasing. A combination of assist device therapy to unload the ventricle while other therapies aiming to regenerate the damaged myocytes (e.g. stem cell therapy, gene therapy) might be a future solution for patients who do not benefit from what we now address as "conventional heart failure surgery".

Key Points

- Patients with increased risk of MR recurrence might benefit from adjunctive measures; these can be directed at the mitral valve leaflets, at the subvalvular apparatus, or at the left ventricle.
- A tailored surgical approach also involves the tricuspid valve and CRT.

13 A Practical Approach to Patients with Functional MR: The Leiden Experience

Patients with heart failure and functional mitral regurgitation should be treated in a multidisciplinary team so that all possible treatment options can be discussed. Patients should receive optimal pharmacological treatment before considering interventional techniques. Initial evaluation should distinguish between an ischaemic or non-ischaemic cause.

For patients with ischaemic MR, the decision to perform surgery will often be guided by revascularization options; if CABG is warranted, the team should consider whether mitral valve surgery should be performed as well. Since ischaemic MR portends a poor prognosis and revascularization alone does not reliably treat MR, we recommend carefully examining the mitral valve and actively searching for ischaemic mitral regurgitation. In patients with MR grade 3+ or 4+, mitral valve repair should be performed. In patients with MR grade 2+ additional examinations are required. MR severity should then be assessed using quantitative techniques to measure ERO and regurgitant volume (which should then be related to LV function to determine the haemodynamic burden of MR in that particular patient). In addition, exercise echocardiography should be considered to examine an increase in MR severity that would warrant mitral valve repair. In patients who cannot perform exercise for physical or medical reasons (e.g. severe left main disease) an intraoperative loading test should be performed.

In patients with non-ischaemic functional MR without other indication for surgery (e.g. LV aneurysm) CRT should be considered, especially with less severe MR, and its results on MR evaluated. When patients persist in heart failure symptoms surgical correction of MR should be considered. The surgical treatment of functional MR has several basic principles. First, a complete and thorough echocardiographic evaluation should be performed, as discussed before. Mitral valve repair should be performed with a complete nonflexible undersized ring; intraoperative TEE should confirm the absence of residual MR, sufficient coaptation length (at least 8 mm) and the absence of mitral stenosis. Long-term outcome is dependent of the extent of preoperative LV remodelling; since there are as yet no proper techniques to determine that extent, we use LV end-diastolic dimension as a cut-off parameter. In patients with LVEDD>65 mm (or >30 mm/m^2 indexed to body surface area), additional techniques are required. We prefer external ventricular restraint using a CorCap device, but as discussed other techniques either directed at the valve, the subvalvular apparatus or the ventricle itself have been used by others with good results.

Additional techniques should also be considered to individualize treatment: complete revascularization in ischaemic patients; tricuspid valve repair based on annular dilatation (tricuspid annulus >40 mm or and indexed value >21 mm/m^2) which is frequently present in non-ischaemic cardiomyopathy; in all patients with LVEF < 30 % we implant an epicardial LV lead to facilitate future CRT.

Our heart failure team has developed a patient-based flow-chart that outlines the different treatment options for heart failure patients (Fig. 10.3). This chart can also be found on http://www.einthoven.nl/Mission!/professional/flowchart_A4_Engels.pdf.

Key Point

- This paragraph provides a practical medico-surgical approach to the patient with heart failure and in which both interventional and non-interventional treatment strategies have been incorporated.

14 Future Directions

One of the major challenges in the field of functional MR remains patient selection: who will benefit from an individualized surgical strategy, and who will not. Imaging techniques are rapidly improving and a further integration of techniques will provide better answers to the questions which patients have already too extensive remodelling and thus will not benefit from current techniques.

Currently eight interventional randomized controlled studies for functional MR are registered (http://clinicaltrials.gov), the majority involving ischaemic MR. Setting up surgical trials is difficult, and strict criteria should be set with regard to patient inclusion, surgical therapy and follow-up. Failing to do so will lead to outcomes that are not unequivocally accepted, as seen in the STICH trial [141]. It is somewhat disappointing that most registered studies do not have strict guidance with regard to the surgical procedure that should be followed; this could again lead to studies reporting on a variety of surgical techniques with ambiguous outcomes. Since survival benefit has not yet been proven for the surgical treatment of functional MR, another drawback of these trials is that only two studies include mortality as an endpoint. Nevertheless, since other important outcomes will be studied (e.g. components of LV reverse remodelling, objective functional improvement and quality of life), outcomes of these trials will add to our knowledge.

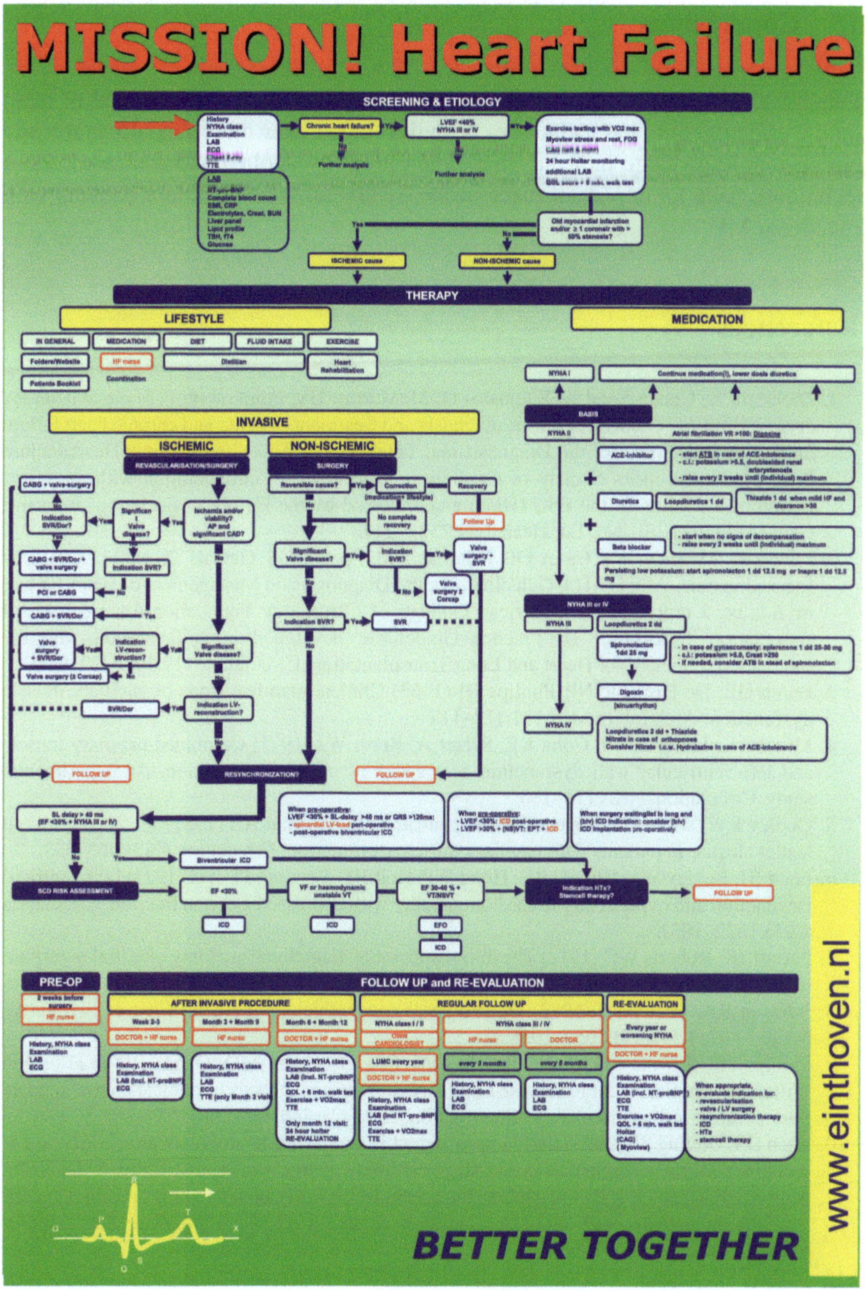

Fig. 10.3 Flow chart used at Leiden University Medical Centre to individualize the analysis and treatment strategy for patients with heart failure

15 Conclusions

Functional MR has tremendous impacts on functional status and survival of heart failure patients. Surgical techniques have developed over more than 15 years, and our current knowledge indicates that, when properly applied and evaluated, these techniques have an important place in the treatment of heart failure patients with functional MR.

References

1. Dickstein K, Cohen-Solal A, Filippatos G, McMurray JJV, Ponikowski P, Poole-Wilson PA et al (2008) ESC Guidelines for the diagnosis and treatment of acute and chronic heart failure 2008: the Task Force for the Diagnosis and Treatment of Acute and Chronic Heart Failure 2008 of the European Society of Cardiology. Developed in collaboration with the Heart Failure Association of the ESC (HFA) and endorsed by the European Society of Intensive Care Medicine (ESICM). Eur Heart J 29:2388–2442
2. Jessup M, Abraham WT, Casey DE, Feldman AM, Francis GS, Ganiats TG et al (2009) 2009 focused update: ACCF/AHA Guidelines for the Diagnosis and Management of Heart Failure in Adults: a report of the American College of Cardiology Foundation/American Heart Association Task Force on Practice Guidelines: developed in collaboration with the International Society for Heart and Lung Transplantation. Circulation 119:1977–2016
3. Burch GE, De Pasquale NP, Phillips JH (1963) Clinical manifestations of papillary muscle dysfunction. Arch Intern Med 112:112–117
4. Mittal AK, Langston M, Cohn KE, Selzer A, Kerth WJ (1971) Combined papillary muscle and left ventricular wall dysfunction as a cause of mitral regurgitation. An experimental study. Circulation 44(2):174–180
5. Godley RW, Wann LS, Rogers EW, Feigenbaum H, Weyman AE (1981) Incomplete mitral leaflet closure in patients with papillary muscle dysfunction. Circulation 63(3):565–571
6. Feild BJ, Baxley WA, Russell RO, Hood WP, Holt JH, Dowling JT et al (1973) Left ventricular function and hypertrophy in cardiomyopathy with depressed ejection fraction. Circulation 47(5):1022–1031
7. Perloff JK, Roberts WC (1972) The mitral apparatus. Functional anatomy of mitral regurgitation. Circulation 46(2):227–239
8. Johnson RA, Palacios I (1982) Dilated cardiomyopathies of the adult (first of two parts). N Engl J Med 307(17):1051–1058
9. Phillips HR, Levine FH, Carter JE, Boucher CA, Osbakken MD, Okada RD et al (1981) Mitral valve replacement for isolated mitral regurgitation: analysis of clinical course and late postoperative left ventricular ejection fraction. Am J Cardiol 48(4):647–654
10. Bach DS, Bolling SF (1995) Early improvement in congestive heart failure after correction of secondary mitral regurgitation in end-stage cardiomyopathy. Am Heart J 129(6):1165–1170
11. Bolling SF, Deeb GM, Brunsting LA, Bach DS (1995) Early outcome of mitral valve reconstruction in patients with end-stage cardiomyopathy. J Thorac Cardiovasc Surg 109(4): 676–682; discussion 682–683
12. Bolling SF, Pagani FD, Deeb GM, Bach DS (1998) Intermediate-term outcome of mitral reconstruction in cardiomyopathy. J Thorac Cardiovasc Surg 115(2):381–386; discussion 387–388
13. Levine RA (2005) Ischemic mitral regurgitation on the threshold of a solution: from paradoxes to unifying concepts. Circulation 112(5):745–758
14. Chaput M, Handschumacher MD, Tournoux F, Hua L, Guerrero JL, Vlahakes GJ et al (2008) Mitral leaflet adaptation to ventricular remodeling: occurrence and adequacy in patients with functional mitral regurgitation. Circulation 118(8):845–852

15. Ahmad RM, Gillinov AM, McCarthy PM, Blackstone EH, Apperson-Hansen C, Qin JX et al (2004) Annular geometry and motion in human ischemic mitral regurgitation: novel assessment with three-dimensional echocardiography and computer reconstruction. Ann Thorac Surg 78(6):2063–2068
16. Flachskampf FA, Chandra S, Gaddipatti A, Levine RA, Weyman AE, Ameling W et al (2000) Analysis of shape and motion of the mitral annulus in subjects with and without cardiomyopathy by echocardiographic 3-dimensional reconstruction. J Am Soc Echocardiogr 13(4):277–287
17. Kaplan SR, Bashein G, Sheehan FH, Legget ME, Munt B, Li XN et al (2000) Three-dimensional echocardiographic assessment of annular shape changes in the normal and regurgitant mitral valve. Am Heart J 139(3):378–387
18. Green GR, Dagum P, Glasson JR, Daughters GT, Bolger AF, Foppiano LE et al (1999) Mitral annular dilatation and papillary muscle dislocation without mitral regurgitation in sheep. Circulation 100(19 suppl):II95–II102
19. Tibayan FA, Rodriguez F, Zasio MK, Bailey L, Liang D, Daughters GT et al (2003) Geometric distortions of the mitral valvular-ventricular complex in chronic ischemic mitral regurgitation. Circulation 108(suppl 1):II116–II121
20. Tibayan FA, Rodriguez F, Langer F, Zasio MK, Bailey L, Liang D et al (2004) Does septal-lateral annular cinching work for chronic ischemic mitral regurgitation? J Thorac Cardiovasc Surg 127(3):654–663
21. Hueb AC, Jatene FB, Moreira LFP, Pomerantzeff PM, Kallás E, de Oliveira SA (2002) Ventricular remodeling and mitral valve modifications in dilated cardiomyopathy: new insights from anatomic study. J Thorac Cardiovasc Surg 124(6):1216–1224
22. Watanabe N, Ogasawara Y, Yamaura Y, Kawamoto T, Toyota E, Akasaka T et al (2005) Quantitation of mitral valve tenting in ischemic mitral regurgitation by transthoracic real-time three-dimensional echocardiography. J Am Coll Cardiol 45(5):763–769
23. Erlebacher JA, Barbarash S (2001) Intraventricular conduction delay and functional mitral regurgitation. Am J Cardiol 88(1):A7, 83–86
24. Kono T, Sabbah HN, Rosman H, Alam M, Jafri S, Goldstein S (1992) Left ventricular shape is the primary determinant of functional mitral regurgitation in heart failure. J Am Coll Cardiol 20(7):1594–1598
25. Sabbah HN, Rosman H, Kono T, Alam M, Khaja F, Goldstein S (1993) On the mechanism of functional mitral regurgitation. Am J Cardiol 72(14):1074–1076
26. White HD, Norris RM, Brown MA, Brandt PW, Whitlock RM, Wild CJ (1987) Left ventricular end-systolic volume as the major determinant of survival after recovery from myocardial infarction. Circulation 76(1):44–51
27. Hauptman PJ, Sabbah HN (2007) Reversal of ventricular remodeling: important to establish and difficult to define. Eur J Heart Fail 9(4):325–328
28. Bursi F, Enriquez-Sarano M, Jacobsen SJ, Roger VL (2006) Mitral regurgitation after myocardial infarction: a review. Am J Med 119(2):103–112
29. Lamas GA, Mitchell GF, Flaker GC, Smith SC, Gersh BJ, Basta L et al (1997) Clinical significance of mitral regurgitation after acute myocardial infarction. Survival and ventricular enlargement investigators. Circulation 96(3):827–833
30. Grigioni F, Enriquez-Sarano M, Zehr KJ, Bailey KR, Tajik AJ (2001) Ischemic mitral regurgitation: long-term outcome and prognostic implications with quantitative Doppler assessment. Circulation 103(13):1759–1764
31. Blondheim DS, Jacobs LE, Kotler MN, Costacurta GA, Parry WR (1991) Dilated cardiomyopathy with mitral regurgitation: decreased survival despite a low frequency of left ventricular thrombus. Am Heart J 122(3 Pt 1):763–771
32. Koelling TM, Aaronson KD, Cody RJ, Bach DS, Armstrong WF (2002) Prognostic significance of mitral regurgitation and tricuspid regurgitation in patients with left ventricular systolic dysfunction. Am Heart J 144(3):524–529
33. Trichon BH, Felker GM, Shaw LK, Cabell CH, O'Connor CM (2003) Relation of frequency and severity of mitral regurgitation to survival among patients with left ventricular systolic dysfunction and heart failure. Am J Cardiol 91(5):538–543

34. Robbins JD, Maniar PB, Cotts W, Parker MA, Bonow RO, Gheorghiade M (2003) Prevalence and severity of mitral regurgitation in chronic systolic heart failure. Am J Cardiol 91(3): 360–362
35. Patel JB, Borgeson DD, Barnes ME, Rihal CS, Daly RC, Redfield MM (2004) Mitral regurgitation in patients with advanced systolic heart failure. J Card Fail 10(4):285–291
36. Bursi F, Enriquez-Sarano M, Nkomo VT, Jacobsen SJ, Weston SA, Meverden RA et al (2005) Heart failure and death after myocardial infarction in the community: the emerging role of mitral regurgitation. Circulation 111(3):295–301
37. Aronson D, Goldsher N, Zukermann R, Kapeliovich M, Lessick J, Mutlak D et al (2006) Ischemic mitral regurgitation and risk of heart failure after myocardial infarction. Arch Intern Med 166(21):2362–2368
38. Agricola E, Ielasi A, Oppizzi M, Faggiano P, Ferri L, Calabrese A et al (2009) Long-term prognosis of medically treated patients with functional mitral regurgitation and left ventricular dysfunction. Eur J Heart Fail 11(6):581–587
39. Rossi A, Dini FL, Faggiano P, Agricola E, Cicoira M, Frattini S et al (2011) Independent prognostic value of functional mitral regurgitation in patients with heart failure. A quantitative analysis of 1256 patients with ischaemic and non-ischaemic dilated cardiomyopathy. Heart 97(20):1675–1680
40. Bonow RO, Carabello BA, Chatterjee K, de Leon AC, Faxon DP, Freed MD et al (2008) 2008 focused update incorporated into the ACC/AHA 2006 guidelines for the management of patients with valvular heart disease: a report of the American College of Cardiology/American Heart Association Task Force on Practice Guidelines (Writing Committee to revise the 1998 guidelines for the management of patients with valvular heart disease): Endorsed by the Society of Cardiovascular Anesthesiologists, Society for Cardiovascular Angiography and Interventions, and Society of Thoracic Surgeons. J Am Coll Cardiol 52:e1–e142
41. Vahanian A, Baumgartner H, Bax J, Butchart E, Dion R, Filippatos G et al (2007) Guidelines on the management of valvular heart disease: The Task Force on the Management of Valvular Heart Disease of the European Society of Cardiology. Eur Heart J 28:230–268
42. Zoghbi WA, Enriquez-Sarano M, Foster E, Grayburn PA, Kraft CD, Levine RA et al (2003) Recommendations for evaluation of the severity of native valvular regurgitation with two-dimensional and Doppler echocardiography. J Am Soc Echocardiogr 16:777–802
43. Marsan NA, Westenberg JJM, Ypenburg C, Delgado V, van Bommel RJ, Roes SD et al (2009) Quantification of functional mitral regurgitation by real-time 3D echocardiography: comparison with 3D velocity-encoded cardiac magnetic resonance. JACC Cardiovasc Imaging 2(11):1245–1252
44. Lebrun F, Lancellotti P, Pierard LA (2001) Quantitation of functional mitral regurgitation during bicycle exercise in patients with heart failure. J Am Coll Cardiol 38(6):1685–1692
45. Lancellotti P, Lebrun F, Piérard LA (2003) Determinants of exercise-induced changes in mitral regurgitation in patients with coronary artery disease and left ventricular dysfunction. J Am Coll Cardiol 42(11):1921–1928
46. Lancellotti P, Troisfontaines P, Toussaint A-C, Piérard LA (2003) Prognostic importance of exercise-induced changes in mitral regurgitation in patients with chronic ischemic left ventricular dysfunction. Circulation 108(14):1713–1717
47. Ennezat PV, Maréchaux S, Huerre C, Deklunder G, Asseman P, Jude B et al (2008) Exercise does not enhance the prognostic value of Doppler echocardiography in patients with left ventricular systolic dysfunction and functional mitral regurgitation at rest. Am Heart J 155(4): 752–757
48. Bach DS, Deeb GM, Bolling SF (1995) Accuracy of intraoperative transesophageal echocardiography for estimating the severity of functional mitral regurgitation. Am J Cardiol 76(7): 508–512
49. Grewal KS, Malkowski MJ, Piracha AR, Astbury JC, Kramer CM, Dianzumba S et al (2000) Effect of general anesthesia on the severity of mitral regurgitation by transesophageal echocardiography. Am J Cardiol 85(2):199–203

50. Aklog L, Filsoufi F, Flores KQ, Chen RH, Cohn LH, Nathan NS et al (2001) Does coronary artery bypass grafting alone correct moderate ischemic mitral regurgitation? Circulation 104(12 suppl 1):I68–I75
51. Rosario LB, Stevenson LW, Solomon SD, Lee RT, Reimold SC (1998) The mechanism of decrease in dynamic mitral regurgitation during heart failure treatment: importance of reduction in the regurgitant orifice size. J Am Coll Cardiol 32(7):1819–1824
52. Hung J, Otsuji Y, Handschumacher MD, Schwammenthal E, Levine RA (1999) Mechanism of dynamic regurgitant orifice area variation in functional mitral regurgitation: physiologic insights from the proximal flow convergence technique. J Am Coll Cardiol 33(2):538–545
53. Dion R, Benetis R, Elias B, Guennaoui T, Raphael D, van Dyck M et al (1995) Mitral valve procedures in ischemic regurgitation. J Heart Valve Dis 4(suppl 2):S124–S129; discussion S129–S131
54. Byrne JG, Aklog L, Adams DH (2000) Assessment and management of functional or ischaemic mitral regurgitation. Lancet 355(9217):1743–1744
55. Mihalatos DG, Gopal AS, Kates R, Toole RS, Bercow NR, Lamendola C et al (2006) Intraoperative assessment of mitral regurgitation: role of phenylephrine challenge. J Am Soc Echocardiogr 19(9):1158–1164
56. Shiran A, Merdler A, Ismir E, Ammar R, Zlotnick AY, Aravot D et al (2007) Intraoperative transesophageal echocardiography using a quantitative dynamic loading test for the evaluation of ischemic mitral regurgitation. J Am Soc Echocardiogr 20(6):690–697
57. Otsuji Y, Kumanohoso T, Yoshifuku S, Matsukida K, Koriyama C, Kisanuki A et al (2002) Isolated annular dilation does not usually cause important functional mitral regurgitation: comparison between patients with lone atrial fibrillation and those with idiopathic or ischemic cardiomyopathy. J Am Coll Cardiol 39(10):1651–1656
58. Kumanohoso T, Otsuji Y, Yoshifuku S, Matsukida K, Koriyama C, Kisanuki A et al (2003) Mechanism of higher incidence of ischemic mitral regurgitation in patients with inferior myocardial infarction: quantitative analysis of left ventricular and mitral valve geometry in 103 patients with prior myocardial infarction. J Thorac Cardiovasc Surg 125(1):135–143
59. Magne J, Pibarot P, Dagenais F, Hachicha Z, Dumesnil JG, Senechal M (2007) Preoperative posterior leaflet angle accurately predicts outcome after restrictive mitral valve annuloplasty for ischemic mitral regurgitation. Circulation 115(6):782–791
60. Lee AP-W, Acker M, Kubo SH, Bolling SF, Park SW, Bruce CJ et al (2009) Mechanisms of recurrent functional mitral regurgitation after mitral valve repair in nonischemic dilated cardiomyopathy: importance of distal anterior leaflet tethering. Circulation 119(19):2606–2614
61. Ciarka A, Braun J, Delgado V, Versteegh M, Boersma E, Klautz R et al (2010) Predictors of mitral regurgitation recurrence in patients with heart failure undergoing mitral valve annuloplasty. Am J Cardiol 106(3):395–401
62. Schuster A, Morton G, Chiribiri A, Perera D, Vanoverschelde J-L, Nagel E (2012) Imaging in the management of ischemic cardiomyopathy special focus on magnetic resonance. J Am Coll Cardiol 59(4):359–370
63. Kim RJ, Wu E, Rafael A, Chen EL, Parker MA, Simonetti O et al (2000) The use of contrast-enhanced magnetic resonance imaging to identify reversible myocardial dysfunction. N Engl J Med 343(20):1445–1453
64. Kaandorp TAM, Bax JJ, Schuijf JD, Viergever EP, van der Wall EE, de Roos A et al (2004) Head-to-head comparison between contrast-enhanced magnetic resonance imaging and dobutamine magnetic resonance imaging in men with ischemic cardiomyopathy. Am J Cardiol 93(12):1461–1464
65. Bax JJ, Van Der Wall EE, Harbinson M (2004) Radionuclide techniques for the assessment of myocardial viability and hibernation. Heart 90(suppl 5):v26–v33
66. Westenberg JJM, Roes SD, Ajmone Marsan N, Binnendijk NMJ, Doornbos J, Bax JJ et al (2008) Mitral valve and tricuspid valve blood flow: accurate quantification with 3D velocity-encoded MR imaging with retrospective valve tracking. Radiology 249(3):792–800
67. Marsan NA, Westenberg JJM, Tops LF, Ypenburg C, Holman ER, Reiber JHC et al (2008) Comparison between tissue Doppler imaging and velocity-encoded magnetic resonance

imaging for measurement of myocardial velocities, assessment of left ventricular dyssynchrony, and estimation of left ventricular filling pressures in patients with ischemic cardiomyopathy. Am J Cardiol 102(10):1366–1372
68. Ellis SG, Whitlow PL, Raymond RE, Schneider JP (2002) Impact of mitral regurgitation on long-term survival after percutaneous coronary intervention. Am J Cardiol 89(3):315–318
69. Tolis GA, Korkolis DP, Kopf GS, Elefteriades JA (2002) Revascularization alone (without mitral valve repair) suffices in patients with advanced ischemic cardiomyopathy and mild-to-moderate mitral regurgitation. Ann Thorac Surg 74(5):1476–1480; discussion 1480–1481
70. Trichon BH (2003) Survival after coronary revascularization, with and without mitral valve surgery, in patients with ischemic mitral regurgitation. Circulation 108(90101):103II–110II
71. Mallidi HR, Pelletier MP, Lamb J, Desai N, Sever J, Christakis GT et al (2004) Late outcomes in patients with uncorrected mild to moderate mitral regurgitation at the time of isolated coronary artery bypass grafting. J Thorac Cardiovasc Surg 127(3):636–644
72. Lam B-K, Gillinov AM, Blackstone EH, Rajeswaran J, Yuh B, Bhudia SK et al (2005) Importance of moderate ischemic mitral regurgitation. Ann Thorac Surg 79(2):462–470; discussion 462–470
73. Wong DR, Agnihotri AK, Hung JW, Vlahakes GJ, Akins CW, Hilgenberg AD et al (2005) Long-term survival after surgical revascularization for moderate ischemic mitral regurgitation. Ann Thorac Surg 80(2):570–577
74. Grossi EA, Crooke GA, DiGiorgi PL, Schwartz CF, Jorde U, Applebaum RM et al (2006) Impact of moderate functional mitral insufficiency in patients undergoing surgical revascularization. Circulation 114(1 suppl):I573–I576
75. Di Mauro M, Di Giammarco G, Vitolla G, Contini M, Iacò AL, Bivona A et al (2006) Impact of no-to-moderate mitral regurgitation on late results after isolated coronary artery bypass grafting in patients with ischemic cardiomyopathy. Ann Thorac Surg 81(6):2128–2134
76. Calafiore AM, Mazzei V, Iacò AL, Contini M, Bivona A, Gagliardi M et al (2008) Impact of ischemic mitral regurgitation on long-term outcome of patients with ejection fraction above 0.30 undergoing first isolated myocardial revascularization. Ann Thorac Surg 86(2):458–464; discussion 464–465
77. Fattouch K, Sampognaro R, Speziale G, Salardino M, Novo G, Caruso M et al (2010) Impact of moderate ischemic mitral regurgitation after isolated coronary artery bypass grafting. Ann Thorac Surg 90(4):1187–1194
78. Kang D-H, Sun BJ, Kim DH, Yun SC, Song J-M, Choo SJ et al (2011) Percutaneous versus surgical revascularization in patients with ischemic mitral regurgitation. Circulation 124(11 suppl 1):S156–S162
79. Bax JJ, Braun J, Somer ST, Klautz R, Holman ER, Versteegh MIM et al (2004) Restrictive annuloplasty and coronary revascularization in ischemic mitral regurgitation results in reverse left ventricular remodeling. Circulation 110(11 suppl 1):II103–II108
80. Mc Gee Jr E, Gillinov A, Blackstone E, Rajeswaran J, Cohen G, Najam F et al (2004) Recurrent mitral regurgitation after annuloplasty for functional ischemic mitral regurgitation. J Thorac Cardiovasc Surg 128(6):916–924
81. Glower DD, Tuttle RH, Shaw LK, Orozco RE, Rankin JS (2005) Patient survival characteristics after routine mitral valve repair for ischemic mitral regurgitation. J Thorac Cardiovasc Surg 129(4):860–868
82. Braun J, Bax JJ, Versteegh MIM, Voigt PG, Holman ER, Klautz RJM et al (2005) Preoperative left ventricular dimensions predict reverse remodeling following restrictive mitral annuloplasty in ischemic mitral regurgitation. Eur J Cardiothorac Surg 27(5):847–853
83. Geidel S, Lass M, Schneider C, Groth G, Boczor S, Kuck KH et al (2005) Downsizing of the mitral valve and coronary revascularization in severe ischemic mitral regurgitation results in reverse left ventricular and left atrial remodeling. Eur J Cardiothorac Surg 27(6):1011–1016
84. Mihaljevic T, Lam B-K, Rajeswaran J, Takagaki M, Lauer MS, Gillinov AM et al (2007) Impact of mitral valve annuloplasty combined with revascularization in patients with functional ischemic mitral regurgitation. J Am Coll Cardiol 49(22):2191–2201

85. Gelsomino S, Lorusso R, De Cicco G, Capecchi I, Rostagno C, Caciolli S et al (2007) Five-year echocardiographic results of combined undersized mitral ring annuloplasty and coronary artery bypass grafting for chronic ischaemic mitral regurgitation. Eur Heart J 29(2): 231–240
86. Gelsomino S, Lorusso R, Capecchi I, Rostagno C, Romagnoli S, Billè G et al (2008) Left ventricular reverse remodeling after undersized mitral ring annuloplasty in patients with ischemic regurgitation. Ann Thorac Surg 85(4):1319–1330
87. Ngaage DL, Daly RC, Rosales G, Sundt TM, Dearani JA, Mullany CJ et al (2008) Mitral regurgitation surgery in heart failure due to ischemic cardiomyopathy: a 24-year experience. J Heart Valve Dis 17(3):251–259; discussion 259–260
88. Crabtree TD, Bailey MS, Moon MR, Munfakh N, Pasque MK, Lawton JS et al (2008) Recurrent mitral regurgitation and risk factors for early and late mortality after mitral valve repair for functional ischemic mitral regurgitation. Ann Thorac Surg 85(5):1537–1542; discussion 1542–1543
89. Braun J, Van de Veire NR, Klautz RJM, Versteegh MIM, Holman ER, Westenberg JJM et al (2008) Restrictive mitral annuloplasty cures ischemic mitral regurgitation and heart failure. Ann Thorac Surg 85(2):430–437
90. Onorati F, Santarpino G, Marturano D, Rubino AS, Pasceri E, Zinzi S et al (2009) Successful surgical treatment of chronic ischemic mitral regurgitation achieves left ventricular reverse remodeling but does not affect right ventricular function. J Thorac Cardiovasc Surg 138(2):341–351
91. Williams ML, Daneshmand MA, Jollis JG, Horton JR, Shaw LK, Swaminathan M et al (2009) Mitral gradients and frequency of recurrence of mitral regurgitation after ring annuloplasty for ischemic mitral regurgitation. Ann Thorac Surg 88(4):1197–1201
92. Fattouch K, Guccione F, Sampognaro R, Panzarella G, Corrado E, Navarra E et al (2009) POINT: Efficacy of adding mitral valve restrictive annuloplasty to coronary artery bypass grafting in patients with moderate ischemic mitral valve regurgitation: a randomized trial. J Thorac Cardiovasc Surg 138(2):278–285
93. Pocar M, Passolunghi D, Moneta A, Di Mauro A, Bregasi A, Mattioli R et al (2010) Baseline left ventricular function and surgical annular stiffening to predict outcome and reverse left ventricular remodeling after undersized annuloplasty for intermediate-degree ischemic mitral regurgitation. J Thorac Cardiovasc Surg 139(6):1529–1538
94. Grossi EA, Woo YJ, Patel N, Goldberg JD, Schwartz CF, Subramanian VA et al (2011) Outcomes of coronary artery bypass grafting and reduction annuloplasty for functional ischemic mitral regurgitation: a prospective multicenter study (Randomized Evaluation of a Surgical Treatment for Off-Pump Repair of the Mitral Valve). J Thorac Cardiovasc Surg 141(1):91–97
95. Gillinov AM, Wierup PN, Blackstone EH, Bishay ES, Cosgrove DM, White J et al (2001) Is repair preferable to replacement for ischemic mitral regurgitation? J Thorac Cardiovasc Surg 122(6):1125–1141
96. Grossi EA, Goldberg JD, LaPietra A, Ye X, Zakow P, Sussman M et al (2001) Ischemic mitral valve reconstruction and replacement: comparison of long-term survival and complications. J Thorac Cardiovasc Surg 122(6):1107–1124
97. Maltais S, Schaff HV, Daly RC, Suri RM, Dearani JA, Sundt TM et al (2011) Mitral regurgitation surgery in patients with ischemic cardiomyopathy and ischemic mitral regurgitation: factors that influence survival. J Thorac Cardiovasc Surg 142(5):995–1001
98. Miller D (2001) Ischemic mitral regurgitation redux—to repair or to replace? J Thorac Cardiovasc Surg 122(6):1059–1062
99. Calafiore AM, Iacò AL, Bivona A, Varone E, Scandura S, Greco P et al (2011) Echocardiographically based treatment of chronic ischemic mitral regurgitation. J Thorac Cardiovasc Surg 141(5):1150–1156.e1
100. Gummert JF, Rahmel A, Bucerius J, Onnasch J, Doll N, Walther T et al (2003) Mitral valve repair in patients with end stage cardiomyopathy: who benefits? Eur J Cardiothorac Surg 23(6):1017–1022; discussion 1022

101. Romano MA, Bolling SF (2004) Update on mitral repair in dilated cardiomyopathy. J Card Surg 19(5):396–400
102. Horii T, Suma H, Isomura T, Nomura F, Hoshino J (2006) Left ventricle volume affects the result of mitral valve surgery for idiopathic dilated cardiomyopathy to treat congestive heart failure. Ann Thorac Surg 82(4):1349–1354; discussion 1354–1355
103. Acker MA, Bolling S, Shemin R, Kirklin J, Oh JK, Mann DL et al (2006) Mitral valve surgery in heart failure: insights from the Acorn Clinical Trial. J Thorac Cardiovasc Surg 132(3):568–577, 577.e1–4
104. Mann DL, Kubo SH, Sabbah HN, Starling RC, Jessup M, Oh JK et al (2012) Beneficial effects of the CorCap cardiac support device: five-year results from the Acorn Trial. J Thorac Cardiovasc Surg 143:1036–1042
105. Braun J, Ciarka A, Versteegh MIM, Delgado V, Boersma E, Verwey HF et al (2011) Cardiac support device, restrictive mitral valve annuloplasty, and optimized medical treatment: a multimodality approach to nonischemic cardiomyopathy. J Thorac Cardiovasc Surg 142:e93–e100
106. Carpentier A (1969) Reconstructive valvuloplasty. A new technique of mitral valvuloplasty. Presse Med 77(7):251–253
107. Duran CG, Ubago JL (1976) Clinical and hemodynamic performance of a totally flexible prosthetic ring for atrioventricular valve reconstruction. Ann Thorac Surg 22(5):458–463
108. Cosgrove DM, Arcidi JM, Rodriguez L, Stewart WJ, Powell K, Thomas JD (1995) Initial experience with the Cosgrove-Edwards Annuloplasty System. Ann Thorac Surg 60(3):499–503; discussion 503–504
109. Tibayan FA, Rodriguez F, Langer F, Liang D, Daughters GT, Ingels NB et al (2004) Undersized mitral annuloplasty alters left ventricular shape during acute ischemic mitral regurgitation. Circulation 110(11 suppl 1):II98–II102
110. Spoor MT, Geltz A, Bolling SF (2006) Flexible versus nonflexible mitral valve rings for congestive heart failure: differential durability of repair. Circulation 114(1 suppl):I67–I71
111. Silberman S, Klutstein MW, Sabag T, Oren A, Fink D, Merin O et al (2009) Repair of ischemic mitral regurgitation: comparison between flexible and rigid annuloplasty rings. Ann Thorac Surg 87(6):1721–1726; discussion 1726–1727
112. Mahmood F, Gorman JH, Subramaniam B, Gorman RC, Panzica PJ, Hagberg RC et al (2010) Changes in mitral valve annular geometry after repair: saddle-shaped versus flat annuloplasty rings. Ann Thorac Surg 90(4):1212–1220
113. Bothe W, Swanson JC, Ingels NB, Miller DC (2010) How much septal-lateral mitral annular reduction do you get with new ischemic/functional mitral regurgitation annuloplasty rings? J Thorac Cardiovasc Surg 140(1):117–121, 121.e1–3
114. De Bonis M, Taramasso M, Grimaldi A, Maisano F, Calabrese MC, Verzini A et al (2011) The GeoForm annuloplasty ring for the surgical treatment of functional mitral regurgitation in advanced dilated cardiomyopathy. Eur J Cardiothorac Surg 40(2):488–495
115. Hung J, Papakostas L, Tahta SA, Hardy BG, Bollen BA, Duran CM et al (2004) Mechanism of recurrent ischemic mitral regurgitation after annuloplasty: continued LV remodeling as a moving target. Circulation 110(11 suppl 1):II85–II90
116. Zhu F, Otsuji Y, Yotsumoto G, Yuasa T, Ueno T, Yu B et al (2005) Mechanism of persistent ischemic mitral regurgitation after annuloplasty: importance of augmented posterior mitral leaflet tethering. Circulation 112(9 suppl):I396–I401
117. Shiota M, Gillinov AM, Takasaki K, Fukuda S, Shiota T (2011) Recurrent mitral regurgitation late after annuloplasty for ischemic mitral regurgitation. Echocardiography 28(2):6
118. De Bonis M, Lapenna E, Verzini A, La Canna G, Grimaldi A, Torracca L et al (2008) Recurrence of mitral regurgitation parallels the absence of left ventricular reverse remodeling after mitral repair in advanced dilated cardiomyopathy. Ann Thorac Surg 85(3):932–939
119. Onorati F, Rubino AS, Marturano D, Pasceri E, Santarpino G, Zinzi S et al (2009) Midterm clinical and echocardiographic results and predictors of mitral regurgitation recurrence following restrictive annuloplasty for ischemic cardiomyopathy. J Thorac Cardiovasc Surg 138(3):654–662

120. Magne J, Pibarot P, Dumesnil JG, Sénéchal M (2009) Continued global left ventricular remodeling is not the sole mechanism responsible for the late recurrence of ischemic mitral regurgitation after restrictive annuloplasty. J Am Soc Echocardiogr 22(11):1256–1264
121. Gelsomino S, van Garsse L, Lucà F, Lorusso R, Cheriex E, Rao CM et al (2011) Impact of preoperative anterior leaflet tethering on the recurrence of ischemic mitral regurgitation and the lack of left ventricular reverse remodeling after restrictive annuloplasty. J Am Soc Echocardiogr 24(12):1365–1375
122. Borger MA, Murphy PM, Alam A, Fazel S, Maganti M, Armstrong S et al (2007) Initial results of the chordal-cutting operation for ischemic mitral regurgitation. J Thorac Cardiovasc Surg 133(6):1483–1492
123. De Bonis M, Lapenna E, La Canna G, Ficarra E, Pagliaro M, Torracca L et al (2005) Mitral valve repair for functional mitral regurgitation in end-stage dilated cardiomyopathy: role of the "edge-to-edge" technique. Circulation 112(9 suppl):I402–I408
124. de Varennes B, Chaturvedi R, Sidhu S, Cote AV, Shan WLP, Goyer C et al (2009) Initial results of posterior leaflet extension for severe type IIIb ischemic mitral regurgitation. Circulation 119(21):2837–2843
125. Kincaid EH, Riley RD, Hines MH, Hammon JW, Kon ND (2004) Anterior leaflet augmentation for ischemic mitral regurgitation. Ann Thorac Surg 78(2):564–568; discussion 568
126. Hvass U, Joudinaud T (2010) The papillary muscle sling for ischemic mitral regurgitation. J Thorac Cardiovasc Surg 139(2):418–423
127. Langer F, Kunihara T, Hell K, Schramm R, Schmidt KI, Aicher D et al (2009) RING+STRING: Successful repair technique for ischemic mitral regurgitation with severe leaflet tethering. Circulation 120(11 suppl):S85–S91
128. Starling RC, Jessup M, Oh JK, Sabbah HN, Acker MA, Mann DL et al (2007) Sustained benefits of the CorCap Cardiac Support Device on left ventricular remodeling: three year follow-up results from the Acorn clinical trial. Ann Thorac Surg 84(4):1236–1242
129. Grossi EA, Patel N, Woo YJ, Goldberg JD, Schwartz CF, Subramanian V et al (2010) Outcomes of the RESTOR-MV trial (randomized evaluation of a surgical treatment for off-pump repair of the mitral valve). J Am Coll Cardiol 56(24):1984–1993
130. Klein P, Braun J, Holman ER, Versteegh MIM, Verwey HF, Dion RAE et al (2012) Management of mitral regurgitation during left ventricular reconstruction for ischemic heart failure. Eur J Cardiothorac Surg 41:74–80
131. Suma H, Isomura T, Horii T, Nomura F (2006) Septal anterior ventricular exclusion procedure for idiopathic dilated cardiomyopathy. Ann Thorac Surg 82(4):1344–1348
132. Suma H, Tanabe H, Uejima T, Isomura T, Horii T (2009) Surgical ventricular restoration combined with mitral valve procedure for endstage ischemic cardiomyopathy. Eur J Cardiothorac Surg 36(2):280–284; discussion 284–285
133. De Bonis M, Lapenna E, Sorrentino F, La Canna G, Grimaldi A, Maisano F et al (2008) Evolution of tricuspid regurgitation after mitral valve repair for functional mitral regurgitation in dilated cardiomyopathy. Eur J Cardiothorac Surg 33(4):600–606
134. Van de Veire NR, Braun J, Delgado V, Versteegh MIM, Dion RA, Klautz RJM et al (2011) Tricuspid annuloplasty prevents right ventricular dilatation and progression of tricuspid regurgitation in patients with tricuspid annular dilatation undergoing mitral valve repair. J Thorac Cardiovasc Surg 141(6):1431–1439
135. Abraham WT, Fisher WG, Smith AL, DeLurgio DB, Leon AR, Loh E et al (2002) Cardiac resynchronization in chronic heart failure. N Engl J Med 346(24):1845–1853
136. Cleland JGF, Daubert J-C, Erdmann E, Freemantle N, Gras D, Kappenberger L et al (2005) The effect of cardiac resynchronization on morbidity and mortality in heart failure. N Engl J Med 352(15):1539–1549
137. Breithardt OA, Sinha AM, Schwammenthal E, Bidaoui N, Markus KU, Franke A et al (2003) Acute effects of cardiac resynchronization therapy on functional mitral regurgitation in advanced systolic heart failure. J Am Coll Cardiol 41(5):765–770

138. St John-Sutton MG, Plappert T, Abraham WT, Smith AL, DeLurgio DB, Leon AR et al (2003) Effect of cardiac resynchronization therapy on left ventricular size and function in chronic heart failure. Circulation 107(15):1985–1990
139. Ghio S, Freemantle N, Scelsi L, Serio A, Magrini G, Pasotti M et al (2009) Long-term left ventricular reverse remodelling with cardiac resynchronization therapy: results from the CARE-HF trial. Eur J Heart Fail 11(5):480–488
140. Ellenbogen KA, Wood MA, Klein HU (2005) Why should we care about CARE-HF? J Am Coll Cardiol 46(12):2199–2203
141. Conte J (2010) An indictment of the STICH trial: "True, true, and unrelated". J Heart Lung Transplant 29(5):491–496

Chapter 11
Percutaneous Approaches to Treat Functional Mitral Regurgitation: Current State of Affairs and Future Perspectives

David Messika-Zeitoun

Abstract Functional mitral regurgitation (FMR) is a common complication of ischemic or dilated cardiomyopathy and portends an adverse prognosis. Undersized annuloplasty using a complete rigid ring is the most common surgical technique performed in patients with FMR but its impact on outcome remained debated. In the recent years, two percutaneous techniques as emerged as a potential alternative to surgery in patients with FMR, the percutaneous annuloplasty via the coronary sinus and the edge-to-edge—MitraClip procedure. Due to both safety (coronary artery compression) and efficacy concerns the coronary sinus approach is almost abandoned. The MitraClip has received the CE approval and thousands of patients have been implanted worldwide. Overall, the MitraClip is associated with functional improvement, MR reduction, and positive left ventricular (LV) remodeling and improvement of ejection fraction. However, robust data regarding survival benefit are still lacking. In addition, the MitraClip does not directly adress the cause of FMR—local LV remodeling and papillary muscle displacement—and in contrast to the surgical edge-to-edge procedure is not associated with an annuloplasty. Many companies are currently working on other devices trying to mimic surgical procedures or on LV reshaping devices. Strong efforts should be directed towards technological improvements but also toward clinical randomized studies clearly demonstrating that these devices improve the outcome of patients with FMR.

D. Messika-Zeitoun (✉)
Department of Cardiology, AP-HP, Cardiovascular Division,
Assistance Publique—Hôpitaux de Paris, Bichat Hospital,
46 rue Henri Huchard, 75018 Paris, France
e-mail: david.messika-zeitoun@bch.aphp.fr

J. Bartunek and M. Vanderheyden (eds.), *Translational Approach to Heart Failure*, DOI 10.1007/978-1-4614-7345-9_11,

1 Introduction

Functional mitral regurgitation (FMR) is a regurgitation that occurs despite a structurally normal mitral valve as a consequence of left ventricular (LV) dysfunction. It is a common feature of either dilated or ischemic cardiomyopathy and the presence and degree of severity of FMR is associated with an increased risk of death and congestive heart failure [1–3]. Mechanisms leading to FMR involve local left ventricular remodeling, mitral valve tenting, annular dilatation, and loss of systolic annular contraction [3]. Despite its high prevalence and its strong association with a poor outcome, whether FMR is a marker or the cause of the observed increased morbidity and mortality is still unclear and surgical treatment of FMR remains debated due to the absence of demonstrated survival benefit and the lack of randomized studies [4–6]. Undersized annuloplasty using a complete rigid ring is the most common surgical technique performed in patients with FMR but both the European Society of Cardiology and American Heart Association/American College of Cardiology gave a IIb recommendation for surgical repair unless the patient should undergo a coronary artery bypass surgery [7, 8]. Furthermore, a significant rate of MR recurrence has been described and several anatomical predictors identified (end-diastolic left ventricular diameter >65 mm, posterior leaflet angle ≥45°, mitral valve coaptation depth ≥11 mm …) [4, 9]. Thus, a percutaneous treatment for FMR, in addition to pharmacological therapy and resynchronization pacing, is highly desirable. The two main approaches that have been developed, the edge-to-edge procedure and the annuloplasty via the coronary sinus, are presented in the present chapter as well as perspectives regarding future percutaneous therapies.

2 Percutaneous Edge-to-Edge Procedure

2.1 *Principle*

The percutaneous edge-to-edge procedure is derived from a surgical technique developed by Alfieri in the early 1990s to treat both organic and functional mitral regurgitation (MR) [10, 11]. The surgical technique consists of the suture of the free edge of the leaflets at the site of the regurgitation and the creation of double valve orifice (Fig. 11.1). This technique, despite debated, has been reported as safe, effective, and durable in experienced hands [12–14]. Percutaneous devices have been subsequently developed to replicate this surgical procedure.

2.2 *Theoretical Concerns*

Several concerns have been raised since the development of this technique. The first concern is the risk of creating mitral stenosis. It has been shown experimentally

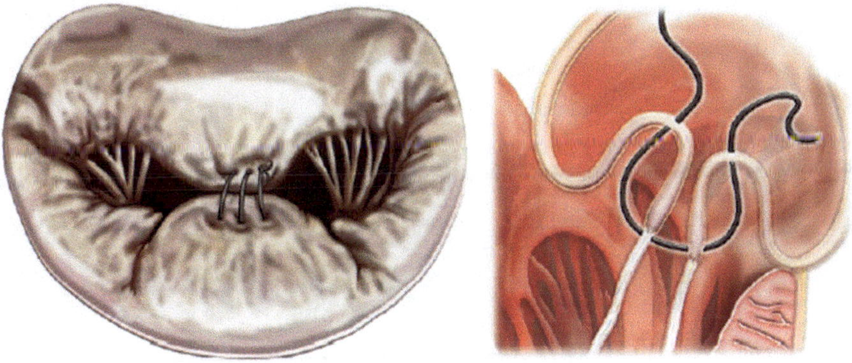

Fig. 11.1 Principle of the surgical edge-to-edge procedure. From [50]

using computational model [15] that hemodynamics are not affected by the double orifice and that valve reserve and exercise response were similar to those treated with conventional repairs [16]. Nevertheless, the suture creates a reduction of the mitral valve area (5.7 ± 1.5 to 3.2 ± 1.2 cm^2 in the EVEREST trial [17]) which had lead to the exclusion of patients with rheumatic MR or those with a valve area <4 cm^2. The second concern is the creation of tension forces on the suture and distortion of the mitral orifice. A large series of explanted clips in 50 patients (67 clips) demonstrated device mechanical integrity up to 5 years and device fibrous encapsulation with extension over adjacent mitral leaflets and tissue bridge formation which adds to structural stability [18]. The third concern is the absence of concomitant annuloplasty. Annuloplasty is the cornerstone of surgical mitral valve repair and is essential in FMR. Annuloplasty improves early and late long-term results of the edge-to-edge surgical repair but is obviously not performed during percutaneous edge-to-edge therapy. Nevertheless, acceptable results have been still achieved without annuloplasty during edge-to-edge surgical repair in selected patients (90 ± 5 % freedom rate of recurrent MR grade >2 and reoperation) [19]. In the future, combined percutaneous edge-to-edge and mitral annuloplasty may further improve and extend indication and results of transcatheter mitral procedure. Finally, the edge-to-edge procedure does not specifically address the anatomic lesion (Neither in organic nor in functional regurgitation). Despite all these limitations, more and more data accumulate regarding the safety and efficacy of the percutaneous edge-to-edge repair.

2.3 *The Devices*

Two systems have been developed, the Mobius (Edwards Lifesciences, Irvine, California) and the MitraClip (Abbott Vascular, Redwood City, California).

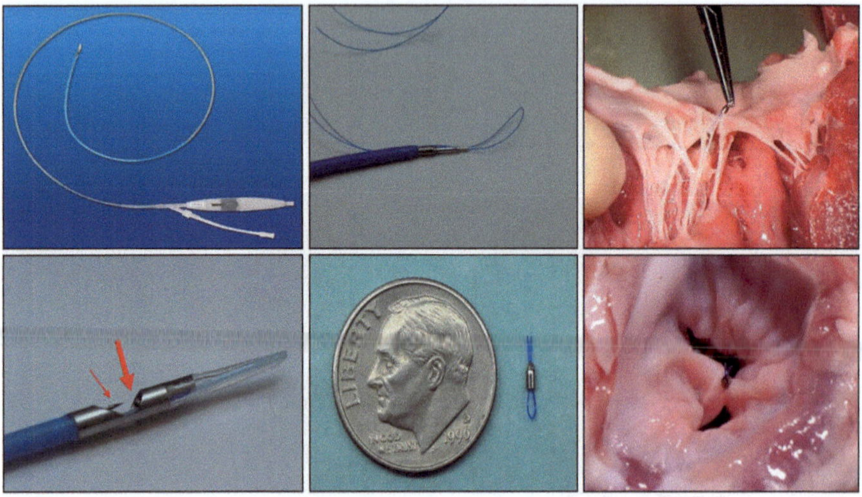

Fig. 11.2 The MOBIUS leaflet repair suture delivery system. The *small arrow* indicates the needle and the *large arrow* the suction port. The suture system is presented on the *bottom* part of the figure (*mid* and *right* part)

The Mobius system. The Edwards catheter contained a suction port which should be directed towards the target leaflet and two needles. Once the leaflet has been captured into the suction port, the needle is advanced through the leaflet. The suction is then discontinued and the suction port redirected toward the opposite leaflet and the process repeated. The two leaflets are finally tied together using a fastener catheter (Fig. 11.2). This device has been evaluated in 15 patients with organic MR and was abandoned due to a limited procedural success rate—at least partially due to the lack of 3D transesophageal echocardiography (TEE) guidance at that time—and limited repair durability [20].

The MitraClip system. The MitraClip device is a MRI-compatible 4-mm-wide cobalt-chromium clip with two arms and two grippers percutaneously delivered via a transferomal venous puncture and 24F venous catheter (22F at the interatrial septum) (Fig. 11.3). The clip arms are opened and closed by a knob on the delivery catheter. The grippers secure the leaflet when the arms are closed. Compared to a suture-based approach, the clip offers a larger surface of coaptation. The MitraClip is implanted through a sequence of standardized steps using a steerable delivery system. The procedure is performed in the catheterization laboratory under general anesthesia using fluoroscopy and TEE guidance and thus requires interventional cardiologist, echocardiographers, and anesthesiologists. Use of three-dimensional TEE has proven to be essential [21] and most of the maneuvering of the system is done under echocardiographic guidance (Fig. 11.4). The transeptal puncture is a crucial step and should be precisely performed at the mid-superior and posterior part of the fossa ovale to allow proper alignment of the delivery system with the

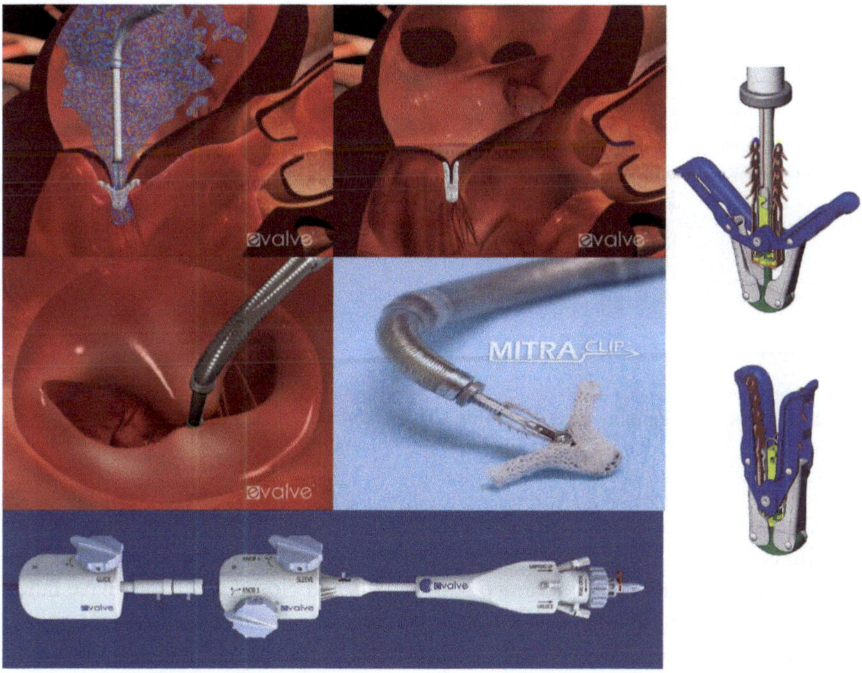

Fig. 11.3 Principle of MitraClip implantation and schematic drawing of the components of the clip. From [22]

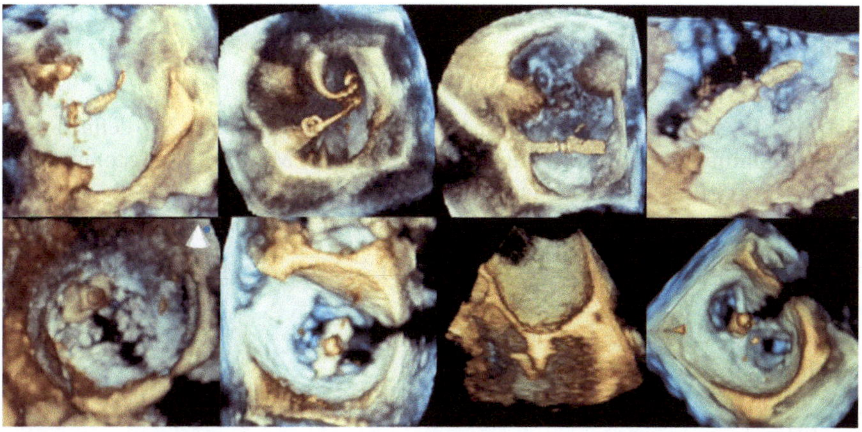

Fig. 11.4 The different steps of MitraClip implantation under three-dimensional transesophageal echocardiography

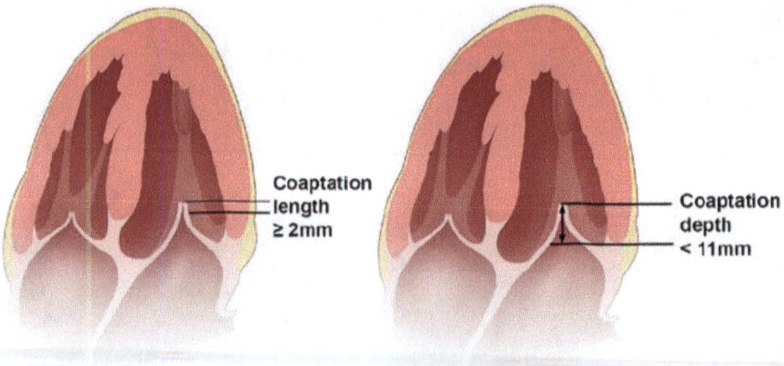

Fig. 11.5 Anatomic eligibility criteria for MitraClip implantation in the EVEREST trial. From [17]

mitral valve. When an adequate perpendicular and central alignment is achieved, the clip is partially opened and passed across the leaflets into the left ventricle. The open clip is then pulled back to grasp both leaflets and closed when they have fallen into the arms. The clip should completely incorporate the disease segment guided by the regurgitant jet. MR reduction is monitored by TEE. One main advantages of this system is its repositionable and retrievable capability. Until the final release, the clip can be easily removed if results are unsatisfactory and repositioned. A second clip is often used to achieve significant MR reduction. MitraClip is the only commercially available percutaneous system with CE approval and thus the following paragraphs are only related to this system.

2.4 Patient Selection

The EVEREST study (endovascular valve edge-to-edge repair) has defined anatomic eligibility criteria for both functional and organic MR [17]. The recommended criteria for FMR are presented in Fig. 11.5:

- Central jets
- Coaptation length >2 mm (some degree of coaptation is needed to capture the leaflets)
- Coaptation depth <11 mm (tenting height)
- Mitral valve orifice >4 cm^2
- Caution in case of short posterior leaflet (<8 mm) or calcification in the grasping area

It is worth noting that patients implanted in the real world such as in the post market registries ACCESS-EU or REALISM, are older, with more comorbidities and that a significant part of them do not fulfill the EVEREST trial criteria.

2.5 Results

After the EVEREST I trial and registry showing the safety, feasibility, and efficacy of MitraClip [17, 22] with immediate and significant hemodynamic improvement [23], the EVEREST II trial was conducted. The EVEREST II trial was a multicenter, randomized controlled trial designed to evaluate the safety and efficacy of endovascular mitral repair vs. conventional open surgical valve repair or replacement for both organic and functional MR [24]. Exclusion criteria were left ventricular ejection fraction (LVEF) ≤25 %, left ventricular end-systolic diameter >55 mm, mitral valve orifice area <4 cm^2 or a recent myocardial infarction. All echocardiograms (before and after implantation) were assessed by an independent echocardiographic core laboratory. Mitral regurgitation was graded according to the American Society of Echocardiography guidelines with the use of quantitative and qualitative criteria [21, 25, 26]. Patients were assigned in a 2:1 ratio to MitraClip repair vs. surgery (repair or replacement). The primary efficacy endpoint was a composite of freedom from death, surgery for mitral valve dysfunction, and MR grade 3 or 4 at 12 months. The primary safety endpoint was a composite of death, myocardial infarction, reoperation for failed MV surgery, non elective cardiovascular surgery for adverse events, stroke, renal failure, deep wound infection, prolonged mechanical ventilation, gastrointestinal complication requiring surgery, septicemia, new onset of permanent atrial fibrillation, and transfusion ≥2 units at 30 days. A total of 279 patients were enrolled. Overall, the study showed a superiority of surgery in term of efficacy with only 4 % of patients with MR grade 3 or 4 compared to 19 % in the MitraClip group ($p<0.001$) and a significant lower need for subsequent surgery (2 % vs. 20 %, $p<0.001$). Overall, primary clinical efficacy was 55 % with the MitraClip and 73 % in the surgical arm ($p=0.007$) (intention-to-treat analysis). On the other side, more major events were observed in the surgical group (48 % vs. 15 %, $p<0.0001$) but were mainly driven by the higher need of blood transfusion and difference didn't reach the statistical difference after exclusion of the need for transfusion (10 % vs. 5 %, $p=0.25$).

Main device-related complications are partial clip detachment requiring surgery or procedure-failure. Leaflet or chordate damages are rare [27] (4 % in EVEREST II [24]). Importantly clip failure seems not to preclude surgical mitral valve repair [18, 28, 29]. However, the EVEREST II trial have shown that the actual repair rate in the 37 patients who underwent surgery after MitraClip was significantly lower than the planned repair rate (92 % vs. 54 %, $p=0.005$) [29]. In addition, among these 37 patients, 11 (30 %) exhibits valve injury (related to the clip procedure in 6 and to difficulty in removing the device in 5). In 5 of these 37 patients (14 %), a valve replacement was performed in part because of mitral valve injury due to MitraClip procedure.

The majority of patients in EVEREST II had organic MR and only 27 % had FMR (in both groups). Subgroup analysis suggest a better outcome in patients older than 70 years, with FMR or LVEF <60 %. Despite being a post-hoc analysis, these results were encouraging. In addition, in the EVEREST High Risk Registry, an arm of the EVEREST II trial which enrolled patients at high risk mainly based on a STS score ≥12 %, 78 patients implanted with the MitraClip (59 % with FMR) were matched to 36 patients, recruited retrospectively, who were not enrolled in the EVEREST trial because they did not meet the anatomic criteria or because of other various reasons [30]. Most of the patients were older than 75 years, had a history of congestive heart failure and coronary artery disease, and more than half had previous cardiac surgery but LVEF was normal in most patients. Implanted patients had a similar 30-day mortality (7.7 % vs. 8.3 %, p=NS) and a better 1 year survival (76 % vs. 55 %, $p<0.05$) as well as a lower rate of hospitalization for congestive heart failure. A majority (78 %) remained free of severe MR (≥grade 3) at 12 months. However, choice of the comparator group was highly debatable, the procedural mortality was high (8 %) and there were also several important methodological concerns.

Since the device has received CE approval, it has gain a rapid expanding experience in Europe with already thousands of patients implanted. In contrast to the EVEREST trial, patients implanted in Europe include a high proportion of high risk patients for surgery and a majority of patients with FMR. In addition, a significant part did not fulfill the stringent EVEREST criteria [31, 32]. Franzen et al. reported among 51 consecutive high-surgical-risk patients (mean logistic EuroSCORE 28±22 and STS score 15±11), two-third with FMR, a 96 % procedural success rate with a single clip (67 %), 2 clips (28 %) or 3 clips (2 %) [31]. MR reduction of at least one grade was observed in almost all patients. There were no procedure-related major adverse events and no in-hospital mortality. These results were confirmed in a larger sample of 104 patients with severe MR not amenable to surgery [32] and by other groups [33–35]. The feasibility and clinical outcome was further evaluated specifically in 50 patients with end-stage heart failure and FMR treated in seven European centers [36]. Left ventricular end-systolic diameter was >55 mm in 78 % of patients and mean EF very low (19±5 %). MR of grade 2 or less was achieved in 92 % and sustained at 6 months in most patients. A concomitant positive effect on LV remodeling and LVEF was observed. There was no procedural death. In a multicenter prospective registry, patients who remained highly symptomatic despite optimal pharmacological therapy and who were nonresponder to cardiac resynchronization therapy (CRT), experienced significant functional improvement, reverse LV remodeling, and LVEF improvement after MitraClip implantation with an acceptable 4 % 30-days mortality [37]. MitraClip implantation in 50 consecutive patients with predominantly FMR resulted in acute hemodynamic improvement and reverse remodeling [27]. These hemodynamic changes were associated with a favorable mid-term outcome. Importantly, none of the patients with successful MitraClip implantation experienced an acute low cardiac output state after the procedure.

The preliminary results regarding the ACCES-EU registry, a multicenter European observational registry, have been presented at the last ESC (2011). Among 529 patients treated, follow-up data at 6 months were available in 257 patients. As other European series, the ACCESS-EU enrolled high-risk patients (mean Euroscore 20 %), highly symptomatic (84 % in NYHA class III/IV) and with low ejection fraction (<40 % in more than half of the patients). The procedure was associated with immediate and sustained functional and hemodynamic improvement and significant MR decrease.

Overall these data show that MitraClip is feasible and safe in patients with FMR who were underrepresented or excluded from EVEREST I and II trials and suggest a possible MR reduction and improved outcome following the procedure. Since survival benefit of surgery in patients with FMR is not demonstrated, in the presence of favorable anatomical characteristics, the MitraClip may be considered in patients with isolated FMR. The decision should be discussed in Heart Team involving clinical cardiologist, imaging specialist, heart failure specialist, surgeon, and anesthesiologist. A randomized study, the COAPT study MitraClip vs. medical therapy, in patients with FMR and total mortality as major criteria of judgment, should start in the United States and Canada in 2012, and will provide elements of answer. Unfortunately, no surgical arm is scheduled.

Key Points

- The MitraClip replicates a surgical procedure but does not involve a mitral annuloplasty which is the cornerstone of surgical mitral valve repair.
- The MitraClip is commercially available and thousands of patients have been already worldwide implanted.
- The EVEREST II trial has demonstrated the safety and feasibility of the procedure but overall lower efficacy than the surgery.
- In contrast to the EVEREST I and II trials, most of the patients implanted in clinical practice in Europe include a high proportions of pts at high risk for surgery and with FMR.
- Main theoretical concerns with the MitraClip are the risk of creating a mitral stenosis, the creation of tension forces on the suture and distortion of the mitral orifice, the absence of concomitant annuloplasty and the feasibility of bail-out surgical mitral valve repair.
- Overall the MitraClip is associated with functional and hemodynamic improvement as well as MR decrease but it favorable impact on survival compared to medical therapy needs to be demonstrated.

3 Coronary Sinus Annuloplasty

3.1 Anatomy of the Coronary Venous System and Principle of Coronary Sinus Annuloplasty

The anatomy of the coronary venous system has gained interest with the development of CRT. It is now well recognized that maximal hemodynamic benefit of CRT may be achieved by an optimal placement of the left ventricular lead, highlighting the importance of a careful evaluation of the coronary venous anatomy. The coronary venous system may also be of great importance for percutaneous mitral annuloplasty in patients with functional MR.

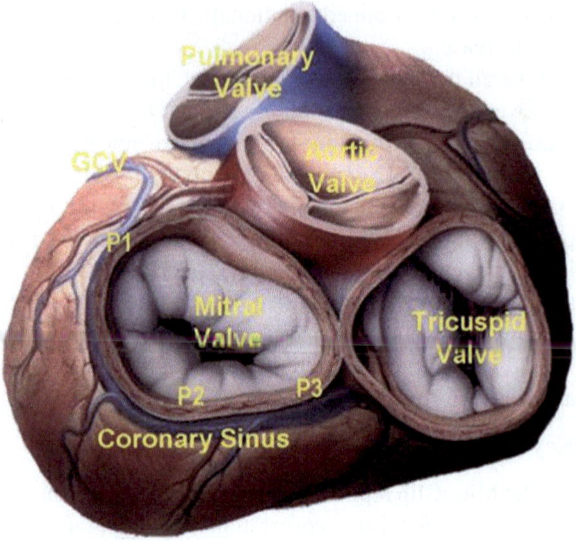

Fig. 11.6 Anatomic view of the base of the heart showing the relationship between the mitral valve annulus and the coronary sinus

The coronary sinus returns blood from most of the left heart. It begins at the termination of the great cardiac vein, and runs through the left atrioventricular junction to terminate into the right atrium. Its diameter at its right atrial mouth varies from 5 to 20 mm and its length from 2 to 5 cm. Its major tributaries are the great cardiac vein, the middle cardiac vein, the veins draining the inferior diaphragmatic surface of the left ventricle, the left marginal veins, the oblique vein of the left atrium, and the small cardiac vein. The anterior interventricular vein originates and runs in the anterior interventricular groove, then courses to the left into the left atrioventricular groove and continues as the great cardiac vein. The great cardiac vein and the coronary sinus have a variable relationship with the coronary arteries and can course either deeply or superficially the circumflex artery. We'll see that these anatomical variations may have important clinical implication for the percutaneous mitral annuloplasty performed via the coronary sinus.

Several devices have been developed exploiting the anatomic proximity of the coronary sinus and of the mitral valve annulus (Fig. 11.6). They are all inserted into the coronary sinus and the great cardiac vein via a venous puncture (cannulation of the coronary sinus is a well established venous access technique) and they all worked on the same principle. They are supposed to shrink the mitral annulus, to increase leaflet coaptation and thus to reduce the regurgitation (Fig. 11.7).

3.2 *The Devices*

Three different systems of percutaneous mitral annuloplasty were evaluated, the Monarc system (Edwards Lifescience, Irvine, California) the Carillon Mitral

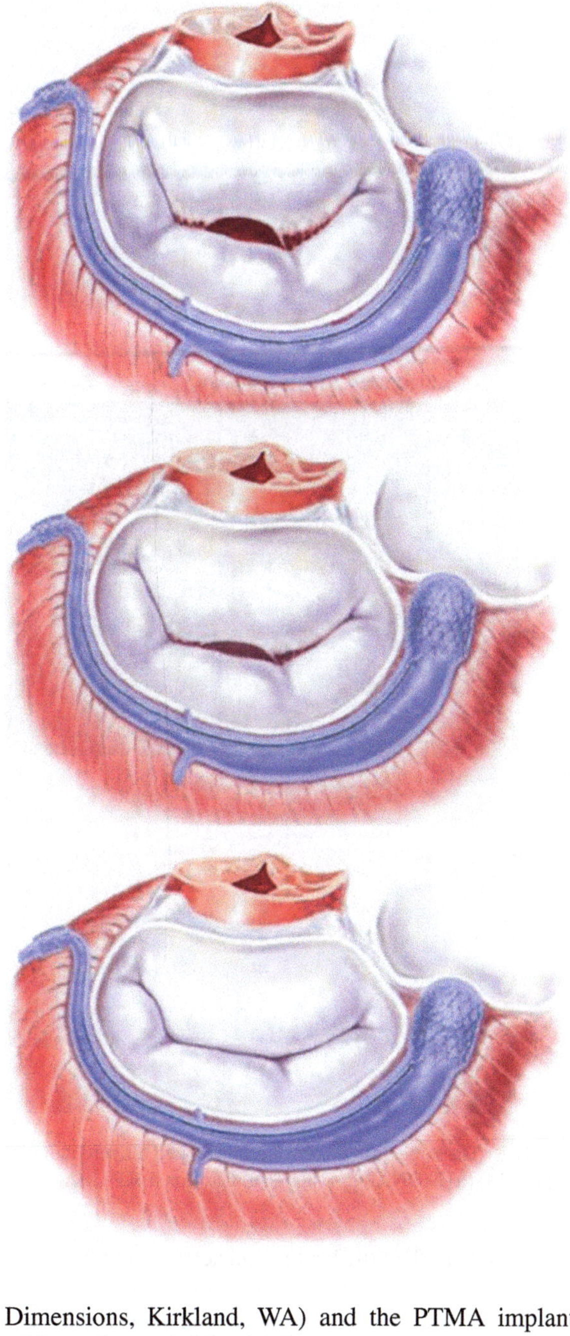

Fig. 11.7 Theoretical effect of the percutaneous mitral annuloplasty via the coronary sinus

Contour System (Cardiac Dimensions, Kirkland, WA) and the PTMA implant system (Viacor, Wilmington, Massachusetts) (Fig. 11.8).

Monarc system. The device consists of two nitinol self-expending stents (proximal and distal) that act as anchors with a connecting spring bridge. A biodegradable

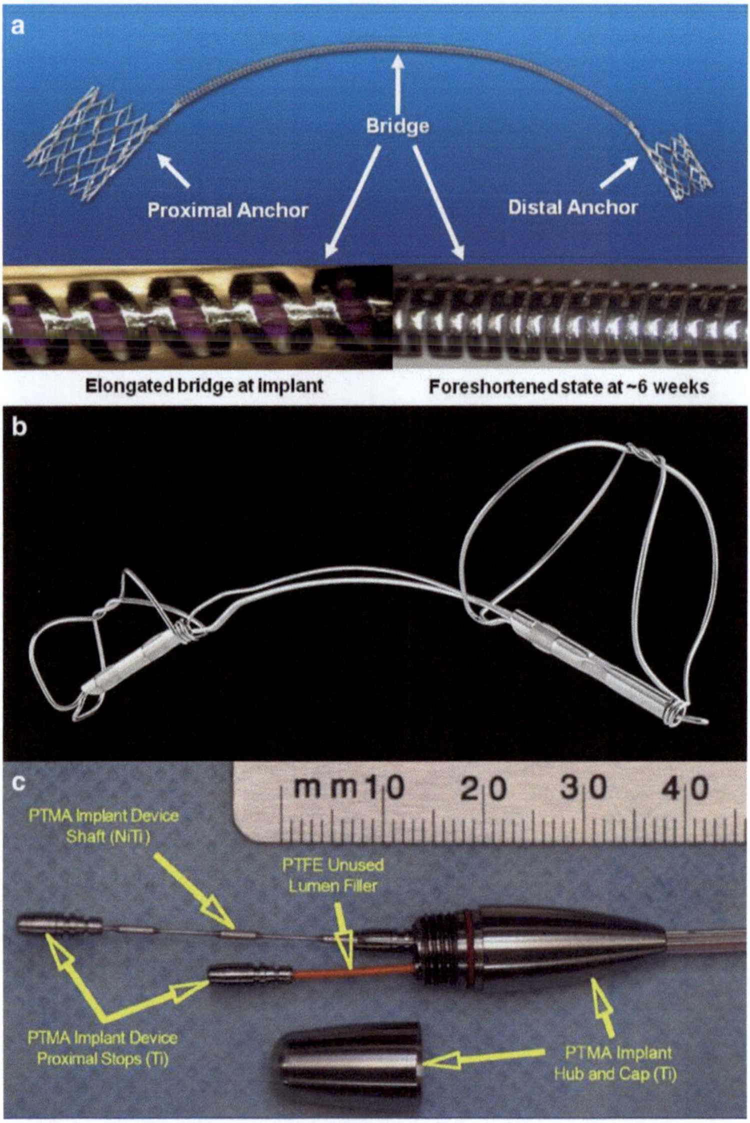

Fig. 11.8 The three different devices developed for percutaneous mitral annuloplasty via the coronary sinus. (**a**) MONARC system, (**b**) Carillon, (**c**) PTMA

suture is wound on the bridge and acts as a temporary spacer to hold the spring open in an elongated state. Over 4–6 weeks, this materiel dissolves and the bridge compresses, shortening the coronary sinus and reducing the septal-lateral dimension. This delay allows the anchors to scar and not to slip as the bridge shortens. Because the MONARC does not have an immediate effect, coronary compressions may be delayed and a systematic 90 days coronary angiography has been recommended.

The device is inserted via the jugular vein using a 12F guide catheter and a 9F delivery catheter. The distal anchor is deployed between the interventricular vein and the great cardiac vein, the proximal anchor in the ostial coronary sinus by retracting the outer restraining sheath. Only a slight tension is applied before deployment of the proximal anchor. In contrast to the two other devices, the MONARC device could not be recaptured and removed once the procedure has started and the distal anchor is delivered.

Carillon Mitral Contour system. The device is composed of two nitinol wire-form anchors, with a nitinol connecting ribbon and is also inserted via the jugular vein. The distal anchor is placed less distal than the two other devices in the great distal vein. Deployment of the distal anchor involves two steps: retraction of the delivery catheter to allow passive expansion of the nitinol wire forms and advancement of the delivery catheter to expand the anchors to their maximum diameter. The anchors were oversized relative to the venous dimensions to apply a circumferential pressure and thereby ensure stable anchoring. A manual tension is applied (4–5 cm) and the proximal anchor is deployed at the ostium of the coronary sinus. The effect is thus immediate both in term of efficacy (immediate assessment of MR reduction) and in term of complications (a coronary angiography is done prior to the definite release of the device). In case of absence of MR reduction or coronary artery compression, another attempt could be made placing the device at a different location or the all system could be recaptured and removed. The procedure was usually made under general anesthesia using a 9F delivery catheter.

PTMA device. The PTMA device is flexible triple lumen catheter placed from a subclavian venous puncture. The distal end is positioned into the anterior interventricular vein. One to three rods (nitinol wire) can be placed into the catheter. The rods are profiled to provide incremental application of stiffness to the posterior mitral annulus. As the Carillon device, effect the PTMA device is immediate and efficacy on the degree of regurgitation as well as potential coronary artery compression can be immediately assessed. Procedures were performed under general anesthesia and TEE guidance using 8F catheters. First, a diagnostic PTMA device was used to determine best size/position of the catheter and number of rods that should be used. In the absence of MR reduction, the device was removed. If significant MR reduction was observed, integrity of coronary arteries was verified (coronary artery angiography) and in the absence of PTMA device instability, the diagnostic catheter was exchanged for the implant PTMA catheter and rods. The proximal end of the device was left outside of the subclavian vein in a subcutaneous pocket.

4 Results

Results regarding efficacy and safety of the three devices have been published in the last 3 years. Results should be analyzed cautiously and were somewhat disappointing due to the small number of patients implanted (approximately 100 patients with the all three devices), the absence of randomization or comparative control group, the limited number of patients with quantitative assessment of MR degree, the occurrence of coronary compression and the raise of theoretical concerns regarding the potential efficacy of the coronary sinus annuloplasty. Importantly, patients with leads into the coronary sinus and thus with biventricular pacing were ineligible for the percutaneous coronary sinus annuloplasty (but a biventricular pacing was performed afterward in several patients).

Monarc system [38]. A total of 72 patients with at least moderate FMR (grade ≥2/4) were enrolled between 2005 and 2007 in 8 participating centers in Canada and Europe (EVOLUTION study). Mean age was 70 years and 82 % were male. FMR was due to ischemic cardiomyopathy if 2/3 of the patients. Mean ejection fraction was 38 ± 10 %. Coronary sinus anatomy was considered suitable for the MONARC device if the diameter of proximal anterior interventricular vein was ≥3 and ≤6 mm, the diameter of the ostium of the coronary sinus was ≥7 and ≤16 mm, and the length from the great cardiac vein between 14 and 18 cm. The device could not be implanted in 13 patients because of excessive tortuosity of the coronary venous anatomy or lack of appropriately sized devices. Measurements were performed using computed tomography and angiography (direct venous angiography). There were two procedure-related complications (two tamponades due to coronary sinus perforation), two device-related complications (myocardial infarction) and eight patients-related complications (cardiovascular deaths due to the severe patients' conditions). Survival free of death, myocardial infarction, and tamponade was 91 % at 30 days and 81 % at 1 year. A systematic coronary angiography was performed at 90 days in 50 of the 59 implanted patients. Despite reinforcement of the suture between the bridge and the proximal anchor (second generation MONARC), separation still occurred in 4 cases (8 %) (Fig. 11.9a). Some degree of coronary artery compression was also noted in 15 patients (30 %). The stenosis severity was ≥50 % in 4 patients (8 %) and 2 of them suffered a myocardial infarction (Fig. 11.9b). External coronary artery compression are observed in patients in whom the coronary sinus/great cardiac vein runs over the marginal/circumflex coronary artery. Unfortunately, this is a very common feature, observed in more than two-third of patients in autopsy studies [39]. This profound course of the marginal—circumflex coronary artery in between the coronary sinus and the mitral annulus can be identified using computed tomography [40–42] allowing pre-procedural screening to exclude patients at risk but was not used in the EVOLUTION study (Fig. 11.10). The device was implanted at intended location in all but 4 patients (55 of the implanted 59 patients, 76 % procedural success rate). Efficacy could be analyzed in approximately half of the patients at 1 year and there was a trend toward functional improvement, reverse left ventricular and left atrial remodeling, mitral annulus diameter reduction and MR reduction (1-grade reduction, from 3/4 to 2/4).

Carillon Mitral Contour system [43, 44]. Forty-eight patients (mean age 65 years, 83 % male) with moderate to severe FMR, in NYHA class II to IV, with left ventricular end-diastolic diameter >55 mm, ejection fraction <40 % in sinus rhythm were enrolled in the AMADEUS trial (CARILLON Mitral Annuloplasty Device

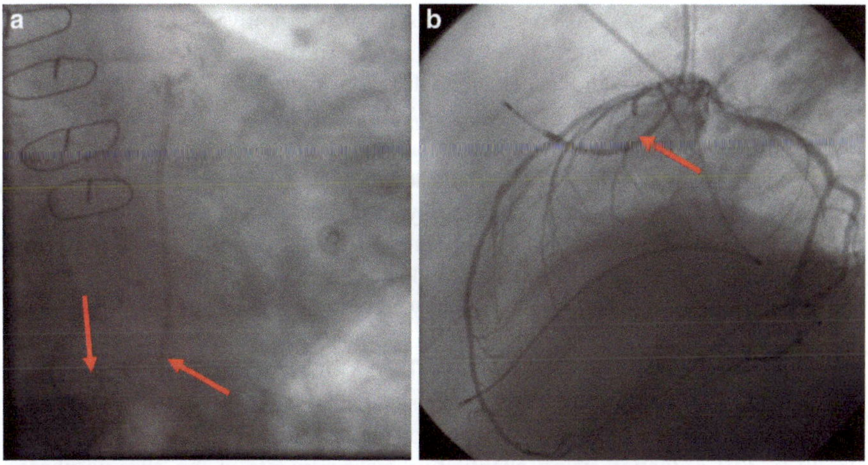

Fig. 11.9 Separation between the bridge and the proximal anchor (**a**) and diagonal compression due to the MONARC device leading to a myocardial infarction (**b**)

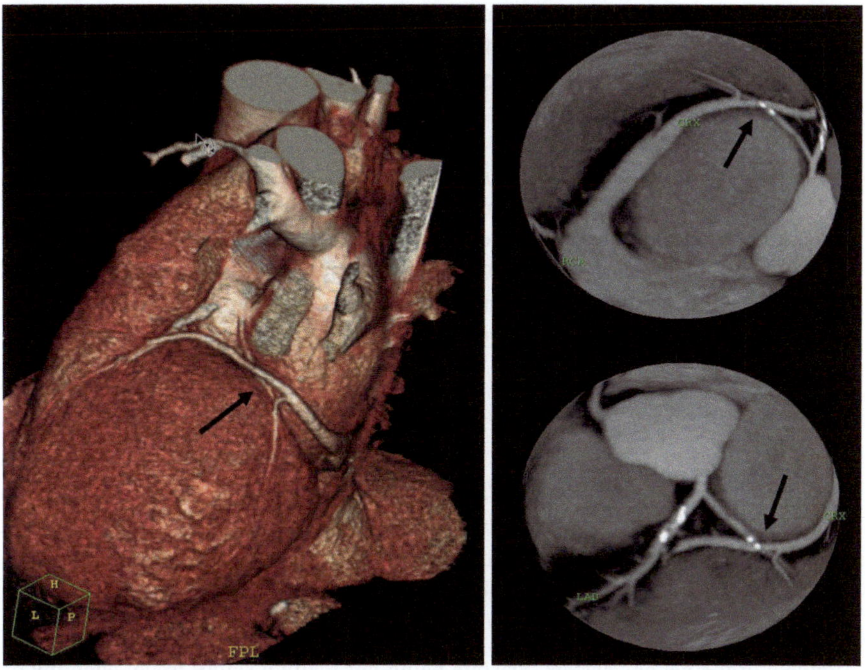

Fig. 11.10 Computed tomography showing the profound course of the circumflex artery between the mitral annulus and the coronary sinus

European Union Study). FMR was due to ischemic cardiomyopathy in 73 % of the patients and mean ejection fraction was 30 ± 8 %. The device was not implanted in 18 patients (63 % procedural success rate due to coronary sinus dissection/perforation ($N=3$), slipping of the distal anchor ($N=3$) or recaptured ($N=10$) because of insufficient MR reduction ($N=4$) or coronary artery compression ($N=6$)). Overall, 11 patients (23 %) had significant arterial compromise as detected using coronary angiography and implants were successfully recaptured without complication in all patients. A second attempt, with the device implanted more proximally, was performed in five patients and resulted in acute MR reduction without coronary artery compression. There was no evidence of late coronary compression in any of the 30 implanted patients. There were three procedure-related coronary sinus dissections in the early phase which resulted in two tamponades. As for the MONARC system, efficacy analysis was only performed in part of the patients and there was a trend toward functional and quality of life improvement, MR reduction (acute MR reduction of one grade and 25–30 % MR reduction using quantitative measurements in the chronic phase), reverse left ventricular remodeling and reduction of the mitral annulus diameter.

PTMA device. Twenty-seven patients (mean age 70 years, 56 % male) from four European and one Canadian centers in NYHA class II/III with grade 2 to 4/4 FMR and LVEF between 20 and 50 % were enrolled between 2006 and 2007. Patients with stent implanted in the proximal circumflex artery or with severe renal insufficiency were excluded. Mean ejection fraction was 36 ± 10 % and FMR was due to ischemic cardiomyopathy in 56 % of patients. In 8 patients, the diagnostic PTMA could not be tested due to unsuccessful venous access ($N=6$), anatomical exclusion ($N=1$) or guidewire perforation ($N=1$). In 6 additional patients, no MR reduction was observed leading to a 48 % procedural success rate (13/27 patients had a successful diagnostic PTMA procedure). Acute MR effect, analyzed in these 13 patients, showed a one-grade reduction overall. The PTMA implant was finally placed in only nine patients (the device was unstable in two patients and could not be delivered in two additional patients) and subsequently removed in four patients during follow-up due to device migration or inefficiency. Only one arterial impingement was observed in the all cohort.

4.1 Theoretical Efficacy Concerns

In addition to safety issues as regard to coronary artery compressions and myocardial infarctions above mentioned, there are several limitations to the coronary sinus annuloplasty common to all these devices.

Anatomy of the venous system. Despite being not really a safety issue, anatomy of the coronary sinus – great cardiac vein is highly variable both in term of diameter and length. Accurate measurements can be performed during the procedure and venous angiography but computed tomography has clearly shown its incremental value as a screening pre-procedural test (Fig. 11.11).

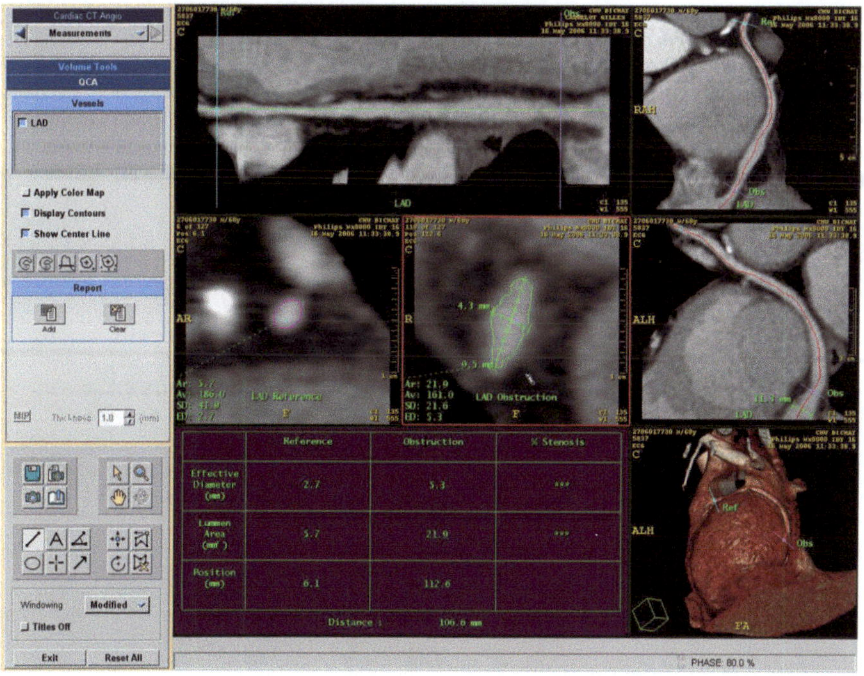

Fig. 11.11 Computed tomography allows precise measurement of the length and diameters of the coronary sinus

Relationship between the coronary sinus and the mitral annulus. The distance between the coronary sinus and the mitral valve annulus was measured in 61 excised cadaveric human hearts [39]. Mean distance was 9.7 ± 3.2 mm and up to 19 mm in some patients. The main finding of this anatomic study was to demonstrate that the coronary sinus lied behind the left atrial wall and not behind the mitral valve annulus (Fig. 11.12). The relationship between the coronary sinus and the mitral valve annulus can also be assessed using CT [42]. In 105 consecutive patients referred for computed tomography coronary angiography, the distance between the coronary sinus and the mitral valve annulus was evaluated at three different levels and the minimal distance was 5.1 ± 2.9 mm. The coronary sinus was located along the left atrial wall, rather than along the mitral valve annulus in the majority of the patients (Fig. 11.13). Even more importantly, the distance between the coronary sinus and the mitral valve annulus was significantly greater in patients with than in patients without severe mitral regurgitation. Thus, the effect of percutaneous mitral annuloplasty devices, if it does exist, may probably be directly related to a shrinking of the left atrial wall and an indirect effect of the mitral valve annulus as well as to a direct mitral annulus shrinking. Nevertheless, in the CARILLON study, the distance between the coronary sinus and mitral annulus plane was not different in responder and nonresponder patients [44].

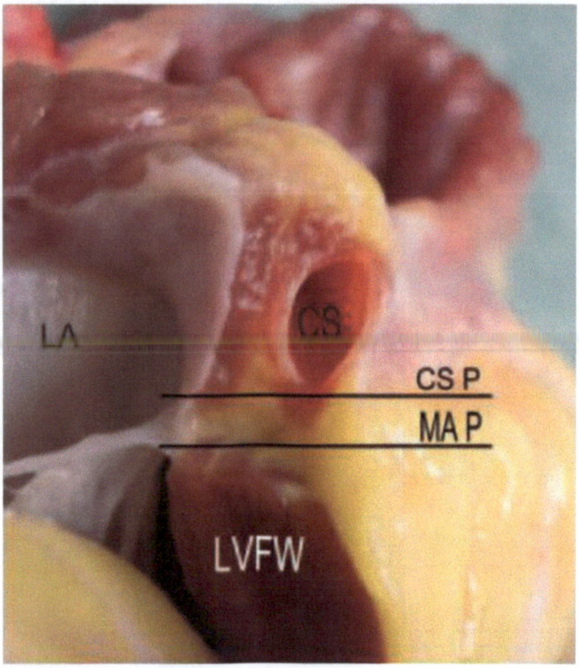

Fig. 11.12 Autopsy study showing that the coronary sinus is not at the level of the mitral annulus but above, behind the left atrial wall. From [40]

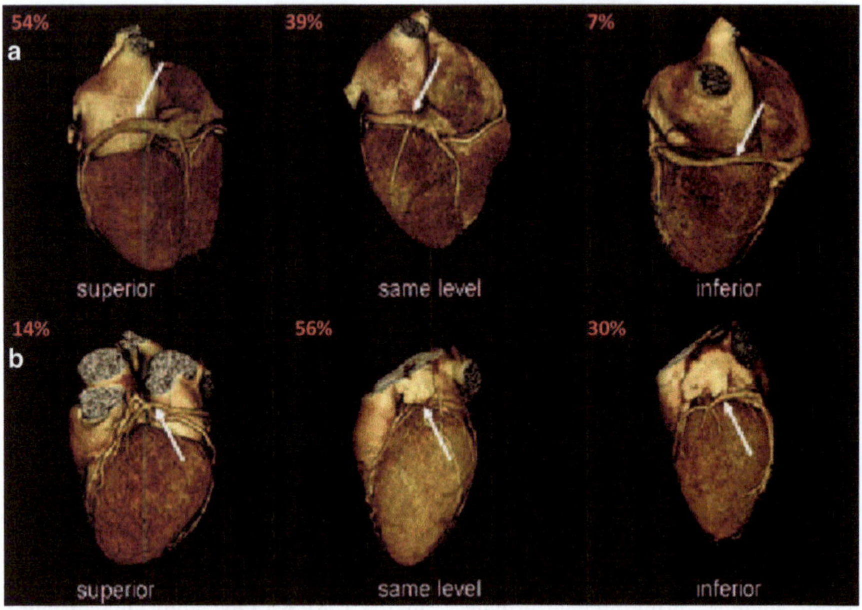

Fig. 11.13 Volume-rendered three-dimensional reconstructions allow a precise evaluation of the position of the coronary sinus (*white arrow*) in relation to the mitral valve annulus. From [42]

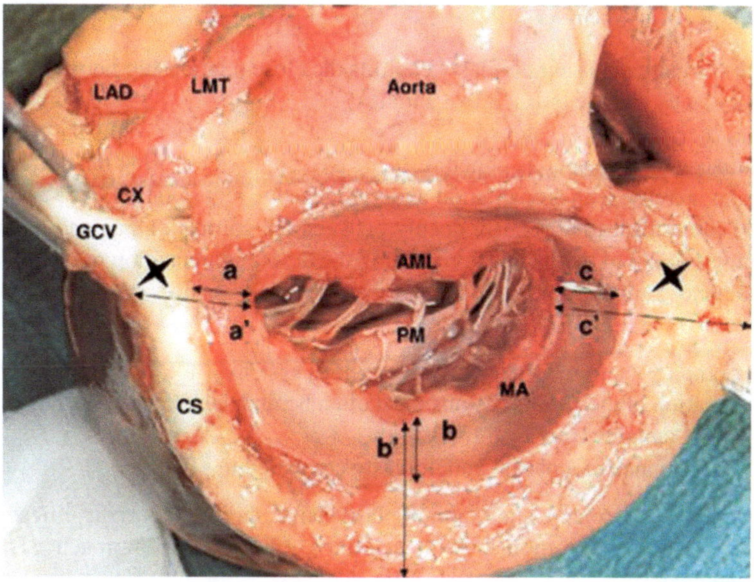

Fig. 11.14 Posterior view from the left atrium in human cadaver (from [45] showing that percutaneous mitral annuloplasty performed via the coronary sinus can only achieve a partial annuloplasty). The *black stars* represent the anchoring points of a percutaneous device (junction between the great coronary vein and coronary sinus; ostium of the coronary sinus)

A partial annuloplasty. The coronary sinus only encircles about two-thirds of the mitral annulus. Our group has compared the degree of annuloplasty that could be achieved using percutaneous devices compared to surgical annuloplasty in ten human cadaver hearts [45]. This study clearly demonstrated that the projection of coronary sinus annuloplasty achieves at best a commissure-to-commissure annuloplasty behind each trigone (Fig. 11.14). Thus, percutaneous annuloplasty via the coronary sinus which mainly modified the posterior annulus with a partial annuloplasty is trying to emulate a procedure already abandoned in the operating room.

Percutaneous annuloplasty and resynchronization therapy. Cardiac resynchronization has been proven to be effective in patients with heart failure reducing both morbidity and mortality as well as the degree of [46–48]. Patients with previous CRT were excluded in trials with all three devices and, on the other side, implantation of devices into the coronary sinus may preclude its use in pacing for resynchronization therapy even it was performed in several patients.

In regard to the risk of coronary compression in 2/3 of patients, the modest despite significant MR reduction rate observed in these studies (but in the absence of control groups), the multiple theoretical efficacy concerns above mentioned, percutaneous mitral annuloplasty using the indirect annuloplasty via the coronary sinus does not seem the most appropriate approach. Two of the three devices have been abandoned and the future of the last one is uncertain.

Key Points

- The coronary sinus annuloplasty exploits the close relationship between the coronary sinus and the mitral valve annulus.
- The three devices developed are inserted into the coronary sinus and the great cardiac vein via a venous puncture. They are supposed to shrink the mitral annulus, to increase leaflet coaptation and to reduce the regurgitation.
- The circumflex artery course deeply between the coronary sinus and the mitral annulus in 2/3 of the patients precluding the device implantation or exposing the patient to compression of the coronary artery compression.
- Several theoretical concerns have been raised
  - Complex anatomy of the coronary venous system.
  - Location of the coronary sinus most often behind the left atrial wall than at the mitral annulus level.
  - Performance of a partial annuloplasty compared to surgery.
- Overall, the coronary sinus annuloplasty have shown important efficacy and safety issues and combined with a limited efficacy, this approach is almost abandoned.

5 Other Percutaneous Techniques: Future Perspectives

Other percutaneous techniques for FMR can be divided into five different categories. The list of devices cited here is not exhaustive and is rapidly evolving.

5.1 Coronary Sinus Annuloplasty

The "cerclage annuloplasty" has not been tried in human [49]. A wire is placed into the coronary sinus than traverse a short segment of the interventricular septum to re-enter the right heart where it is exchanged for a suture. Tension is applied to cinch the mitral valve and secured with a locking device.

5.2 Direct Annuloplasty

Direct annuloplasty imitates surgical annuloplasty and overcomes several limitations of indirect annuloplasty via the coronary sinus but requires an arterial access and the procedure is much more technically challenging. This technology is in early development.

The Mitralign Percutaneous Annuloplasty System (Mitralign, Tewksbury, MA) mimics surgical suture annuloplasty and aims to plicate the dilated posterior mitral valve annulus in patients with FMR. The Mitralign system approaches the posterior

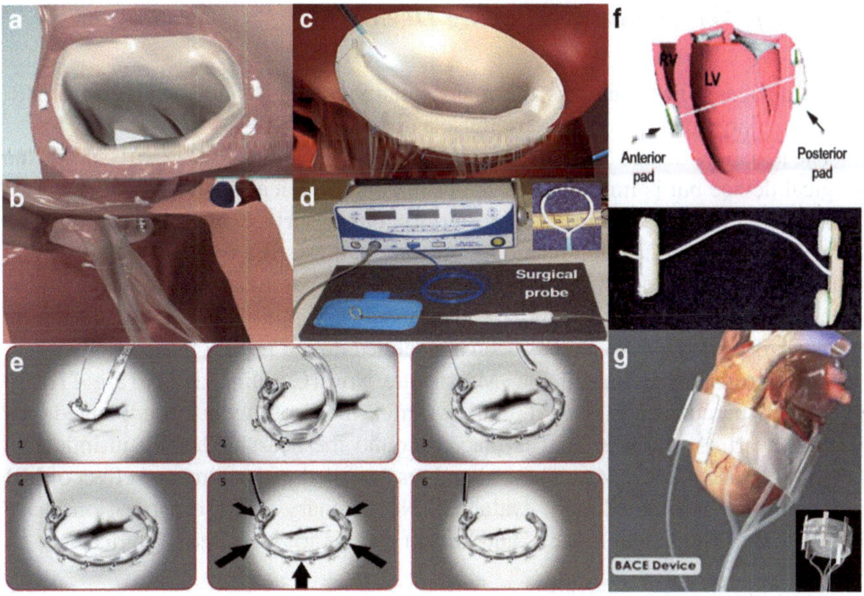

Fig. 11.15 Other percutaneous techniques. (**a, b**) Mitralign Percutaneous Annuloplasty System (Mitralign, Tewksbury, MA), (**c**) AccuCinch device (Guided Delivery Systems, SantaClara, CA), (**d**) QuantumCor Endovascular Device (QuantumCor, San Clemente, CA), (**e**) CardioBand (Valtech, Or Yehuda, Israel), (**f**) iCoapsys device (Myocor, Inc., Maple Grove, Minn), (**g**) Mardil-BACE (Mardil, Inc., Morrisville, North Carolina)

mitral annulus via the left ventricle. A two-arm (bident) catheter places two pairs of connected pledgets through the mitral annulus at the P1 and P3 locations which are tethered and put into tension to decrease the annulus circumference, and the achieved mitral annulus plication is locked in place (Fig. 11.15a, b). This device has been already employed in humans.

The AccuCinch device (Guided Delivery Systems, SantaClara, CA) also performes a direct annuloplasty via a retrograde approach across the aortic valve. A small adjustable ring of anchors interlinked with a cable is implanted percutaneously into the left ventricular muscle below the mitral valve (Fig. 11.15c). First in man implantations have been performed.

The QuantumCor Endovascular Device (QuantumCor, San Clemente, CA) applies radiofrequency energy via an end-loop catheter placed around the mitral annulus into the left atrium via a transeptal puncture. The energy is designed to induce collagen shrinkage and annular reduction (Fig. 11.15d). The ReCor (ReCor, Paris, France) device delivers high-intensity focused ultrasound on the mitral annylus to induce tissue heating and collagen shrinkage. The development of this device is stopped.

The CardioBand (Valtech, Or Yehuda, Israel) performed a percutaneous transeptal mitral ring annuloplasty secured from trigone to trigone with miniature anchors (Fig. 11.15e). The system should be soon evaluated in human.

5.3 Left Ventricular Reshaping Devices

These devices aim to address the main pathophysiological mechanism of FMR, annular enlargement, and papillary muscle displacement.

The iCoapsys device (Myocor, Inc., Maple Grove, Minn) (Fig. 11.15f) mimic the surgical device but is implanted using a subxiphoid pericardial access sheath. Two fixation pads placed anteriorly and posteriorly on the surface of the left ventricle are connected through a cable. Tensioning the cable draws the two pads together and thus compresses the left ventricle. Feasibility of the percutaneous iCoapsys procedure has been demonstrated animal studies and recently initial human implants have been performed. This device has been abandoned due to insufficient resources.

The Mardil-BACE (Mardil, Inc., Morrisville, North Carolina) device (Fig. 11.15g) is not truly percutaneous since it requires a mini-thoracotomy but is implanted on a beating heart. A silicone band is placed around the heart with built-in inflatable chambers placed on the MA. These chambers are filled with saline and effect of MR reduction can be immediately evaluated. No coronary artery compressions have been observed in animal models, and human experience has already started.

5.4 Percutaneous Neochordae

A strong effort is placed on the development of percutaneous implantation of neochordae.

5.5 Mitral Valve Replacement

Several devices are currently developed to perform direct percutaneous mitral valve replacement (The Endovalve-Herrmann prosthesis (Endovalve, Inc., Princeton, New Jersey), CardiAQ (CardiAQ Valve Technologies, Inc., Winchester, Massachusetts)…). These systems are still at the experimental level but human implantations are soon expected.

5.6 Mitral Annuloplasty Ring

Companies are also currently working on rings similar to those used during surgical mitral repair that could be implanted surgically and adjusted percutaneously or fully percutaneously (Adjustable Annuloplasty Ring (MitralSolutions, Fort Lauderdale, Florida), Dynamic annuloplasty Ring System (MiCardia, Inc., Irving, California)…).

The list above presented in not exhaustive and list of devices tested or evaluated is rapidly evolving and growing. In the setting of FMR, it is crucial to respond to two independent questions. The first step would be to demonstrate that the devices reduce the degree of MR not only acutely but also on the mid-long term. The second step would be to demonstrate that the treatment of FMR improve the outcome of patients with FMR which is the final aim of all these treatment. To date, the answers to these questions are only partial and demonstration that FMR is a cause and not a marker of increased morbidity and mortality has to be made. Future studies using medical devices should be randomized against optimal medical therapy including CTR and ideally against surgical annuloplasty. Only the answers to these two questions would improve the care we deliver to our patients. It is likely that the combination of devices with different target reproducing that can be made during surgery will be needed. No doubt that these combined strategies will even more complicate the demonstration of their usefulness but are essential. An additional major issue would be to define the optimal population target that would benefit from percutaneous device therapy. Surgical series have identified potential predictors of MR improvement based on LV or mitral valve apparatus measurements. It is possible that some patients are seen to late in the course of the disease and will not benefit from any therapy. Appropriate identification of the subgroups of patients with FMR who may potentially benefit from percutaneous therapy is crucial. We are living a rapidly moving and very exciting time but we should keep in mind that our final aim is to improve the care of our patients. This would not be possible without careful research programs involving not only engineers and interventional cardiologists but also surgeons, imaging specialists, and clinical cardiologist.

6 Conclusion

The field of percutaneous mitral repair is evolving rapidly but percutaneous approaches to MR remain largely investigational. Percutaneous edge-to-edge has been shown to be not inferior to surgery in the EVEREST trial but mainly enrolled patients with organic MR. Whether, it improves survival in patients with FMR still needs to be demonstrated and a randomized trial (MitraClip vs. medical therapy) should start this year. Indirect annuloplasty via the coronary sinus has shown both important efficacy and safety issues and does not seem a good approach. Anatomy of the mitral valve apparatus and pathophysiology of FMR (from a mechanical point of view) is much more complex than aortic stenosis and as for conventional surgery, a combination of more than one transcatheter technique or procedure will most likely be needed to achieve satisfactory results. A randomized trial should compare the efficacy of these devices vs optimal medical therapy with or without CRT and ideally vs surgical annuloplasty.

7 Sources of Further Information

The references are, to the best of our knowledge, up to date at the time of the redaction of the current chapter but publications are rapidly increasing and the readers should be encouraged to keep updated. In addition, we try to provide descriptions and illustrations of the current devices as clear and precise as we could but nice cartoons are available on the websites of most companies.

References

1. Grigioni F, Enriquez-Sarano M, Zehr K, Bailey K, Tajik A (2001) Ischemic mitral regurgitation: long-term outcome and prognostic implications with quantitative Doppler assessment. Circulation 103:1759–1764
2. Lancellotti P, Troisfontaines P, Toussaint AC, Pierard LA (2003) Prognostic importance of exercise-induced changes in mitral regurgitation in patients with chronic ischemic left ventricular dysfunction. Circulation 108(14):1713–1717
3. Yiu S, Enriquez-Sarano M, Tribouilloy C, Seward J, Tajik A (2000) Determinants of the degree of functional mitral regurgitation in patients with systolic left ventricular dysfunction: a quantitative clinical study. Circulation 102:1400–1406
4. Braun J, van de Veire NR, Klautz RJ, Versteegh MI, Holman ER, Westenberg JJ et al (2008) Restrictive mitral annuloplasty cures ischemic mitral regurgitation and heart failure. Ann Thorac Surg 85(2):430–436; discussion 436–7
5. Mihaljevic T, Lam BK, Rajeswaran J, Takagaki M, Lauer MS, Gillinov AM et al (2007) Impact of mitral valve annuloplasty combined with revascularization in patients with functional ischemic mitral regurgitation. J Am Coll Cardiol 49(22):2191–2201
6. Wu AH, Aaronson KD, Bolling SF, Pagani FD, Welch K, Koelling TM (2005) Impact of mitral valve annuloplasty on mortality risk in patients with mitral regurgitation and left ventricular systolic dysfunction. J Am Coll Cardiol 45(3):381–387
7. Vahanian A, Baumgartner H, Bax J, Butchart E, Dion R, Filippatos G et al (2007) Guidelines on the management of valvular heart disease: the Task Force on the Management of Valvular Heart Disease of the European Society of Cardiology. Eur Heart J 28(2):230–268
8. Nishimura RA, Carabello BA, Faxon DP, Freed MD, Lytle BW, O'Gara PT et al (2008) ACC/AHA 2008 guideline update on valvular heart disease: focused update on infective endocarditis: a report of the American College of Cardiology/American Heart Association Task Force on Practice Guidelines: endorsed by the Society of Cardiovascular Anesthesiologists, Society for Cardiovascular Angiography and Interventions, and Society of Thoracic Surgeons. Circulation 118(8):887–896
9. Magne J, Pibarot P, Dagenais F, Hachicha Z, Dumesnil JG, Senechal M (2007) Preoperative posterior leaflet angle accurately predicts outcome after restrictive mitral valve annuloplasty for ischemic mitral regurgitation. Circulation 115(6):782–791
10. Maisano F, Schreuder JJ, Oppizzi M, Fiorani B, Fino C, Alfieri O (2000) The double-orifice technique as a standardized approach to treat mitral regurgitation due to severe myxomatous disease: surgical technique. Eur J Cardiothorac Surg 17(3):201–205
11. Maisano F, Torracca L, Oppizzi M, Stefano PL, D'Addario G, La Canna G et al (1998) The edge-to-edge technique: a simplified method to correct mitral insufficiency. Eur J Cardiothorac Surg 13(3):240–245; discussion 245–6
12. Brinster DR, Unic D, D'Ambra MN, Nathan N, Cohn LH (2006) Midterm results of the edge-to-edge technique for complex mitral valve repair. Ann Thorac Surg 81(5):1612–1617
13. De Bonis M, Lapenna E, La Canna G, Ficarra E, Pagliaro M, Torracca L et al (2005) Mitral valve repair for functional mitral regurgitation in end-stage dilated cardiomyopathy: role of the "edge-to-edge" technique. Circulation 112(9 Suppl):I402–I408
14. De Bonis M, Lorusso R, Lapenna E, Kassem S, De Cicco G, Torracca L et al (2006) Similar long-term results of mitral valve repair for anterior compared with posterior leaflet prolapse. J Thorac Cardiovasc Surg 131(2):364–370
15. Maisano F, Redaelli A, Pennati G, Fumero R, Torracca L, Alfieri O (1999) The hemodynamic effects of double-orifice valve repair for mitral regurgitation: a 3D computational model. Eur J Cardiothorac Surg 15(4):419–425
16. Hori H, Fukunaga S, Arinaga K, Yoshikawa K, Tayama E, Aoyagi S (2008) Edge-to-edge repair for mitral regurgitation: a clinical and exercise echocardiographic study. J Heart Valve Dis 17(5):476–484

17. Feldman T, Kar S, Rinaldi M, Fail P, Hermiller J, Smalling R et al (2009) Percutaneous mitral repair with the MitraClip system: safety and midterm durability in the initial EVEREST (Endovascular Valve Edge-to-Edge REpair Study) cohort. J Am Coll Cardiol 54(8):686–694
18. Ladich E, Michaels MB, Jones RM, McDermott E, Coleman L, Komtebedde J et al (2011) Pathological healing response of explanted MitraClip devices. Circulation 123(13): 1418–1427
19. Maisano F, Vigano G, Blasio A, Colombo A, Calabrese C, Alfieri O (2006) Surgical isolated edge-to-edge mitral valve repair without annuloplasty: clinical proof of the principle for an endovascular approach. EuroIntervention 2(2):181–186
20. Webb JG, Maisano F, Vahanian A, Munt B, Naqvi TZ, Bonan R et al (2009) Percutaneous suture edge-to-edge repair of the mitral valve. EuroIntervention 5(1):86–89
21. Silvestry FE, Rodriguez LL, Herrmann HC, Rohatgi S, Weiss SJ, Stewart WJ et al (2007) Echocardiographic guidance and assessment of percutaneous repair for mitral regurgitation with the Evalve MitraClip: lessons learned from EVEREST I. J Am Soc Echocardiogr 20(10):1131–1140
22. Feldman T, Wasserman HS, Herrmann HC, Gray W, Block PC, Whitlow P et al (2005) Percutaneous mitral valve repair using the edge-to-edge technique: six-month results of the EVEREST Phase I Clinical Trial. J Am Coll Cardiol 46(11):2134–2140
23. Siegel RJ, Biner S, Rafique AM, Rinaldi M, Lim S, Fail P et al (2011) The acute hemodynamic effects of MitraClip therapy. J Am Coll Cardiol 57(16):1658–1665
24. Feldman T, Foster E, Glower DD, Kar S, Rinaldi MJ, Fail PS et al (2011) Percutaneous repair or surgery for mitral regurgitation. N Engl J Med 364(15):1395–1406
25. Zoghbi WA, Enriquez-Sarano M, Foster E, Grayburn PA, Kraft CD, Levine RA et al (2003) Recommendations for evaluation of the severity of native valvular regurgitation with two-dimensional and Doppler echocardiography. J Am Soc Echocardiogr 16(7):777–802
26. Foster E, Wasserman HS, Gray W, Homma S, Di Tullio MR, Rodriguez L et al (2007) Quantitative assessment of severity of mitral regurgitation by serial echocardiography in a multicenter clinical trial of percutaneous mitral valve repair. Am J Cardiol 100(10): 1577–1583
27. Gaemperli O, Moccetti M, Surder D, Biaggi P, Hurlimann D, Kretschmar O et al (2012) Acute haemodynamic changes after percutaneous mitral valve repair: relation to mid-term outcomes. Heart 98(2):126–132
28. Argenziano M, Skipper E, Heimansohn D, Letsou GV, Woo YJ, Kron I et al (2010) Surgical revision after percutaneous mitral repair with the MitraClip device. Ann Thorac Surg 89(1):72–80; discussion p 80
29. Glower D, Ailawadi G, Argenziano M, Mack M, Trento A, Wang A et al (2012) EVEREST II randomized clinical trial: predictors of mitral valve replacement in de novo surgery or after the MitraClip procedure. J Thorac Cardiovasc Surg 143(4 Suppl):S60–S63
30. Whitlow PL, Feldman T, Pedersen WR, Lim DS, Kipperman R, Smalling R et al (2012) Acute and 12-month results with catheter-based mitral valve leaflet repair: the EVEREST II (Endovascular Valve Edge-to-Edge Repair) High Risk Study. J Am Coll Cardiol 59(2): 130–139
31. Franzen O, Baldus S, Rudolph V, Meyer S, Knap M, Koschyk D et al (2010) Acute outcomes of MitraClip therapy for mitral regurgitation in high-surgical-risk patients: emphasis on adverse valve morphology and severe left ventricular dysfunction. Eur Heart J 31(11): 1373–1381
32. Rudolph V, Knap M, Franzen O, Schluter M, de Vries T, Conradi L et al (2011) Echocardiographic and clinical outcomes of MitraClip therapy in patients not amenable to surgery. J Am Coll Cardiol 58(21):2190–2195
33. Pleger ST, Mereles D, Schulz-Schonhagen M, Krumsdorf U, Chorianopoulos E, Rottbauer W et al (2011) Acute safety and 30-day outcome after percutaneous edge-to-edge repair of mitral regurgitation in very high-risk patients. Am J Cardiol 108(10):1478–1482

34. Tamburino C, Ussia GP, Maisano F, Capodanno D, La Canna G, Scandura S et al (2010) Percutaneous mitral valve repair with the MitraClip system: acute results from a real world setting. Eur Heart J 31(11):1382–1389
35. Van den Branden BJ, Swaans MJ, Post MC, Rensing BJ, Eefting FD, Jaarsma W et al (2012) Percutaneous edge-to-edge mitral valve repair in high-surgical-risk patients: do we hit the target? JACC Cardiovasc Interv 5(1):105–111
36. Franzen O, van der Heyden J, Baldus S, Schluter M, Schillinger W, Butter C et al (2011) MitraClip(R) therapy in patients with end-stage systolic heart failure. Eur J Heart Fail 13(5):569–576
37. Auricchio A, Schillinger W, Meyer S, Maisano F, Hoffmann R, Ussia GP et al (2011) Correction of mitral regurgitation in nonresponders to cardiac resynchronization therapy by MitraClip improves symptoms and promotes reverse remodeling. J Am Coll Cardiol 58(21):2183–2189
38. Harnek J, Webb JG, Kuck KH, Tschope C, Vahanian A, Buller CE et al (2011) Transcatheter implantation of the MONARC coronary sinus device for mitral regurgitation: 1-year results from the EVOLUTION phase I study (Clinical Evaluation of the Edwards Lifesciences Percutaneous Mitral Annuloplasty System for the Treatment of Mitral Regurgitation). JACC Cardiovasc Interv 4(1):115–122
39. Maselli D, Guarracino F, Chiaramonti F, Mangia F, Borelli G, Minzioni G (2006) Percutaneous mitral annuloplasty: an anatomic study of human coronary sinus and its relation with mitral valve annulus and coronary arteries. Circulation 114(5):377–380
40. Choure AJ, Garcia MJ, Hesse B, Sevensma M, Maly G, Greenberg NL et al (2006) In vivo analysis of the anatomical relationship of coronary sinus to mitral annulus and left circumflex coronary artery using cardiac multidetector computed tomography: implications for percutaneous coronary sinus mitral annuloplasty. J Am Coll Cardiol 48(10):1938–1945
41. Mao S, Shinbane JS, Girsky MJ, Child J, Carson S, Oudiz RJ et al (2005) Coronary venous imaging with electron beam computed tomographic angiography: three-dimensional mapping and relationship with coronary arteries. Am Heart J 150(2):315–322
42. Tops LF, Van de Veire NR, Schuijf JD, de Roos A, van der Wall EE, Schalij MJ et al (2007) Noninvasive evaluation of coronary sinus anatomy and its relation to the mitral valve annulus: implications for percutaneous mitral annuloplasty. Circulation 115(11):1426–1432
43. Schofer J, Siminiak T, Haude M, Herrman JP, Vainer J, Wu JC et al (2009) Percutaneous mitral annuloplasty for functional mitral regurgitation: results of the CARILLON Mitral Annuloplasty Device European Union Study. Circulation 120(4):326–333
44. Siminiak T, Hoppe UC, Schofer J, Haude M, Herrman JP, Vainer J et al (2009) Effectiveness and safety of percutaneous coronary sinus-based mitral valve repair in patients with dilated cardiomyopathy (from the AMADEUS trial). Am J Cardiol 104(4):565–570
45. Lansac E, Di Centa I, Al Attar N, Messika-Zeitoun D, Raffoul R, Vahanian A et al (2008) Percutaneous mitral annuloplasty through the coronary sinus: an anatomic point of view. J Thorac Cardiovasc Surg 135(2):376–381
46. Breithardt OA, Sinha AM, Schwammenthal E, Bidaoui N, Markus KU, Franke A et al (2003) Acute effects of cardiac resynchronization therapy on functional mitral regurgitation in advanced systolic heart failure. J Am Coll Cardiol 41(5):765–770
47. van Bommel RJ, Marsan NA, Delgado V, Borleffs CJ, van Rijnsoever EP, Schalij MJ et al (2011) Cardiac resynchronization therapy as a therapeutic option in patients with moderate-severe functional mitral regurgitation and high operative risk. Circulation 124(8):912–919
48. Ypenburg C, van Bommel RJ, Borleffs CJ, Bleeker GB, Boersma E, Schalij MJ et al (2009) Long-term prognosis after cardiac resynchronization therapy is related to the extent of left ventricular reverse remodeling at midterm follow-up. J Am Coll Cardiol 53(6):483–490
49. Kim JH, Kocaturk O, Ozturk C, Faranesh AZ, Sonmez M, Sampath S et al (2009) Mitral cerclage annuloplasty, a novel transcatheter treatment for secondary mitral valve regurgitation: initial results in swine. J Am Coll Cardiol 54(7):638–651
50. Maisano F, La Canna G, Colombo A, Alfieri O (2011) The evolution from surgery to percutaneous mitral valve interventions: the role of the edge-to-edge technique. J Am Coll Cardiol 58(21):2174–2182

Chapter 12
Tailored Approach to Functional Mitral Regurgitation

Martin Penicka and Frank Van Praet

Abstract Functional (ischemic or non-ischemic) mitral regurgitation (MR) is highly prevalent in patients with systolic heart failure and its presence is associated with worse long-term survival, independently of other baseline characteristics and degree of LV dysfunction. Patients with moderate to severe MR show a twofold increase in mortality and a fourfold increase in hospitalizations for worsening heart failure. This chapter reviews current causal therapeutic approaches to treat functional MR with focus on an individually tailored strategy.

Functional (ischemic or non-ischemic) mitral regurgitation (MR) is highly prevalent in patients with systolic heart failure and its presence is associated with worse long-term survival, independently of other baseline characteristics and degree of LV dysfunction [1–7]. Several studies have reported that 30 % of patients with chronic systolic heart failure had echocardiography evidence of moderate-to-severe (grades 3/4 and 4/4) MR [1, 2, 4–7]. The presence of significant MR is an independent predictor of survival regardless of etiology of the heart failure, degree of left ventricular (LV) dilation or ejection fraction [2–5, 7]. Patients with moderate-to-severe MR show a twofold increase in mortality and a fourfold increase in hospitalizations for worsening heart failure. Less severe MR (grades 2/4 and 2+/4, effective regurgitant orifice between 20 and 30 mm^2) has also been associated with reduced survival [5, 8]. This suggests that even moderate MR should receive attention and therapeutic consideration. It is surprising and disappointing that despite the ominous prognosis associated with MR in heart failure, there are almost no randomized trials described in the literature. The published evidence consists of single-center, observational,

M. Penicka, M.D., Ph.D. (✉)
Cardiovascular Centre, OLV Hospital, Aalst, Belgium
e-mail: martin.penicka@olvz-aalst.be

F. Van Praet, M.D.
Department of Cardiovascular and Thoracic Surgery, OLV Hospital, Aalst, Belgium

J. Bartunek and M. Vanderheyden (eds.), *Translational Approach to Heart Failure*, DOI 10.1007/978-1-4614-7345-9_12, © Springer Science+Business Media New York 2013

often retrospective, and at best, propensity matched studies. Therefore, therapeutic recommendations are based mostly on personal experience, expert consensus, or pathophysiologic insights into the mechanism of functional MR; hence, it is challenging to provide evidence-based therapeutic guidance. This chapter will focus on an individually tailored approach to therapeutic management of functional MR in chronic systolic heart failure.

1 Causal Therapy of Functional MR: Pathophysiology-Based Approach

The most important mechanism of functional MR is LV remodeling. LV dilatation with increased sphericity or more localized post-infarction remodeling leads to a displacement of papillary muscles. This causes stretching of the chordae which leads to redistribution and increase of tethering forces, resulting in incomplete leaflet coaptation and MR [7]. Mitral annulus-related factors and closing forces play a lesser role (Fig. 12.1). Figure 12.2 shows the typical echocardiography appearance of a mitral valve in functional MR, which is characterized by restricted systolic leaflet motion (Carpentier type IIIb) and tenting of the anterior leaflet.

Functional MR is a complication of systolic heart failure resulting from LV remodeling. Onset of MR induces a vicious circle; MR leads to LV volume overload, which then leads to LV remodeling, which in turn leads to MR. Chronic volume overload is associated with structural and functional alterations of cardiomyocytes and the extracellular matrix [9]. Within a time frame of months to years, these changes progress to an irreversible stage characterized by loss of cardiomyocytes and "replacement" fibrosis. This suggests that causal therapy for

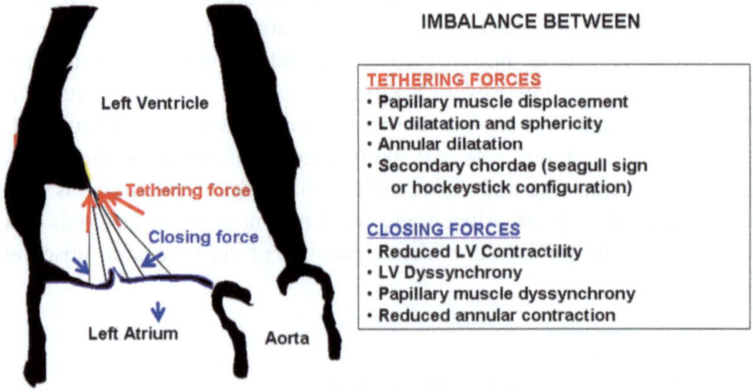

Fig. 12.1 Interplay between tethering and closing forces. Functional MR (Carpentier type IIIb) is a valvular dysfunction secondary to myocardial disease. An imbalance between closing and tethering forces is the underlying mechanism of the disorder

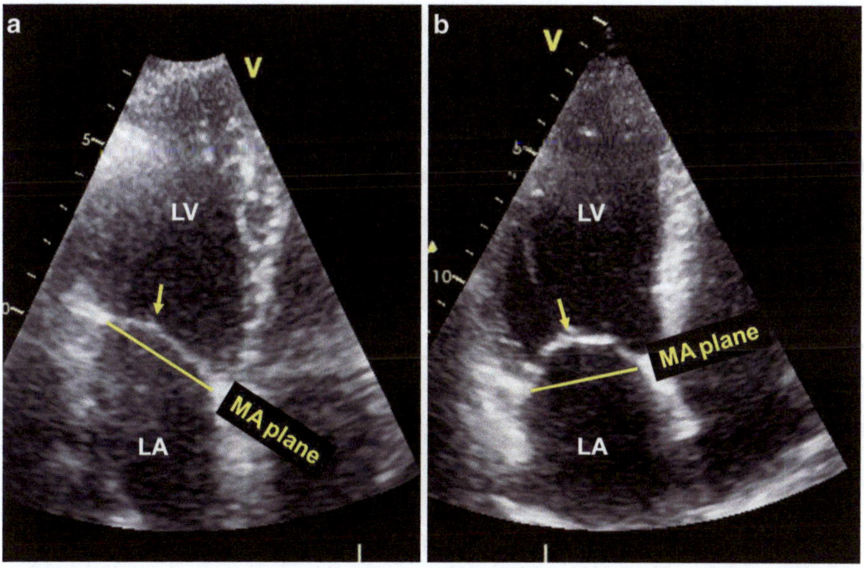

Fig. 12.2 An example of a typical echocardiography appearance of a normal mitral valve (**a**) and distorted mitral valve geometry leading to functional MR (**b**). In healthy individuals with a normal left ventricle (**a**), mitral valve leaflets are "flat" with the coaptation point (*arrow*) almost at the level of the mitral annulus (MA) plane. In contrast, in a dilated LV with functional MR (**b**), the leaflets are pulled toward the LV apex due to the stretching of chordae, which results in tenting of the anterior leaflet and restrictive systolic motion of the posterior leaflet with the coaptation point (*arrow*) displaced apically and posterolaterally. *LA* left atrium, *LV* left ventricle, *MA* mitral annulus

functional MR should be targeted toward reverse LV remodeling; additionally, the treatment should be delivered promptly, before progression to an irreversible stage. Reverse LV remodeling is associated not only with decreased MR but also with a reduction of heart failure hospitalizations and improved survival. Figure 12.3 shows an overview of therapeutic interventions associated with reverse LV remodeling in systolic heart failure.

2 Pharmacological Therapy

The first step is to optimize heart failure medication including beta blockers, ACE inhibitors or ATR blockers, and aldosterone blockers; the importance of this step should not be underestimated.

Unless contraindicated, every patient with systolic LV dysfunction, regardless of the presence of MR, should receive the maximal tolerated dosage of these drugs with a target resting heart rate of 60 bpm, a systolic blood pressure of 110 mmHg and a NT-proBNP less than 1,000 pg/mL. Optimal heart failure therapy has been shown to improve prognosis and reduce heart failure hospitalizations. Moreover, in

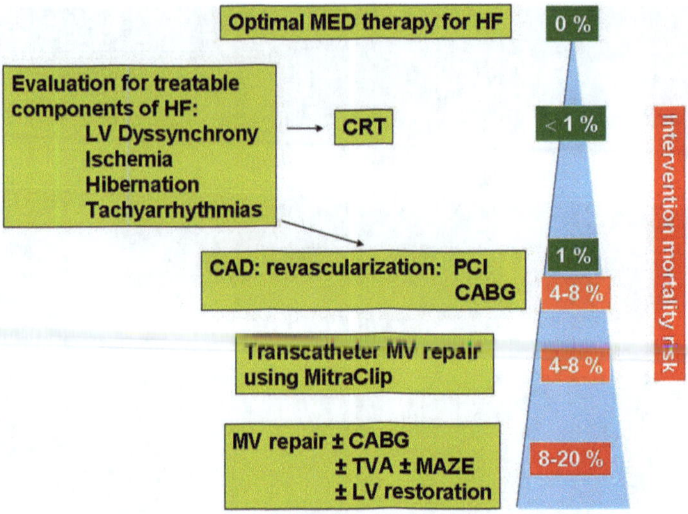

Fig. 12.3 An overview of therapeutic interventions associated with reverse LV remodeling in systolic heart failure. The *left* side of the panel shows treatable components of systolic heart failure, which should be promptly identified and treated. The *right* side of the panel shows acute mortality risk associated with each therapeutic intervention

Table 12.1 Assessment of therapeutic effects on systolic heart failure

	Therapy success	Therapy failure
Mortality	Alive	Dead
HF hospitalization	–	+
NYHA functional class	I–II	>II
NT-proBNP, pg/mL	<1,000	≥1,000
LV filling pressures	Normal or slightly ↑	> Mild elevation
Reverse LV remodeling	+	–
Functional MR	Rest: ERO < 20 (≤2/4)	Rest: ERO ≥ 20 (>2/4)
ERO, mm^2 (grade)	Exercise: ERO increase < 13 (≤2+/4)	Exercise: ERO increase ≥ 13 (>2+/4)

EFO effective regurgitant orifice, ↑ elevated

selected patients, significant reverse LV remodeling has been demonstrated with MR reductions of 1–2 echocardiography grades, on average [10–15]. It is noteworthy, that on an individual basis, the prediction of response to pharmacological therapy is challenging and many patients continue to have moderate or severe MR even after optimization of medication [15, 16]. Favorable effects can be expected mostly in patients with of the large extent of myocardial viability, without extensive LV remodeling, and in the absence of significant dyssynchrony [17–19]. The response to therapy should be evaluated after 3 months. Table 12.1 shows clinical and echocardiography characteristics of favorable responses, as well as therapy failure. Those who respond to therapy should be ambulatory, in NYHA class I or II, without signs of fluid retention, have low NT-proBNP and normal biventricular filling pressures (impaired relaxation transmitral flow pattern, normal systolic pulmonary artery pressure and preserved respiratory variation of inferior vena cava diameter). Furthermore, echocardiography needs to demonstrate both reverse LV remodeling (reduction in LV diameters, volumes, and increased ejection fraction) and decreased MR down to the level of mild to moderate. It should be noted that stabilization of LV remodeling alone, without actual improvement, should not be viewed as successful therapy. Reduction of MR needs to be seen both at rest and during appropriate exercise levels, which reflect the daily routines of individual patients. Decreased MR at rest, with a huge increase during low-level exercise, should be regarded as treatment failure. In nonresponders, other suitable therapeutic options should be considered, even at the expense of increased intervention-related risks.

3 Cardiac Resynchronization Therapy

In advanced systolic heart failure, LV dyssynchrony is very prevalent and its onset is associated with functional deterioration and a poor prognosis [20–22]. LV dyssynchrony globally, but specifically between papillary muscles, has been shown to be a very important contributory mechanism of functional MR [23–25]. Correction of LV dyssynchrony, by cardiac resynchronization therapy (CRT), has been associated with improved survival paralleled by reverse LV remodeling and reduction of MR [18, 25–28]. Several studies have demonstrated that reverse LV remodeling and resynchronization of contraction of papillary muscles are the main mechanisms underlying improvement in MR following CRT [23–25, 27–29]. On average, a decrease in MR by 1–2 echocardiography degrees can be expected [30–32]. A significant reduction of MR, at rest, has been observed immediately after CRT, and is attributed to resynchronization of the left ventricle and papillary muscles, with an acute recruitment of LV contractility and thus, an increase in closing forces acting on the mitral valve [25, 28, 29, 33]. In our study, despite a significant decrease in MR at rest, CRT failed to attenuate immediate exercise-induced MR [28]. During a 3 month follow-up, CRT was shown to lead to significant reverse LV remodeling paralleled by a further reduction in MR at rest, as well as by a significant attenuation of exercise-induced MR (Fig. 12.4). Hence, the late, exercise-induced, reduction of MR and its dynamic component is strongly related to reverse LV remodeling [28, 31]. It is worth noting that the amount of MR decrease correlates with the extent of reverse remodeling and an improved prognosis during mid-term follow-up [33]. In contrast, persistent moderate (or greater) MR several months after CRT has been shown to be predictive of poor outcomes [33]. So it seems that an acute decrease in MR leads to reverse LV remodeling, which in turn leads to late decreases in MR. Furthermore, patients likely to experience beneficial effects are those individuals with significant myocardial viability and dyssynchrony [18, 24, 28, 34]. Effects of CRT should be evaluated within 3 months. In nonresponders (Table 12.1), the optimization of pharmacological therapy and CRT (AV and VV delay) can be attempted with a

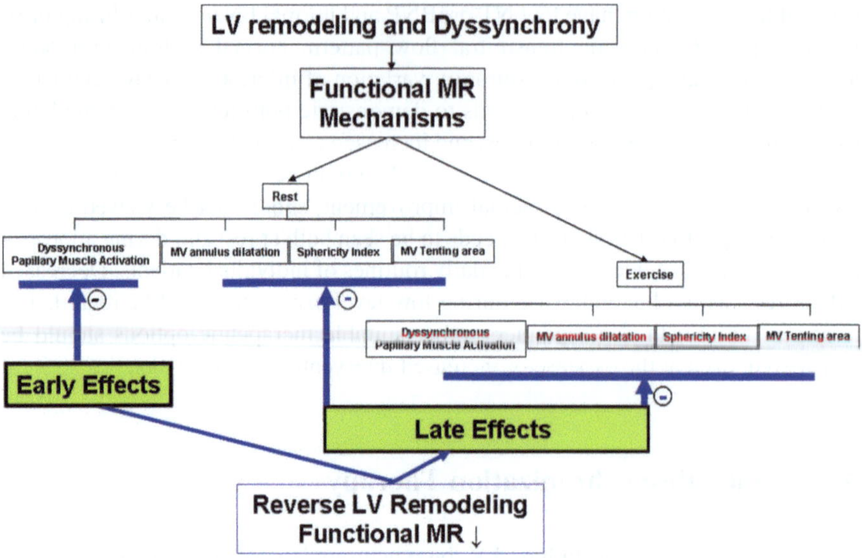

Fig. 12.4 The potential mechanisms responsible for reduction of MR after CRT. Dyssynchronous activation of the papillary muscles and a more spherical ventricle with mitral valve leaflets tethering and tenting, all contribute to MR. In the acute phase post-CRT implantation, MR is reduced thanks to resynchronization whereas in the chronic phase, not only resynchronization but also reverse LV remodeling contributes to the improvement in MR

complete reassessment after another 3 months. Alternatively, there should be a timely consideration of other suitable therapeutic methods, such as mitral valve repair.

4 Transcatheter Mitral Valve Repair Using MitraClip

Outcome of pharmacological therapy with or without CRT often remains unsatisfactory with many nonresponders. Functional MR has been shown to persist in 20–25 % of CRT patients and, in an additional 10–15 % may actually get worse after CRT [32]. Therefore, other therapeutic modalities need to be considered. Transcatheter implantation of a MitraClip device (Abbot, USA) has recently emerged as a valuable, alternative, MR treatment (for a detailed description of these technique see chapter 11). Two recent studies have investigated MitraClip therapy in patients with severe systolic heart failure and significant functional MR (≥2/4) [35, 36]. MitraClip implantation was shown to be feasible and safe with a 30-day mortality between 4 and 6 % [35, 36]. During a follow-up of 6–12 months, the MitraClip was associated with a reduction of MR, an improvement of NYHA class and significant reverse LV remodeling [35, 36]. The average reduction of MR achieved by MitraClip was 2 echocardiography grades, which left the majority of patients with mild to moderate residual MR (grades 1+/4, 2/4). This confirms the lower efficiency of MitraClip to reduce MR compared to surgical mitral valve annuloplasty, where the residual 2/4 grade MR is considered to be an unacceptable result. Nevertheless, these studies suggest, that even moderate reduction of MR is sufficient to induce significant reverse LV remodeling, which in turn leads to reduction of MR with favorable clinical outcomes. Of note, in around 50 % of patients, implantation of two clips during the same procedure was necessary to achieve the desired effect on MR [35]. Taken together, the data from several studies suggest that the implantation of MitraClip could be safely performed in patients who (1) failed to response to pharmacological therapy and/or CRT, (2) have moderate-to-severe residual MR, (3) suitable mitral valve anatomy, and (4) a prohibitive surgical risk.

5 Myocardial Revascularization

Myocardial revascularization, in the form of percutaneous coronary intervention (PCI), does not improve the natural history of moderate-to-severe functional MR. This was demonstrated by Pastorius, who examined long-term outcomes in 711 patients who had undergone PCI [37]. On the other hand, surgical myocardial revascularization (CABG) seems to be more promising. In a recent large randomized trial (STICH) and many observational studies, CABG, when compared to pharmacological therapy, has been associated with reduced cardiovascular mortality and decreased hospitalizations for heart failure [38, 39]. The greatest benefit of CABG has been observed in patients with less extensive pre-CABG LV remodeling and a low-degree dyssynchrony [17, 18, 39–41]. It is worth noting that several studies have demonstrated a close association between regression of functional MR post-CABG and reverse LV remodeling, suggesting the critical role of myocardial viability [24, 42, 43]. We recently investigated preoperative predictors of unrepaired moderate (grades 2/4 and 2+/4) functional MR improvement in 121 patients with ischemic LV dysfunction (ejection fraction 35 ± 10 %) undergoing isolated CABG [24]. MR was assessed pre-CABG and at 12 months post-CABG. This study has demonstrated that greater myocardium viability and the absence of dyssynchrony between papillary muscles were the main independent predictors of long-term MR improvement after isolated CABG. Reduced MR was paralleled by reverse LV remodeling and associated with improved mitral valve geometry. This confirms that LV functional recovery of viable myocardium is necessary to reduce tethering forces, increase closing forces and subsequent restoration of mitral valve function. Of note, extensive LV dilation prior to CABG and persistent high-degree dyssynchrony post-CABG do not allow viable myocardium to recover contractile function and reverse LV remodeling fails to occur despite revascularization [17, 18].

Several authors have also observed that factors, other than global LV factors, play an important, independent, role in the development of functional MR. For example, local LV remodeling with apical and posterior displacement of papillary muscles has been shown to be a major determinant of the degree of MR, and is independent of global LV dilation [44–48]. In corroborating these findings, our study showed that the degree of viability and absence of dyssynchrony in the segments adjacent to papillary muscles are also very important factors associated with reduction of functional MR after CABG [24]. The likely explanation is local reverse LV remodeling that ameliorates displacement of papillary muscles and reduces the mitral valve tenting area, along with synchronous contraction of papillary muscles with increased closing forces. Other authors have shown that the extent of mitral valve deformation significantly contributes to the severity of functional MR [49–52]. In non-ischemic dilated cardiomyopathy, the mitral valve tenting area has been shown to be strongly correlated with the degree of MR, functional status, and plasma BNP [49]. Moreover, tenting area has been also independently associated with mortality and hospitalizations [49].

This suggests that pre-CABG assessment of LV dilation, segmental viability and dyssynchrony, and mitral valve geometry may provide guidance as to whether or not to perform concomitant mitral valve annuloplasty in patients with systolic heart failure undergoing CABG.

6 Mitral Valve Surgery Using Restrictive Mitral Valve Annuloplasty

Restrictive mitral valve annuloplasty (MVA) is an effective approach to reduce functional MR. However, there have been no randomized trials, to date, which compare survival benefits of MVA to pharmacological therapy or myocardial revascularization alone. Based on the observational studies, several conclusions can be drawn. Functional MR is highly prevalent in patients undergoing CABG and its presence is associated with worse long-term survival, which is independent of other baseline characteristics and degree of LV dysfunction [53–57]. While severe MR is not usually improved by revascularization alone [55–57], changes in cases of moderate MR, in response to revascularization, are highly variable [24]. Patients with unrepaired even moderate MR have greater early and long-term mortality than similar patients without MR [53, 58]. Likewise, many patients show progression of MR during follow-up, despite revascularization [24, 58]. Hence, one might presume that, in patients with moderate-to-severe functional MR, mitral valve repair combined with CABG would offer an improved prognosis. However, several recent studies have failed to demonstrate a long-term survival benefit of combined procedures compared to CABG alone [54, 55, 59–61]. Besides the use of an imperfect surgical strategy, the failure of MVA to improve survival could also be attributed to the high recurrence rate of MR despite initially successful repair and higher perioperative mortality of combined procedures compared to CABG alone [43, 55, 57, 59, 62–65]. Braun et al. reported restrictive MVA (downsizing of two ring sizes) outcomes in 100 patients with functional MR undergoing CABG [66]. At 4.3 years of follow-up, restrictive MVA was associated with symptomatic improvement, reverse LV remodeling, low MR recurrence (15 %) and mortality (18 %) rates [66]. It is noteworthy, that these favorable results were observed only in patients with preoperative less extensive LV remodeling (LV end-diastolic diameter ≤ 65 mm). Keeping with this line, De Bonis and Kang showed that MR recurrence, after repair, parallels the absence of reverse LV remodeling, and hence, the absence of myocardial viability [43, 67]. In 54 patients with severe MR and LV dysfunction undergoing CABG with MVA, the presence of myocardial viability (more than five segments) was associated with long-term survival benefits [68]. As previously shown, extensive LV dilation prior to CABG and persistent high-degree dyssynchrony post-CABG may hinder reverse LV remodeling and thus, the durability of MVA [17, 18]. This underscores the importance of myocardium-related factors such as viability, dyssynchrony, and remodeling as outcome predictors for MVA. Apart from global LV-related factors, patients with severely distorted mitral valve geometry pre-MVA are likely to experience recurrent MR after successful MVA with a negative impact on 3-year survival [52, 64].

Taken together, these studies suggest that a failing LV will benefit from relief of chronic volume overload imposed by severe MR. MVA can be performed safely with low perioperative mortality. Moreover, MVA is associated with long-term reverse LV remodeling and low MR recurrence rates. The critical issue is the selection of suitable candidates.

7 Tailored Approach to Functional MR

The selection, sequence, and amount of intervention should be tailored according to individual characteristics of the patient (Fig. 12.3). It is important to realize that the majority of patients with chronic systolic heart failure are high-risk elderly who commonly have other cardiac comorbidities and may present after having undergone repeated percutaneous or surgical myocardial revascularizations [69]. Hence, the logical approach is to begin with less risky procedures (optimizing pharmacological therapy plus selective CRT). If the primary treatment fails to meet the desired outcome, only then would it be time to move on to interventions associated with higher mortality risks (Fig. 12.3, right side). LV dyssynchrony is a deadly, but treatable, complication of systolic heart failure. Because of that, every suitable patient should undergo implantation of a CRT-D early in the disease course. Moreover, the presence of CRT often allows further up-titration of dosages of heart failure medication, which increases the chances of a favorable response. Optimizing pharmacological therapy, plus or minus CRT, is a safe initial strategy, which is also frequently effective and sufficient to improve LV remodeling, MR and the patient's prognosis. Responders are mostly patients with less advanced heart failure with little elapsed time from the first diagnosis, non-ischemic cardiomyopathy, less extensive LV remodeling, and significant myocardial viability. Response to therapy should be evaluated as early as 3 months (Table 12.1). In the absence of reverse LV remodeling and a reduction of MR, the therapy should be intensified or other therapeutic modalities should be considered, taking into account the severity of the underlying heart failure and perioperative risk (Fig. 12.3).

Table 12.2 When is it too late to perform mitral valve repair

Myocardium-related factors
HF duration ≥5 year or LVEDd > 65–70 mm for ischemic CMP
≥8 year for or LVEDd > 75–80 mm for non-ischemic CMP
Nonviable myocardium
Fixed pulmonary hypertension and/or refractory RV failure
Peak VO_2 max < 14 mg/kg/min
Systolic blood pressure < 80 mmHg
Multiorgan failure
Serum sodium < 135 mmol/L
Creatinine > 2.5 mg/dL
Elevated serum bilirubin
Cachexia

CMP cardiomyopathy, *LVEDd* left ventricular end-diastolic diameter, *RV* right ventricular

Patients with advanced "terminal" heart failure are usually beyond the horizon for mitral valve repair. These are patients with a severely dilated nonviable left ventricle, severe refractory pulmonary hypertension and right-sided heart failure, very low peak oxygen consumption (with or without signs of multiorgan failure) (Table 12.2). Such patients would more likely benefit from the implantation of an assist-device or heart transplantation, rather than from MVA.

In less advanced (stage C) heart failure, mitral valve repair should be considered. High-risk nonresponders to medication and/or CRT with severe MR and a prohibitive surgical risk can benefit from percutaneous mitral valve repair using MitraClip [35, 36]. Nonresponders with a lower perioperative risk can benefit from surgical MVA, which provides more effective and stable mitral valve repair than percutaneous approaches. If available, a minimally invasive access, without a sternotomy, is preferable.

It is worth noting that some patients should be immediately considered for an early aggressive approach including CABG and/or MVA. These are the patients with significant angina pectoris or myocardial ischemia, left main or proximal LAD disease, extensive hibernating myocardium or severe mitral valve tethering.

Once heart surgery has been scheduled, the next critical question is the selection of individuals who will benefit from isolated CABG, and thus will avoid the increased perioperative risk associated with concomitant MVA. Severe functional MR is not usually improved by revascularization alone and persistent MR, after isolated CABG, may hinder contractile LV function recovery and reverse LV remodeling [55–57]. Therefore, in cases of severe functional MR, the current expert consensus [70, 71] recommends concomitant restrictive MVA at the time of CABG. Table 12.3 shows the clinical and echocardiography pro and con characteristics for

Table 12.3 Key clinical and echocardiography points for decision making regarding surgical mitral valve repair in patients with systolic heart failure of ischemic and non-ischemic origin

	Ischemic cardiomyopathy		Non-ischemic cardiomyopathy	
	MV repair +	MV repair -	MV repair +	MV repair -
Functional MR	Severe (rest or exercise)	Stable moderate	Severe (rest or exercise)	Stable moderate
Perioperative mortality risk, %	<5	≥5	<5	≥5
CABG	+	–	Not applicable	Not applicable
LVEDd, mm	≤60 (♀), ≤65 (♂)	>60 (♀), >65 (♂)	≤70 (♀), ≤75 (♂)	>70 (♀), >75 (♂)
LVEDd (mm) and myocardial viability	EDd 61–65 (♀), 66–70 (♂) + Viable myocardium	EDd 61–65 (♀), 66–70 (♂) + Nonviable myocardium	EDd 71–75 (♀), 76–80 (♂) + Viable myocardium	EDd 71–75 (♀), 76–80 (♂) + Nonviable myocardium
Myocardial viability	≥5 segments EF ≥ 10 % at DSE	<5 segments EF < 10 % DSE	≥5 segments EF ≥ 10 % at DSE	<5 segments EF < 10 % DSE
LV ejection fraction, %	≥30	<30	Not applicable	Not applicable
Duration of HF, year	<5	≥5	<8	≥8

DSE dobutamine stress echocardiography, *HF* heart failure, *LVEDd* left ventricular end-diastolic diameter

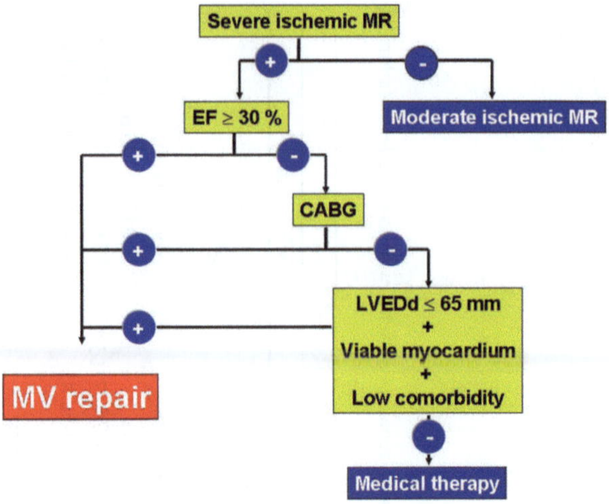

Fig. 12.5 Decision making regarding MVA in patients with severe functional MR in ischemic cardiomyopathy: the key characteristics associated with favorable clinical outcomes and durability of mitral valve repair

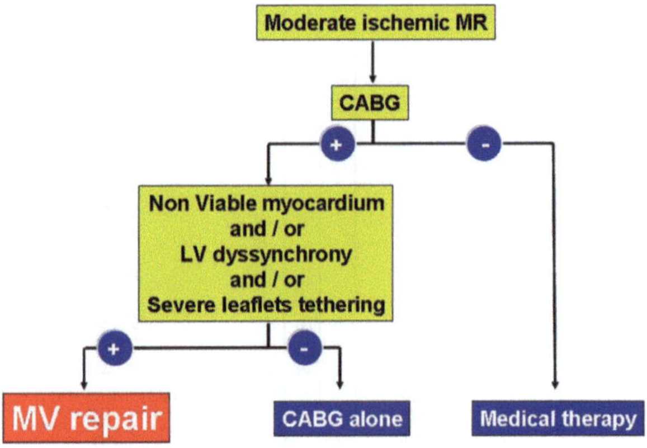

Fig. 12.6 Decision making regarding MVA in patients with moderate functional MR undergoing CABG

performing MVA in patients with ischemic and non-ischemic cardiomyopathy and functional MR. MVA should be considered in patients with severe MR undergoing concomitant CABG and with a low prevalence of comorbidities. Patients who will likely experience long-term benefit from MVA are those with a less dilated left ventricle, higher LV ejection fractions, and significant myocardial viability (Fig. 12.5). All patients with significant LV dyssynchrony undergoing CABG should receive CRT either before or soon after CABG. This recommendation is based on a recent study which showed that in the majority of patients, CABG alone is insufficient to eliminate pre-CABG dyssynchrony [18, 72]. Moreover, persistent post-CABG dyssynchrony hampers LV functional recovery and reduction of MR, which negatively impacts the prognosis [18, 72].

On the other hand, in patients with moderate functional MR undergoing CABG, the indication for concomitant mitral valve repair is highly controversial. Based on the findings of our and other studies, a practical approach for the management of patients with moderate MR undergoing CABG can be proposed (Fig. 12.6) [17, 18, 23–25, 42, 43, 45–52]. In patients with a potential for LV functional recovery (i.e., significant myocardial viability, which includes the papillary muscles, without significant LV remodeling and LV dyssynchrony) and without a high-degree of mitral valve tethering, we have observed that favorable changes in MR after isolated CABG appear to be fairly predictable, with a majority (93 %) of individuals showing MR improvement following revascularization alone. Reduction in MR is accompanied by alleviation of symptoms, reverse LV remodeling, and improved long-term outcomes. In all other combinations (i.e., absence of viable myocardium, presence of high-degree LV remodeling, LV dyssynchrony, or significant mitral valve deformation), which represents roughly 2/3 s of patients, changes in MR, after isolated CABG, are unpredictable, suggesting that concomitant MVA may be necessary [24, 42].

8 Conclusions

Functional MR is caused by disease of the left ventricle with secondary distortion of mitral valve geometry. There is also strong evidence that the severity of LV disease and not the degree of MR is the major determinant of survival. Hence, causal therapy to manage MR should primarily address the underlying mechanism leading to the disease of the left ventricle and induce reverse LV remodeling. Optimal heart failure therapy, CRT, myocardial revascularization, percutaneous mitral valve repair using MitraClip or surgical MVA are all associated with reverse LV remodeling and reduction of MR. Timing and selection of interventions should be tailored to individual characteristics. All treatable components of heart failure, such as LV dyssynchrony, ischemia, hibernation, or tachyarrhythmias, should be promptly identified and treated. In the majority of patients, onset of reverse LV remodeling will be accompanied by reduction of MR with diminishing LV volume overload, which in turn will lead to additional reverse LV remodeling with further long-term reduction of MR. Having said that, it is clear, that patients with the potential for reverse LV remodeling, i.e., those with the significant myocardial viability, will gain the greatest benefit from all of the above mentioned therapeutic modalities. The effects of each therapy should be continuously monitored and in the absence of a favorable response, other therapeutic options should be promptly considered and delivered before LV dysfunction progresses to an irreversible stage. On a similar note, authors of this chapter believe, that performing mitral valve repair early in the disease course, i.e., in patients with dynamic MR, can be more effective than waiting until development of late advanced disease, i.e., severe fixed MR. In conclusion, despite the lack of randomized studies, results of observational studies are promising and appear to suggest that, in selected patients, functional MR is a treatable complication of systolic heart failure provided that appropriate therapeutic interventions occur early in the disease course.

References

1. Allen LA, Felker GM (2008) Advances in the surgical treatment of heart failure. Curr Opin Cardiol 23(3):249–253
2. Koelling TM et al (2002) Prognostic significance of mitral regurgitation and tricuspid regurgitation in patients with left ventricular systolic dysfunction. Am Heart J 144(3):524–529
3. Mehra MR et al (2008) Surgery for severe mitral regurgitation and left ventricular failure: what do we really know? J Card Fail 14(2):145–150
4. Robbins JD et al (2003) Prevalence and severity of mitral regurgitation in chronic systolic heart failure. Am J Cardiol 91(3):360–362
5. Trichon BH et al (2003) Relation of frequency and severity of mitral regurgitation to survival among patients with left ventricular systolic dysfunction and heart failure. Am J Cardiol 91(5):538–543
6. Patel JB et al (2004) Mitral regurgitation in patients with advanced systolic heart failure. J Card Fail 10(4):285–291
7. Levine RA, Schwammenthal E (2005) Ischemic mitral regurgitation on the threshold of a solution: from paradoxes to unifying concepts. Circulation 112(5):745–758
8. Grigioni F et al (2001) Ischemic mitral regurgitation: long-term outcome and prognostic implications with quantitative Doppler assessment. Circulation 103(13):1759–1764
9. Gaasch WH, Meyer TE (2008) Left ventricular response to mitral regurgitation: implications for management. Circulation 118(22):2298–2303
10. Stevenson LW et al (1987) Effects of afterload reduction (diuretics and vasodilators) on left ventricular volume and mitral regurgitation in severe congestive heart failure secondary to ischemic or idiopathic dilated cardiomyopathy. Am J Cardiol 60(8):654–658
11. Hamilton MA et al (1991) Sustained reduction in valvular regurgitation and atrial volumes with tailored vasodilator therapy in advanced congestive heart failure secondary to dilated (ischemic or idiopathic) cardiomyopathy. Am J Cardiol 67(4):259–263
12. Kizilbash AM et al (1998) Effects of afterload reduction on vena contracta width in mitral regurgitation. J Am Coll Cardiol 32(2):427–431
13. Capomolla S et al (2000) Beta-blockade therapy in chronic heart failure: diastolic function and mitral regurgitation improvement by carvedilol. Am Heart J 139(4):596–608
14. Lowes BD et al (1999) Effects of carvedilol on left ventricular mass, chamber geometry, and mitral regurgitation in chronic heart failure. Am J Cardiol 83(8):1201–1205
15. Kotlyar E et al (2004) The impact of baseline left ventricular size and mitral regurgitation on reverse left ventricular remodelling in response to carvedilol: size doesn't matter. Heart 90(7):800–801
16. Woo GW et al (2005) Ventricular reverse remodeling and 6-month outcomes in patients receiving cardiac resynchronization therapy: analysis of the MIRACLE study. J Interv Card Electrophysiol 12(2):107–113
17. Bax JJ et al (2004) Extensive left ventricular remodeling does not allow viable myocardium to improve in left ventricular ejection fraction after revascularization and is associated with worse long-term prognosis. Circulation 110(11 Suppl 1):II18–II22
18. Penicka M et al (2007) Severe left ventricular dyssynchrony is associated with poor prognosis in patients with moderate systolic heart failure undergoing coronary artery bypass grafting. J Am Coll Cardiol 50(14):1315–1323
19. Cleland JG et al (2003) Myocardial viability as a determinant of the ejection fraction response to carvedilol in patients with heart failure (CHRISTMAS trial): randomised controlled trial. Lancet 362(9377):14–21
20. Bader H et al (2004) Intra-left ventricular electromechanical asynchrony. A new independent predictor of severe cardiac events in heart failure patients. J Am Coll Cardiol 43(2):248–256
21. Grines CL et al (1989) Functional abnormalities in isolated left bundle branch block. The effect of interventricular asynchrony. Circulation 79(4):845–853

22. Xiao HB, Brecker SJ, Gibson DG (1992) Effects of abnormal activation on the time course of the left ventricular pressure pulse in dilated cardiomyopathy. Br Heart J 68(4):403–407
23. Kanzaki H et al (2004) A mechanism for immediate reduction in mitral regurgitation after cardiac resynchronization therapy: insights from mechanical activation strain mapping. J Am Coll Cardiol 44(8):1619–1625
24. Penicka M et al (2009) Predictors of improvement of unrepaired moderate ischemic mitral regurgitation in patients undergoing elective isolated coronary artery bypass graft surgery. Circulation 120(15):1474–1481
25. Ypenburg C et al (2008) Mechanism of improvement in mitral regurgitation after cardiac resynchronization therapy. Eur Heart J 29(6):757–765
26. Cleland JG et al (2005) The effect of cardiac resynchronization on morbidity and mortality in heart failure. N Engl J Med 352(15):1539–1549
27. Ypenburg C et al (2007) Acute effects of initiation and withdrawal of cardiac resynchronization therapy on papillary muscle dyssynchrony and mitral regurgitation. J Am Coll Cardiol 50(21):2071–2077
28. Madaric J et al (2007) Early and late effects of cardiac resynchronization therapy on exercise-induced mitral regurgitation: relationship with left ventricular dyssynchrony, remodelling and cardiopulmonary performance. Eur Heart J 28(17):2134–2141
29. Breithardt OA et al (2003) Acute effects of cardiac resynchronization therapy on functional mitral regurgitation in advanced systolic heart failure. J Am Coll Cardiol 41(5):765–770
30. Sitges M et al (2009) Long-term effect of cardiac resynchronization therapy on functional mitral valve regurgitation. Am J Cardiol 104(3):383–388
31. St John Sutton MG et al (2003) Effect of cardiac resynchronization therapy on left ventricular size and function in chronic heart failure. Circulation 107(15):1985–1990
32. Ypenburg C et al (2009) Long-term prognosis after cardiac resynchronization therapy is related to the extent of left ventricular reverse remodeling at midterm follow-up. J Am Coll Cardiol 53(6):483–490
33. Verhaert D et al (2012) Impact of mitral regurgitation on reverse remodeling and outcome in patients undergoing cardiac resynchronization therapy. Circ Cardiovasc Imaging 5(1):21–26
34. Ypenburg C et al (2007) Impact of viability and scar tissue on response to cardiac resynchronization therapy in ischaemic heart failure patients. Eur Heart J 28(1):33–41
35. Auricchio A et al (2011) Correction of mitral regurgitation in nonresponders to cardiac resynchronization therapy by Mitraclip improves symptoms and promotes reverse remodeling. J Am Coll Cardiol 58(21):2183–2189
36. Franzen O et al (2011) MitraClip(R) therapy in patients with end-stage systolic heart failure. Eur J Heart Fail 13(5):569–576
37. Pastorius CA, Henry TD, Harris KM (2007) Long-term outcomes of patients with mitral regurgitation undergoing percutaneous coronary intervention. Am J Cardiol 100(8):1218–1223
38. Velazquez EJ et al (2011) Coronary-artery bypass surgery in patients with left ventricular dysfunction. N Engl J Med 364(17):1607–1616
39. Chareonthaitawee P et al (2005) Revascularization in severe left ventricular dysfunction: the role of viability testing. J Am Coll Cardiol 46(4):567–574
40. Bonow RO et al (2011) Myocardial viability and survival in ischemic left ventricular dysfunction. N Engl J Med 364(17):1617–1625
41. Allman KC et al (2002) Myocardial viability testing and impact of revascularization on prognosis in patients with coronary artery disease and left ventricular dysfunction: a meta-analysis. J Am Coll Cardiol 39(7):1151–1158
42. Campwala SZ et al (2005) Factors affecting regression of mitral regurgitation following isolated coronary artery bypass surgery. Eur J Cardiothorac Surg 28(1):104–108
43. Kang DH et al (2006) Mitral valve repair versus revascularization alone in the treatment of ischemic mitral regurgitation. Circulation 114(1 Suppl):I499–I503
44. Otsuji Y et al (2002) Isolated annular dilation does not usually cause important functional mitral regurgitation: comparison between patients with lone atrial fibrillation and those with idiopathic or ischemic cardiomyopathy. J Am Coll Cardiol 39(10):1651–1656

45. He S et al (1997) Integrated mechanism for functional mitral regurgitation: leaflet restriction versus coapting force: in vitro studies. Circulation 96(6):1826–1834
46. Kono T et al (1992) Left ventricular shape is the primary determinant of functional mitral regurgitation in heart failure. J Am Coll Cardiol 20(7):1594–1598
47. Yiu SF et al (2000) Determinants of the degree of functional mitral regurgitation in patients with systolic left ventricular dysfunction: a quantitative clinical study. Circulation 102(12):1400–1406
48. Komeda M et al (1997) Geometric determinants of ischemic mitral regurgitation. Circulation 96(9 Suppl):II128–II133
49. Karaca O et al (2011) Tenting area reflects disease severity and prognosis in patients with non-ischaemic dilated cardiomyopathy and functional mitral regurgitation. Eur J Heart Fail 13(3):284–291
50. Donal E et al (2009) Mitral regurgitation in dilated cardiomyopathy: value of both regional left ventricular contractility and dyssynchrony. Eur J Echocardiogr 10(1):133–138
51. Sadeghpour A et al (2008) Echocardiographic evaluation of mitral geometry in functional mitral regurgitation. J Cardiothorac Surg 3:54
52. Lee AP et al (2009) Mechanisms of recurrent functional mitral regurgitation after mitral valve repair in nonischemic dilated cardiomyopathy: importance of distal anterior leaflet tethering. Circulation 119(19):2606–2614
53. Schroder JN et al (2005) Impact of mitral valve regurgitation evaluated by intraoperative transesophageal echocardiography on long-term outcomes after coronary artery bypass grafting. Circulation 112(9 Suppl):I293–I298
54. Trichon BH et al (2003) Survival after coronary revascularization, with and without mitral valve surgery, in patients with ischemic mitral regurgitation. Circulation 108(Suppl 1): II103–II110
55. Gillinov AM et al (2001) Is repair preferable to replacement for ischemic mitral regurgitation? J Thorac Cardiovasc Surg 122(6):1125–1141
56. Aklog L et al (2001) Does coronary artery bypass grafting alone correct moderate ischemic mitral regurgitation? Circulation 104(12 Suppl 1):I68–I75
57. Kim YH et al (2005) Ischemic mitral regurgitation: revascularization alone versus revascularization and mitral valve repair. Ann Thorac Surg 79(6):1895–1901
58. Lam BK et al (2005) Importance of moderate ischemic mitral regurgitation. Ann Thorac Surg. 79(2):462–470; discussion 462–470
59. Mihaljevic T et al (2007) Impact of mitral valve annuloplasty combined with revascularization in patients with functional ischemic mitral regurgitation. J Am Coll Cardiol 49(22):2191–2201
60. Wu AH et al (2005) Impact of mitral valve annuloplasty on mortality risk in patients with mitral regurgitation and left ventricular systolic dysfunction. J Am Coll Cardiol 45(3):381–387
61. Ryden T et al (2001) The importance of grade 2 ischemic mitral regurgitation in coronary artery bypass grafting. Eur J Cardiothorac Surg 20(2):276–281
62. Kuwahara E et al (2006) Mechanism of recurrent/persistent ischemic/functional mitral regurgitation in the chronic phase after surgical annuloplasty: importance of augmented posterior leaflet tethering. Circulation 114(1 Suppl):I529–I534
63. Zhu F et al (2005) Mechanism of persistent ischemic mitral regurgitation after annuloplasty: importance of augmented posterior mitral leaflet tethering. Circulation 112(9 Suppl):I396–I401
64. Magne J et al (2007) Preoperative posterior leaflet angle accurately predicts outcome after restrictive mitral valve annuloplasty for ischemic mitral regurgitation. Circulation 115(6):782–791
65. McGee EC et al (2004) Recurrent mitral regurgitation after annuloplasty for functional ischemic mitral regurgitation. J Thorac Cardiovasc Surg 128(6):916–924
66. Braun J et al (2008) Restrictive mitral annuloplasty cures ischemic mitral regurgitation and heart failure. Ann Thorac Surg 85(2):430–446; discussion 436–447

67. De Bonis M et al (2008) Recurrence of mitral regurgitation parallels the absence of left ventricular reverse remodeling after mitral repair in advanced dilated cardiomyopathy. Ann Thorac Surg 85(3):932–939
68. Pu M et al (2003) Importance of ischemic and viable myocardium for patients with chronic ischemic mitral regurgitation and left ventricular dysfunction. Am J Cardiol 92(7):862–864
69. Nieminen MS et al (2006) EuroHeart Failure Survey II (EHFS II): a survey on hospitalized acute heart failure patients: description of population. Eur Heart J 27(22):2725–2736
70. Vahanian A et al (2007) Guidelines on the management of valvular heart disease: The Task Force on the Management of Valvular Heart Disease of the European Society of Cardiology. Eur Heart J 28(2):230–268
71. Bonow RO et al (2008) 2008 Focused update incorporated into the ACC/AHA 2006 guidelines for the management of patients with valvular heart disease: a report of the American College of Cardiology/American Heart Association Task Force on Practice Guidelines (Writing Committee to Revise the 1998 Guidelines for the Management of Patients With Valvular Heart Disease): endorsed by the Society of Cardiovascular Anesthesiologists, Society for Cardiovascular Angiography and Interventions, and Society of Thoracic Surgeons. Circulation 118(15):e523–e661
72. Pokushalov E et al (2011) Coronary artery bypass grafting with and without concomitant epicardial cardiac resynchronization therapy in patients with ischemic cardiomyopathy: a randomized study. Heart Surg Forum 13(3):E177–E184

Chapter 13
Revascularization and Left Ventricular Reconstruction in a Patient with Ischemic Heart Failure: to STICH or not to STICH?

Marisa Di Donato

Abstract The present chapter addresses the management of ischemic heart failure (HF) patients after the release of the Surgical Treatment for Ischemic Heart Failure (STICH) trial results. The STICH trial is a multicenter, international, randomized, non-blinded trial that started in 2002.

The trial presents several flaws and has been largely criticized, therefore the question "to STICH or not to STICH" that reminds us of Shakespeare, still remains clinically relevant and the management of ischemic HF still represents a challenge.

Enrollment criteria, patient's evaluation, patient selection, and imaging modalities are reviewed and discussed in the present chapter at the light of the results interpretation. One important issue, i.e., the "equipoise" of the investigator (equivalent risks and benefits) was introduced for ethical reasons but varying physician threshold for equipoise in the treatment assignment were permitted therefore, the characteristics of enrolled pts showed wide diversities in the 2,137 pts enrolled across the 127 participating, located in 27 countries, reflecting the experience of cardiologists and surgeons, the volume of operations in severely depressed cardiac function patients etc. This represents one major limitation/bias of the trial.

M. Di Donato, M.D. (✉)
Department Surgical and Medical Critical Care Medicine, University of Florence, Via dei Fossi 12, Florence 50123, Italy
e-mail: marad@tin.it

J. Bartunek and M. Vanderheyden (eds.), *Translational Approach to Heart Failure*, DOI 10.1007/978-1-4614-7345-9_13, © Springer Science+Business Media New York 2013

Coronary artery disease (CAD) is the most common substrate for heart failure in industrialized countries; it represents the underlying because of heart failure (HF) in nearly 65 % of patients [1]. The prevalence, incidence, rate of hospitalization for chronic HF have increased in the past 30 years and it is likely that it will continue to increase because of the increasing number of elderly patients in the general population and the improved survival of patients after acute myocardial infarction (MI). It has been demonstrated that HF patients with CAD have a much worse prognosis than patients with idiopathic cardiomyopathy after adjustment for baseline variables [2, 3]. These findings emphasize the importance of accurate differentiation between ischemic and non-ischemic causes of HF and the potential role of revascularization in patients with ischemic cardiomyopathy. Current working models for HF as the Cardio-renal model (Excessive salt and water retention), the hemodynamic model (pump failure and excessive vasoconstriction) and the neurohormonal model (over expression of biologically active molecules able of exerting unfavorable effects on the heart and circulation) may all be necessary but not sufficient to explain all causes of disease progression in the failing heart. The biomechanical model for HF described by Mann and coworkers helps to explain the progression of HF independently of the neurohormonal status of the patient [4]. In fact, current medical therapy, acting against neurohormonal activation tends to slow progression but fails to arrest the process of remodeling.

The biomechanical model focuses on LV size and geometry abnormalities as being responsible for progression of the disease. Geometric changes lead to structural abnormalities of the myocytes and of the myocardium, which worsen cardiac function and increase neurohormonal activation; this may make the cardiovascular system less responsive to normal homeostatic control mechanisms [5].

The management of patients with ischemic HF with or without angina is a challenge because of the lack of randomized controlled trials (RCTs) in this population; there are three important management alternatives in patients with CAD and HF: pharmacological treatment, electrophysiological devices (Cardiac Resynchronization Therapy, CRT), and revascularization strategies. CRT device implantation seems very promising, as confirmed by the recently released European Society of Cardiology (ESC) guidelines [6, 7]; medical treatment has improved however, the prognosis of pts affected by ischemic HF remains extremely poor [8]. Recognition of the importance of LV remodeling and the negative impact of akinetic or dyskinetic myocardium on LV size and performance has led to surgical intervention specifically targeting those factors, beyond coronary revascularization. But, despite the improvements in surgery technology and surgical skills that has widened the indications for cardiac surgery; a comprehensive strategy that includes surgery often is not used.

The detection of myocardial viability should be included in the diagnostic workup of HF patients with known CAD. Several prospective and retrospective studies and meta-analyses have consistently shown improved LV function and survival in patients with ischemic but viable myocardium, who subsequently underwent revascularization [9]. Conversely, patients without viability will not benefit from revascularization; moreover, patients with a severely dilated LV have a low likelihood of showing improvement in LVEF even in the presence of substantial viability [10].

Surgical ventricular reconstruction (SVR) represents the surgical approach aiming to restore (bring back to normal) the dilated, distorted LV cavity in order to improve function. It implies the knowledge and understanding of the remodeling infrastructure, the structural changes leading to geometry abnormalities, the role of compensatory, remote muscle and of stretching mechanisms leading to electrical disadvantages [11].

SVR is not a single procedure in that it includes coronary grafting and mitral repair if needed; its advantages in clinical status, cardiac function improvement and survival have been extensively evaluated and confirmed in several observational studies [12–17]. The possibility of combining myocardial revascularization with SVR to reverse LV remodeling has been addressed in a few RCTs.

The encouraging results obtained with SVR and its physiological appealing represent the rationale of the prospective randomized STICH trial designed to address many of the key concepts summarized above and aiming to validate the safety and efficacy of the procedure, in addition to coronary artery bypass grafting (CABG) and optimal medical therapy for HF and CAD.

The Surgical Treatment for Ischemic Heart Failure (STICH) trial is a multicenter, international, randomized, non-blinded, National Heart, Lung, and Blood Institute-funded trial performed in 127 clinical sites in 26 countries [18]. It is based on two specific primary hypotheses in patients with LV dysfunction who have CAD amenable to surgical revascularization: (1) Hypothesis one: CABG with optimal medical therapy improves long-term survival compared with medical therapy alone, and (2) Hypothesis two: in patients with anterior LV dysfunction, CABG and SVR to achieve more normal LV size and geometry, improves survival free of subsequent hospitalization compared to CABG alone. The eligibility criteria included LVEF ≤ 35 %, coronary anatomy suitable for revascularization, and willingness to consent to the entire study protocol, including SVR, if eligible.

Results for hypothesis one reported that there was no significant difference between medical therapy alone and medical therapy plus CABG with respect to the primary end point of death from any cause [19]. One can conclude that with the results of the STICH trial *hypothesis one*, we should be comfortable with the notion that, in general, surgery is not superior to optimal medical therapy for ischemic left ventricular dysfunction. However, secondary end points were in favor of CABG alone and the authors conclude that 5-year results of the study provide support for coronary bypass surgery on heart-failure patients with coronary disease, even though CABG did not beat medical therapy alone in the primary analysis of the trial.

Results for *hypothesis two* reported that adding SVR to coronary bypass was not associated with greater improvement in symptoms, exercise tolerance, or with a reduction in the rate of death or hospitalization for cardiac causes [18].

One can conclude that with the results of STICH trial hypothesis two, we should be comfortable that SVR added to CABG in ischemic dilated cardiomyopathy does not increase either the operative or the late mortality. However, the authors conclude that STICH shows that "widespread application of SVR to patients with ischemic cardiomyopathy is not warranted." To tell the truth one should reasonably conclude that both primary STICH trial hypotheses failed!

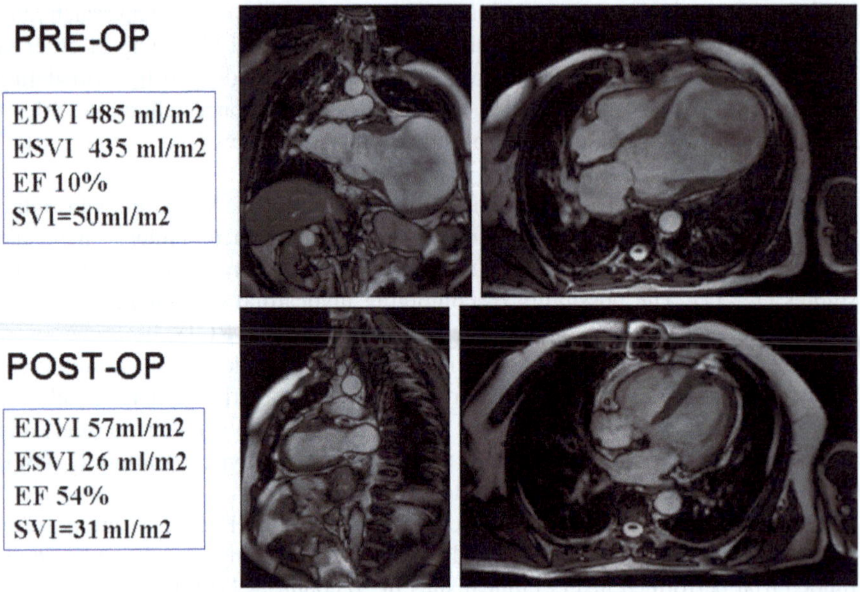

Fig. 13.1 Shows a CMR imaging study pre- and post-SVR operation in a patient with post-infarction extreme dilatation of the left ventricle and severe pump dysfunction. Two chamber view on the left and four chamber view on the right are shown. Notice the improvement in EF (from 10 to 50 %), the dramatic reduction of ESV (from 435 to 26 mL/m^2) and the almost normalized ventricular shape in 4CH view

There has been a great expectation from the STICH trial on the part of the cardiology and cardiac surgery community because of the clinical need to clarify what is the best therapy for pts with ischemic cardiomyopathy, reduced pump function, and signs of heart failure.

The two objectives to be conclusively clarified by the STICH trial were: (1) the role of revascularization in CAD and HF and (2) the efficacy and safety of ventricular reconstruction associated to CABG compared to CABG alone in patients with ischemic dilated cardiomyopathy.

Owing to the fact that both STICH trial hypothesis failed, cardiologists and surgeons still remain with their uncertainties.

And the patient? An interesting editorial by Kieser [20] argued that, if on the basis of the STICH results, we negate ventricular reconstruction to a pts with post-infarction extreme LV dilatation and poor LV pump function, aware that CABG alone is enough to cure him, we would give him/her the wrong treatment. Figure 13.1 shows an example of such patient pre- and postoperatively.

In this chapter we will try to explain why the results of the STICH trial hypothesis two have been that far from expectations of cardiologists and surgeons with long experience of the disease and of the surgical treatment.

Enrollment criteria, patient selection, and imaging modalities are reviewed and discussed in the present chapter at the light of STICH results interpretation.

1 Patient Enrollment

The STICH original protocol required that pts were eligible for the trial if they had EF < 35 % and symptoms of HF as detected by NYHA functional class ≥2. During the trial the need of HF symptoms was retracted so that the only criterion for eligibility remained EF ≤ 35 %.

Moreover, eligibility for STICH required that all patients will be further evaluated for appropriateness of SVR. This includes evidence of absent viability in the anterior wall, LVESVI ≥60 mL/m^2, and asynergy ≥35 % of the anterior wall (either akinetic or dyskinetic). Figure 13.2 shows the inclusion criteria as for the protocol (left) and the criteria adopted after liberalization (right). Less than 50 % of the enrolled patients had symptoms of advanced HF whilst more than 50 % had angina in advanced Canadian class; 13 % did not have had myocardial infarction; the extent and severity of the scar was unknown; ESVI was less than 60 mL/m^2 in more than one third of the enrolled population.

Key Point

- Many changes in the protocol have been requested and accepted during enrollment period therefore, the STICH population is mostly affected by ischemia rather than by heart failure and this can explain the success of CABG alone in reducing LV size and improving wall motion (hibernated myocardium).

2 Ventricular Geometry

LV anterior myocardial infarction may leave a spectrum of LV size and shape abnormalities (Fig. 13.3) depending on infarct size, collateral circulation, cellular matrix abnormalities, and other cellular and metabolic factors [21, 22]. Figure 13.3 shows

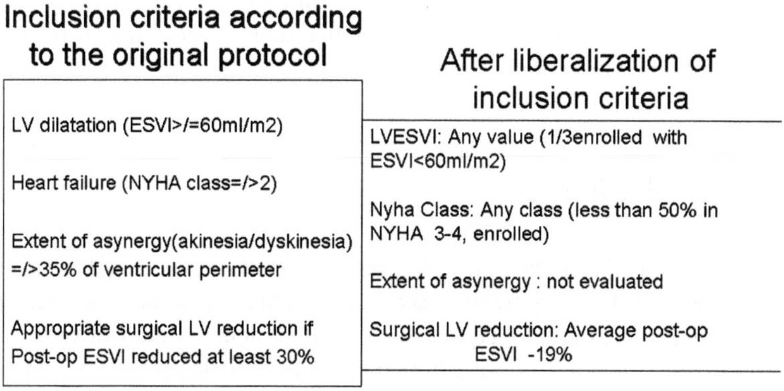

Fig. 13.2 Shows the inclusion criteria as in the original protocol and the criteria after liberalization, as patients were actually included

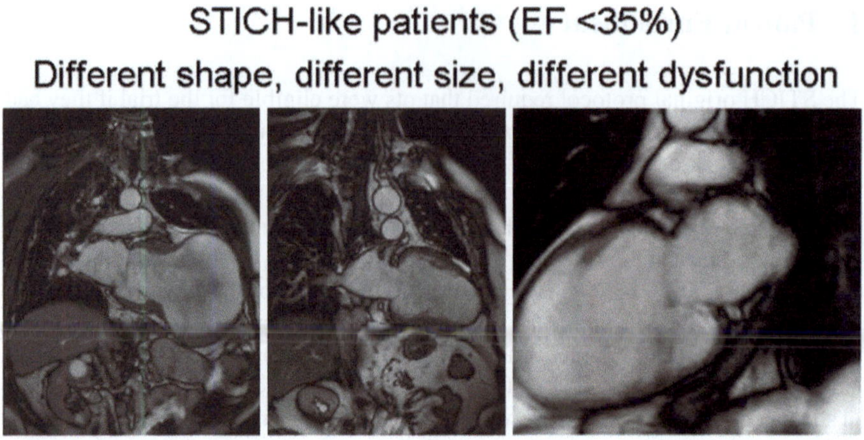

EDVI (ml/m2)	485	132	228
ESVI (ml/m2)	435	95	204
EF (ml/2)	10	29	11
SVI(ml/m2)	50	37	24

Fig. 13.3 Shows three patients with previous anterior myocardial infarction (MI), to emphasize the spectrum of size and shape abnormalities following MI. The three patients have an EF below 35 %, but their ventricular size and shape are very different and different could be the results obtained with SVR. Unfortunately, we do not know whom of these patients have been enrolled in the STICH trial

examples of three pts with previous anterior MI, all with a reduction in EF below 35 %; their ventricular size and shape abnormalities make these pts very diverse one from the other and also different can be the surgical approach; we do not know and probably, we will never know, whom of these patients has been enrolled in the trial.

Key Point

- Patient selection limited to the baseline EF, in addition measured by transthoracic Echo, makes the enrolled population extremely diverse and even more difficult the interpretation of the trial results.

3 Patient Selection

During enrollment, the Stich trial relied heavily on the clinical judgment of the physician to ensure that the potential risks and benefits to patients were equivalent. Varying physician threshold for equipoise in the treatment assignment were permitted, therefore the characteristics of enrolled pts showed wide diversities in the 2,137 pts enrolled across the 127 participating sited in 27 countries. Figure 13.4 shows changes in ESVI in pts randomized in the trial to receive SVR [18] compared with a nonrandomized series of STICH like pts with EF $\leq$ 35 % operated by SVR in a

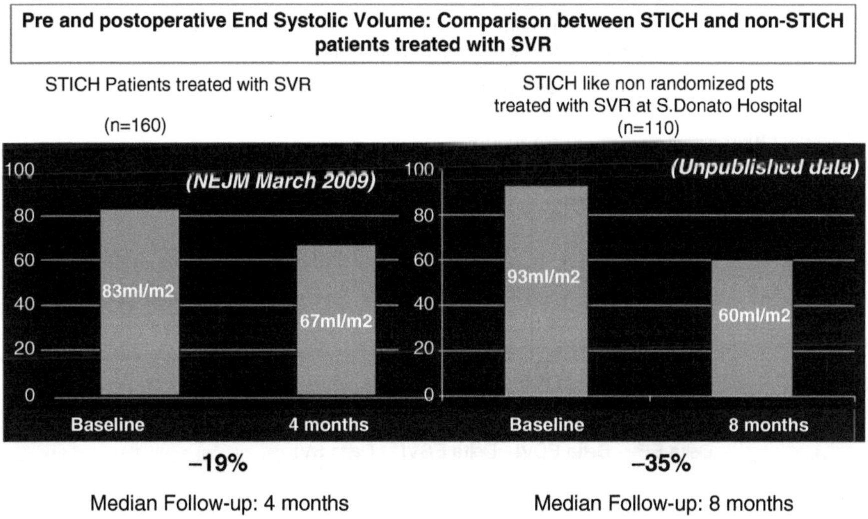

Fig. 13.4 Shows end systolic volume changes following SVR. *Left*: 160 patients enrolled in the STICH trial and randomized to receive SVR. *Right*: a series of 110 pts not enrolled in the trial and treated with SVR at San Donato Hospital, Italy. ESVI reduction at 8 months is almost double than that achieved at 4 months in the STICH population

single Italian Hospital, participating in the trial. The results are significantly different because, in our opinion, patients are different. As reported by Shroyer in his recent editorial [23] the variations in STICH patient selection would have been examined by comparing enrolled patients with screened and not enrolled pts, directly; unfortunately, a registry with randomized and screened-nonrandomized pts is not available for STICH and this is a serious limitation.

At San Donato Hospital during the STICH enrollment period (2001–2008) STICH eligible but not enrolled patients have been compared with eligible and enrolled patients, treated with ventricular reconstruction (unpublished data). There were 142 STICH like pts with baseline EF $\leq$35 %; 27 were randomized in STICH hypothesis 2 (since they were eligible for SVR); 12 were randomized to receive SVR and 115 were screened, nonrandomized and operated by SVR.

Figure 13.5 shows hemodynamic changes at 8 months follow-up in randomized (black bars) and nonrandomized patients (Open bars). The differences are highly significant and show that in nonrandomized pts the reduction in EDVI and ESVI and the improvement in EF are greater and very similar to the average reported series either from our or other Centers [13, 15, 24, 25], Fig. 13.6.

It appears evident that the study physician enrolled and randomized only the pts for whom he/she was not sure between risks and benefits and excluded the majority of pts for whom he/she was sure to give them a clear benefit with SVR.

Key Point

- Baseline LV geometry and function impact the decision and the surgical outcome of SVR

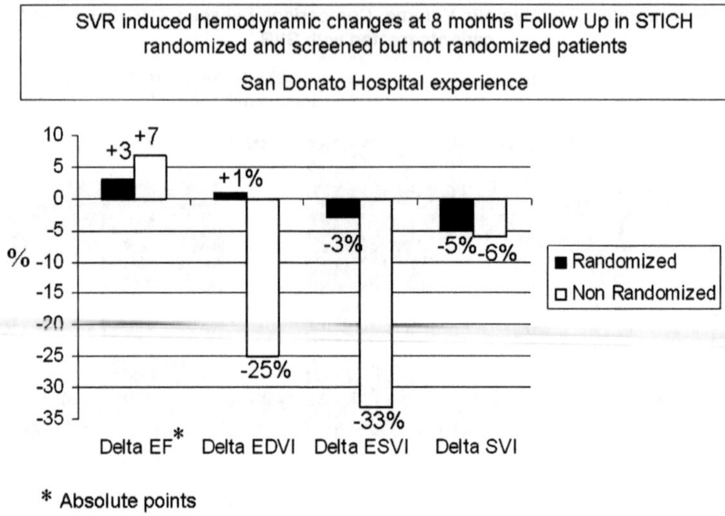

Fig. 13.5 Shows the comparison between patients screened and randomized to receive SVR and patients screened but not randomized patients who received SVR at San Donato Hospital, Italy, during the enrollment period. The improvement in hemodynamics is much greater in screened and nonandomized patients (*white bars*). This is the evidence that investigators randomized only the pts for whom they were not sure between risks and benefits (Equipose in the treatment assignment!)

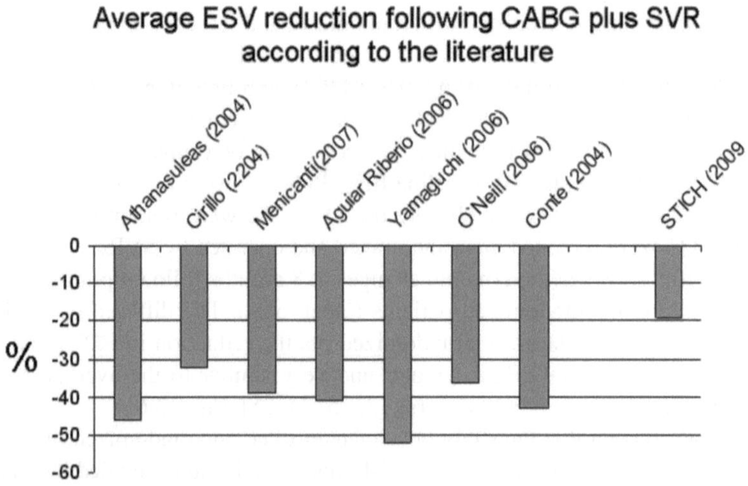

Fig. 13.6 Shows the average ESVI reduction following SVR, as reported in the literature. The STICH ESVI reduction is by far the smallest. This result may reflect the bias selection as described in Fig. 13.5

4 LV Reconstruction (Surgical Modalities)

In the original protocol there is no definition or description of the technique of SVR. The only reference is the following: "certification of surgeon for performing SVR required evidence of consistent postoperative decrease in LV volume in five consecutive surviving patients." An ESVI reduction of at least 30 % was considered a goal of a correct LV reconstruction; however, the results showed that this goal was not achieved since the average reduction of ESVI in the STICH trial is 19 % that is much smaller than the values reported in the literature by most of the surgeons [13, 15, 24, 25]. The improvement in ejection fraction was also very small (from 21 to 27 % in CABG plus SVR and from 21 to 25 % in CABG alone) and more importantly the postoperative ESVI was still too large in both arms, well beyond the threshold of mortality risk which is 60 mL/m^2. Both groups in fact remain at identical risk and show the same mortality rate and the same rate of hospitalization (the two primary end points of the STICH trial hypothesis two).

These STICH results are similar to those of classical resection of an apical aneurysm followed by linear suturing, overlapping, or plicature, as described by Cooley and associates in 1958 [26] but the results obtained with SVR both in terms of pump function improvement and volume reduction were expected to be much better. Therefore, an important question arise: was the surgical technique inadequate or was the patient selection wrong in the STICH trial?

In our opinion both technical inadequacy and wrong selection of patients play a role.

In a recent paper [27] Dor strongly argued that surgical treatment of ischemic failing ventricles needs an extensive diagnostic work up because "it is impossible to cure a patient if we do not know the pathophysiology of the disease" (i.e., the cause of the disease that according to Dor is the myocardial scar triggering the remodeling process). In the STICH population such extensive work up was not requested and we do not have any information on the presence, the extent and the transmurality of the post-infarction scar. By the way, the STICH population not even has myocardial infarction in a consistent percentage of cases!

Dor describes a quite large series of patients with extremely severe ischemic failing ventricles operated of LV reconstruction at the Cardiothoracic Center of Monaco who had been excluded from the trial because they met the exclusion criteria [18, 27].

A large area of ischemic but viable myocardium requires CABG, as opposed to a large irreversibly scarred wall, which requires ventricular surgery and Dor objected that revascularization can be beneficial in scarred myocardium, especially when it involves 40 % or more of the perimeter of the failing ventricle: this is what left ventricular reconstruction is intended to treat.

Figure 13.7 shows a patient operated at San Donato Hospital, Italy who had preoperative Magnetic Resonance with Gadolinium late enhancement (GLE) to assess the extent and the transmurality of the scar. The figure shows a very large and transmural scar in this patient and, in agreement with Dor, we object that revascularization can improve the contractility of such antero-septal scarred wall.

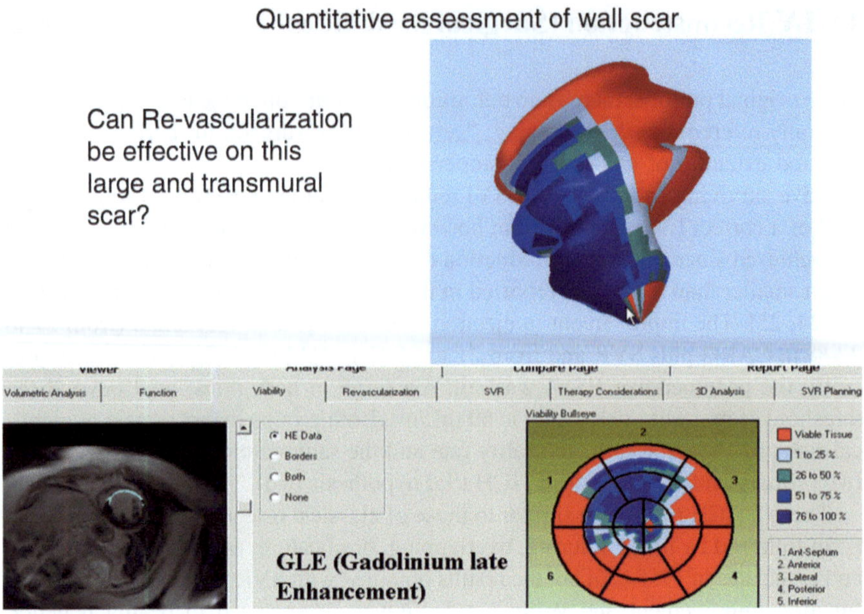

Fig. 13.7 An example of CMR study with dedicated cardiac function software analysis (Chase Medical, Richardson, Texas). The scar is seen as *dark blue* in the antero-septal region in 3D image (*right*) and in bulls eyes presentation (*bottom, right*). *Bottom left*: the gadolinium late enhancement (*white*) in short axis view is shown. See text for discussion

Key Point

- Technical surgical modalities have not been well defined in the STICH protocol nor were the patients' characteristics and the pump function abnormalities.

5 Volume Reduction and Residual LV Cavity Shape

5.1 Open Problems: Is the Resual LV Size or LV Shape the Key of Success of SVR in Post-infarction Patients?

The volume of the LV cavity to be left after the SVR procedure is not well defined, yet. Surgeons are afraid to leave too a small cavity for the acute effect of low cardiac output and for the late diastolic restrictive dysfunction that may occur as Burkhoff and Wechsler predicted on the basis of mathematical, experimental observations [28].

Dor introduced in 1998 the use of a balloon sizer just with the purpose of leaving an adequate diastolic chamber and Menicanti refined the sizing technique using a sizing and shaper device to give a more elliptical shape to the residual ventricle [29]. In the STICH trial surgeons were free to use sizing devices but judging from the large residual volumes of the Stich pts there is no way that the residual cavity was too small.

The importance of the LV residual shape is not well defined, as well. We must recognize that there is a misleading circulating message difficult to overcome, i.e., that SVR transforms a soccer-ball shape into a basket-ball shape; in other words that SVR changes the ventricle from spherical to elliptical [11]. Unfortunately, this has never been demonstrated; rather, if we quantitate sphericity index either as axis or volume ratio we obtain an increase in sphericity post-SVR, since the procedure shortens the long axis more than the short axis. More importantly, in dilated ischemic cardiomyopathy, as opposite to non-ischemic dilated cardiomyopathy, baseline sphericity index is not increased, being the elongation of the ventricle the first geometric change following anterior MI [30]. The apical shape deformation is instead frequently observed after anterior MI and its reconstruction with the elliptical device is an important goal since gives a more conical shape to the new apex [30]. We believe that the conical shape of the new apex, although apex cannot always recuperate its torsion, can improve the direction of intracavitary flow towards the outflow tract, thus improving cardiac performance. However, this issue is still debated and further studies are needed to clarify whether volume or shape of the post-SVR LV cavity play the major role to give benefit to the patient.

Conversely, the residual end systolic volume has been demonstrated to impact survival following SVR and an ESVI cut-off value >60 mL/m^2 postoperatively has been found to be predictive of an adverse outcome [31].

6 Patient Selection for Post-infarction Ventricular Surgery

An extensive and accurate preoperative work with imaging studies is necessary for patient selection, treatment planning, and results evaluation of SVR. Among the options Cardiac Magnetic Resonance (CMR) is the best since it provides the surgeon with all the necessary information for planning an effective, comprehensive surgery tailored to the patient's individual need [32, 33] and all the information can be obtained in a single examination taking less than 1 h.

For a correct indication it is important that cardiologists, radiologists, and surgeons closely cooperate to improve knowledge about patient selection and to achieve an optimal surgical outcome. First indication is clinical: i.e., signs and symptoms of heart failure in post-infarction patients with LV dilatation and reduced pump function; second, the left ventricle must be carefully evaluated using coronary angiography (ventricular angiography in Right and Left anterior oblique projections) or complete echocardiographic study (in 4CH, 2CH, parasternal long and short axis views, or with CMR study). The objective, with any imaging technique, for patient selection, treatment planning and follow-up is to assess the following parameters:

- Internal dimensions of the ventricle (diastolic and systolic diameters) in mm
- Ventricular volumes (both in diastole and in systole) in mL/m^2

- Ejection fraction %
- Thickness in mm and thickening of the wall as systo-diastolic % change
- Extent of asynergic area in respect to the entire LV perimeter
- Status of the remote regions (Normal, Hypokinetic, Akinetic, Dyskinetic)
- Presence or absence of viability (Echo Dobutamine or stress CMR)
- Presence or absence of mitral regurgitation
- Mitral annulus size and the left atrium size
- Right ventricular function

Key Point

- The presence of post-MI scar, symptoms or signs of HF and an accurate study of LV function are all mandatory for patient selection.

7 Evaluation of Asynergic Areas

The term asynergy means wall motion abnormality and includes hypokinesia, akinesia, and dyskinesia. Patients with either akinetic or dyskinetic scar benefit from SVR and the extent of asynergy rather than the type of asynergy is related to outcome following SVR [34]. The regions to be surgically excluded should be carefully evaluated for wall motion and thickening. Wall motion assessment can be accomplished by LV angiography, echocardiography, nuclear scintigraphic methods, and CMR, as previously reported.

Echo has several limitations: (1) the LV apex is not adequately seen when the ventricle is enlarged, as it is in dilated ischemic cardiomyopathy (2) the endocardial border often is not clearly seen and this accounts for intra and interobserver variability in measuring LV volumes and EF (3) many pts have comorbidities that make the echo images suboptimal, like obstructive pulmonary disease, obesity etc. [35]. Nuclear scintigraphic methods display endocardial border motion in planar views (with radionuclide angiography, labeling the blood pool) or the myocardium, including endocardial and epicardial visualization with gated SPECT examination. However, such studies require the use of radioactive tracers and are not available in all the cardiac centers.

CMR (despite not available everywhere and contraindicated if claustrophobia, or implantable cardioverter defibrillator are present), offers the advantage of a more accurate determination of LV volumes and EF, as it shows the epicardial and endocardial border from the base to the apex in a 3D view and it allows the most comprehensive evaluation with highly accurate and reproducible measurements in one single session [33]. The greatest usefulness of CMR is the detection of the myocardial scar with the GLE. A predictor of myocardial viability is the ratio of the thickness of tissue exhibiting late contrast enhancement in a segment to the total LV wall thickness in that segment. Segments with nearly transmural extent of late contrast enhancement are highly unlikely to show recovery of function following revascularization [32].

Recently, newer software dedicated to LV function analysis are becoming commercially available; with these methods, a semi-automated assessment of regional wall motion, of the extent of normal and abnormal contracting myocardium and of the percentage of the scarred tissue are easily obtained. With the development of tissue Doppler imaging technique and the 2D-based speckle or endocardial border tracking analysis [36, 37] it is nowadays possible to measure systolic and diastolic deformation either longitudinally or radially. With the analysis of untwisting it is possible to obtain information on diastolic function, at least on rapid filling.

Key Point

- CMR is the best cardiac function imaging study, but dedicated softwares for LV analysis need to be implemented. The analysis of cardiac function with new tissue Doppler, speckle tracking, and endocardial border tracking analysis has to be validated for the specific aim of LV reconstruction.

8 Status of Remote Regions

The quantification of the remote regions is essential to determine if a patient is a candidate for a SVR procedure and these regions are often not evaluated by conventional imaging studies. Following anterior MI remote regions may show hypokinesia or even akinesia due to critical coronary disease in the right or left circumflex coronary artery (hibernated myocardium) or remote myocardium may be dysfunctional in the absence of coronary stenosis, because of the high local tension that reduces shortening [38].

In a recent paper Dor proposed a careful evaluation of the diastolic volume of the contractile area and found that if this is greater than 45–50 mL/m^2, an efficient contractile cavity can be rebuilt [27].

The volume of the contractile area strictly correlates with the diastolic residual volume of the ventricle. Several years ago we demonstrated that in pts with anterior infarction due to single left anterior descending artery, regions remote from the scar may show severe asynergy in the absence of ischemic insult and that they significantly improve after LV reconstruction when the burden imposed by the scar on the wall is released, by scar exclusion [38].

Nowadays, the detection of scar in remote regions by GLE may predict unsatisfactory pump improvement and higher mortality rate following SVR. A significant scarring in a myocardial segment precludes in fact, the likelihood of postoperative contractile recovery of that segment. If GLE is not available or if uncertainties exist on the recovery of function, the diagnostic assessment needs to be completed with Dobutamine stress echo, to search for viable myocardium and to estimate the risk of surgery.

9 Right Ventricular Function

Analysis of right ventricular function (at least with visual inspection) should be part of patient evaluation, to determine if dysfunction is mild, moderate, or severe. The measure of tricuspid plane systolic excursion (TAPSE) may help in quantifying right ventricular dysfunction being a TAPSE less than 14 mm considered a marker of poor outcome, associated with higher operative mortality and therefore considered a contraindication to SVR. Finally, for a complete and correct assessment of surgical risk the presence and the severity of associate mitral regurgitation (MR) cannot be disregarded. Functional MR is a major component of LV dysfunction, causing pulmonary hypertension and LV volume overload, which in turn potentiates LV remodeling, a major determinant of the outcome of LV dysfunction. Ischemic mitral regurgitation conveys adverse prognosis, doubling mortality after myocardial infarction (MI), in chronic heart failure, and after surgical or catheter revascularization. It is common and increases mortality even when it is mild, with a graded relationship between severity and reduced survival [39, 40].

Key Point

- A correct risk evaluation includes: The extent and transmurality of the scar: the status of remote regions and of residual contractility; the analysis of right ventricular function; the presence and the severity of concomitant mitral regurgitation.

10 Coronary Revascularization in Ischemic Cardiomyopathy and Heart Failure

The role of CABG in the treatment of patients with CAD and heart failure has been more and more emphasized by clinical practice although there are no recent randomized trials supporting the superiority of CABG vs. medical therapy.

In three landmark clinical trials in the 1970s, recommendations supported the use of CABG to disabling symptoms of angina, particularly among high risk subgroups with extensive CAD [41, 42]. These trials excluded patients with severe left ventricular dysfunction (patients with an ejection fraction of <35 %).

Furthermore, medical therapy at that time consisted mainly in nitrates and surgeons did not approach patients with cardiac dysfunction, as they do more and more nowadays, thanks to the improved technical and anaesthesiologic skills. Moreover, in the early eighties percutaneous revascularization became the new revascularization therapy that widespread all over the countries and that in many circumstances is considered the first choice of revascularization. The STICH trial, designed in 2000 did not address PCI as revascularization option and this is another important limitation of the trial that does not reflect the current clinical practice. Ischemic Heart Failure (STICH) trial was designed to evaluate the role of cardiac surgery in the treatment of patients with CAD and left ventricular systolic dysfunction. A major hypothesis of the trial was that CABG plus intensive medical therapy based on current guidelines, as compared with medical therapy alone, would reduce mortality.

Between July 2002 and May 2007, a total of 1,212 patients with an ejection fraction of 35 % or less and CAD amenable to CABG were randomly assigned to medical therapy alone (602 patients) or medical therapy plus CABG (610 patients). The primary outcome was the rate of death from any cause. Major secondary outcomes included the rates of death from cardiovascular causes and of death from any cause or hospitalization for cardiovascular causes.

The conclusions were: In this randomized trial, there was no significant difference between medical therapy alone and medical therapy plus CABG with respect to the primary end point of death from any cause. Patients assigned to CABG, as compared with those assigned to medical therapy alone, had lower rates of death from cardiovascular causes and of death from any cause or hospitalization for cardiovascular causes.

As discussed in previous chapters, the STICH trial has suffered from multiple flaws and the conclusions derived by the hypothesis one are forced towards the benefits of revascularization, in our opinion, underestimating the fact that the primary hypothesis failed. These results were published in 2011, 1 year later than the Task Force on Myocardial Revascularization of the ESC and the European Association for Cardio-Thoracic Surgery (EACTS) [43] advised the creation of a Heart Team that serves the purpose of a balanced multidisciplinary decision process about revascularization in patients with CAD and heart failure. Guidelines stated that additional input may be needed from general practitioners, anaesthesiologists, geriatricians, or intensivists to address decisions in patients with angina and/or heart-failure symptoms, poor cardiac function, and other comorbidities. The task force reached a consensus that SVR combined with CABG can be considered as a surgical option in selected patients affected by ischemic heart failure and LV dysfunction mainly in centers with a high level of surgical expertise. This recognition with a level of evidence 1B, is valid for patients with CHF and systolic LV dysfunction (EF $\leq$ 35 %), presenting predominantly either with anginal symptoms or with HF symptoms.

In particular, these guidelines stated that CABG with SVR may be considered in patients with LVESV index >60 mL/m^2 and scarred LAD territory. In a previous paper we demonstrated that post-operative value of ESVI ($\geq$60 mL/m^2) significantly affects survival in ischemic patients operated of CABG plus SVR at San Donato Hospital, Italy, confirming the ESVI predictive value of adverse outcome [31]. The task force stated that SVR can be added to CABG if the LV is enlarged beyond 60 mL/m^2 at end systole, thus recognizing the predictive value of end systolic volume in pts with ischemic LV pump dysfunction and the importance of reducing ESVI to less than 60 mL/m^2 to improve prognosis.

They conclude that "...choosing to add SVR to CABG should be based on a careful evaluation of patients, including symptoms (HF symptoms should be predominant over angina), measurements of LV volumes, assessment of the transmural extent of myocardial scar tissue, and should be performed only in centers with a high level of surgical expertise." In this context, MRI is the standard imaging technique to assess myocardial anatomy, regional and global function, viability, and, more importantly, infarct size and percentage of transmurality determined by late gadolinium enhancement. The Task force gave therefore little recognition to the STICH trial results in the clinical practice and recognized that in the STICH trial ESVI reduction was much smaller than that reported in several observational studies thus raising concerns about the extent of the SVR procedure that was applied in the STICH trial.

To conclude, although extensively criticized the STICH trial has the merit of having enrolled a large number of ischemic population evaluated with several imaging modalities that represent the substratum for several sub-studies and potential future researches. If ever possible, the trial should be redesigned taking care to compare homogeneous pts with post-infarction dilated failing ventricle, due to extreme remodeling, large wall scar, and symptoms of advanced heart failure.

Presently, we do not think that the STICH data are generalizable and caution should be used in negating SVR plus/minus CABG to a patient that presents with:

- Dilated ischemic failing ventricle (EDVI $\geq$ 100 mL/m^2 and ESVI $\geq$ 60 mL/m^2)
- Signs and symptoms of HF (NYHA class >2)
- Transmural infarction and/or absence of myocardial viability
- Extent of asynergy either akinetic or dyskinetic greater than 35–40 %
- Ejection Fraction below 35 %

11 Future Trends for Coronary Revascularization and Ventricular Surgery in Heart-Failure Patients

Despite the orientation of the last task force concerning the applicability of the SVR to patients with anterior myocardial scar and enlarged ESVI (>60 mL/m^2) we must recognize that at present, there is no general consensus on the indication of adding SVR to CABG to patients with CAD and heart failure. The STICH trial results not only do not reflect the current clinical practice but more importantly, the authors insist to negate the usefulness of adding SVR to CABG in any clinical condition. Therefore, we cannot be satisfied neither by the trial conduction nor by the trial results interpretation.

We would need a process that combines evidence-based medicine and guidelines (that honestly are very few) that give special consideration to the practice experience through a scoring process and for this purpose we wish it will be possible to organize a technical panel as it has been done for coronary revascularization appropriateness [43].

12 Sources of Further Information

Patel MR, Spertus JA, Brindis RG, et al. ACCF proposed method for evaluating the appropriateness of cardiovascular imaging. J Am Coll Cardiol. 2005;46:1606–13.

King, SB, Aversano, T, Ballard WL, et al. ACCF/AHA/SCAI 2007 update of the clinical competence statement on cardiac interventional procedures: a report of the American College of Cardiology Foundation/American Heart Association/American College of Physicians Task Force on Clinical Competence and Training. J Am Coll Cardiol. 2007;50:82–108.

Eagle KA, Guyton RA, Davidoff R, et al. ACC/AHA 2004 guideline update for coronary artery bypass graft surgery: summary article: a report of the American College of Cardiology/American Heart Association Task Force on Practice Guidelines (Committee to Update the 1999 Guidelines for Coronary Artery Bypass Graft Surgery). J Am Coll Cardiol. 2004;44:e213–310.

References

1. Gheorghiade M, Sopko G, De Luca L et al (2006) Navigating the crossroads of coronary artery disease and heart failure. Circulation 114:1202–1213
2. Felker GM, Thompson RE, Hare JM et al (2000) Underlying causes and long-term survival in patients with initially unexplained cardiomyopathy. N Engl J Med 342:1077–1084
3. Felker GM, Shaw LK, O'Connor CM (2002) A standardized definition of ischemic cardiomyopathy for use in clinical research. J Am Coll Cardiol 39:210–218
4. Mann DL, Bristow MR (2005) Mechanisms and models in heart failure. The bio-mechanical model and beyond. Circulation 111:2837–2849
5. Mann DL, Deswal A, Bozkurt B, Torre-Amione G (2002) New therapeutics for chronic heart failure. Annu Rev Med 53:59–74
6. Abraham WT, Fisher WG, Smith AL et al (2002) Cardiac resynchronization in chronic heart failure. N Engl J Med 346:1845–1853
7. Dickstein K, Vardas PE, Auricchio A et al (2010) An update of the 2008 ESC Guidelines for the diagnosis and treatment of acute and chronic heart failure and the 2007 ESC guidelines for cardiac and resynchronization therapy. Eur Heart J 31:2677–2687
8. Levy D, Kenchaiah S, Larson MG et al (2002) Long term trends in the incidence of and survival with heart failure. N Engl J Med 347(18):1397–1402
9. Allman KC, Shaw LJ, Hachamovitch R, Udelson JE (2002) Myocardial viability testing and impact of revascularization on prognosis in patients with coronary artery disease and left ventricular dysfunction: a meta-analysis. J Am Coll Cardiol 39:1151–1158
10. Bax JJ, Schinkel AF, Boersma E et al (2004) Extensive left ventricular remodeling does not allow viable myocardium to improve in left ventricular ejection fraction after revascularization and is associated with worse long-term prognosis. Circulation 110S(Suppl II):II18–II22
11. Buckberg GD (2004) Overview: ventricular restoration—a surgical approach to reverse ventricular remodelling. Heart Fail Rev 9:233–239
12. Dor V, Sabatier M, Montiglio F et al (2004) Endoventricular patch reconstruction in ischemic failing ventricle. A single center with 20 years experience. Advantages of magnetic resonance imaging assessment. Heart Fail Rev 9:269–286
13. Athanasuleas CL, Buckberg GD, Stanley AW, et al.; Restore Group (2004) Surgical ventricular restoration in the treatment of congestive heart failure due to post-infarction ventricular dilation. J Am Coll Cardiol 44(7):1439–1445
14. Conte JV (2004) Surgical ventricular restoration: techniques and outcomes. Congest Heart Fail 10:248–251

15. Menicanti L, Castelvecchio S, Ranucci M et al (2007) Surgical therapy for ischemic heart failure: single-center experience with surgical anterior ventricular restoration. J Thorac Cardiovasc Surg 134(2):433–441
16. Sartipy U, Albage A, Lindblom D (2005) The Dor procedure for left ventricular reconstruction. Ten-year clinical experience. Eur J Cardiothorac Surg 27:1005–1010
17. Sartipy U, Albåge A, Lindblom D (2007) Improved health-related quality of life and functional status after surgical ventricular restoration. Ann Thorac Surg 83:1381–1388
18. Jones RH, Velazquez EJ, Michler RE, Sopko G, Oh JK, O'Connor CM, Hill JA, Menicanti L, Sadowski Z, Desvigne-Nickens P, Rouleau JL, Lee KL (2009) Coronary bypass surgery with or without surgical ventricular reconstruction. N Engl J Med 360:1705–1717
19. Velazquez EJ, Lee KL, Deja MA et al (2011) Coronary-artery bypass surgery in patients with left ventricular dysfunction. N Engl J Med 364:1607–1616
20. Kieser TM (2009) The left ventricle: to reconstruct or not – lessons from the STICH trial. J Thorac Cardiovasc Surg 138(3):784
21. Cohn PF, Ferrari R, Sharpe N (2000) Cardiac remodelling concepts and clinical implications: a consensus paper from an international forum on cardiac remodeling. J Am Coll Cardiol 35:569–582
22. Libby P, Lee RT (2000) Matrix matters. Circulation 102:1874–1876
23. Shroyer ALV, Collins JF, Grover FL (2010) Evaluating clinical applicability: the STICH trial's findings. J Am Coll Cardiol 56:508–509
24. Di Donato M, Toso A, Maioli M et al (2001) Intermediate survival and predictors of death after surgical ventricular restoration. Semin Thorac Cardiovasc Surg 13:468–475
25. Ribeiro GA, Cledicyon E, da Costa M, Lopes M et al (2006) Left ventricular reconstruction benefits patients with ischemic cardiomyopathy and non-viable myocardium. Eur J Cardiothorac Surg 29:196–201
26. Cooley DA, Collins HA, Morris GC Jr, Chapman DW (1958) Ventricular aneurysm after myocardial infarction; surgical excision with use of temporary cardiopulmonary bypass. JAMA 167:557–560
27. Dor V, Civaia F, Alexandrescu C, Sabatier M, Montiglio F (2011) Favorable effects of left ventricular reconstruction in patients excluded from the Surgical Treatments for Ischemic Heart Failure (STICH) trial. J Thorac Cardiovasc Surg 141:905–916
28. Burkhoff D, Wechsler AS (2006) Surgical ventricular remodeling: a balancing act on systolic and diastolic properties. J Thorac Cardiovasc Surg 132:459–463
29. Menicanti L, Di Donato M (2002) The Dor procedure: what has changed after fifteen years of clinical practice? J Thorac Cardiovasc Surg 124(5):886–890
30. Di Donato M, Dabic P, Castelvecchio S et al (2006) Left ventricular geometry in normal and post-anterior myocardial infarction patients: sphericity index and 'new' conicity index comparisons. Eur J Cardiothorac Surg 29(Suppl 1):S225–S230
31. Di Donato M, Castelvecchio S, Menicanti L (2010) End-systolic volume following surgical ventricular reconstruction impacts survival in patients with ischaemic dilated cardiomyopathy. Eur J Heart Fail 12:375–381
32. Kim RJ, Wu E, Rafael A et al (2000) The use of contrast-enhanced magnetic resonance imaging to identify reversible myocardial dysfunction. N Engl J Med 343:1445–1453
33. Lloyd GS, Buckberg GD, Restore group (2006) Use of cardiac magnetic resonance imaging in surgical ventricular restoration. Eur J Cardiothorac Surg 295:S216–S224
34. Di Donato M, Sabatier M, Dor V, Toso A, Maioli M, Fantini F (1997) Akinetic versus dyskinetic postinfarction scar: relation to surgical outcome in patients undergoing endoventricular circular patch plasty repair. J Am Coll Cardiol 29:1569–1575
35. Schiller N, Shah P, Crawford M et al (1989) Recommendations for quantitation of the left ventricle by two-dimensional echocardiography. American Society of Echocardiography Committee on Standards, Subcommittee on Quantitation of Two-dimensional Echocardiograms. Am Soc Echocardiogr 2:358–367

36. Artis NJ, Oxborough DL, Williams G, Pepper CB, Tan LB (2008) Two-dimensional strain imaging: a new echocardiographic advance with research and clinical applications. Int J Cardiol 123:240–248
37. Reisner SA, Lysyansky P, Agmon Y et al (2004) Global longitudinal strain: a novel index of left ventricular systolic function. J Am Soc Echocardiogr 17:630–633
38. Di Donato M, Sabatier M, Toso A et al (1995) Regional myocardial performance of non-ischemic zones remote from anterior wall left ventricular aneurysm. Effects of aneurysmectomy. Eur Heart J 1:1285–1292
39. Lamas GA, Mitchell GF, Flaker GC et al (1997) Survival and Ventricular Enlargement Investigators. Clinical significance of mitral regurgitation after acute myocardial infarction. Circulation 96:827–833
40. Grigioni F, Enriquez-Sarano M, Zehr KJ et al (2001) Ischemic mitral regurgitation: long-term outcome and prognostic implications with quantitative Doppler assessment. Circulation 103:1759–1764
41. Alderman EL, Fisher LD, Litwin P et al (1983) Results of coronary artery surgery in patients with poor left ventricular function (CASS). Circulation 68:785–795
42. Yusuf S, Zucker D, Peduzzi P et al (1994) Effect of coronary artery bypass graft surgery on survival: overview of 10-year results from randomised trials by the Coronary Artery Bypass Graft Surgery Trialists Collaboration. Lancet 344:563–570 [Erratum, Lancet 1994;344:1446.]
43. Wijns W, Kolh P, Danchin N et al (2010) Guidelines on myocardial revascularization: the Task Force on Myocardial Revascularization of the European Society of Cardiology (ESC) and the European Association for Cardio-Thoracic Surgery (EACTS). Eur Heart J 31:2501–2555

Part IV
When Every Therapy Fails

Chapter 14
Cardiac Arrest and Refractory Cardiogenic Shock

Koen De Decker

Abbreviations

AHA	American Heart Association
AMI	Acute myocardial infarction
BIVAD	Biventricular assist device
BNP	Brain natriuretic peptide
CA	Cardiac arrest
CPB	Cardiopulmonary bypass
CPR	Cardiopulmonary resuscitation
CS	Cardiogenic shock
ECMO	Extracorporeal membrane oxygenation
ICU	Intensive care unit
INTERMACS	Interagency Registry for Mechanically Assisted Circulatory Support
IRA	Infarct-related artery
LVAD	Left ventricular assist device
MODS	Multiorgan dysfunction syndrome
PCCS	Postcardiotomy cardiogenic shock
PCI	Percutaneous coronary intervention
RVAD	Right ventricular assist device
TAH	Total artificial heart
VAD	Ventricular assist device

K. De Decker (✉)
Department of Anesthesiology and Intensive Care, OLV Hospital, Aalst, Belgium
e-mail: Koen.De.Decker@olvz-aalst.be

J. Bartunek and M. Vanderheyden (eds.), *Translational Approach to Heart Failure*, 357
DOI 10.1007/978-1-4614-7345-9_14, © Springer Science+Business Media New York 2013

Abstract Cardiogenic shock is a serious condition that still has high mortality rates, despite the improvements with early revascularisation. In the most severe cases mechanical support is used to reverse shock and preserve other organ functions. Historically, intraaortic balloon pump counterpulsation was the first device that was used, later on followed by ECLS and ventricular assist devices. In this chapter we describe the outcomes of percutaneous mechanical circulatory support in cardiogenic shock and circulatory arrest as well as their complications.

1 Introduction

When observing incidence, etiology, and outcomes of cardiogenic shock (CS), hardly any randomized data can be found besides those of the SHOCK trial [1]. As for other causes of CS (postcardiotomy, acute decompensation of chronic heart failure, myocarditis, etc.), most data come from large registries. Acute myocardial infarction (AMI), together with its mechanical complications, was responsible for almost 90 % of CS cases.

When resistant to inotropes and intra-aortic balloon pump (IABP) counterpulsation, more powerful mechanical circulatory support is the only remaining option in order to reverse shock and to prevent or treat secondary organ failure. In the last 2 decades cannulas and oxygenators have become more biocompatible and pumps have become much smaller, more implantable, and their material more durable. Several devices were used in order to support (1) patients with mechanical cardiac complications, either ischemic or nonischemic (postcardiotomy, myocarditis, acutely decompensating chronic heart failure, valvular heart disease, acute post-transplant rejection, or toxic/metabolic derangements due to drug overdose or other causes), (2) patients with refractory arrhythmias, (3) patients undergoing high risk percutaneous coronary intervention (PCI), or (4) young post-cardiac arrest patients.

We will focus on short-term, percutaneous mechanical support in cardiac arrest (CA), infarct-related and postcardiotomy CS, refractory to all medical therapy. The use of implantable assist devices and total artificial heart is discussed elsewhere.

2 Refractory Cardiogenic Shock

2.1 Introduction

The incidence of CS after AMI has been rather stable between 1975 and the late 1980s, averaging 7.5 % in a series of more than 13,000 patients [2]. Since the 1990s there was a decline, resulting in an overall CS incidence (1975–2005) of 6.6 % as shown in Fig. 14.1 [2]. Before talking about mechanical support, one should not

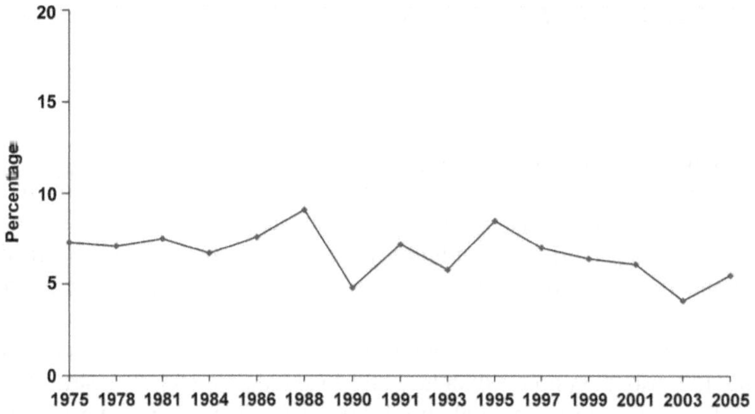

Fig. 14.1 Trends in incidence rates of cardiogenic shock in patients with acute myocardial infarction (AMI) [2]

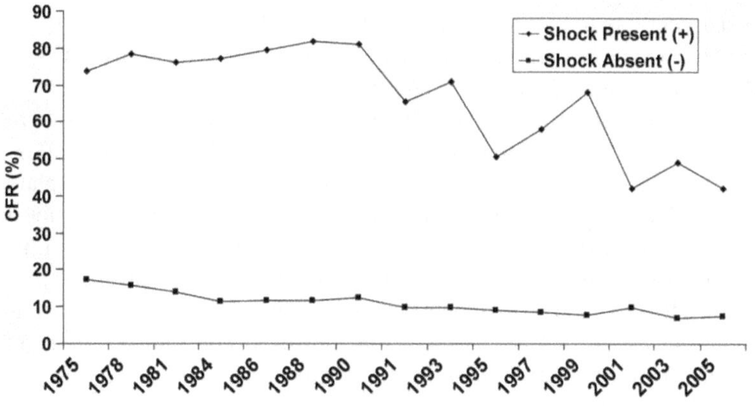

Fig. 14.2 Trends in hospital case-fatality rates in patients with AMI according to the presence of cardiogenic shock [2]

forget that early revascularization is the cornerstone of therapy. This was demonstrated in a randomized setting by the previously mentioned SHOCK trial [1]. There was a trend to increased survival at 30 days in the group that was revascularized, which became significant at 6 months (50.3 % vs. 63.1 %; $p = 0.027$) and at 6 years of follow-up (19.6 % vs. 32.8 %; $p = 0.02$) [3]. When observing the evolution of the case-fatality rate, a decline was seen from around 75 to 40 %, as illustrated in Fig. 14.2 [2]. Data from the National Registry for Myocardial Infarction (NRMI) show that in some subgroups, e.g., revascularized patients under the age of 75 treated by means of PCI, mortality dropped below 30 % [4]. So there remains a substantial group of patients that might benefit from mechanical support.

2.2 *Infarct-Related Cardiogenic Shock*

2.2.1 Intra-aortic Balloon Pump

IABP counterpulsation was the first type of mechanical support, besides cardiopulmonary bypass (CPB) systems, and was introduced some 50 years ago [5]. It has long been the golden standard for mechanical support in different indications: refractory angina pectoris, postcardiotomy low cardiac output syndrome, mechanical complications of AMI and CS. Through inflation of the balloon in diastole, it will induce augmentation of diastolic blood pressure and as a consequence increased coronary perfusion pressure. But there is no active blood volume displacement. The deflation just prior to systole will induce afterload reduction for the heart. For a long time IABP was the most commonly used form of mechanical circulatory support in CS with an American Heart Association (AHA) class I recommendation [6]. This is mainly based on the results of large registries and observational studies (Table 14.1, [7]) and there are hardly any randomized data to support this.

In the shock registry, IABP was used in 52 % of the patients and it resulted in a significant decrease in mortality rates (50 % vs. 72 %; $p<0.0001$) [8]. The second NRMI is one of the largest databases, containing over 23,000 cases of CS, with an overall mortality rate of 70 % [9]. IABP was used in 7,268 patients (31 %) and resulted in a significant mortality reduction (67 % vs. 49 %) in the subgroup of patients, treated with thrombolysis. However, in the PCI group, no difference in outcomes was observed (45 % vs. 47 % mortality). This is probably explained by the fact that IABP counterpulsation increases the effects and results of fibrinolytic therapy. A recent retrospective cohort study of 437 consecutive patients illustrated also an effect on long-term survival [10]. Randomized data, however, are scarce. In the TACTICS trial [11] 57 patients were included and there was a 21 % mortality reduction (43 % vs. 34 %), which was however not statistically significant ($p = 0.027$). Unfortunately this study was stopped early, due to enrollment problems. The latter were caused by a bias towards the IABP group and the unwillingness to give thrombolytics alone. A small ($n = 45$), single-center, randomized pilot trial [12] compared the use of IABP with medical treatment in patients treated with PCI of the infarct-related artery (IRA). The addition of IABP did not result in a significant hemodynamic improvement (by means of cardiac index) or a reduction in multiorgan dysfunction syndrome (MODS), although brain natriuretic peptide (BNP) levels were significantly lower. In 2009 a Dutch group [7] identified seven randomized trials and nine cohort studies of IABP therapy in, respectively, STEMI patients and STEMI patients with CS. In the nine observational trials ($n=10{,}529$) there was a significant ($p<0.0001$) improvement in the 30-day survival in patients with IABP that received thrombolysis, but a 6 % worse 30-day survival in patients that underwent primary PCI, as shown in Fig. 14.3 ($p<0.0008$). The authors concluded that the improved survival in the thrombolysis cohort was due to selection bias and confounding variables secondary to younger age, whereas the worse survival in the PCI cohort could be explained by the patients being sicker and also the longer ischemic times in some patients before transfer to a primary PCI center.

Table 14.1 Characteristics of cohort studies of IABP therapy in STEMI complicated by cardiogenic shock [7]

Study	No. of patients	Type of reperfusion	Setting	Period	Cardiogenic shock definition	Mean age (years)		Male sex (%)	
						IABP	Control	IABP	Control
Moulopoulos et al. [22]	49	No reperfusion	Single center	<1985	SysRR ≤80, urine output <20 mL/h, clinical signs of hypoperfusion	60	61	85	87
Stomel et al. [23]	64	Thrombolysis/rescue PCI	Single center	1985–1991	SysRR ≤80 unresponsive to fluids CI ≤2.0 L/min/m², PCWP ≥18 mmHg, clinical signs of hypoperfusion	66[a]	66[a]	45*	62*
Kovack et al. [24]	46	Thrombolysis/rescue PCI	Multicenter	1985–1995	SysRR ≤90 unresponsive to fluids, CI ≤2.2 L/min/m², clinical signs of hypoperfusion	62	64	59	63
Bengtson et al. [25]	200	Thrombolysis/rescue PCI	Single center	1987–1988	≥30 min sysRR <90 unless IABP/pressors, CI ≤2.2 L/min/m² and PCWP ≥18, clinical signs of hypoperfusion	64	67	–	–
Waksman et al. [26]	41	Thrombolysis/rescue PCI	Single center	1989	SysRR ≤90 unresponsive to fluids, clinical signs of hypoperfusion	66	68	70	71

(continued)

Table 14.1 (continued)

Study	No. of patients	Type of reperfusion	Setting	Period	Cardiogenic shock definition	Mean age (years)		Male sex (%)	
						IABP	Control	IABP	Control
GUSTO-I [27]	310	Thrombolysis/rescue PCI	Multicenter	1990–1993	SysRR ≤90 unresponsive to fluids, CI ≤2.2 L/min/m^2, clinical signs of hypoperfusion	64	68	68	62
NRMI-2 [28][b]	8,671	Thrombolysis/rescue PCI or primary PCI	Multicenter	1994–1998	SysRR ≤90 unresponsive to fluids, clinical signs of hypoperfusion	67*	74*	61*	51*
SHOCK registry [29]	856	Thrombolysis/rescue PCI	Multicenter	1995–2000	SysRR ≤90 unresponsive to fluids, CI ≤2.2 L/min/m^2, clinical signs of hypoperfusion	65[a],*	72[a],*	67[a],*	60[a],*
AMC CS cohort [20, 21]	292	Primary PCI	Single center	1997–2005	SysRR ≤90 unresponsive to fluids, CI ≤2.2 L/min/m^2, clinical signs of hypoperfusion	65	62	68	66

IABP intra-aortic balloon pump, *STEMI* ST-elevation myocardial infarction, *sysRR* systolic blood pressure (mmHg), *NR* not reported, *CI* cardiac index, *PCI* percutaneous coronary intervention, *LV* left ventricle

*$p<0.05$

[a]Calculated from the extracted data

[b]The NRMI-2 study reported about a thrombolysis and a primary PCI cohort

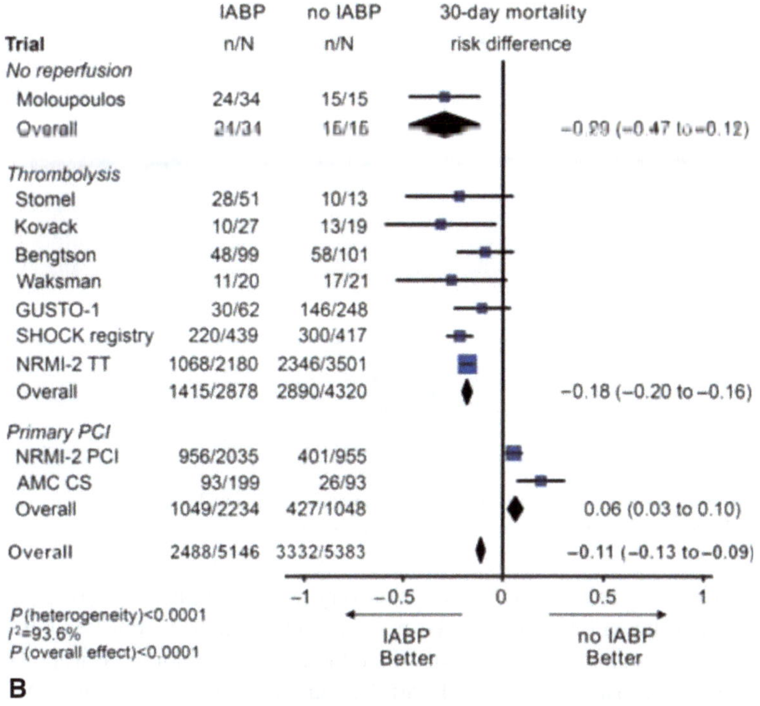

Fig. 14.3 Risk differences in 30-day mortality for individual studies, for each type of reperfusion therapy, and for the overall analysis [7]

Their challenge of the guideline was followed by a Cochrane review [13] that included six eligible and two ongoing studies out of 1,410 references, evaluating IABP use in patients with infarct-related CS. Three trials compared IABP to standard treatment and three to percutaneous left ventricular assist devices (LVADs). Of the 190 included patients, 105 were treated with IABP. The other 85 patients served as controls, of which 45 were treated with LVADs. There were no differences in all-cause 30-day mortality (hazard ratio of 1.04).

In summary, IABP counterpulsation is frequently used in CS and without any doubt it is also the least expensive form of mechanical support. However, in the era of early revascularization (mainly PCI) its level I recommendation for use in cardiogenic shock has become questionable.

2.2.2 Percutaneous Ventricular Assist Device

The use of IABP requires a certain residual level of left ventricular function. In contrast with newer technologies, that generate active volume displacement, it is unable to provide the support needed to reverse the most severe cases of CS. Extracorporeal membrane oxygenation (ECMO) and several percutaneous ventricular assist devices (pVADs) have been used in order to facilitate high risk PCI cases

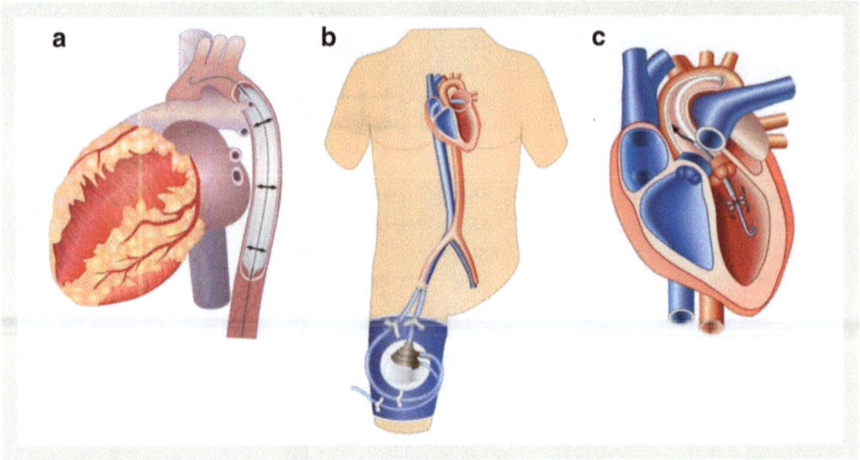

Fig. 14.4 Schematic drawings of current percutaneous mechanical support devices: (**a**) intra-aortic balloon pump (IABP); (**b**) TandemHeart; (**c**) Impella [14]

or as bridging therapy in CS, either to recovery or to definitive therapy (long-term VAD or transplantation). Over the years, numerous devices were tested but only a few made it to commercialization, of which the Impella (Abiomed Europe GmbH, Aachen, Germany) and the TandemHeart (Cardiac Assist Inc., Pittsburgh, PA, USA) are best known (Fig. 14.4, [14]). The technical features of both devices are listed in Table 14.2 [15].

Most published data come from case reports or case series and only three controlled studies met the strict inclusion criteria of a meta-analysis [16]. The Impella (Abiomed Europe GmbH, Aachen, Germany) has a 5 L and a 2.5 L version. Only the latter was studied in a small ($n = 25$), randomized trial [17]. In this safety study the Impella 2.5 was compared to IABP support in CS. Cardiac index after 30 min of support, which was the primary outcome parameter, was significantly increased. Overall 30-day mortality was equal in both groups (46 %).

In a multicenter, randomized trial, another device called the TandemHeart was compared ($n = 19$) with IABP support [18]. The pVAD increased cardiac index and mean arterial blood pressure significantly. The decrease in pulmonary capillary wedge pressure was also statistically significant. Overall 30-day mortality and serious adverse events were not significantly different between the two groups. The same device was compared with IABP support in 41 CS cases of a single center [19]. The outcome data were similar to the previous trial. Hemodynamics, with cardiac power index as the primary outcome parameter, was improved more effectively by VAD support. Again, no survival benefit (45 % vs. 43 % mortality; $p = 0.86$) could be illustrated and complications like severe bleeding or limb ischemia were encountered more frequently after VAD support.

Although pVADs provide superior hemodynamic support, they did not improve early survival. Therefore the authors of the meta-analysis [16] concluded that pVADs cannot be recommended as first choice in the management of cardiogenic shock.

Table 14.2 Comparison of IABP and currently available pVADs for cardiogenic shock [15]

	IABP	TandemHeart pVAD	Impella 2.5 recover system	ECMO
Pump mechanism	Pneumatic	Centrifugal	Axial flow	Centrifugal flow
Insertion	Retrograde 7–9F balloon catheter into descending aorta via femoral artery	21F inflow cannula into left atrium via femoral vein and transseptal puncture and 15/17F outflow cannula into femoral artery	12F catheter (13F sheath) placed retrograde across the aortic valve via femoral artery	18–31F inflow cannula into the right atrium via femoral vein and 15–22F outflow cannula into descending aorta via femoral artery
Difficulty of insertion	+	++++	+++	++
Degree of support	+ (⇑ CO by 0.5 L/min)	+++ (⇑ CO by 3.5–4 L/min)	++ (⇑ CO by 2.5 L/min)	++++ (⇑ CO to >4.5 L/min)
Cardiac power output[a]	+	+++	++	++++
Time for implantation	10 min	25–65 min	11–25 min	10–15 min
Limb ischemia	+	+++	++	+++
Hemolysis	0	++	++++	+++
Bleeding risks	+	+++	++	++++
Contraindications	Moderate–severe AI/aortic stenosis, coagulopathy, severe sepsis	Peripheral arterial disease (may be placed with antegrade sideport for limb perfusion), RV failure	LV thrombus, ventricular septal defect, severe aortic stenosis, RV failure, peripheral arterial disease	Contraindication to anticoagulation, irreversible brain injury, terminal disease

AI aortic insufficiency, *CO* cardiac output, *ECMO* extracorporeal membrane oxygenation, *IABP* intra-aortic balloon pump, *LV* left ventricular, *pVAD* percutaneous ventricular assist device, *RV* right ventricular

[a]Cardiac power output, measured in watts, is defined as the mean arterial pressure (MAP) multiplied by CO divided by 451. It takes into account the need for adequate MAPs as well as CO for adequate end-organ perfusion and has prognostic utility in predicting mortality in cardiogenic shock associated with ischemic and nonischemic cardiomyopathy

The largest published (non-randomized) series investigated 117 CS patients [20]. Again, a significant improvement of hemodynamic variables was seen, resulting in significant decreases in creatinine and lactic acid levels. Thirty-day mortality was 40.2 %, which was comparable with the data from the randomized trials, however in a sicker cohort of patients with more comorbidities. Eighty-two percent of patients had IABP support prior to pVAD implantation.

The Impella 5.0 L might have a place in univentricular failure, as suggested by a rare analysis comparing ECMO and microaxial flow pumps [21]. In 58 patients, there were no differences in weaning percentage (Impella 41 % vs. ECMO 47 %), 30-day mortality (Impella 38 % vs. ECMO 44 %), or the proportion of patients discharged home (Impella 59 % vs. ECMO 41 %). The authors reserve ECMO for patients with biventricular failure or combined respiratory and circulatory failure. This was however a retrospective analysis, the etiology of cardiogenic shock was distributed differently and duration of support was rather short (46 and 63 h, respectively). An explanation for the absence of improved survival might be the timing of implantation. A close relationship was seen between the depth of CS and survival in another form of CS (postcardiotomy patients), suggesting that earlier implantation may improve outcome [22].

Unless large randomized trials confirm results in the future, the replacement of IABP by pVADs in refractory (infarct-related) cardiogenic shock cannot be given a high class of recommendation.

2.2.3 Extracorporeal Membrane Oxygenation

Since the first successful ECMO implantation in 1972 [23], numerous reports on ECMO have been published. Three indications for ECMO in ischemic heart disease have been studied: (1) support during high risk PCI; (2) in patients with cardiogenic shock as a bridge to revascularization, a bridge to recovery, a bridge to transplantation, or a bridge to bridge (where the ECMO is later replaced by an implantable VAD); (3) as rescue therapy in patients with ongoing cardiopulmonary resuscitation (CPR) for cardiac arrest (CA). In the latter case veno-arterial ECMO is often used as a “bridge to decision” (where post-ECMO management depends on neurological outcome). The main benefit of ECMO in comparison with IABP and pVADs is that it can produce higher flow rates (5 L and more). Only the 5 L version of the Impella comes close, but the support with ECMO can be continued for a longer period of time. Furthermore, the option of adding an oxygenator to the circuit allows for (quick) correction of hypoxia.

For several reasons it is difficult to compare outcome data. As stated before, randomized data are lacking. Furthermore infarct-related CS is probably the subgroup of patients in which mechanical support was least discussed separately. This in contrast with patients suffering from cardiac arrest, postcardiotomy shock, or even smaller subgroups (e.g., myocarditis and posttransplant CS). For this reason we will discuss the data on ECMO use in cardiac arrest and postcardiotomy separately. The data on infarct-related cardiogenic shock, discussed in this paragraph, were extracted out of case series with mixed etiology of CS.

Table 14.3 ECMO in postinfarct cardiogenic shock—overview of results of larger cohorts

	Number of CS		Weaned (%)		Survival to discharge (%)	
Author	Total	AMI	Total	AMI	Total	AMI
Combes [31]	81	16	43 (53.1 %)	6 (37.5 %)	34 (42 %)	5 (31.2 %)
Vanzetto [32]	100	32	33 (33 %)	?	20 (20 %)	?
Liden [33]	52	19	26 (50 %)	?	24 (46 %)	?
Chung [34]	134	53	68 (50.7 %)	?	57 (42.5 %)	27 (51 %)
Loforte [35]	73	12	44[a] (60 %)	7 (58 %)	33 (45 %)	5 (42 %)
Sakamoto [36]	98	98	54 (55 %)		32 (32.5 %)	

[a]Forty-seven patients survived ECMO but three were bridged to a long-term VAD

The outcome data of relevant and reliable studies were nicely presented in a systematic review on percutaneous ECMO [24] and another review article by Allen et al. [25]. In the systematic review 84 studies (out of 3,289 eligible studies published between 1966 and 2005) met the inclusion criteria. Among these studies, there were 52 groups of patients with cardiogenic shock ($n=533$), 54 groups of patients with cardiac arrest ($n=675$), and 5 with both ($n=286$). The weaning rates overall, in CS, and in CA were 76.8 %, 82.8 %, 71.5 % and survival to discharge was possible in 40 %, 51.6 %, and 44.9 %, respectively. There was however significant statistical heterogeneity among the studies and the presence of publication bias was suggested. We combined the data of the largest trials (>50 patients), cited in both reviews, with those of later publications on ECMO support in CS in Table 14.3 [26–31]. In only four of these reports the outcome of infarct-related CS patients, supported with ECMO, was mentioned. Weaning rates are around 50 % and survival to discharge was achieved in 30–40 % of the cases.

Only a few publications report on the use of mechanical support in the subpopulation of post-AMI CS. A review article by Garatti et al. [32] grouped 17 studies. The mean weaning and survival rates were 58.5 % and 40 %, respectively. The patients in this trial were younger and in worse hemodynamic condition, when compared to the SHOCK trial cohort, but it needs to be said that data regarding time from symptom onset to revascularization and/or LVAD support are often missing. Taking these considerations in mind, the authors conclude that (percutaneous) LVAD support gave no survival improvement in infarct-related CS compared with early reperfusion therapy alone or in combination with IABP.

Sheu et al. [33] compared a group of 1,650 STEMI patients (of which 219 developed cardiogenic shock; 13.3 %) with 920 historic controls (of which 115 developed cardiogenic shock; 12.5 %). The incidence of profound shock (defined as systolic blood pressure remaining <75 mmHg under IABP and inotropic support) was similar in both groups (21.7 % vs. 21 %; $p>0.5$), but only the patients in the study cohort (enrolled between August 2002 and December 2009) were allowed to be converted to ECMO in the cathlab. Thirty-day mortality almost halved in the profound shock group (72 % vs. 39.1 %; $p=0.008$). More or less the same outcome data are seen in two smaller series of 21 [34] and 20 patients [35]. Weaning rates were 81.5 % and 70 %, respectively, and survival to discharge was 59.3 % and 50 %, respectively.

Randomized data on ECMO use in CS are missing. Nevertheless a few general trends can be recognized in case series: around 50 % of patients can be weaned of ECMO with survival to discharge rates that average 40 %. A few groups manage to do better, although the number of included patients is usually small. A Swedish group [28] achieved a 48 % overall survival group in 52 CS patients supported with ECMO. In the non-cardiotomy group ($n = 19$; 36 %), the long-term survival was 63 %. At Penn State University [36], ten patients were supported for an average of 5.8 days with the Centrimag (Levitronix LLC, Waltham, MA) ECMO. Survival in this group was 60 %.

In summary half of the patients can be weaned and around 40 % of the patients survive to discharge. These numbers, as previously shown, are not very different from the ones with pVADs, although the latter were less studied in this field. The only just conclusion to be drawn is that we need data from randomized trials, analogue to the data from the CESAR trial [37] that studied the use of (veno-venous) ECMO in refractory respiratory failure.

2.3 *Postcardiotomy Cardiogenic Shock*

Postcardiotomy shock was, in contrast with infarct-related CS, evaluated more frequently as a separate subgroup. The incidence is ranging from 0.5 to 5 % [38, 39], but IABP and/or inotropic support will allow weaning from CPB in most cases. Like in infarct-related shock, IABP is still seen as the primary form of support in most centers. Outcome is usually worse than in other subsets of CS, averaging around 25 % survival [39]. In approximately 1 % of postcardiotomy cardiogenic shock (PCCS) cases, the only alternative for CPB withdrawal is the initiation of ECMO or the implantation of a VAD. The use of the latter has declined in the last decade because of the technological improvements with pVADs and ECMO. When to change from IABP to VADs is not always clear. The group from Berlin developed an IABP score (0–5 points) that predicts survival [40]. In patients with a high risk score, the implantation of a VAD should be considered.

Some 15 publications report on the use of Impella, before a multicenter trial [41] studied the use of the Impella 5.0 L (Impella Cardiosystems GmbH, Aachen, Germany) in PCCS. Sixteen patients were observed with a mean duration of support of 3,7 days. Recovery was obtained in 93 % of the patients. The largest study investigating the use of the TandemHeart postcardiotomy [42] included 11 patients of which eight could be weaned and six patients survived to discharge.

Percutaneous VADs were also used in special subsets of PCCS patients. For instance, both Impella [43] and TandemHeart [44] have been used as a bridge to recovery for right ventricular dysfunction after heart transplantation. In a case of severe cardiac allograft rejection the Impella 2.5 and the TandemHeart were even combined with a good patient outcome [45].

In the review by Allen et al. [25], 15 case series on postcardiotomy ECMO support are cited. Only six of these series contain more than 20 patients. Overall, survival ranged from 19 to 67 % with irreversible cardiac failure and multiple organ failure being the most common causes of death [25]. In the largest cohort [46], 219 patients out of 18,150 (1.2 %) required postoperative ECMO support. Arterial cannulation was done into the ascending aorta in 159 patients (72.6 %). Weaning was successful after a mean support duration of 2,8 days in 134 patients (61 %) and survival to discharge (after a mean of 30 days) was 24 %. After 5 years 37 of these patients (74 %) were alive.

In a more recent report [47], 517 adults with PCCS were supported with ECMO. Support was established through thoracic cannulation in 60.8 % of the cases and mean support duration was 3,28 days. Weaning was successful in 63.3 % of the patients and 24.8 % survived to discharge. After 5 years, 13.7 % of patients were still alive (just over half of those that survived to discharge). Several other large case series [48–50] included 51, 72, and 110 patients, respectively, and their results are in correlation with those of the previous studies. They reported weaning rates of 52, 56, and 61 % with survival to discharge rates of 33, 40, and 42 %. It is also noteworthy that the benefits of ECMO seem controversial after a 7-day support [50].

In recent series, using Centrimag support, even higher weaning and discharge rates were achieved. Akay et al. [51] supported 22 patients of which 12 were initiated after circulatory arrest in the intensive care unit (ICU) and 10 in the operation room (OR) at the time of CPB weaning. In the latter group 70 % of the patients survived. In another small cohort of 15 patients, supported with the levitronix pump, 12 patients (80 %) were weaned and 7 (46.6 %) were discharged [52].

These data are in contrast with the findings of the Cleveland Clinic [53], where three groups were compared (one with biomedical pump and affinity oxygenator; one with a biomedicus pump and Quadrox D oxygenator; and one with the Rotaflow pump and the Quadrox D oxygenator). Although oxygenator durability was significantly better, they report poor outcomes (27.3 %, 27.3 %, and 33.3 %, respectively). Some comments however need to be made [54]. Only two patients were bridged to VADs, and this was in an high volume center. Secondly, only 17 patients received central ECMO cannulation, meaning that most patients probably received ECMO support after a postoperative evolution towards CS in the ICU. Both items illustrate that early initiation of ECMO support is extremely important, as suggested before.

Like pVADS ECMO is also used in more specific forms of PCCS (right ventricular failure post-LVAD implantation [55, 56], posttransplant right ventricular failure, or primary graft failure [57, 58]).

3 Cardiac Arrest

Mechanical circulatory support has been studied as well for out-of-hospital arrest as in-hospital CA. Because of the uncertainty of neurological outcome, bridging with ECMO to decision, recovery, or bridge to VAD is usually preferred. The data on the use of mechanical support during or immediately after CPR show mixed survival percentages, as most series are very small. In the previously cited review article by Allen et al. [25] survival ranges from 0 to 88 %. If we look at the cited CA series in this review, including >50 patients, survival averages 30 %. In a meta-analysis [59] 141 publications were retrieved when searching the literature. Of these, 11 patient series and 9 case reports were included in the meta-analysis, containing 135 individual cases. The median age was 46 years with a median support time of 54 h. AMI was the leading cause of the arrest and the overall survival to discharge was 40 %. Survival was better in younger patients (<40 years), in patients with shorter support times, and especially after early implantation (<30 min of manual CPR). Although major (esp. neurologic) complications are thought to be high, they are poorly described in the evaluated publications.

Several other large series were published afterwards. In a propensity matched analysis of 406 adult witnessed in-hospital arrests [60], 85 patients were supported with ECMO once CPR lasted more than 10 min. Survival to discharge with minimal neurologic impairment (34 %) was significantly higher (OR 0.17; 95 % confidence interval, 0.04–0.68; $p=0.012$) in the ECMO group, especially in cases with cardiac origins. An analysis of ECPR cases in the ELSO registry [61] from 1992 to 2007 retrieved 297 ECPR cases in 295 patients. Median age was 52 years and the arrest was of cardiac origin in 221 patients (75 %). Survival to discharge was 27 % and brain death occurred in 61 patients (28 %) of the nonsurvivors. In two propensity match analyses from the same group [62, 63] data of 59 patients, supported with ECMO for witnessed in-hospital cardiac arrest of cardiac origin after more than 10 min of CPR, were evaluated. The ECMO supported patients had a higher survival to discharge and a better 1-year survival [62]. When making comparisons in patients with return of spontaneous beating between ECMO support and conventional CPR, no difference in survival to discharge was seen (29 % vs. 22 %, respectively; $p=0.394$).

The survival data of the latter three studies are comparable (somewhere between 25 and 30 %); this in contrast with the outcome data of ECMO-treated patients after out-of-hospital arrest. In a single-center Japanese series of 77 patients [64], approximately 50 % ($n=39$) were out-of-hospital arrests. All outcome data were better in the in-hospital CA group: shorter interval times until the start of ECMO support (25 vs. 59 min; $p<0.001$), higher weaning rates (61 % vs. 36 %; $p = 0.027$), higher 30-day survival (34 % vs. 13 %; $p = 0.03$), and a higher rate of favorable neurologic outcome (26 % vs. 10 %; $p = 0.07$). After multivariate regression analysis no difference in 30-day survival (odds ratio 0.94; $p=0.67$) or 1-year survival (odds ratio 0.99; $p=0.95$) was seen.

When combining all Japanese publications [65] on the use of ECMO in out-of-hospital CA (1983–2008), 1,282 cases were found in 105 reports. Overall survival to discharge was 29.1 % compared to 26.7 for 516 cases (after exclusion of accidental hypothermia cases). In-depth review of 139 cases (of which 88 with arrest of cardiac origin) came up with overall survival to discharge rates of 62.6 and 48.2 % of good neurologic recovery. This is in sharp contrast with the data from a French trial [66] where only 2 out 51 patients (4 %) treated with ECMO after out-of-hospital CA were alive at 28 days. Causes of death were MOF (47 %), brain death (20 %), and refractory hemorrhagic shock (14 %), and 90 % of patients died within 48 h. Possible explanations for the discrepancy are differences in CPR (automatic chest compression), longer no-flow episodes, and a longer interval to the initiation of ECMO in comparison with the Japanese study (>20 min difference).

It is unclear whether there is a cutoff in duration of CPR before extracorporeal rescue. Certainly in children very long episodes of CPR with good outcome after ECMO escape have been described [67]. Based on the poor results several French societies agreed to make an algorithm [68] that excludes ECMO as rescue therapy if a patient was >5 min in no-flow or experienced >100 min of low-flow (with and $ETCO_2$ <10 mmHg after 20 min of CPR).

4 How to Improve Outcomes?

4.1 Prediction of Success, Patient Selection, and Timing

Probably one of the most difficult issues is patient selection and the timing of initiation of mechanical support. Efforts should be made to implant in the "window of opportunity" and to prevent the implantation in futile situations, thereby prolonging the process of dying. An estimation of the chances of survival or the potential for myocardial recovery is important for this.

Although there is a large variation in the used (combination of) clinical, hemodynamical, or laboratory parameters in order to predict outcomes, most experts in the field agree to implant before significant myocardial injury or end-organ damage has developed. In a group of 185 ECMO patients [69] all sorts of cardiogenic shock (and respiratory failure) were included and 21 % of patients were in cardiac arrest, 21.6 % were stable, and 56.8 % were in CS. Mean ECMO support was 4,7 days and weaning was successful in 68 patients (36.7 %) with 38 (20.5 %) being discharged home. Weaning success was significantly lower and early death percentage significantly higher in those in severe shock, with the use of IABP before implantation as an exponent of this.

The early use of cardiac biomarkers in order to predict recovery was studied but did not appear to be useful [70]. In postcardiotomy shock, CKMB index after 48 h can be a predictor of mortality on ECMO support [71]. Others [72] identified age >70 years (p=0.05), duration of support (p=0.017), urine output within initial 24 h (p=0.041), and low cardiac function at institution of support (p=0.004) as risk factors for hospital mortality.

Given the aging of our population, one final point that should be taken into account with regard to patient selection is the elderly population. In chronic heart failure there is more and more literature on the use of VADs as destination therapy in patients that are no longer eligible for transplantation. In acute heart failure, there's hardly any literature on the use of (temporary) mechanical support in older people. In a Japanese series [73] of 91 patients, supported with percutaneous ECMO, 19 patients were older than 75. There was no significant difference in weaning or in survival to discharge and they were able to save the life of almost half of these patients. It is however dangerous to extrapolate these data, since this is a single study indicating elderly benefit in a similar way from ECMO. One possible explanation is the low amount of patients with postcardiotomy support, who usually do worse than other cardiac failure patients [74]. None of the three postcardiotomy ECMO cases in the Japanese cohort survived.

4.2 Percutaneous Devices as a Bridge to Decision

The indications for mechanical circulatory support were classically divided into "bridge to transplantation," "bridge to recovery," or "destination therapy." In the latest decade new terms like "bridge to candidacy" or "bridge to decision" were introduced [75]. The implantation of an ECMO circuit or pVADs reestablishes an appropriate cardiac output and provides time to perform revascularization or to assess neurological status, before deciding on the indications for more complicated assist systems. The latter case is often referred to as a "bridge to bridge." An additional advantage of ECMO is that conversion to an implantable VAD can be done without switching to conventional CPB [76].

Several of the above-described systems have been used as a bridge to an implantable VAD (or directly to heart transplant). The Impella LP 5.0 [77], the TandemHeart [78, 79], and ECMO [80, 81] all have been used for this purpose. In the largest series, which also had the longest follow-up period [80], 131 patients were bridged with ECMO. Thirty-five percent was weaned, 4 % was transplanted, 40 % died, and 21 % (28/131) underwent subsequent VAD implantation. Half of the latter group became long-time survivors with a mean follow-up of 39 months. Besides the previously mentioned advantages of ECMO, the potential for a longer duration of support is becoming very important, given the increased waiting time to transplant (even after High Urgency Request). With the Centrimag levitronix pump, support times up to 6 months have been described [82].

On the one hand the use of percutaneous VADs in the bridge to bridge indication selects patients in a very high risk cohort, thereby preventing moribund of being implanted with expensive devices. Already in 1999 the group of Michigan [81] showed that the 1-year (actuarial) survival from the time of LVAD implant was not statistically different between those patients primarily implanted with an LVAD and those implanted after they survived through ECLS support (75 % vs. 71 %; $p<0.05$). On the other hand, we must conclude that the use of (percutaneous) mechanical support before the implantation significantly worsens survival. If we look at the 1-year actuarial survival of the Michigan cohort from the initiation of mechanical support, survival was significantly lower than in the ECMO group (43 % vs. 75 %). These data are comparable with those recently published by a Japanese group [83]. Survival at 3 years after LVAD implantation was 38 % in patients with preoperative (percutaneous) mechanical support vs. 64 % in those without preoperative mechanical support ($p = 0.015$). Although survival on LVAD was better in those without preoperative devices, the survival rates after transplantation were similar.

Besides the fact that there's a better selection of those shock patients eligible for long-term VAD support, the use of the "bridging" concept also induced a shift from biventricular to univentricular (left-sided) support. In a French group of 71 CS patients implanted between 1996 and 2006 without the pre operative use of percutaneous support, the majority (79 %) required biventricular assist device (BIVAD) support [84]. As previously shown in case reports [33], the early implantation of ECMO (in the catheterization lab) is possible. In one trial [85] ECMO was even initiated before revascularization in the cathlab.

4.3 Technological Improvement

The industry continues to improve its products. ECMO circuits are more and more miniaturized, making interhospital transport possible. The Cardiohelp system (Maquet, Hirrlingen, Germany) is an example of this [86]. Another new feature is the magnetically levitated pump, resulting in lower levels of hemolysis, which allows the pump to run for several weeks [87].

Several other devices (Luo-Ye VAD, Cancion, and PulseCath iVAC) have been investigated [88–90]. The PulseCath iVAC 3 L (PulseCath BV, Amsterdam, Netherlands), at present, can only be placed after cutdown of the subclavian artery. A longer percutaneous version (designed for femoral approach) is under development and awaiting CE mark. This may be a promising device for the future, but no randomized data are published yet. The Chinese device [88] was used in 17 postcardiotomy patients of which 8 were weaned (47.1 %) and 7 discharged (41.2 %). The MOMENUM study [89] investigated acute decompensating chronic heart failure patients with hemodynamic variables as primary outcome parameter. Its use resulted in decreased wedge pressures and increased stroke work.

The PulseCath iVAC device was already used for postcardiotomy right ventricular failure after insertion through the pulmonary artery trunk [91].

4.4 Complications

Although less invasive than the implantable VADs, percutaneous devices and ECMO support also have their complication. Infection, bleeding, and limb ischemia are the common reported complications, as depicted in Fig. 14.5 for pVADs [16]. Reported outcomes and complications in pVAD or ECMO support are summarized in Table 14.4. Unfortunately, there is a large inconsistency in the reporting of complications. Patients with percutaneous support are especially prone to vascular complications. In a trial, investigating the TandemHeart [19], 7 out 21 patients suffered from limb ischemia. In contrast, in the larger series published by Kar et al. [20], only 4 out of 117 patients (3.4 %) developed limb ischemia. But in this series, routine use of peripheral angiography before cannula selection was performed as well as the use of antegrade cannulas for distal perfusion. In a series of 174 ECMO

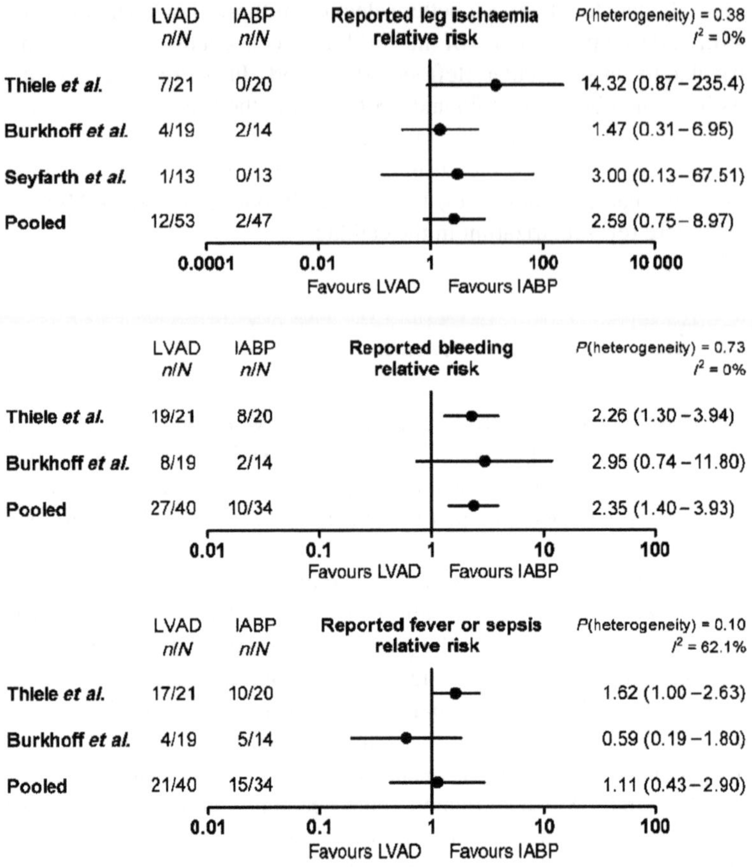

Fig. 14.5 Relative risk of adverse events in meta-analysis of percutaneous ventricular assist devices (pVADs) [16]

patients, of which 143 with arterial cannulation, vascular complications were observed in 17 patients (10 %). In two cases this led to limb amputation [92]. It is noteworthy to say that in all but one of these patients 6F single lumen sheaths were inserted along the arterial cannula in the distal direction of the femoral artery in order to preserve limb perfusion (Fig. 14.6). In the larger French series, ECMO support was complicated by limb ischemia in 19 % of the patients in the Grenoble cohort [27] and 18.5 % in the series at La Pitié (3/21 central ECMO and 12/60 peripheral ECMO) [26]. However, limb ischemia did not seem to impact on the observed mortality rates (both in the TandemHeart study and in the ECMO group). Vascular complications are hardly reported with the Impella, probably due to its smaller catheter size in comparison with the other two devices (13 vs. 15–17 Fr).

It has to be further investigated whether hemolysis is a significant problem associated with Impella use [16]. In ECMO patients the same was true, but since the introduction of low resistance gas exchange devices and the newer generation

Table 14.4 Outcome and complication rate in pVAD and ECMO trials for pVAD (A) and ECMO (B)

(A) pVAD	Seyfarth [19]	Burkhoff [20]	Thiele [21]	Kar [22]	Lamarche (pVAD)[26]	(ECMO)[26]		
Amount of patients	12	19	21	117	19	32		
Median support duration	23 h	2,5 days	3,5 days	5,8 days	63,3 h	46,3 h		
Median VAD flow			3.4 L	3.29 L	3.7 L	4 L		
Weaning percentage		6 (32 %)		70 (59.8 %)	12 (41.4 %)	15 (46.9 %)		
Bridge to LVAD/TX		7 (36 %)/0		31 (26.4 %)/5 (4.2 %)	8 (27.6 %)/0	6 (18.8 %)/3(9.4 %)		
Dead on support	3 (25 %)	6 (32 %)	4 (19 %)					
30-Day mortality		9 (47 %)	9 (43 %)	47 (40.2 %)	11 (37.9 %)	14 (43.8 %)		
Hospital discharge	6 (50 %)	10 (52.6 %			17 (5.86 %)	13 (40.6 %)		
Distal leg ischemia	1 (8 %)	4 (21.1 %)	7 (33 %)	4 (3.41 %)	0	5 (15.6 %)		
Thrombo-embolic event		0 (0 %)	0		1 (3.4 %)	6 (18.8 %)		
Thrombocytopenia		0 (0 %)	8 (38 %)		1 (3.4 %)			
Neurologic dysfunction/ stroke		6 (31.6 %)		8 (6.83 %)				
Systemic infection/sepsis		4 (21.2 %)	17 (81 %)	35 (29.9 %)		3 (9 %)		
Technical failure	0	1 (5.3 %)						
Bleeding	0	8 (42.1 %)	19 (90 %)					
Hepatic dysfunction		3 (15.8 %)	4 (19 %)	31 (26.4 %)[a]				
Renal dysfunction		4 (21.1 %)	4 (19 %)	31 (26.4 %)[a]				
(B) ECMO	Combes [31][b]	Vanzetto [32]	Chung [34]	Loforte [35]	Sakamoto [36]	Doll [65]	Rastan [73]	Hsu [74]
Amount of patients	81	100	134	83	98	219	517	51
Median support duration	7–4 days[b]	57 h	5,1 days	10,9 days	68,9 h	2,8 days	3,28 days	7,5 days
Weaning percentage		33	68 (50.7 %)	44 (60.2 %)	54 (55.1 %)	133 (61.5 %)	327 (63.3 %)	27 (53 %)
Bridge to LVAD/TX	6 (7.4 %)/8 (9.8 %)			3 (4.1 %)/0		8 (4 %)/4 (2 %)		
Dead on support	38 (46.9 %)	40		26 (35.6 %)				

(continued)

Table 14.4 (continued)

Hospital discharge	34 (42 %)	20	57 (42.5 %)	33 (45.2 %)	32 (32.7 %)	52 (24 %)	128 (24.8 %)	17 (33 %)
Technical failure		13	4 (3 %)			48 (22 %)		
Bleeding	27 (33.3 %)	49		37 (44.6 %)[c]				
Need for reintervention						136 (62 %)	425 (82.2 %)	
Neurologic dysfunction	7 (8.6 %)	10				34 (16 %)		3 (5.9 %)
Stroke	7 (8.6 %)	6	17 (12.7 %)		3 (3 %)	24 (11 %)	90 (17.4 %)	
Thrombo-embolic event	7 (8.6 %)	19						
Hemolysis		10						
Thrombocytopenia		9						
Hepatic dysfunction				30 (36.1 %)	17 (17.3 %)			
Renal dysfunction		69		27(32.5 %)	17 (17.3 %)	127 (58 %)	336 (65 %)	38 (75 %)
Dialyze	49 (60.5 %)	20		38 (45.8 %)		122 (56 %)		
Cardiac tamponade				37 (44.6 %)[d]				
Cannulation site infection	10 (16.6 %)				23 (23.5 %)[e]			
Systemic infection/sepsis		9	120 (89.6 %)	11 (13.3 %)	4 (4.1 %)	52 (24 %)		
Distal leg ischemia	15 (18.5 %)	19	4 (3 %)	4 (4.8 %)	7 (7.1 %)	28 (13 %)	28/141 (19.9 %)	8 (15.7 %)
Pulmonary edema	5 (6.2 %)							

Thiele described: 1 case (0.85 %) of atrial perforation. Burkhoff described: cannulation site infection in 3 (15.8 %); hemolysis (free hemoglobin >40) in 1 (5.3 %); right ventricular failure in 1 (5.3 %); cardiac tamponade in 2 (10.5 %); deep venous thrombosis in 2 (10.5 %); arrhythmia in 11 (57.9 %)

[a]Thirty-one cases of multiple organ failure

[b]Seven days in survivors and 4 days in nonsurvivors

[c]Bleeding and tamponade combined

[d]21/81 patients were treated with central ECMO

[e]All cannula site complications

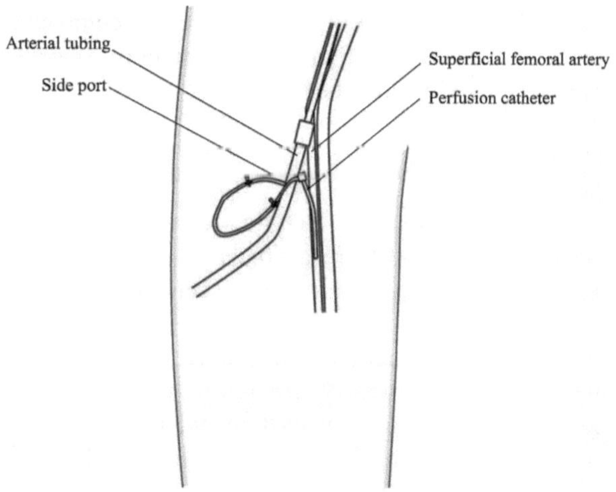

Fig. 14.6 Antegrade limb perfusion by a catheter in the femoral artery, that is connected with the side port of the arterial tubing of the extracorporeal membrane oxygenation (ECMO) circuit [31]

centrifugal problems, hemolysis is lower and prolonged and safer use is possible [93–95].

A specific ECMO-related problem is the distention of the left ventricle and secondary pulmonary edema. Five out of 81 patients developed this complication in the Paris cohort (of which four with peripheral ECMO). This can be prevented or treated in several ways. Cannulation of the pulmonary artery or bi-atrial cannulation can prevent this problem, but this of course is only possible in case of an open chest. Percutaneous options that may help are the transseptal catheter decompression [96] but also IABP and more recently pVADs have been used for this purpose [97–99].

Mortality in these patients is mostly correlated with progressive shock states and multiple organ failure, both of which favor infections and sepsis (in those surviving the initial shock). However, in rare cases death can directly be associated with mechanical support. Massive thrombus formation (as well in the aorta as in the pulmonary artery), whether or not with secondary embolization, has been described during ECMO support [100].

5 Summary

Acute deterioration of chronic heart failure, AMI, and cardiac surgery can all lead to life threatening CS or CA. The largest outcome improvement in the last decades was obtained by early revascularization of AMI patients. Nevertheless mortality remains high in CS (30–40 %). It is in this subset of patients that mechanical circulatory support is often used.

IABP counterpulsation is frequently used and without any doubt it is also the least expensive form of mechanical support. However, in the era of early revascularization (mainly PCI) its level I recommendation for use in cardiogenic shock has become questionable. In parallel pVADs were investigated as an alternative in the first line treatment of infarct-related CS and PCCS. The current evidence shows no outcome benefit over IABP, although hemodynamics were improved. Therefore pVADs need to be evaluated in a large, randomized clinical trial with hard outcomes.

The same counts for ECMO. Although more frequently used than pVADs, randomized data in CS are lacking; this in contrast to the use of veno-venous ECMO in respiratory failure. Furthermore comparisons between ECMO and pVAD are scarce and show no difference in survival. Although more invasive and more prone to complications than IABP or pVAD, the use of ECMO has several advantages: higher flows than most pVADs (with the exception of the Impella 5.0 [101]), the possibility to improve oxygenation, and the ability for longer support. The latter is due to more biocompatible materials, improved oxygenator, and pump technology (e.g., magnetically levitated pumps).

In acute heart failure, the timing of implantation is often postponed to a later time point, as severe CS cases are frequently bridged with ECMO (or pVADs). This prevents the more expensive, implantable VADs to be implanted in futile situations.

The most important (and difficult) decision remains patient selection and the timing of implantation. Earlier implantation becomes generally accepted and seems to improve outcome. But without large, multicenter, randomized trials it will remain difficult to make standardized algorithms that (preoperatively) predict patient risk and make firm recommendations for the type of device and the time of implantation.

References

1. Hochman JS et al (1999) Early revascularization in acute myocardial infarction complicated by cardiogenic shock. N Engl J Med 341:625–634
2. Goldberg RJ, Spencer FA, Gore JM, Lessard D, Yarzebski J (2009) Thirty-year trends (1975–2005) in the magnitude of, management of, and hospital death rates associated with cardiogenic shock in patients with acute myocardial infarction: a population-based perspective. Circulation 119:1211–1219
3. Hochman JS et al (2006) Early revascularization and long-term survival in cardiogenic shock complicating acute myocardial infarction. JAMA 295:2511–2515
4. Babaev A et al (2005) Trends in management and outcomes of patients with acute myocardial infarction complicated by cardiogenic shock. JAMA 294:448–454
5. Kantrowitz A et al (1968) Initial clinical experience with intraaortic balloon pumping in cardiogenic shock. JAMA 203:113–118
6. Antman EM et al (2004) ACC/AHA guidelines for the management of patients with ST-elevation myocardial infarction—executive summary: a report of the American College of Cardiology/American Heart Association Task Force on Practice Guideline. Circulation 110:588–636
7. SJauw KD et al (2009) A systematic review and meta-analysis of intra-aortic balloon pump therapy in ST elevation myocardial infarction: should we change the guidelines? Eur Heart J 30:459–468

8. Sanborn TA et al (2000) Impact of thrombolysis, intra-aortic balloon pump counterpulsation, and their combination in cardiogenic shock complicating acute myocardial infarction: a report from the SHOCK Trial Registry. Should we emergently revascularize Occluded Coronaries for cardiogenic shock? J Am Coll Cardiol 36(3 Suppl A):1123–1129
9. Barron HV et al (2001) The use of intra-aortic balloon counterpulsation in patients with cardiogenic shock complicating acute myocardial infarction: data from the National Registry for Myocardial Infarction 2. Am Heart J 141(6):933–939
10. Valk SD et al (2011) Encouraging survival rates in patients with acute myocardial infarction treated with an intra-aortic balloon pump. Neth Heart J 19:112–118
11. Ohman EM et al (2005) Thrombolysis and counterpulsation to improve survival in myocardial infarction complicated by hypotension and suspected cardiogenic shock or heart failure: results of the TACTICS Trial. J Thromb Thrombolysis 19(1):33–39
12. Prodzinsky R et al (2010) Intra-aortic balloon counterpulsation in patients with acute myocardial infarction complicated by cardiogenic shock: the prospective, randomized IABP SHOCK Trial for attenuation of multiorgan dysfunction syndrome. Crit Care Med 38:152–160
13. Unverzagt S et al (2011) Intra-aortic balloon pump counterpulsation (IABP) for myocardial infarction complicated by cardiogenic shock. Cochrane Database Syst Rev 6(7):CD007398
14. Thiele H, Allam B, Chatellier G, Schuler G, Lafont A (2010) Shock in AMI: the Cape Horn for trials. Eur Heart J 31:1828–1835
15. Basra SS, Loyalka P, Kar B (2011) Current status of percutaneous ventricular assist devices for cardiogenic shock. Curr Opin Cardiol 26:548–554
16. Cheng JM et al (2009) Percutaneous left ventricular assist devices vs. intra-aortic balloon pump counterpulsation for treatment of cardiogenic shock: a meta-analysis of controlled trials. Eur Heart J 30:2102–2108
17. Seyfarth M et al (2008) A randomized clinical trial to evaluate the safety and efficacy of a percutaneous left ventricular assist device versus intra-aortic balloon pumping for treatment of cardiogenic shock caused by myocardial infarction. J Am Coll Cardiol 52:1584–1588
18. Burkhof D et al (2006) A randomized multicenter clinical study to evaluate the safety and efficacy of the TandemHeart percutaneous ventricular assist device versus conventional therapy with intraaortic balloon pumping for treatment of cardiogenic shock. Am Heart J 152:469.e1–e8
19. Thiele H et al (2005) Randomized comparison of intra-aortic balloon support with a percutaneous left ventricular assist device in patients with revascularized acute myocardial infarction complicated by cardiogenic shock. Eur Heart J 26:1276–1283
20. Kar B, Gregori ID, Basra SS, Idelchik GM, Loyalka P (2011) The percutaneous ventricular assist device in severe refractory cardiogenic shock. J Am Coll Cardiol 57:688–696
21. Lamarche Y et al (2011) Comparative outcomes in cardiogenic shock patients managed with Impella microaxial pump or extracorporeal life support. J Thorac Cardiovasc Surg 142:60–65
22. Potapov EV et al (2010) Prediction of survival in patients with cardiogenic shock and multiorgan failure treated with biventricular assist device. ASAIO J 56:273–278
23. Hill JD et al (1972) Prolonged extracorporeal oxygenation for acute post-traumatic respiratory failure (shock-lung syndrome). Use of the Bramson membrane lung. N Engl J Med 286(12):629–634
24. Nichol G, Karmy-Jones R, Salerno C, Cantore L, Becker L (2006) Systematic review of percutaneous cardiopulmonary bypass for cardiac arrest or cardiogenic shock states. Resuscitation 70:381–394
25. Allen S, Holena D, Mccunn M, Kohl B, Sarani B (2011) A review of the fundamental principles and evidence base in the use of extracorporeal membrane oxygenation (ECMO) in critically ill adult patients. J Intensive Care Med 26(1):13–26
26. Combes A et al (2008) Outcomes and long-term quality-of-life of patients supported by extracorporeal membrane oxygenation for refractory cardiogenic shock. Crit Care Med 36:1404–1411

27. Vanzetto G et al (2009) Percutaneous extracorporeal life support in acute severe hemodynamic collapses: single-centre experience in 100 consecutive patients. Can J Cardiol 25(6):179–186
28. Liden H, Wiklund L, Haraldsson A, Berglin E, Hultman J, Dellgren G (2009) Temporary circulatory support with extra corporeal membrane oxygenation in adults with refractory cardiogenic shock. Scand Cardiovasc J 43(4):226–232
29. Chung SY et al (2012) Outcome of patients with profound cardiogenic shock after cardiopulmonary resuscitation and prompt extracorporeal membrane oxygenation support. A single-center observational study. Circ J 76(6):1385–1392
30. Loforte A et al (2012) Peripheral extracorporeal membrane oxygenation system as salvage treatment of patients with refractory cardiogenic shock: preliminary outcome evaluation. Artif Organs 36(3):E53–E61
31. Sakamoto S, Taniguchi N, Nakajima S, Takahashi A (2012) Extracorporeal life support for cardiogenic shock or cardiac arrest due to acute coronary syndrome. Ann Thorac Surg 94(1):1–7
32. Garatti A et al (2007) Mechanical circulatory support for cardiogenic shock complicating acute myocardial infarction: an experimental and clinical review. ASAIO J 53:278–287
33. Sheu JJ et al (2010) Early extracorporeal membrane oxygenator-assisted primary percutaneous coronary intervention improved 30-day clinical outcomes in patients with ST-segment elevation myocardial infarction complicated with profound cardiogenic shock. Crit Care Med 38:1810–1817
34. Kim H et al (2012) Efficacy of veno-arterial extracorporeal membrane oxygenation in acute myocardial infarction with cardiogenic shock. Resuscitation 83(8):971–975
35. Chung ES et al (2011) Results of extracorporeal membrane oxygenation (ECMO) support before coronary reperfusion in cardiogenic shock with acute myocardial infarction. Korean J Thorac Cardiovasc Surg 44:273–278
36. Aziz TA et al (2010) Initial experience with CentriMag extracorporal membrane oxygenation for support of critically ill patients with refractory cardiogenic shock. J Heart Lung Transplant 29:66–71
37. Peek G et al (2009) Efficacy and economic assessment of conventional ventilator support versus extracorporeal membrane oxygenation for severe adult respiratory failure (CESAR): a multicenter randomized controlled trial. Lancet 374(9698):1351–1363
38. Golding LA (1991) Postcardiotomy mechanical support. Semin Thorac Cardiovasc Surg 3(1):29–32
39. Sylvin EA, Stern DR, Goldstein DJ (2010) Mechanical support for postcardiotomy cardiogenic shock: has progress been made? J Card Surg 25:442–454
40. Hausmann H et al (2002) Prognosis after the implantation of an intra-aortic balloon pump in cardiac surgery calculated with a new score. Circulation 106:I203–I206
41. Griffith BP et al (2013) The RECOVER I: a multicenter prospective study of Impella 5.0/LD for postcardiotomy circulatory support. J Thorac Cardiovasc Surg 145(2):548–554
42. Pitsis AA et al (2007) Feasibility study of a temporary percutaneous left ventricular assist device in cardiac surgery. Ann Thorac Surg 84(6):1993–1999
43. Bennett MT et al (2010) The use of the Impella RD as a bridge to recovery for right ventricular dysfunction after cardiac transplantation. Innovations (Phila) 5(5):369–371
44. Brinkman WT et al (2009) Role of a percutaneous ventricular assist device in decision making for a cardiac transplant program. Ann Thorac Surg 8:1462–1467
45. Rajagopal V, Steahr G, Wilmer CI, Raval NY (2010) A novel percutaneous mechanical biventricular bridge to recovery in severe cardiac allograft rejection. J Heart Lung Transplant 29:93–95
46. Doll N et al (2004) Five-year results of 219 consecutive patients treated with extracorporeal membrane oxygenation for refractory postoperative cardiogenic shock. Ann Thorac Surg 77:151–157

47. Rastan AJ et al (2010) Early and late outcomes of 517 consecutive adult patients treated with extracorporeal membrane oxygenation for refractory postcardiotomy cardiogenic shock. J Thorac Cardiovasc Surg 139:302–311
48. Hsu PS et al (2010) Extracorporeal membrane oxygenation for refractory cardiogenic shock after cardiac surgery: predictors of early mortality and outcome from 51 adult patients. Eur J Cardiothorac Surg 37:328–333
49. Wu MY et al (2009) Postcardiotomy extracorporeal life support in adults: the optimal duration of bridging to recovery. ASAI0 J 55:608–613
50. Wu MY et al (2010) Using extracorporeal life support to resuscitate adult postcardiotomy cardiogenic shock: treatment strategies and predictors of short-term and midterm survival. Resuscitation 81:1111–1116
51. Akay MH, Gregoric ID, Radovancevic R, Cohn WE, Frazier OH (2011) Timely use of a CentriMag heart assist device improves survival in postcardiotomy cardiogenic shock. J Card Surg 26:548–552
52. Russo CF et al (2010) Veno-arterial extracorporeal membrane oxygenation using Levitronix centrifugal pump as bridge to decision for refractory cardiogenic shock. J Thorac Cardiovasc Surg 140:1416–1421
53. Pokersnik JA, Buda T, Bashour A, Gonzalez-STawinski GV (2012) Have changes in EMO technology impacted outcomes in adult patients developing postcardiotomy cardiogenic shock? J Card Surg 27:246–252
54. Rao V (2012) Defying death: an new ECMO technology improve the outcomes of postcardiotomy shock? J Card Surg 27:253–254
55. Haneya A et al (2011) Successful use of temporary right ventricular support to avoid implantation of biventricular long-term assist device: a transcutaneous approach. ASAIO J 57:274–277
56. Loforte A, Montalto A, Della Monica PL, Musumeci F (2010) Simultaneous temporary CentriMag right ventricular assist device placement in HeartMate II left ventricular assist system recipients at high risk of right ventricular failure. Interact Cardiovasc Thorac Surg 10:847–850
57. Leprince P et al (2005) Peripheral extracorporeal membrane oxygenation (ECMO) in patients with posttransplant cardiac graft failure. Transplant Proc 37:2879–2880
58. Kittleson MM et al (2011) Heart transplant recipients supported with extracorporeal membrane oxygenation: outcomes from a single-center experience. J Heart Lung Transplant 30(11):1250–1256
59. Cardarelli MG, Young AJ, Griffith B (2009) Use of extracorporeal membrane oxygenation for adults in cardiac arrest (E-CPR): a meta-analysis of observational studies. ASAIO J 55:581–586
60. Shin TG et al (2011) Extracorporeal cardiopulmonary resuscitation in patients with inhospital cardiac arrest: a comparison with conventional cardiopulmonary resuscitation. Crit Care Med 39:1–7
61. Thiagarajan RR et al (2009) Extracorporeal membrane oxygenation to support cardiopulmonary resuscitation in adults. Ann Thorac Surg 87:778–785
62. Chen YS et al (2008) Cardiopulmonary resuscitation with assisted extracorporeal life-support versus conventional cardiopulmonary resuscitation in adults with in-hospital cardiac arrest: an observational study and propensity analysis. Lancet 372:554–561
63. Lin JW et al (2010) Comparing the survival between extracorporeal rescue and conventional resuscitation in adult in-hospital cardiac arrests: propensity analysis of three-year data. Resuscitation 81:796–803
64. Kagawa E et al (2010) Assessment of outcomes and differences between in- and out-of-hospital cardiac arrest patients treated with cardiopulmonary resuscitation using extracorporeal life support. Resuscitation 81:968–973
65. Morimura N et al (2011) Extracorporeal cardiopulmonary resuscitation for out-of-hospital cardiac arrest: a review of the Japanese literature. Resuscitation 82:10–14

66. Le Guen M et al (2011) Extracorporeal life support following out-of-hospital refractory cardiac arrest. Crit Care 15:R29
67. Kelly RB, Porter PA, Meier AH, Myers JL, Thomas NJ (2005) Duration of cardiopulmonary resuscitation before extracorporeal rescue: how long is not long enough? ASAIO J 51:665–667
68. Riou B et al (2009) Recommendations sur les indications de l'assistance circulatoire dans le traitement des arrest cardiaques réfractaires. Ann Fr An Rean 28:182–186
69. Lee SH, Chung CH, Lee JW, Jung SH, Choo SJ (2012) Factors predicting early- and long-term survival in patients undergoing extracorporeal membrane oxygenation (ECMO). J Card Surg 27:255–263
70. Luyt CE et al (2012) Usefulness of cardiac biomarkers to predict cardiac recovery in patients on extracorporeal membrane oxygenation support for refractory cardiogenic shock. J Crit Care 27(5):524.e7–e14
71. Zhang R et al (2006) Creatine kinase isoenzyme MB relative index as predictor of mortality on extracorporeal membrane oxygenation support for postcardiotomy cardiogenic shock in adult patients. Eur J Cardiothorac Surg 30:617–620
72. Murashita T et al (2004) Outcome of the perioperative use of percutaneous cardiopulmonary support for adult cardiac surgery: factors affecting hospital mortality. Artif Organs 28(2):189–195
73. Saito S et al (2007) Is extracorporeal life support contraindicated in elderly patients? Ann Thorac Surg 83:140–145
74. Franke UFW (2007) Invited commentary. Ann Thorac Surg 83:145
75. Stewart GC, Givertz MM (2012) Mechanical circulatory support for advanced heart failure. Patients and technology in evolution. Circulation 125:1304–1315
76. Haneya A et al (2012) Ventricular assist device implantation in patients on percutaneous extracorporeal life support without switching to conventional cardiopulmonary bypass system. Eur J Cardiothorac Surg 41(6):1366–1370
77. Samoukovic G, Rosu C, Giannetti N, Cecere R (2009) The Impella LP 5.0 as a bridge to long-term circulatory support. Interact Cardiovasc Thorac Surg 8:682–683
78. Idelchik GM et al (2008) Use of the percutaneous left ventricular assist device in patients with refractory cardiogenic shock as a bridge to long-term left ventricular assist device implantation. J Heart Lung Transplant 27:106–111
79. Gregoric ID et al (2008) The TandemHeart as a bridge to a long-term axial-flow left ventricular assist device. Tex Heart Inst J 35(2):125–129
80. Hoefer D et al (2006) Outcome evaluation of the bridge to bridge concept in patients with cardiogenic shock. Ann Thorac Surg 82:28–34
81. Pagani FD et al (1999) Extracorporeal life support to left ventricular assist device bridge to heart transplant. A strategy to optimize survival and resource utilization. Circulation 100(Suppl II):206–210
82. Barbone A et al (2012) 6 months of "temporary" support by Levitronix left ventricular assist device. Artif Organs 36(7):639–642
83. Toda K et al (2012) Impact of preoperative percutaneous cardiopulmonary support on outcome following left ventricular assist device implantation. Circ J 76:88–95
84. Kirsch M et al (2008) Impact of preoperative hemodynamic support on early outcome in patients assisted with paracorporeal Thoratec ventricular assist device. Eur J Cardiothorac Surg 34:262–267
85. Lee MS, Pessegueiro A, Tobis J (2008) The role of extracorporeal membrane oxygenation in emergent percutaneous coronary intervention for myocardial infarction complicated by cardiogenic shock and cardiac arrest. J Invasive Cardiol 20:E269–E272
86. Philipp A et al (2011) First experience with the ultra compact mobile extracorporeal membrane oxygenation system cardiohelp in interhospital transport. Interact Cardiovasc Thorac Surg 12:978–981
87. Potapov EV, Krabatsch T, Venturo HO, Htzer R (2011) Advances in mechanical circulatory support: year in review. J Heart Lung Transplant 30(5):487–493

88. Xiao XJ et al (2009) The short-term pulsatile ventricular assist device for postcardiotomy cardiogenic shock: a clinical trial in China. Artif Organs 33(4):373–377
89. Zile MR et al (2010) Progressive improvement in cardiac performance with continuous flow augmentation (aortic flow therapy) in patients hospitalized with severe heart failure: results of the Multicenter Trial of the Orqis Medical Cancion System for the Enhanced Treatment of Heart Unresponsive to Medical Therapy (MOMENTUM). J Heart Lung Transplant 29:86–92
90. Niclauss L, Segesser LK (2011) PulseCath iVAC 3LTM hemodynamic performance for simple assisted flow. Interact Cardiovasc Thorac Surg 12(6):912–913
91. Arrigoni SC, Kuijpers M, Mecozzi G, Mariani MA (2011) PulseCath as a right ventricular assist device. Interact Cardiovasc Thorac Surg 12:891–894
92. Bisdas T et al (2011) Vascular complications in patients undergoing femoral cannulation for extracorporeal membrane oxygenation support. Ann Thorac Surg 92:626–631
93. Toomasian JM, Barlett RH (2011) Hemolysis and ECMO pumps in the 21st century. Perfusion 26(1):5–6
94. Byrnes J et al (2011) Hemolysis during cardiac extracorporeal membrane oxygenation: a case-control comparison of roller pumps and centrifugal pumps in a pediatric population. ASAIO J 57(5):456–461
95. Yu K et al (2011) Clinical evaluation of two different extracorporeal membrane oxygenation systems: a single center report. Artif Organs 35(7):733–737
96. Schwartz MF, Smith F, Byrum CJ, Alfieris GM (2012) Transseptal catheter decompression of the left ventricle during extracorporeal membrane oxygenation. Pediatr Cardiol 33:185–187
97. Vlasselaers D, Desmet M, Desmet L, Meyns B, Dens J (2006) Ventricular unloading with a miniature axial flow pump in combination with extracorporeal membrane oxygenation. Intensive Care Med 32:329–333
98. Koeckert MS, Jorde UP, Naka Y, Moses JW, Takayama H (2011) Impella LP 2.5 for left ventricular unloading during venoarterial extracorporeal membrane oxygenation support. J Card Surg 26:666–668
99. Anastasiadis K, Chalvatzoulis O, Antonitsis P, Tossios P, Papakonstantinou C (2011) Left ventricular decompression during peripheral extracorporeal membrane oxygenation support with the use of the novel iVAC pulsatile paracorporeal assist device. Ann Thorac Surg 92:2257–2259
100. Leontiadis E, Koertke H, Bairaktaris A, Koerfer R (2010) Thrombosis of the ascending aorta during mechanical circulatory support in a patient with cardiogenic shock. Interact Cardiovasc Thorac Surg 11:510–511
101. Engström AE et al (2011) The Impella 2.5 and 5.0 devices for ST-elevation myocardial infarction patients presenting with severe and profound cardiogenic shock: the Academic Medical Center intensive care unit experience. Crit Care Med 39:2072–2079

Chapter 15
Left Ventricular Assist Devices: From Bridge to Transplant to Destination Therapy

Lars H. Lund

Abstract In heart failure, neurohormonal antagonists, cardiac resynchronization therapy, and implantable cardioverter defibrillators have improved prognosis dramatically but have also increased the number of patients living with advanced refractory heart failure with poor prognosis and quality of life. For these patients, heart transplantation improves symptoms and prognosis, but organ supply is limited and waiting times are increasing.

Therefore, left ventricular assist devices (LVADs) are well suited to fill the growing need for advance heart failure therapy. LVADs are used to bridge patients to transplantation or increasingly as destination therapy. With improved technology, patient selection, and patient care, 1-year survival in properly selected patients has increased from 50 % to nearly 90 % over the last decade.

However, LVADs are still underutilized. The main reason is lack of awareness among referring cardiologists. This chapter will review LVAD therapy and patient selection from the cardiologist's perspective.

1 Background: Advanced Heart Failure—A Growing Pandemic

Heart Failure (HF) is a growing pandemic with high morbidity and mortality. The incidence in Western countries is approximately 0.5 % annually [1–3]. The prevalence of known HF is approximately 2–3 % [4, 5] and of undiagnosed HF estimated at another 2 %. At age 40, the lifetime risk of HF is one in five [6] and a diagnosis

L.H. Lund, M.D., Ph.D. (✉)
Department of Medicine, Karolinska Institutet, 171 77 Stockholm, Sweden

Department of Cardiology, Karolinska University Hospital, 171 77 Stockholm, Sweden
e-mail: Lars.Lund@karolinska.se

J. Bartunek and M. Vanderheyden (eds.), *Translational Approach to Heart Failure*,
DOI 10.1007/978-1-4614-7345-9_15, © Springer Science+Business Media New York 2013

of HF entails higher mortality than a diagnosis of cancer [7], with 1-year mortality ranging from 5 % to over 75 % depending on HF severity [8–11]. HF is a major source of disability, and is the most common cause of hospitalization in patients over age 65, accounting for over 20 % of all hospitalizations in this patient group [7], and HF accounts for 2 % of all healthcare expenditures [12]. With improving survival after myocardial infarction and in HF, the prevalence of HF has increased and is projected to continue to increase [8, 13]. Finally, the prevalence of HF increases with age [8] and the proportion of the Western population over age 65 is projected to increase from 12 % in the year 2000 to 20 % in the year 2030 [14]. Thus we are heading toward an enormous public health epidemic of HF.

While HF with preserved ejection fraction (HFPEF) is becoming increasingly recognized, HF with reduced ejection fraction (HFREF) is still more common, more severe, and associated with higher morbidity and mortality, especially cardiac related [15]. HFPEF is mainly a disease of the elderly, there is no evidence-based therapy, and patients are, with rare exceptions, not candidates for left ventricular assist device (LVAD) or heart transplantation (HTx). This chapter will focus on HFREF and for the remainder of this chapter references to HF will entail HFREF only.

Advanced HF affects 10 % of the HF population and is associated with a dismal quality of life, recurrent hospitalizations and a mortality of up to 50 % at 1 year [8–10, 16]. The proportion of HF patients that become truly refractory are estimated at up to 5 % [5]. Medical arms in LVAD trials have generally been inotrope dependent and have had 1-year mortalities of over 75 % [17, 18].

These gloomy figures may be surprising in light of the remarkable success of evidence-based interventions for cardiovascular disease and HF over the last decades. Between 1970 and 2000, Western population-wide life expectancy increased by 6 years, more than 4 of which were attributed to reduced cardiovascular mortality [19]. Since the 1980s, randomized controlled trials in HFREF have demonstrated that drugs (angiotensin converting enzyme [ACE] inhibitors, β-blockers, aldosterone antagonists and angiotensin receptor blockers [ARBs]) and electrical device therapy (cardiac resynchronization therapy [CRT] and implantable cardioverter defibrillator [ICD]) reduce mortality by 10–40 % [12, 20]. Indeed, mortality in HF has declined consistently between 1950 and 2000 [2, 21]. However, since 2000, improvements in prognosis may be leveling off [22, 23]. Furthermore, the success of above interventions are keeping patients with advanced HF alive and increasing the patient pool with severe HF. For the 5–10 % of HF patients with advanced disease, the outlook today is poor [5, 24].

Thus, there is a great unmet need for interventions in severe HF. Public awareness and perception of the prevalence and dangers of cardiovascular disease are much lower than of cancer, and the US National Institutes of Health (NIH) estimated 2011 research spending on heart disease was 1.3 Billion USD, only about 1/4 of the 5.8 Billion USD spent on cancer (http://report.nih.gov/rcdc/categories/; accessed 18 January 2012). Patients with HF underestimate their risk of death and are unlikely to enquire for additional interventions or resources from society [25, 26]. Physicians are less likely to share prognostic information with patients when there is uncertainty [27], such as in advanced HF. If properly informed of their prognosis and options, patients prefer LVAD implantation if their expected mortality is within 6–12 months or their activity is limited to less than one block [28]. HTx is a great option for patients with advanced HF who qualify, but the number of transplants worldwide continue to decrease from a peak of 4,500 in the mid-1990s to just over 3,000 today [29]. Waiting lists are growing, organs are increasingly going to patients on high-urgency lists, and in many countries the hopes for receiving a heart if not inotrope or mechanical device dependent are small to nil, especially in larger blood group 0 patients. Even for those who do receive a heart, quality of life and prognosis is imperfect; the 50 % 10-year survival after HTx has improved only marginally over the last 10 years [29].

In contrast, mechanical circulatory support (MCS) and specifically LVAD technology, patient selection, patient care, and cost-effectiveness are continually improving. The near 90 % survival at 1 year is now approaching that after HTx. The number of HTx patients that are bridged with an LVAD is increasing [29]. Patients still generally prefer HTx over permanent LVAD (destination therapy), but for patients who do not qualify for HTx, destination therapy is an increasingly attractive option and it is not inconceivable that it will be preferred over HTx in the future. Thus, LVADs are set become standard of care in advance heart failure [5, 24, 30–32]. Yet, LVAD therapy has still to gain widespread acceptance and penetrate the cardiology field, and is severely underutilized, with up to 300,000 theoretical candidates in the US alone [5]. In all patients with reduced EF who remain in NYHA III-IV despite optimal medical therapy and CRT/ICD, an LVAD should be considered a potential treatment option.

Key Points

- Advanced refractory HF is a growing epidemic.
- LVADs are underutilized. The main reason is lack of awareness among internists and cardiologists.
- All patients with reduced EF and NYHA III-IV should be assessed for LVAD candidacy. Most will not be candidates but many will be.

Further Information

- The growing HF epidemic: [1, 7, 8, 19]
- LVAD underutilization: [5, 24, 32]

2 History, Technology, and Outcomes

2.1 LVAD History

Following the development of experimental models in the early twentieth century, the earliest type of MCS was the cardiopulmonary bypass, first used in 1953 by Gibbon [33]. Failure to wean patients off cardiopulmonary bypass provided an impetus for designing more sophisticated systems for use over days rather than hours. In 1961, Clauss et al. published experience with arterial counterpulsation [34], the basis for the current intra-aortic balloon pump, and already in 1963, Liotta implanted the first true LVAD, for management of post-cardiotomoy shock after valve surgery [35]. The patient was supported for 10 days and myocardial function recovered.

The US National Heart, Lung and Blood Institute (NHLBI) total artificial heart (TAH) program, initiated in 1964, and extension to an LVAD program, in 1972, set the stage for the development of longer-term, durable devices. In 1969, Cooley—allegedly covertly—implanted the first TAH, developed by DeBakey and Liotta. This provided 64 h of support until transplantation [36]. Heart transplantation, first performed by Barnard in 1967 but widely accepted after the introduction of cyclosporine-based immunosuppression in 1980, introduced a need to keep patients alive while awaiting an organ and provided a growing demand for MCS.

Since then numerous types of devices for different but overlapping purposes have been developed. Durable mechanical support, the vast majority in the LVAD configuration [37], have been implanted in over 30,000 patients worldwide, and LVADs are the focus of this chapter. The TAH, such as the CardioWest (SynCardia Systems Inc.) or Abiocor (Abiomed Inc.) consists of two volume displacement chambers that actually replace the native left and right ventricles, which are removed, and is used for patients with severe biventricular failure as a bridge to transplant. Extracorporeal volume displacement pumps, such as the Thoratec Inc. PVAD, Abiomed Inc. AB5000 or Berlin Heart Inc. Excor can be used a left or right VAD or with two concurrent devices, as a BiVAD, as a bridge to decision, recovery or transplant also in patients with severe, generally biventricular, failure. Increasingly however, patients with the most severe heart failure (INTERMACS 1, see below) or even cardiac arrest are being rescued with bridge to decision strategies using short-term devices such as the Centrimag (Thoratec Inc.), CadioHelp (Maquet Inc.), or TandemHeart (CardiacAssist Inc.), which are magnetically levitated extracorporeal centrifugal continuous flow pumps that can be used as VADs in any configuration or as extracorporeal membrane oxygenation (ECMO) for weeks to months. All these systems can be used in the short (days) to medium (months) term to rescue severe biventricular failure or cardiac arrest, and this indication receives a IC recommendation from the European Society of Cardiology (ESC) guidelines [12]. However, they serve only as a bridge to more definitive therapy, such as HTx or an implantable durable LVAD. Short- and medium-term support will not be discussed further in this chapter.

Key Points

- Mechanical circulatory support was pioneered in the 1950s
- Wide acceptance of heart transplantation in the 1980s introduced a need to keep patients alive while awaiting an organ

Further Information

- LVAD history: [32]

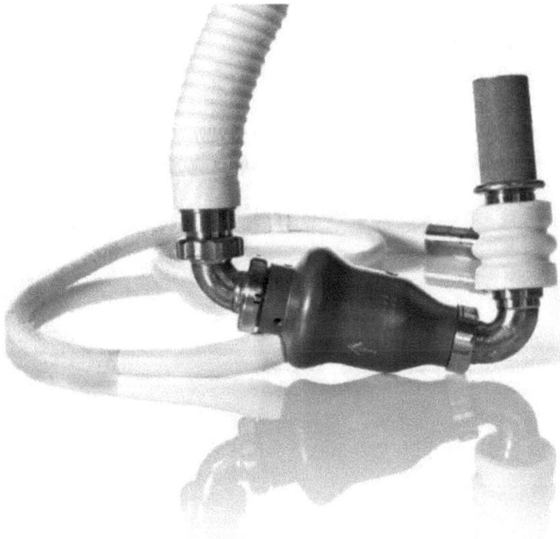

Fig. 15.1 Thoratec HeartMate II. With permission, Thoratec Inc.

2.2 *LVAD Technology*

Early LVAD designs utilized biocompatible polymer materials and bladder and pusher-plate designs learned from artificial valve and TAH development. In 1984, the Novacor, the first electrically powered implantable device successfully bridged a patient to HTx [38], in 1988, patients with implantable LVADs were discharged to wait for a donor heart, and in 1991, the first HeartMate vented electric (VE) was implanted in a patient who survived 503 days before suffering an embolic stroke [39]. In 1994, the HeartMate VE LVAD was the first implantable device to receive approval from the US Food and Drug Administration (FDA) as a bridge to transplantation and in 2002 it was approved for destination therapy.

The HeartMate VE and XVE and the Novacor were first generation volume displacement pumps, with pusher plates and inflow and outflow valves. They were bulky, placed in the abdomen, and required air vents and compliance chambers. Second and third generation LVADs utilize impeller or centrifugal rotary motor designs that are mechanically, magnetically or hydro-suspended, and provide continuous/axial flow. Generally, the pump is connected to the LV apex via an inflow cannula and to the ascending aorta via an outflow cannula. There is a driveline from the pump that exits the skin through the abdomen and connects to an external controller, which in turn connects to a power source (Figs. 15.1, 15.2, 15.3, 15.4, 15.5, and 15.6).

The second generation devices include the HeartMate II (Thoratec Inc.), the Jarvik 2000 (Jarvik Heart Inc.), and the MicroMed-DeBakey (MicroMed Inc.). They have an internal impeller rotor that is suspended by contact, blood immersed bearings. Third generation devices are so called because of a "non-contact" bearing

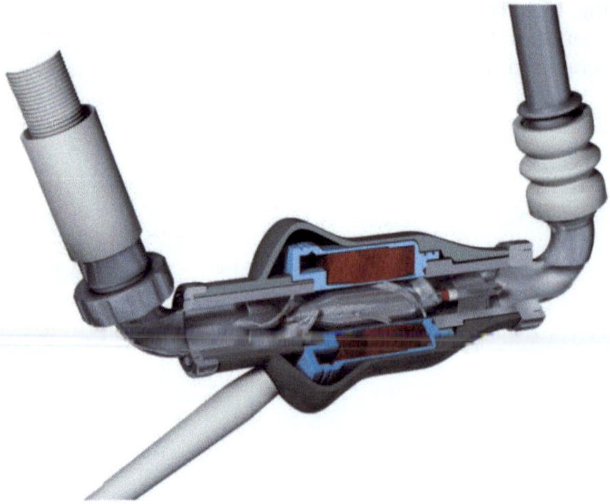

Fig. 15.2 Thoratec HeartMate II internal view. With permission, Thoratec. Inc.

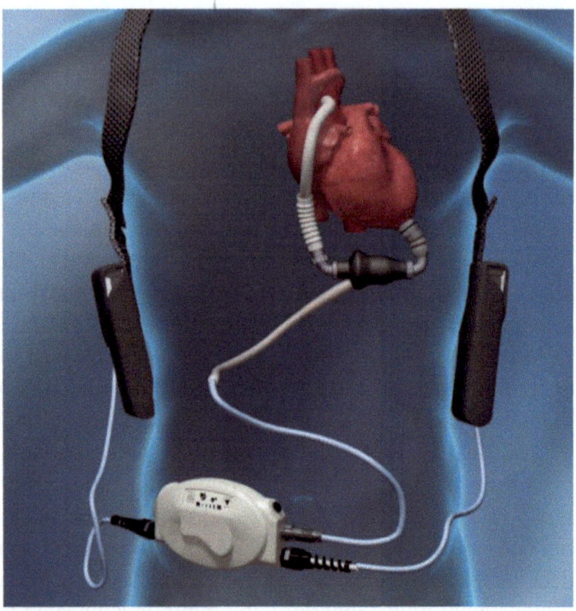

Fig. 15.3 Thoratec HeartMate II in situ. With permission, Thoratec Inc.

design. The rotor is magnetically and hydrodynamically levitated which eliminates all contact bearings and thus reduces potential friction and wear. Examples include the HeartWare HVAD and the DuraHeart (Terumo Heart Inc.) which utilize centrifugal rotors, and the Berlin Heart Incor which utilizes and impeller. The term "bearing-less" is often applied to third generation devices but this is technically incorrect and merely as matter of semantics [40], and whether third generation design improves outcomes has yet to be shown.

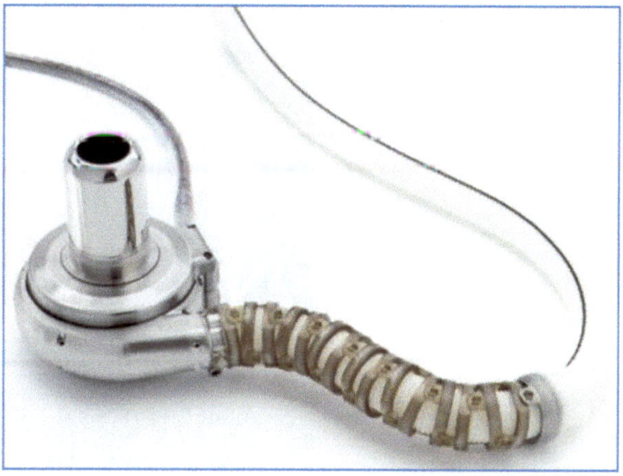

Fig. 15.4 HeartWare HVAD. With permission, HeartWare Inc.

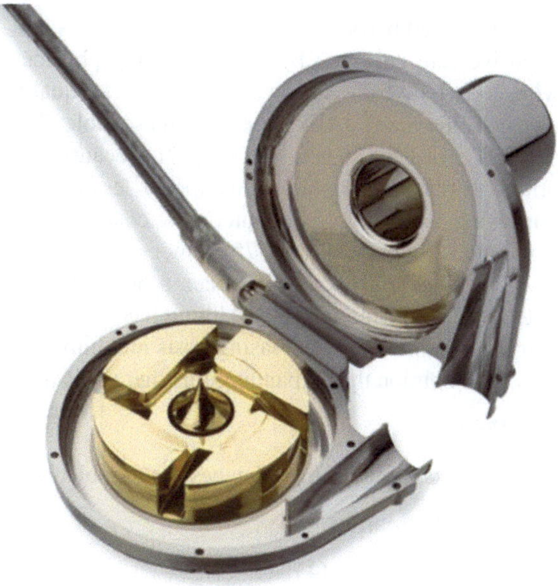

Fig. 15.5 HeartWare HVAD internal components. With permission, HeartWare Inc.

Because they have non-pulsatile flow, second and third generation LVADs were initially viewed with skepticism. However, their smaller size, limited blood contacting area, fewer moving parts, and lack of valves, air vents and compliance chambers provide for longer durability with lower risk for thrombus formation, thromboembolism, infection and malfunction, minimizes complications and allow support for many years and potentially decades. Continuous flow LVADs are now standard of care and the devices currently most used today, the Thoratec HeartMate II and Heartware HVAD, have been implanted in over 13,000 (number from Thoratec, Inc.) and 2,000 patients (number from Heartware, Inc.), respectively. The history and technology of LVADs have been reviewed in greater detail [40–46].

Fig. 15.6 HeartWare HVAD in situ. With permission, HeartWare Inc.

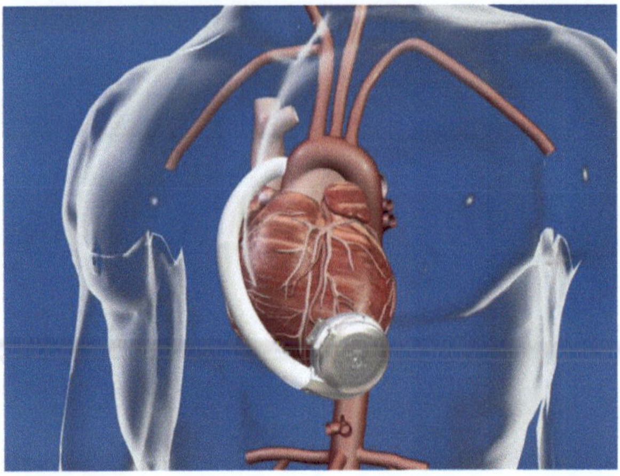

A perceived barrier to extending LVAD use is cost. The high up front device and intensive care costs are by many referring physicians considered prohibitive, but with good long-term survival with improved quality of life, the cost per quality-adjusted life year (QALY) becomes reasonable. The best estimates suggest a cost per QALY of US $36,000–86,000 [47]. Because of the limited duration of support, bridge to transplant applications appear less cost-effective [48]. With continually improving technology and outcomes, cost-effectiveness is expected to increase. Continuous flow LVADs are 75 % more cost-effective than older pulsatile LVADs [49] and since 2001, there has been a 50 % decrease in hospital costs associated with LVAD implantation [50]. Although costs may still be prohibitive by strict standards, the continually decreasing costs and improving outcomes, many in the field are of the opinion that expanding this therapy is justified [51, 52].

Key Points

- Modern continuous flow devices are durable for many years

Further Information

- LVAD technology: [41, 43, 44]

2.3 LVAD Outcomes

Over the last decade, outcomes after LVAD placement have improved dramatically, due to improved technology, patient selection and care. Operative mortality in well-selected patients has improved to about 5–10 % [53, 54] and 1-year overall survival has improved from about 50 % [17, 18, 55] to over 80 % in unselected patients in INTERMACS [37] and approaching 90 % in well-selected patients in recent series [54, 56–66].

The perioperative period is crucial, with the vast majority of deaths occurring prior to hospital discharge [10]. The most important complications perioperatively are multi-organ failure, neurologic or peripheral embolic events, bleeding, infection and sepsis (which increase the risk for stroke), and acute RV failure (see below) [67, 68]. In the longer term, complications include embolic or hemorrhagic stroke, the progression of preexisting or de novo development of RV failure or aortic insufficiency, human leukocyte antigen (HLA) sensitization, renal insufficiency, device failure or infection requiring transplantation, explantation or replacement, acquired von Willebrand syndrome, gastrointestinal arteriovenous malformation and bleeding, and psychological maladjustment [18, 54, 55, 58, 68–75]. Perioperative and long-term complications are minimized by careful patients selection and monitoring [24].

Key Points

- LVADs improve survival, symptoms, and quality of life. One-year survival after LVAD has increased from 50 to 80–90 % in 1 decade
- The main complications are pump thrombus, thromboembolism, bleeding, infection, and RV failure

Further Information

- Selected bridge to transplant studies: [54, 57, 61, 62, 65, 66]
- Selected destination therapy studies: [17, 18, 60, 63]
- Fourth INTERMACS Report: [37]
- Improvements in quality of life: [18, 76]

3 Who Should Get an LVAD and When

3.1 LVAD Aims

The aims of LVAD implantation are bridge-to-transplant (BTT), destination therapy (DT), or bridge-to-recovery (BTR). When outcomes with LVAD and/or future candidacy for transplant are less certain, the terms bridge-to-candidacy (BTC) or bridge-to-decision (BTD) are often used. For short-term extracorporeal devices used in cardiac arrest or critical cardiogenic shock (INTERMACS 1; see below), the terms BTD or bridge-to-bridge (BTB) may be used.

LVADs evolved as BTT therapy. Patients were in actual or impending cardiogenic shock and generally supported with multiple inotropes and an intra-aortic balloon pump [9, 77–80], the equivalent of INTERMACS 1–2 (see below). These patients are increasingly being treated with short-term extracorporeal devices with BTD or BTB aims. Furthermore, with improving device technology, surgical skill and LVAD patient management, patients awaiting transplant are being implanted at increasingly earlier stages [24]. About 45 % of LVAD implants are with a stated BTT aim, 45 % as BTC and 10 % as DT, and a handful with a stated BTR aim [37, 81]. BTT patients are or are expected to become too sick for transplant, are expected to die prior to transplant, or have contraindications to transplant that can be reversed by an LVAD, such as renal failure or vasodilator-resistant elevations in pulmonary vascular resistance. Of patients transplanted, 20–30 % have an LVAD or other MCS [29]. This proportion is expected to increase and is already much higher at many centers at many centers this figure is much higher.

Since the landmark REMATCH [17] and HeartMate II DT [60] trials and with improving device technology and long-term LVAD patient management, DT represents a growing share of implants and offers the greatest potential for improvement in HF morbidity and mortality. BTR has been reproducibly achieved in some centers with specific protocols but is rare [82–85], and it is very rarely an a priori stated aim.

Clinical trials and regulatory approvals have involved clear dichotomization of BTT vs. DT, but increasingly this distinction is becoming blurred, and a better term may be simply long-term therapy or BTD or BTC. In DT patients, contraindications to HTx such as elevated PVR or renal failure may be reversed, a treated cancer may remain free of recurrence, or suspected HTx caveats such as smoking or drug or alcohol dependence may be treated or prove unfounded. Up to 17 % of DT patients subsequently undergo HTx [10]. Conversely, BTT patients may experience such improvement in quality of life with an LVAD that they elect to forego HTx, whereas, presenting difficult ethical dilemmas, others may develop contraindications making them ineligible for HTx, and/or complications leading to a poor quality of life and requests to have the device turned off [86]. While recovery is rare, it may occur in non-ischemic cardiomyopathy, and occasionally even in ischemic cardiomyopathy [82–85]. Finally, some patients developing complications requiring device explants may have incomplete but adequate recovery to sustain life and may be able to forego transplant or a new device implant.

Key Points

- LVADs evolved as BTT but are increasingly used as DT
- Increasingly, the BTT/DT distinction is less clear and many patients receive an LVAD as a "bridge to candidacy"

Further Information

- LVAD aims: [32]
- LVAD use: Fourth INTERMACS Report [37]

3.2 *LVAD Indications: Is the Patient Sick Enough?*

Prior to considering an LVAD, an assessment of potentially reversible causes of cardiomyopathy must be made. Echocardiography should rule out valvular disease. It is unlikely that revascularization would be beneficial in chronic ischemic cardiomyopathy [87], even with viable myocardium [88], but select patients may benefit and should be evaluated with cardiac MR or a nuclear study. Treatable and reversible cardiomyopathy usually presents acutely, in patients considered for short-term MCS. Endomyocardial biopsy is most strongly indicated in acute presentations [89] but should be considered also in chronic non-ischemic cardiomyopathy.

After reversible causes of cardiomyopathy have been ruled out, an assessment of the severity of HF must be made in order to determine prognosis *without* LVAD implantation and thus the need for an LVAD. Historically, outcomes with an LVAD were poor and implant criteria were based on subjective assessment of HF severity. Patients were in severe acute or chronic HF with NYHA class IV, inotrope dependence and actual or impending cardiogenic shock and multi-organ failure [9, 77–80]. With improving outcomes and with larger proportions receiving DT, we are moving toward implantation in a less ill and more stable patient cohort. Now, the most critically ill are bridged with short-term MCS, the inotrope dependent are suitable for LVAD, and the stable NYHA III-IV patient is assessed with the peak VO_2, composite prognostic scores and a series of high-risk markers. However, indications are changing rapidly (see below) and vary depending on clinical setting, center, and region.

Key Points

- LVAD implantation is moving from the most critically ill (INTERMACS 1) to more stable patients (INTERMACS 2–4)

Further Information

- LVAD use: [32, 37]

3.3 LVAD Indications: Guidelines

Compared to the numerous randomized trials for drug and electrical device therapy in HF, there is a paucity of randomized controlled data for LVAD therapy. Therefore, guidelines have been slow and cautious to incorporate recommendations on LVAD therapy, which may have contributed to slow acceptance in the broader cardiology field. For BTT, there are no randomized trials. For DT, there is only on trial that randomized an LVAD (HeartMate XVE) vs. usual care (REMATCH) [17] and one other that randomized the HeartMate II vs. the HeartMate XVE [60], and these two trials are the foundation for major society guidelines, approval from the US FDA, and reimbursement policies from the US Center for Medicare and Medicaid Services (CMS) (Table 15.1).

Key Points

- Guidelines from major societies provide recommendations but there is no consensus on specific implant criteria

Further Information

- Guidelines: Table 15.1

Table 15.1 Professional society and regulatory agency guidelines

	Recommendation	Criteria
BTT		
ACC/AHA	Not graded [20, 111]	Not stated
ESC	I—B [165]	End-stage HF despite optimal pharmacological and device treatment
		≥1 of: EF < 25 % and peak VO_2 < 12 mL/kg/min; ≥3 HF hospitalizations in last 12 months; iv inotrope dependence; progressive organ dysfunction; deteriorating right ventricular function
HFSA	B [166]	Refractory to medical circulatory support
ISHLT	I—C [102]	If need increased dose of inotropes or additional agent. To enable HTx if high PVR
FDA	NA	HM II approved for risk of imminent death from nonreversible LV failure. April 2008, http://www.accessdata.fda.gov/cdrh_docs/pdf6/P060040b.pdf
CMS	NA	Not specified. https://www.cms.gov/transmittals/downloads/R68NCD.pdf, accessed 9 February 2012
DT		
ACC/AHA	IIa—B [20, 111]	Refractory end-stage HF and estimated 1-year mortality >50 %
ESC	IIa—B [165]	Same as for BTT
HFSA	B [166]	Refractory to conventional therapy, in particular those who cannot be weaned from iv inotropic support
ISHLT	IB [102]	Long-term inotrope dependent
FDA	NA	HM II approved for NYHA IIIB/IV end-stage LV failure with optimal medical therapy for 45 of the last 60 days. January 2010, available at http://www.fda.gov/MedicalDevices/ProductsandMedicalProcedures/DeviceApprovalsandClearances/Recently-ApprovedDevices/ucm201473.htm
CMS	NA	NYHA IV and EF < 25 % and optimal medical therapy for 45 of the last 60 days or IABP for 7 days or iv inotropes for 14 days and peak VO_2 < 14 unless IABP, inotropes, or unable to perform the test. CMS Administrative file CAG-00119R2, 9 November 2010, available at http://www.cms.gov

ACC: American college of Cardiology
AHA: American Heart Association
ESC: European Society of Cardiology
HFSA: Heart Failure Society of America
ISHLT: International Society for Heart and Lung Transplantation
FDA: (US) Food and Drug Administration
CMS: (US) Centers for Medicare & Medicaid Services

Table 15.2 INTERMACS classification

Level	Description	Implants[a] (%)	Strategy[b]
1	Critical cardiogenic shock	30	Short-term MCS
2	Progressive decline	40	LVAD BTT or DT
3	Stable but inotrope dependent	15	LVAD BTT or DT
4	Recurrent advanced HF	10	LVAD DT
5	Exertion intolerant	2	Assess prognosis with risk scores
6	Exertion limited	1	Assess prognosis with risk scores
7	Advanced NYHA III	2	Assess prognosis with risk scores
Overall		100, $n = 1{,}092$	

From reference [81]
[a]Primary LVAD implants June 2006—March 2009
[b]Author recommendation

3.4 LVAD Indications and Timing: INTERMACS

The US Interagency Registry for Mechanically Assisted Circulatory Support (INTERMACS, http://www.intermacs.org) is an important effort to consolidate experience in the MCS field and has facilitated patient selection. It is a US registry with 128 active sites and 6,091 patients entered to date who have received a long-term MCS device for a HF indication, as a VAD in the left (LVAD), right (RVAD), or biventricular (BiVAD) configuration or as a TAH (http://www.intermacs.org, accessed 23 January 2012). INTERMACS classifies patients into 7 levels of HF severity (Table 15.2). INTERMACS level 1 are too unstable to do well with an LVAD implant and should be bridged with a short-term MCS device. INTERMACS 2–3 are inotrope dependent have an indication for an LVAD for BTT or DT based on INTERMACS classification alone.

The most difficult assessment is for INTERMACS 4. Up to 40 % of stable HTx-listed patients destabilize to require high-urgency HTx or emergency LVAD [90]. Earlier implantation, before RV and multi-organ failure, leads to better outcomes (see below). This is a favored strategy for DT. Yet, LVADs are still associated with 5–10 % perioperative mortality [53, 54] and considerable morbidity and cost, and a HTx-listed patient in good clinical status and a short estimated waiting time may be better served by conservative management.

An emerging issue in BTT patients is whether to implant an LVAD before the institution of chronic inotrope support, a decision that depends on the relative effects of inotropes and LVADs on survival up to and after HTx. Survival on the waiting list depends on the likelihood of being transplanted within a reasonable time [91]. A vast majority of patients implanted to date have been inotrope dependent [17, 18, 54, 55, 58, 68–71, 79, 92]. Inotrope dependence is associated with more than 50 % mortality at 6 months [93] and the medical arm in REMATCH [17] and INTrEPID [18] had 76 % and 89 % mortality at 1 year respectively. However, in HTx-listed patients protected with a defibrillator, inotropes may improve or preserve organ function and clinical status until HTx [94, 95], and pre-HTx inotropes do not impair post-HTx prognosis [96]. A pre-HTx LVAD is associated with the complications of the LVAD itself, may provoke HLA sensitization which can impact heart transplant candidacy, and entails re-sternotomy at the time of HTx. In the ISHLT registry, patients with pre-HTx pulsatile LVAD fared worse post-HTx but this may not be the case for continuous flow LVADs [29]. Furthermore, this registry analysis does not account for selection bias, era of implant, patient characteristics, and other confounding factors. In fact, other studies suggest a neutral [68, 97, 98] or favorable [69, 70, 79, 99, 100] effect of pre-HTx LVAD on post-HTx outcomes.

Furthermore, many patients on inotropes eventually need an LVAD anyway, for successful bridging to transplantation [101]. One attempt at withdrawing inotropes may be attempted [102] but the need for repeat or chronic inotropes should prompt consideration for LVAD implantation. Timing also depends on aim. For inotrope-dependent DT candidates, LVAD implantation should not be deferred, as chronic inotrope use does not prolong survival. It is also important to recognize that poor tolerance of evidence-based pharmacologic therapy, repeat hospitalizations, escalating inotrope or even pressor needs, or end organ dysfunction, are more important integrated criteria for LVAD than single hemodynamic parameters [103]. Most importantly, outcomes are better for stable patients entering an operative procedure than for subjects who are in extremis.

INTERMACS 5–7 currently have insufficient for an LVAD based on INTERMACS level alone. These patients are not hospitalized or dependent on continuous or recurrent infusion of inotropes and should be evaluated by the well-validated peak VO_2, Heart Failure Survival Score (HFSS), and Seattle Heart Failure Model (SHFM) and assessed for unfavorable prognostic markers.

This author's proposed indications for LVAD are listed in Table 15.3

Key Points

- INTERMACS classification is the first step in assessing LVAD candidacy
- INTERMACS 1 should receive short-term MCS as a bridge to decision
- INTERMACS 2–4 are currently proper LVAD candidates
- INTERMACS 5–7 have insufficient indication based on INTERMACS alone. Use other risk assessment tools (peak VO_2, HFSS, SHFM, see below)
- Most but not all LVAD candidates are inotrope dependent
- The criteria for BTT are stricter than for DT

Further Information

- INTERMACS: website http://www.intermacs.org; [32, 37, 104]

3.5 LVAD Indications: The Peak VO_2, Composite Scores, and Poor Prognostic Markers in HF

The peak VO_2 is the single best predictor of prognosis in patients with moderate-severe HF and has long been used in transplant selection. It was derived in a transplant-referred population in 1991 [105], has since been validated in numerous settings [106–109] including the elderly [110] and is now a standard criterion for HTx selection in patients who are not dependent on inotropes or MCS [12, 102, 111]. However, it may not be obtainable in patients unable to perform a maximal

Table 15.3 Proposed indications for LVAD

Strong indication. Generally INTERMACS 2–3. Bridge to transplant or destination. *All* must apply	
Reversible causes of cardiomyopathy ruled out	
Maximal tolerated medical therapy and CRT/ICD if indicated	
NYHA IV[a]	
LVEF ≤ 25 %	
Inotrope dependence for 14 days *or* IABP for 7 days *or* peak VO_2 < 12 mL/kg/min	
Moderate indication. Generally INTERMACS 4–7. More often destination than bridge to transplant[b]. *All* must apply	
Reversible causes of cardiomyopathy ruled out	
Maximal tolerated medical therapy and CRT/ICD if indicated	
NYHA IIIB or IV	
LVEF ≤ 30 %	
Objectively assessed poor prognosis by	
Peak VO_2 < 14 mL/kg/min *or*	
Moderate or High-risk HFSS *or*	
1-year survival < 80 % by the SHFM *or*	
High-risk markers[c]	
Potential future indications. *All* must apply	
NYHA III	
LVEF ≤ 40 %	
Objectively assessed moderately poor prognosis by	
Peak VO_2 < 16 mL/kg/min *or*	
Moderate risk HFSS *or*	
1-year survival < 90 % by the SHFM	
Indication to enable HTx. *Either* must apply	
Irreversible PVR > 5–6 Woods units, secondary to chronic HF and expected to reverse after LVAD	
GFR < 25–30 mL/min/1.73 m^2, secondary to chronic HF and likely to improve after LVAD	
Rarely: other contraindications to HTx that may be reversed during LVAD support: BMI > 35, provide cardiac support during treatment of active Hepatitis C, cancer treatment	
Uncertain suitability for HTx based on psychosocial or compliance issues that can be evaluated and/or improved during LVAD support. LVAD implant considered bridge to decision	
Conversion from short-term MCS to long-term LVAD	
Patients with a short-term MCS in bridge to decision or bridge to bridge setting	

[a]If not on inotropes or an IABP, NYHA IV for 45 out of the last 60 days

[b]Patients listed for HTx generally require a worse clinical status (inotrope dependence) than patients considered for destination therapy. The former group would generally not receive LVAD on a moderate indication since the risks of LVAD outweigh the benefits as HTx before severe deterioration is possible, whereas the latter derive no benefit from deferring LVAD implantation

[c]High-risk markers in Table 15.8

exercise test, and it may not be readily available in community settings and presents a barrier for general cardiologists who otherwise might refer patients for HTx or LVAD. Furthermore, it may not perform reliably in women [112] and in contemporary HF populations, treated with β-blockers [113] and CRT and/or ICD [114].

The HFSS is a composite score consisting of seven strong independent predictors, including the peak VO_2 [115]. It was derived and validated in

Table 15.4 Prognostic markers and risk

	High risk	Medium risk	Low risk
Peak VO_2 mL/kg/min	≤10	10.1–14	>14
1-year survival [114]	65 %	77 %	87 %
HFSS score	≤7.19	7.20–8.09	≥8.10
1-yearr survival [109]	60 %	72 %	89 %
SHFM score	2	1	0
1-year survival [109]	58 %	76 %	93 %

transplant-referred patients and has since been validate in numerous settings. The HFSS performs better than the peak VO_2 alone in the modern era of drug [113] and electrical device treatment [114] and should be used instead of the peak VO_2 alone. The main drawback is that it still requires the peak VO_2, which may not be readily available at all hospitals. The peak VO_2 and the HFSS have been validated in the elderly [110] and are thus suitable for selection for DT LVAD.

The SHFM includes 20 variables and provides a risk score and corresponding estimates of 1- and 5-year survival in HF. The SHFM was derived from clinical drug trials in moderate HF [11] but predicts prognosis (discriminates) also in severe HF [116], HTx-referred patients [109], in REMATCH LVAD patients and controls with adjustment for inotropic, IABP and ventilator support [117], and has been used as a comparison vs. actual LVAD outcomes [118, 119]. However, in severe HF, it underestimates mortality risk (calibrates poorly) [116, 119, 120]. The main practical drawback is that it requires some laboratory variables not routinely obtained.

The peak VO_2, HFSS, and SHFM apply mainly to stable patients who are not treated with inotropes, i.e., INTERMACS 5–7. For patients who have recently been treated with inotropes or receive intermittent levosimendan infusions, these variables should be assessed at least 2 weeks after the most recent treatment. The peak VO2, HFSS and SHFM risk categories and corresponding prognosis are listed in Table 15.4.

The HFSS and SHFM are recommended in the assessment of INTERMACS 5–7 patients but are still uncommonly used. A major reason may be the perceived complexity. The HFSS requires a calculation based on the published formula (Table 15.5), and to facilitate this we use a simple Microsoft Excel sheet with the formula entered. The SHFM can be easily calculated on the web (http://depts.washington.edu/shfm/; screen shot in Fig. 15.7). Calculating these score may take a few extra minutes but is well worth the trouble considering the extra prognostic information and the otherwise very large investment that goes into an LVAD assessment and implantation.

There are numerous additional variables that predict prognosis in HF, including markers of functional status organ failure [103] and recent hospitalizations [121]. Several of these are useful in assessing the prognosis in severe HF without LVAD implantation and should be assessed in conjunction with the peak VO_2, HFSS, and SHFM (Table 15.6).

This authors proposed indications are listed in Table 15.7 and an algorithm for LVAD selection is presented in Fig. 15.8.

Table 15.5 How to calculate the heart failure survival score (HFSS)

Variables in the model	Coefficient	Example	Example result
Ischemic etiology, no = 0, yes = 1	×0.6931	1	0.6931
Resting heart rate, bpm	×0.0216	70	1.512
LVEF, %	×−0.0464	22	−1.0208
Mean arterial blood pressure, mmHg	×−0.0255	80	−2.04
Intraventricular conduction delay (QRS ≥ 0.12 s, regardless of pacing), no = 0, yes = 1	×0.6083	1	0.6083
Peak VO_2 (mL/min/kg)	×−0.0546	12.2	−0.66612
Serum Na (mmol/L)	×−0.047	137	−6.439
HFSS			Absolute value of sum of above: 7.35 (medium risk)

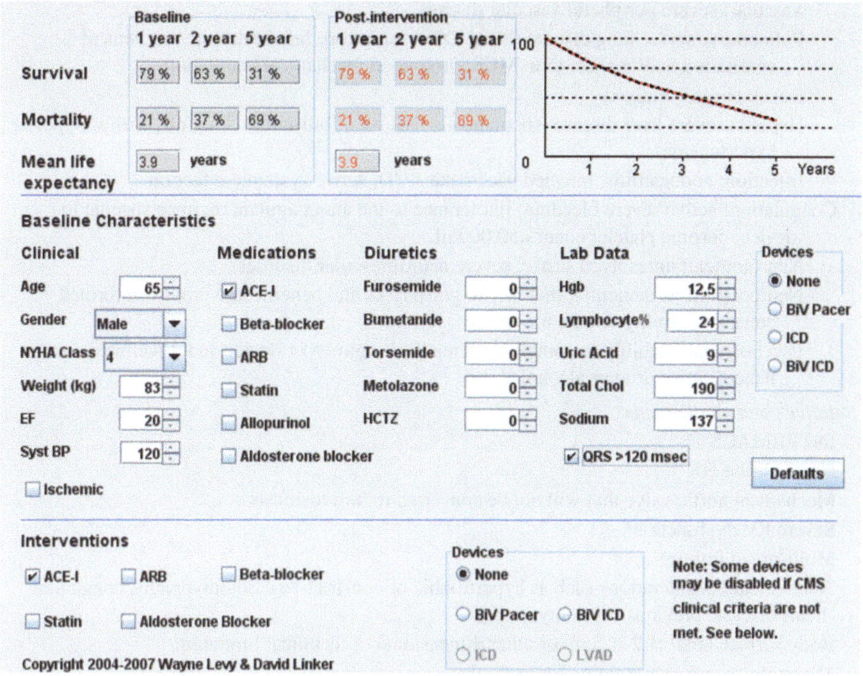

From http://depts.washington.edu/shfm/app.php, accessed 27 January 2012, with permission

Fig. 15.7 Screen shot of the Seattle heart failure model (SHFM)

Table 15.6 Risk factors for mortality in severe HF than increase the need for an LVAD

Walk <1 block without dyspnea
Sodium <136 mEq/L
Serum urea nitrogen >40 mg/dL (15 mmol/L) *or* Creatinine >1.8 mg/dL (160 ≤ mol/L)
Cannot tolerate ACEI/ARB/β-blocker
Furosemide dose >1.5 mg/kg/d
HF hospital admission <6 months
CRT nonresponder
Hematocrit <35 %

From reference [103]

Table 15.7 Proposed contraindications for LVAD

Absolute contraindications

- Acute cardiogenic shock or arrest with uncertain neurologic status[a]
- Severe multi-organ failure[a]
- Irreversible contraindication to HTx if destination or recovery is not the aim
- Right HF not secondary to left HF (consider RVAD)
- Moderate or severe aortic insufficiency that will not be corrected
- LV thrombus that will not be removed
- Ventricular septal defect that will not be repaired
- Coexisting illness with life expectancy <2 years
- Severe comorbidity, for example
  - Metastatic or advanced cancer
  - Vascular: severe peripheral vascular disease
  - Pulmonary: severe lung disease (home O2); respiratory failure despite mechanical ventilation and/or short-term MCS; prolonged mechanical ventilation
  - Renal: chronic dialysis
  - Hepatic: severe liver disease (spontaneous INR >2.5; bilirubin >5 mg/dL; cirrhosis; portal hypertension)
  - Infection: endocarditis, infected pacemaker/ICD, active systemic infection
- Coagulation: active severe bleeding; Intolerance to the anticoagulant regimen specific to device; chronic platelet count <50,000/μL
  - Neurological: unresolved stroke; severe neuromuscular disorder
  - Neurocognitive: dementia; Inability to grasp risks and benefits and provide informed consent; inability to care for device
  - Psychosocial: inability to comply with medical regimen or device and driveline maintenance; active drug or alcohol abuse

Relative contraindications

- INTERMACS 1[a]
- Non-systolic HF
- Mechanical aortic valve that will not be converted to bioprosthesis
- Severe RV dysfunction[a]
- Multi-organ failure[a]
- Anatomical considerations such as hypertrophic or constrictive cardiomyopathy, congenital heart disease, previous cardiomyoplasty
- Body surface area <1.2–1.5 m^2 or other dimensional or technical limitation
- Moderate-severe comorbidity, for example
  - Pulmonary: moderate-severe lung disease (FVC, FEV1, or CO diffusion capacity <50 % predicted)
  - Renal: moderate-severe renal disease; creatinine >3.5 mg/dL; GFR < 30 mL/min/1.73 m^2; acute renal failure requiring dialysis[a]
  - Hepatic: moderate liver disease
  - Infection: local infection or significant risk for infection
  - Endocrine: diabetes with retinopathy, neuropathy, foot ulcers, or very poor glycemic control
  - Coagulation: platelet count <150,000/μL; HIT confirmed by antibody and serotonin release assays
  - Neurological: previous moderate-severe stroke; moderate-severe neuromuscular disorder
  - Psychosocial: limitation inability of patient or companion to maintain LVAD operation and interpret alarms
- Poor social support, poor access to transportation, telephone

[a]These patients may be considered for short-term MCS

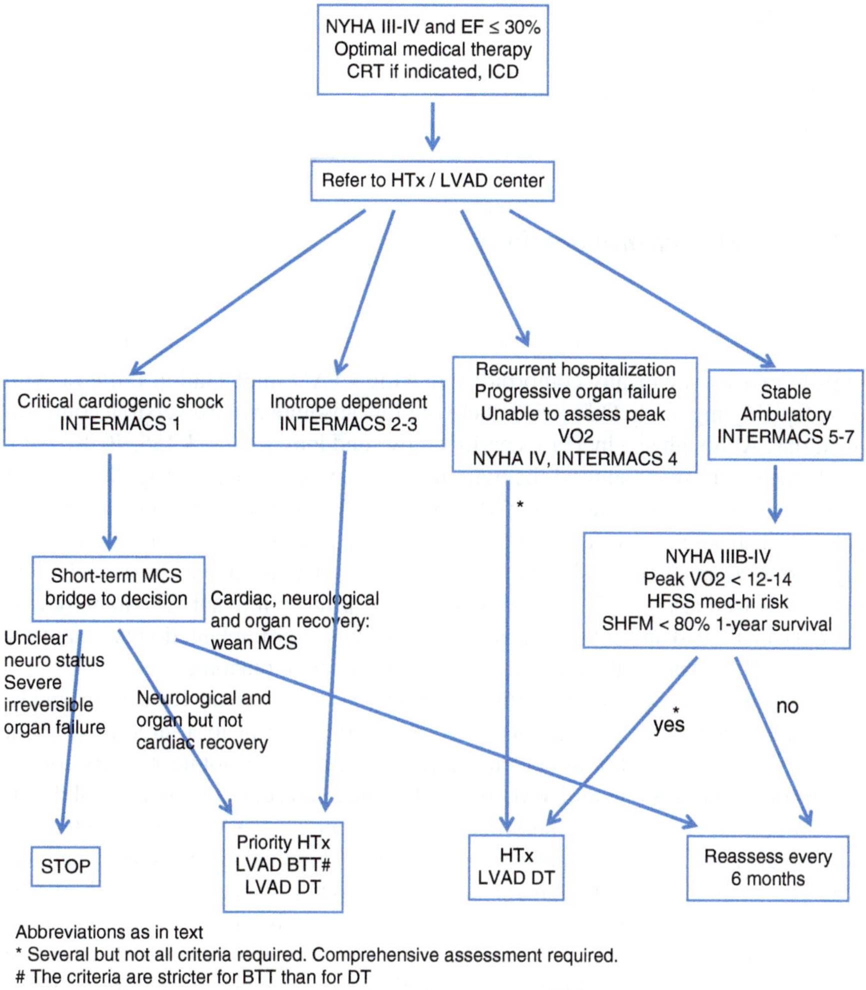

Fig. 15.8 LVAD selection algorithm

Key Points

- In INTERMACS 5–7 patients, consider LVAD for patients with EV ≤ 25 % and peak VO_2 < 12–14 mL/kg/min, medium- to high-risk HFSS and/or SHFM estimated 1-year survival <80 % (Fig. 15.8).
- Future indications may be NYHA III and EF ≤ 40 % and peak VO_2 < 14–16 mL/kg/min.
- The SHFM was derived from clinical drug trials and may underestimate risk in severely ill patients.

Further Information

- Peak VO_2: [105–110].
- HFSS: [110, 113–115].
- SHFM: [11, 109, 116–120].

3.6 LVAD Contraindications

Once a potential indication has been established, the team should assess potential contraindications, listed in Table 15.7. These are either noncardiac morbidity limiting life expectancy or any comorbidity making LVAD implantation futile or with unacceptably high risk. Otherwise, there are few absolute and irreversible contraindications. Although age increases perioperative and long-term risk [55, 70, 81, 122, 123], one recent study suggest that with improved management, the age >70 cohort do not have worse outcomes than <70 years [64]. The decision to implant and LVAD depends instead on a careful and detailed selection process and optimal timing, taking into account the extensive available published data available for the selection process as well as strategies to optimize patients prior to implant. The main reason patients are denied an LVAD or have poor outcomes after implantation are that they are referred too late, with numerous risk factors for poor outcome.

In the general population, routine screening is controversial for certain conditions, e.g., cancer, but should generally be performed prior to a large investment such as an LVAD. Conditions detected during screening may not necessarily constitute a contraindication to an LVAD but will require careful evaluation. An abdominal ultrasound to rule out abdominal aortic aneurysm (AAA) in patients with peripheral vascular disease or age ≥60 and an ankle brachial index (ABI) in patients with known or suspected peripheral vascular disease or diabetes mellitus should be performed [41]. Patients with prior stroke should have a head CT to assess extent of disease and patients with cerebrovascular, coronary or peripheral artery disease, and patients over age 50 should have a carotid ultrasound. Patients with prior stroke, a family history of Alzheimer's or age >65 should undergo a rudimentary neurocognitive assessment such as the mini mental status exam. Screening for breast cancer (mammography), cervical cancer (cytology), colorectal cancer (colonoscopy), lung cancer in smokers (chest CT), and prostate cancer (prostate-specific antigen (PSA)) should be performed. Serology for human immunodeficiency virus, hepatitis B, and hepatitis C should be performed. Finally, immunization against seasonal influenza and pneumococcus should be performed in LVAD candidates.

Key Points

- The main contraindication is concurrent terminal disease or multi-organ failure
- There is no absolute age limit but few patients are over 75 years old and higher age is associated with worse outcomes after LVAD

Further Information

- Contraindications: [41]

3.7 LVAD Selection: Is the Patient too Sick and How Do We Optimize?

Once a potential LVAD indication has been established and absolute and irreversible contraindications have been ruled out, begins the work of refining selection and if the decision to implant an LVAD is made, optimizing the patient prior to implant. LVAD indications depend on risk *without* LVAD implantation, whereas the selection process entails assessing risk *with* LVAD implantation [104]. Improved patient selection over the last decade is a major reason for improved outcomes. Selection is a complex process, requiring a multidisciplinary team of cardiologists, cardiac surgeons, anesthetists, percussionists, LVAD nurses and coordinators, and social workers. Work-up includes echocardiography with detailed analysis of RV function, right heart catheterization, extensive laboratory testing, and a complete psychosocial assessment. For BTT patients, a complete transplant work-up should be performed prior to LVAD implantation.

The most important predictors of poor outcomes with LVAD implantation are poor RV function, renal failure, liver failure, respiratory failure, and poor nutritional and functional status. The most important preoperative steps to improve outcomes are to avoid the most critically ill (INTERMACS 1), minimizing RV afterload and preload, optimizing coagulation and renal, liver and respiratory function, as well as judicious prophylactic antibiotics [41]. Table 15.8 lists variables that should be assessed, the values that portend increased risk at LVAD implantation, and strategies and objectives for further optimization prior to LVAD implantation. These risk factors are derived from numerous studies of single variables and multivariable composite scores that are associated with especially high risk. These data have been derived mainly in the patient cohorts receiving first generation pulsatile devices but should be considered also prior to second or third generation LVAD implant. Also, many variables are moving hemodynamic targets which should be optimized but even when optimized may reflect underlying high-risk pathology.

Key Points

- Timing is critical—many patients are referred to late, with too irreversible contraindication such as right-sided HF

Further Information

- Timing and selection: [24, 32, 41, 104]

Table 15.8 LVAD selection: check list for work-up and assessing risk factors for poor outcome and strategies for optimization

Risk factor/diagnostics	Management/goal	References
Age[a, b]	Age alone not contraindication but risk increases with age >50. Implantation in age >75 is rarely considered. Carotid Doppler if age >50. Abdominal ultrasound for AAA if age >60 or PAD	[55, 64, 70, 81, 122, 123, 130, 133, 146]
Gender[b]	Female gender generally higher risk and less acceptance of LVAD therapy	[140, 142, 143, 152, 156, 167]
Anatomical considerations		
BSA < 1.2[b]	Contraindication	
BSA < 1.5[b]	Increased risk	[140, 143, 152]
Previous thoracic or abdominal surgery[a, b]	Increases risk. Chest and/or abdominal CT	[41, 130, 131, 143]
Previous CABG	Chest CT to locate bypass grafts	
Functional status		
Pre-op cardiac arrest or CPR[a, b]		[130, 139]
INTERMACS level 1[a]	Bridge with short-term MCS in BiVAD or ECMO configuration	[81]
Emergent implant[a, b]	Avoid emergent implant, bridge with short-term MCS if necessary	[41, 130, 156]
Pre-op short-term MCS[a, b]	Associated with increased overall and RV failure risk at LVAD implant but is preferred over emergent LVAD implant. Use short-term MCS to optimize organ function and prophylactically for RV	[81, 130, 132, 139, 143, 145, 152]
Pre-op IABP[b]	Associated with increased risk but use if necessary	[143, 145, 156]
Poor SHFM score[a]	Optimize organ function	[118]
Lactate > 3 mg/dL[a]		[130]
LDH > 500 U/L[a, b]		[130, 139]
Hemodynamics		
HR > 100/min[a]		[130]
SBP ≤ 96[b]	Aim for SBP 80–90 or according to symptoms	[143]
Cardiogenic shock[a]	Optimize with drugs or short-term MCS	[81]
CI ≤ 2.2[b]		[136, 139, 140, 143, 156]
Low SVO_2[b]		[143, 151]
Pulmonary edema[b]		[151]
PCWP > 25–30[a]	Inotropes, diuretics, short-term LVAD	[41]
mPAP < 25 mmHg[a, b]		[10, 139, 140, 143, 152, 153, 168]
PVR > 4[b]	May increase risk of RV failure but is also an indication for LVAD as BTT	[41, 145, 146, 169]
TPG > 15[b]		[41, 169]

(continued)

Table 15.8 (continued)

Risk factor/diagnostics	Management/goal	References
RVSWI[c] < 300 mmHg × mL/m^2 [b]		[41, 139, 140, 143, 152, 168]
CVP > 20 mmHg[a, b]	Pulmonary vasodilators, Inotropes, hemofiltration, diuretics, short-term RVAD. Aim for CVP 15	[41, 131, 132, 136, 143, 146, 155, 168, 169]
Higher NT-proBNP[b]		[136]
Vasopressor need[a, b]	Assess for SIRS, consider short-term MCS. If necessary, use vasopressin (pulmonary vasodilator) rather than noradrenaline	[41, 139]
Inotrope need[a, b]	Associated with worse outcomes but if needed, improves outcomes	[10, 81, 130, 136, 139, 145, 151]
LV		
Coronary artery disease[a, b]	May increase overall LVAD risk and if RV ischemia, increases risk of RV failure. Also, perform carotid Doppler	[41, 130]
Acute myocardial infarction in LAD distribution/LV apex	Delay LVAD if possible	
Non-ischemic etiology[b]		[152]
Myocarditis[b]		[140]
Higher LVEF and lower LVEDD[b]		[144]
Ventricular septal defect	Repair	
Moderate-severe AI	Correct with bioprosthesis or oversowing. AI may be underestimated pre-op due to high LV filling pressures	[41]
Mechanical aortic valve	Replace with bioprosthesis or oversowing	
Moderate-severe mitral stenosis	Replace with bioprosthesis	[41]
Mechanical mitral valve	Not contraindication but increases risk of thrombosis. Consider increased anti-coagulation post-op	[41, 170]
RV	Pulmonary vasodilators (nitric oxide, sildenafil, prostaglandins), Inotropes, ultrafiltration or dialysis, diuretics, preoperative or concurrent prophylactic short-term RVAD	[81]
Severe TR[b]	Concurrent tricuspid valve annuloplasty of moderate-severe TR	[53, 136, 171]
TAPSE < 7.5[b]		[172]
RV short/long axis ratio >0.55–0.60[b]		[136]
RVEDD/LVEDD ratio >0.72[b]		[173]
RVEDV > 200 mL[b]		[41]
RVESV < 177 mL[b]		[41]
High RV wall thickness[b]		[151]
Pulmonary	Repeat spirometry if suspect poor values due to inability to cooperate	[77]

(continued)

Table 15.8 (continued)

Risk factor/diagnostics	Management/goal	References
Mechanical ventilation[a, b]	Strong predictor of RV failure and overall poor outcomes. Consider bridge to decision with short-term MCS	[130–132, 139, 143, 152, 153, 155, 156]
FVC < 50 % predicted[a]	Relative contraindication	[41]
FEV1 < 50 % predicted[a]	Relative contraindication	[41]
CO diffusion capacity <50 % predicted[a]	Relative contraindication	[41]
Renal	Improve cardiac output and reduce CVP: Inotropes, vasopressors, short-term MCS	[127, 128]
Creatinine >2.5 md/dL (>220 μmol/L)[a, b]		[41, 130, 139, 143]
GFR < 50 mL/min/1.73 m^2 [a]		
BUN > 51 mg/dL (>18 nmol/L)[a, b]	Aim for BUN < 40 mg/dL	[10, 130, 139, 155]
Urine output <30 mL/h[a, b]	Inotropes, diuretics, short-term MCS	[131]
Renal replacement therapy[a, d]	Associated with increased risk but use to optimize volume status and organ function	[139]
Hepatic	Liver failure is often secondary to RV failure and increases risk of post-op RV failure. Assess and optimize RV. Assess MELD score. Screen liver with ultrasound	[134, 135]
AST > 45 U/L (0.75 μkat/L)[a, b]		[10, 139, 153]
ALT > 70 U/L (1.2 μkat/L)[a, b]		[41, 153]
Total bilirubin >2.5 mg/dL (43 μmol/L[a, b])		[41, 133, 139, 141, 143, 156]
Ascites		[133]
Cirrhosis	Contraindication. Liver biopsy if unsure diagnosis	
Portal hypertension	Contraindication	
Gastrointestinal		
Active serious GI bleed	Contraindication	
History of GI bleed[a]	Increases risk. Perform EGD and colonoscopy	[41]
Hematology		
Hematocrit <34 %[a]	As indicated, erythropoietin, oral or iv iron, transfusion to hematocrit >30 % is controversial	[10, 130]
Preoperative RBC transfusions[a, b]	Minimize	[130]
Coagulation	Fresh frozen plasma as needed Aspirin and clopidogrel/prasugrel/ticagrelor in patients with recent stents is controversial	
Spontaneous INR > 1.1 or warfarin treatment[a, b]	Discontinue warfarin; if necessary bridge with heparin/LMWH. Avoid vitamin K reversal because this disrupts long-term warfarin titration. Use prothrombin complex concentrate for reversal as needed	[10, 136, 143, 146]

(continued)

Table 15.8 (continued)

Risk factor/diagnostics	Management/goal	References
PTT	Measure	
Platelet count <148,000/μL[a, b]	Transfusion controversial. Screen for HIT	[10, 130, 139, 143]
Preoperative platelet transfusions		[130]
HIT	If platelets <148,000/μL, decline of >20 %, or thrombosis while receiving heparin perform HIT diagnostics. If HIT confirmed, consider bivalirudin or argatroban	[41]
Infection	Perioperative prophylactic antibiotics according to local flora and resistance patterns. Assess and optimize risk factors listed below	[41, 174]
Infective endocarditis	Contraindication to LVAD. Treat	
Infected pacemaker/ICD	Contraindication to LVAD. Treat	
Active systemic infection	Contraindication to LVAD. Treat	[24]
Localized infection	Treat and delay LVAD implant if possible	[41]
Fever	Assess and delay LVAD implant if possible	
WBC > 10,000–13,000[a, b]	Assess	[130, 139, 143, 146, 155]
CRP > 8 mg/dL[a, b]		[130, 136]
Prolonged intubation[a]	Bridge with short-term MCS	
Pre-op indwelling catheters[a]	replace if >36 h	[41]
Poor dental status[a]	Dental evaluation including panorex images	[41]
Nasal Staph aureus carriage[a]	Local treatment (mupirocin 2 % nasal ointment the evening before and twice per day for 5 days)	[41]
Urinary tract infection[a]	Treat	[41]
Skin lesions[a]		[41]
Immunosuppression[a]	Consider measuring immunoglobulins	[41]
Endocrine		
Diabetes, hyperglycemia[a, b]	HBa1c < 70 mmol/mol, glucose < 11 mmol/L/200 mg/dL	[41, 139]
Thyroid function	TSH	
Nutrition	Nutritional support, including enteric feeding tube	
BMI < 22[a]		[175]
Albumin <3.3 g/dL[a, b]		[10, 139, 143]
Pre-albumin <15 mg/dL[a]		[176]
Total cholesterol <130 mg/dL[a]		[41]
Obesity		
BMI > 40	Contraindication. Dietician, exercise training; goal <35	[41]
Peripheral arterial disease[a]	Abdominal ultrasound for AAA if age >60 or PAD. ABI if claudication or diabetes	[41]
Neurological		
Previous stroke[a, b]	Carotid ultrasound, head CT	[41, 139]

(continued)

Table 15.8 (continued)

Risk factor/diagnostics	Management/goal	References
Carotid stenosis >70 %	Asymptomatic: LVAD prior to carotid intervention Previous stroke: consider intervention prior to LVAD	[177–179]
Neurocognitive condition that interferes with care of device or driveline	Contraindication	
Psychosocial		[41, 180, 181]
Current drug or alcohol abuse	Contraindication. Consider rehabilitation	
Psychiatric or psychosocial conditions that interfere with compliance or care for device and driveline	Contraindication	
Lack of support	Relative contraindication. Enlist next of kin. Ensure transport, grounded electricity, telephone service, insurance as needed	

This table is meant as a practical guide for which data should be collected, how the data affect risk, and how they should be managed

Variables in this table are from extensive review of the literature. Some variable are independent predictors whereas other are only univariate predictors

Abbreviations as in text or conventionally used

[a]Increases overall risk

[b]Increases risk of RV failure

[c]RVSWI: right ventricular stroke work index = ([mPAP–CVP] × CI × 1,000)/HR. Example: ([40–20] × 2.0 × 1,000)/80 = 500 mmHg mL/beat/m^2. To convert to g/m^2: multiply by 0.0136. Example 500 mmHg mL/beat/m^2 = 6.8 g/m^2

[d]Inotropes, IABP, short-term MCS, renal replacement therapy are associated with worse outcomes because they are markers of severity, but if they are needed, their use is associated with improved outcomes

3.8 LVAD Selection: Overall Risk

There are numerous individual predictors of poor operative outcome including age [55, 70, 122, 123], female gender [55], diabetes [55] prior cardiac surgery [70, 124], preexisting right heart failure [122], respiratory failure and septicemia [122], preoperative ECMO [125] or mechanical ventilation [55], renal dysfunction [55, 125–128], elevated blood urea nitrogen [124], coagulopathy and lower platelet and higher white blood cell counts [55], and worse INTERMACS levels [59, 129]. Paradoxically, INTERMACS 3 may have better prognosis than 1–2 but also 4–7 [81], which may be statistical chance or reflect that INTERMACS 3 patients are more aggressively optimized prior to implantation. Absence of preoperative inotropes is associated with better outcomes [130] although one study suggested the reverse [10] which may reflect intolerance to inotropes due to arrhythmia.

In addition, there are several risk scores that predict overall outcomes. The Lietz-Miller destination therapy risk score (DTRS) analyzed 45 baseline parameters and outcomes in DT patients in the post-REMATCH era. Laboratory, hemodynamic, and clinical predictors generated a score that divided candidates into low, medium, and high-risk strata [10]. Klotz el al. analyzed 100 preoperative parameters in a variety of device recipients and found 34 univariate and 13 multivariate risk factors for intensive care unit mortality. They devised a score with high-, medium-, and low-risk strata [130]. The Columbia University/Cleveland Clinic risk factor selection scale (RFSS) [131] and revised screening scale (RSS) [132] analyzed predictors in BTT recipients, and Holman et al. in the INTERMACS database [133]. General risk scores such as the Model for End-stage Liver Disease (MELD) [134, 135] and the Simplified Acute Physiology Score II (SAPS II) [136] also predict post-LVAD outcomes.

These studies and risk models have several important limitations. They were derived mainly in patients receiving first generation pulsatile devices and where there is independent prospective validation in continuous flow patients, these risk scores may no longer be valid [137] and may overestimate risk. Furthermore, they do not consider underrepresented populations such as women, African Americans, and those who due to body size limitations were ineligible for the larger first generation devices. Comorbidities such as diabetes or severe cachexia or obesity were underrepresented but are known to fare worse and may preclude transplant. Psychosocial factors and outcomes are not considered. Recidivism of drug and/or alcohol and return to work are unknown. Finally, data is available only on short-term and not longer-term outcomes.

The SHFM predicts mortality in HF and can be used to determine LVAD indication (see above). The preoperative SHFM score also predicts outcomes after LVAD implant [118], better than the Lietz-Miller, Columbia, INTERMACS and APACHE II (Acute Physiology and Chronic Health Evaluation II) scores [138], and can be used to identify patients at high risk of poor post-LVAD outcomes and to optimize timing of implantation. Thus in INTERMACS 5–7, the SHFM can be used to determine indication, whereas in INTERMACS 1–4, it can be used to assess postoperative outcomes.

Key Points

- There are numerous risk markers and risk scores for potential LVAD implantation
- LVAD implantation risk and outcomes can be assessed prior to implant. Taking the time and effort to properly assess risk is mandatory prior to embarking on this expensive therapy
- The decision to implant an LVAD is a multidisciplinary team decision requiring careful attention to patient preferences and input from at least cardiologist, cardiac surgeon, anesthetist, LVAD nurse/coordinator, and social worker

Further Information

- LVAD selection and risk scores reviewed: [24]

3.9 LVAD Selection: RV Failure

In the long term, LV unloading and decreases in LV filling pressures and subsequently pulmonary vascular resistance (PVR) often lead to improved RV function after LVAD. But in the early postoperative period, numerous complex mechanisms may contribute to RV failure. These include sudden increases in cardiac output, leading to increased venous return and thus RV preload, septal shift causing increased RV wall stress, and increased pulmonary vasoreactivity in the setting of cardiopulmonary bypass, blood transfusions, and inflammation, leading to increased RV afterload [139].

The incidence of RV failure, generally defined as need for an RV assist device or inotropic support for >14 days, ranges from 7 to 50 % depending on definition and study [55, 79, 80, 136, 139–146]. RV failure leads to organ failure and underfilling of the LV and the pump, with potential for arrhythmia and cardiogenic shock. It increases bleeding, liver and renal failure, and prolongs hospitalization. Perioperative mortality increases from 19 to 43 % and survival both to and after HTx becomes worse [139, 145], although the increased risk is primarily in the perioperative period and chronic RV failure post-LVAD may not impair successful bridging to transplantation [147].

RV failure can be decreased by preoperative optimization of nutrition, hemodynamics, and organ function and minimization of RV preload, with parenteral nutrition, inotropes and IABP. Other steps to lower the risk of RV failure include perioperative minimization of bleeding and transfusion needs, effective coronary perfusion and avoidance of cardioplegia, avoidance of surgical RV injury and RV distension, prophylactic RVAD [148, 149] and inotropes, tricuspid annuloplasty, early cessation of positive pressure ventilation and RV afterload reduction with nitric oxide [80, 150] nitroprusside, and perhaps prostanoids, endothelin receptor antagonists, and phosphodiesterase inhibitors.

For those accustomed to HTx selection, assessing RV failure risk post-LVAD is counterintuitive. A key favorable prognostic factor is the ability of the RV to generate pressure and forward flow; thus high pulmonary artery pressure (PAP) is favorable whereas high central venous pressure (CVP) and preoperative RV failure and large tricuspid regurgitation are detrimental. Numerous predictors of RV failure have been identified [136, 139–144, 151–155]. Interpretation of these data is again clouded by the fact that most publications identified only univariate predictors, describe exclusively [69, 80, 140–142, 151–153, 156] or mostly first generation devices [55, 139, 146] and lack validation. Although RV failure appears less common with second generation devices [54, 58], there are also fewer parameters to predict it [157].

Key Points

- RV failure is a common contraindication—refer early
- The risk of RV failure can be assessed with risk markers and scores
- Assess risk of RV failure prior to implant and use planned, prophylactic RV support if risk is deemed high

Further Information

- RV failure risk markers and scores, reviewed: [24]

4 Future Directions

The main technical directions for the future include even smaller size devices for ease of implantation and reduction of complications (e.g., the Thoratec HeartMate III and HeartMate X and the Heartware MVAD and others [40, 43, 158, 159]), the use of two separate continuous flow LVADs as an implantable rather than extracorporeal BiVAD [160, 161], and importantly, the development of fully implantable systems, with no external components and energy transmission via transcutaneous energy transfer (TET) [162]. The main limitation for patients' quality of life is the driveline and the external components, and the driveline and its long-term risk of infection is the main factor limiting truly permanent LVAD support. The LionHeart (Arrow Inc.) was a totally implantable LVAD with TET technology but was abandoned because of technical problems. More novel technology developed by e.g., WiTricity Inc. in partnership with Thoratec Inc. make TET a potential reality in the near future.

However, improved technology is only one aspect of the future. LVAD therapy is at a pivotal point of gaining widespread acceptance. This field has traditionally been one of pioneering and visionary surgeons. Now is the time for the LVAD field to become part of the broader cardiology field. Improved technology, patient selection and perioperative and long-term patient care has led to improved outcomes, wider indications, and rapid growth in the number of implants [24, 163]. But LVADs are still underutilized [5, 51]. Real and perceived risks of complications and high costs have kept LVAD therapy from gaining widespread acceptance among cardiologists [51]. Technical developments and increasing volumes will bring down device costs, but continued improved selection is necessary to improve cost-effectiveness further [49–52]. This will be accomplished by rigorous patient selection and care, rigorous clinical research and reporting to registries (INTERMACS [37], IMACS [164], EUROMACS), and increased collaboration between surgeons and cardiologists and multidisciplinary LVAD teams.

Key Points

- LVAD technology will continue to improve.
- The next technological steps will be smaller devices and TET.
- TET and totally implantable systems without external components will take LVAD therapy to the next level, reducing infection and dramatically improving quality of life.
- LVAD cost will continue to decline and cost-effectiveness will continue to improve.
- Novel technology may make LVAD therapy temporarily more expensive.

- LVADs are underutilized. The main reason is lack of awareness among referring cardiologists.
- For LVAD therapy to gain widespread acceptance and become widely available, cardiologists need to become more involved in the field.
- Rigorous clinical and registry based research needs to be conducted.

Further Information

- LVAD utilization, resource allocation, and cost-effectiveness: [5, 51, 52]

5 Disclosures

The author has received research funding to author's institution, consulting fees and/or speakers' fees from Thoratec Inc. and HeartWare Inc., and is principal investigator of the SEE—HF registry, a prospective study of screening HF patients for markers of severe HF and need for HTx and/or LVAD, sponsored by Thoratec, Inc.

References

1. Roger VL, Go AS, Lloyd-Jones DM et al (2012) Heart disease and stroke statistics—2012 update: a report from the American Heart Association. Circulation 125(1):e2–e220
2. Levy D, Kenchaiah S, Larson MG et al (2002) Long-term trends in the incidence of and survival with heart failure. N Engl J Med 347(18):1397–1402
3. Loehr LR, Rosamond WD, Chang PP, Folsom AR, Chambless LE (2008) Heart failure incidence and survival (from the Atherosclerosis Risk in Communities study). Am J Cardiol 101(7):1016–1022
4. Roger VL, Go AS, Lloyd-Jones DM et al (2011) Heart disease and stroke statistics—2011 update: a report from the American Heart Association. Circulation 123(4):e18–e209
5. Miller LW (2011) Left ventricular assist devices are underutilized. Circulation 123(14): 1552–1558; discussion 1558
6. Lloyd-Jones DM, Larson MG, Leip EP et al (2002) Lifetime risk for developing congestive heart failure: the Framingham Heart Study. Circulation 106(24):3068–3072
7. Jessup M, Brozena S (2003) Heart failure. N Engl J Med 348(20):2007–2018
8. Lund LH, Mancini D (2004) Heart failure in women. Med Clin North Am 88(5):1321–1345; xii
9. Warner-Stevenson L (2006) The evolving role of mechanical circulatory support in advanced heart failure. In: Frazier O, Kirklin J (eds) ISHLT monograph series 1, mechanical circulatory support. Maryland Heights, Missouri, USA, pp 181–203
10. Lietz K, Long JW, Kfoury AG et al (2007) Outcomes of left ventricular assist device implantation as destination therapy in the post-REMATCH era: implications for patient selection. Circulation 116(5):497–505
11. Levy WC, Mozaffarian D, Linker DT et al (2006) The seattle heart failure model: prediction of survival in heart failure. Circulation 113(11):1424–1433
12. Dickstein K, Cohen-Solal A, Filippatos G et al (2008) ESC Guidelines for the diagnosis and treatment of acute and chronic heart failure 2008 the task force for the diagnosis and treatment of acute and chronic heart failure 2008 of the European Society of Cardiology.

Developed in collaboration with the heart failure association of the ESC (HFA) and endorsed by the European Society of Intensive Care Medicine (ESICM). Eur J Heart Fail 10(10):933–989
13. McCullough PA, Philbin EF, Spertus JA, Kaatz S, Sandberg KR, Weaver WD (2002) Confirmation of a heart failure epidemic: findings from the resource utilization among congestive heart failure (REACH) study. J Am Coll Cardiol 39(1):60–69
14. CDC (2003) Trends in aging—United States and worldwide. MMWR Morb Mortal Wkly Rep 52(6):101–104; 106
15. Henkel DM, Redfield MM, Weston SA, Gerber Y, Roger VL (2008) Death in heart failure: a community perspective. Circ Heart Fail 1(2):91–97
16. Deng MC (2004) Orthotopic heart transplantation: highlights and limitations. Surg Clin North Am 84(1):243–255
17. Rose EA, Gelijns AC, Moskowitz AJ et al (2001) Long-term mechanical left ventricular assistance for end-stage heart failure. N Engl J Med 345(20):1435–1443
18. Rogers JG, Butler J, Lansman SL et al (2007) Chronic mechanical circulatory support for inotrope-dependent heart failure patients who are not transplant candidates: results of the INTrEPID Trial. J Am Coll Cardiol 50(8):741–747
19. Lenfant C (2003) Shattuck lecture—clinical research to clinical practice—lost in translation? N Engl J Med 349(9):868–874
20. Hunt SA, Abraham WT, Chin MH et al (2009) 2009 focused update incorporated into the ACC/AHA 2005 Guidelines for the Diagnosis and Management of Heart Failure in Adults: a report of the American College of Cardiology Foundation/American Heart Association Task Force on Practice Guidelines: developed in collaboration with the International Society for Heart and Lung Transplantation. Circulation 119(14):e391–e479
21. Roger VL, Weston SA, Redfield MM et al (2004) Trends in heart failure incidence and survival in a community-based population. JAMA 292(3):344–350
22. Chen J, Normand SL, Wang Y, Krumholz HM (2011) National and regional trends in heart failure hospitalization and mortality rates for Medicare beneficiaries, 1998–2008. JAMA 306(15):1669–1678
23. Curtis LH, Greiner MA, Hammill BG et al (2008) Early and long-term outcomes of heart failure in elderly persons, 2001–2005. Arch Intern Med 168(22):2481–2488
24. Lund LH, Matthews J, Aaronson K (2010) Patient selection for left ventricular assist devices. Eur J Heart Fail 12(5):516–520
25. Allen LA, Yager JE, Funk MJ et al (2008) Discordance between patient-predicted and model-predicted life expectancy among ambulatory patients with heart failure. JAMA 299(21):2533–2542
26. Remme WJ, McMurray JJ, Rauch B et al (2005) Public awareness of heart failure in Europe: first results from SHAPE. Eur Heart J 26(22):2413–2421
27. Parascandola M, Hawkins J, Danis M (2002) Patient autonomy and the challenge of clinical uncertainty. Kennedy Inst Ethics J 12(3):245–264
28. Stewart GC, Brooks K, Pratibhu PP et al (2009) Thresholds of physical activity and life expectancy for patients considering destination ventricular assist devices. J Heart Lung Transplant 28(9):863–869
29. Stehlik J, Edwards LB, Kucheryavaya AY et al (2010) The registry of the international society for heart and lung transplantation: twenty-seventh official adult heart transplant report—2010. J Heart Lung Transplant 29(10):1089–1103
30. Fang JC (2009) Rise of the machines—left ventricular assist devices as permanent therapy for advanced heart failure. N Engl J Med 361(23):2282–2285
31. Felker GM, Rogers JG (2006) Same bridge, new destinations rethinking paradigms for mechanical cardiac support in heart failure. J Am Coll Cardiol 47(5):930–932
32. Stewart GC, Givertz MM (2012) Mechanical circulatory support for advanced heart failure: patients and technology in evolution. Circulation 125(10):1304–1315
33. Kirklin J, Frazier O (2006) Developmental history of mechanical circulatory support. In: Frazier O, Kirklin J (eds) ISHLT monograph series, mechanical circulatory support. Maryland Heights, Missouri, USA. pp 1–9

34. Clauss RH, Birtwell WC, Albertal G et al (1961) Assisted circulation. I. The arterial counterpulsator. J Thorac Cardiovasc Surg 41:447–458
35. DeBakey ME (1971) Left ventricular bypass pump for cardiac assistance. Clinical experience. Am J Cardiol 27(1):3–11
36. Cooley DA, Liotta D, Hallman GL, Bloodwell RD, Leachman RD, Milam JD (1969) Orthotopic cardiac prosthesis for two-staged cardiac replacement. Am J Cardiol 24(5):723–730
37. Kirklin JK, Naftel DC, Kormos RL et al (2012) The Fourth INTERMACS Annual Report: 4,000 implants and counting. J Heart Lung Transplant 31(2):117–126
38. Portner P, Oyer P, McGregor C (1985) First human use of an electrically powered implantable ventricular assist system. Artif Organs 9:36
39. Frazier OH (1994) First use of an untethered, vented electric left ventricular assist device for long-term support. Circulation 89(6):2908–2914
40. Nguyen D, Thourani V (2010) Third-generation continuous flow left ventricular assist devices. Innovations 5(4):250–258
41. Slaughter MS, Pagani FD, Rogers JG et al (2010) Clinical management of continuous-flow left ventricular assist devices in advanced heart failure. J Heart Lung Transplant 29(4 suppl):S1–S39
42. Lahpor JR (2009) State of the art: implantable ventricular assist devices. Curr Opin Organ Transplant 14(5):554–559
43. Pagani FD (2008) Continuous-flow rotary left ventricular assist devices with "3rd generation" design. Semin Thorac Cardiovasc Surg 20(3):255–263
44. Patel CB, Alexander KM, Rogers JG (2010) Mechanical circulatory support for advanced heart failure. Curr Treat Options Cardiovasc Med 12(6):549–565
45. Sheikh FH, Russell SD (2011) HeartMate(R) II continuous-flow left ventricular assist system. Expert Rev Med Devices 8(1):11–21
46. Caccamo M, Eckman P, John R (2011) Current state of ventricular assist devices. Curr Heart Fail Rep 8(2):91–98
47. Hutchinson J, Scott DA, Clegg AJ et al (2008) Cost-effectiveness of left ventricular-assist devices in end-stage heart failure. Expert Rev Cardiovasc Ther 6(2):175–185
48. Moreno SG, Novielli N, Cooper NJ (2012) Cost-effectiveness of the implantable HeartMate II left ventricular assist device for patients awaiting heart transplantation. J Heart Lung Transplant 31:450–458
49. Rogers JG, Bostic RR, Tong KB, Adamson R, Russo M, Slaughter MS (2012) Cost-effectiveness analysis of continuous-flow left ventricular assist devices as destination therapy. Circ Heart Fail 5(1):10–16
50. Slaughter MS, Bostic R, Tong K, Russo M, Rogers JG (2011) Temporal changes in hospital costs for left ventricular assist device implantation. J Card Surg 26(5):535–541
51. Westaby S, Taggart D (2012) Inappropriate restrictions on life saving technology. Heart 98(15):1117–1119
52. Slaughter MS, Rogers JG (2012) Editorial commentary: determining the cost-effectiveness of mechanical circulatory support. J Heart Lung Transplant 31(5):448–449
53. Pal JD, Klodell CT, John R et al (2009) Low operative mortality with implantation of a continuous-flow left ventricular assist device and impact of concurrent cardiac procedures. Circulation 120(11 suppl):S215–S219
54. Miller LW, Pagani FD, Russell SD et al (2007) Use of a continuous-flow device in patients awaiting heart transplantation. N Engl J Med 357(9):885–896
55. Deng MC, Edwards LB, Hertz MI et al (2005) Mechanical circulatory support device database of the international society for heart and lung transplantation: third annual report—2005. J Heart Lung Transplant 24(9):1182–1187
56. Lahpor J, Khaghani A, Hetzer R et al (2010) European results with a continuous-flow ventricular assist device for advanced heart-failure patients. Eur J Cardiothorac Surg 37:357–361

57. Pagani FD, Miller LW, Russell SD et al (2009) Extended mechanical circulatory support with a continuous-flow rotary left ventricular assist device. J Am Coll Cardiol 54(4):312–321
58. Esmore D, Kaye D, Spratt P et al (2008) A prospective, multicenter trial of the VentrAssist left ventricular assist device for bridge to transplant: safety and efficacy. J Heart Lung Transplant 27(6):579–588
59. INTERMACS (2009) http://www.uab.edu/ctsresearch/intermacs/statisticalsummaries.htm
60. Slaughter MS, Rogers JG, Milano CA, Russel SD, Conte JV, Feldman D, Sun B, Tatooles AJ, Delgado RM III, Long JW, Wozniak TC, Ghumman W, Farrrar DJ, Frazier OH, HeartMate II Investigators (2009) Advanced heart failure treated with continous-flow left ventricular assist device. N Engl J Med 361(23):2241–2251
61. Strueber M, O'Driscoll G, Jansz P, Khaghani A, Levy WC, Wieselthaler GM (2011) Multicenter evaluation of an intrapericardial left ventricular assist system. J Am Coll Cardiol 57(12):1375–1382
62. Starling RC, Naka Y, Boyle AJ et al (2011) Results of the Post-U.S. Food and Drug Administration-Approval Study with a continuous flow left ventricular assist device as a bridge to heart transplantation a prospective study using the INTERMACS (interagency registry for mechanically assisted circulatory support). J Am Coll Cardiol 57(19):1890–1898
63. Park SJ, Milano CA, Tatooles AJ et al (2012) Outcomes in advanced heart failure patients with left ventricular assist devices for destination therapy. Circ Heart Fail 5(2):241–248
64. Adamson RM, Stahovich M, Chillcott S et al (2011) Clinical strategies and outcomes in advanced heart failure patients older than 70 years of age receiving the HeartMate II left ventricular assist device: a community hospital experience. J Am Coll Cardiol 57(25):2487–2495
65. John R, Naka Y, Smedira NG et al (2011) Continuous flow left ventricular assist device outcomes in commercial use compared with the prior clinical trial. Ann Thorac Surg 92(4): 1406–1413; discussion 1413
66. Aaronson KD, Slaughter MS, Miller LW et al (2012) Use of an intrapericardial, continuous flow, centrifugal pump in patients awaiting heart transplantation. Circulation 125(25):3191–3200
67. Holman WA, Kirklin JK (2006) Outcomes after mechanical circulatory support. In: Frazier OH, Kirklin JK (eds) ISHLT Monograph Series, vol 1. Maryland Heights, Missouri, USA. pp 137–154
68. Holman WL, Pae WE, Teutenberg JJ et al (2009) INTERMACS: interval analysis of registry data. J Am Coll Surg 208(5):755–761; discussion 761–752
69. Frazier OH, Rose EA, McCarthy P et al (1995) Improved mortality and rehabilitation of transplant candidates treated with a long-term implantable left ventricular assist system. Ann Surg 222(3):327–336; discussion 336–328
70. Frazier OH, Rose EA, Oz MC et al (2001) Multicenter clinical evaluation of the HeartMate vented electric left ventricular assist system in patients awaiting heart transplantation. J Thorac Cardiovasc Surg 122(6):1186–1195
71. Goldstein DJ (2003) Worldwide experience with the MicroMed DeBakey Ventricular Assist Device as a bridge to transplantation. Circulation 108(suppl 1):II272–II277
72. Cowger J, Pagani FD, Haft JW, Romano MA, Aaronson KD, Kolias TJ (2010) The development of aortic insufficiency in left ventricular assist device-supported patients. Circ Heart Fail 3(6):668–674
73. Meyer AL, Malehsa D, Bara C et al (2010) Acquired von Willebrand syndrome in patients with an axial flow left ventricular assist device. Circ Heart Fail 3(6):675–681
74. Uriel N, Pak SW, Jorde UP et al (2010) Acquired von Willebrand syndrome after continuous-flow mechanical device support contributes to a high prevalence of bleeding during long-term support and at the time of transplantation. J Am Coll Cardiol 56(15):1207–1213
75. Eckman PM, John R (2012) Bleeding and thrombosis in patients with continuous-flow ventricular assist devices. Circulation 125(24):3038–3047
76. Rogers JG, Aaronson KD, Boyle AJ et al (2010) Continuous flow left ventricular assist device improves functional capacity and quality of life of advanced heart failure patients. J Am Coll Cardiol 55(17):1826–1834

77. Aaronson KD, Patel H, Pagani FD (2003) Patient selection for left ventricular assist device therapy. Ann Thorac Surg 75(6 suppl):S29–S35
78. Stevenson LW, Shekar P (2005) Ventricular assist devices for durable support. Circulation 112(9):e111–e115
79. Potapov EV, Loforte A, Weng Y et al (2008) Experience with over 1000 implanted ventricular assist devices. J Card Surg 23(3):185–194
80. Goldstein DJ, Oz MC, Rose EA (1998) Implantable left ventricular assist devices. N Engl J Med 339(21):1522–1533
81. Kirklin JK, Naftel DC, Kormos RL et al (2010) Second INTERMACS annual report: more than 1,000 primary left ventricular assist device implants. J Heart Lung Transplant 29(1):1–10
82. Birks EJ, Tansley PD, Hardy J et al (2006) Left ventricular assist device and drug therapy for the reversal of heart failure. N Engl J Med 355(18):1873–1884
83. Mancini DM, Beniaminovitz A, Levin H et al (1998) Low incidence of myocardial recovery after left ventricular assist device implantation in patients with chronic heart failure. Circulation 98(22):2383–2389
84. Maybaum S, Mancini D, Xydas S et al (2007) Cardiac improvement during mechanical circulatory support: a prospective multicenter study of the LVAD Working Group. Circulation 115(19):2497–2505
85. Liden H, Karason K, Bergh CH, Nilsson F, Koul B, Wiklund L (2007) The feasibility of left ventricular mechanical support as a bridge to cardiac recovery. Eur J Heart Fail 9(5):525–530
86. Simon JR (2008) Case study. "Doctor, will you turn off my LVAD?" Commentary. Hastings Cent Rep 38(1):14–15
87. Velazquez EJ, Lee KL, Deja MA et al (2011) Coronary-artery bypass surgery in patients with left ventricular dysfunction. N Engl J Med 364(17):1607–1616
88. Bonow RO, Maurer G, Lee KL et al (2011) Myocardial viability and survival in ischemic left ventricular dysfunction. N Engl J Med 364(17):1617–1625
89. Cooper LT, Baughman KL, Feldman AM et al (2007) The role of endomyocardial biopsy in the management of cardiovascular disease: a scientific statement from the American Heart Association, the American College of Cardiology, and the European Society of Cardiology Endorsed by the Heart Failure Society of America and the Heart Failure Association of the European Society of Cardiology. Eur Heart J 28(24):3076–3093
90. Mokadam NA, Ewald GA, Damiano RJ Jr, Moazami N (2006) Deterioration and mortality among patients with United Network for Organ Sharing status 2 heart disease: caution must be exercised in diverting organs. J Thorac Cardiovasc Surg 131(4):925–926
91. Kamiya H, Koch A, Sack FU et al (2008) Who needs 'bridge' to transplantation in the presence of the eurotransplant high-urgency heart transplantation program? Eur J Cardiothorac Surg 34(6):1129–1133; discussion 1134–1125
92. Frazier OH, Myers TJ, Westaby S, Gregoric ID (2003) Use of the Jarvik 2000 left ventricular assist system as a bridge to heart transplantation or as destination therapy for patients with chronic heart failure. Ann Surg 237(5):631–636; discussion 636–637
93. Stevenson LW (2003) Clinical use of inotropic therapy for heart failure: looking backward or forward? Part II: chronic inotropic therapy. Circulation 108(4):492–497
94. Upadya S, Lee FA, Saldarriaga C et al (2004) Home continuous positive inotropic infusion as a bridge to cardiac transplantation in patients with end-stage heart failure. J Heart Lung Transplant 23(4):466–472
95. Zemljic G, Bunc M, Yazdanbakhsh AP, Vrtovec B (2007) Levosimendan improves renal function in patients with advanced chronic heart failure awaiting cardiac transplantation. J Card Fail 13(6):417–421
96. Taylor DO, Edwards LB, Boucek MM et al (2007) Registry of the international society for heart and lung transplantation: twenty-fourth official adult heart transplant report—2007. J Heart Lung Transplant 26(8):769–781

97. Morgan JA, John R, Rao V et al (2004) Bridging to transplant with the HeartMate left ventricular assist device: The Columbia Presbyterian 12-year experience. J Thorac Cardiovasc Surg 127(5):1309–1316
98. Nativi JN, Drakos SG, Kucheryavaya AY et al (2011) Changing outcomes in patients bridged to heart transplantation with continuous- versus pulsatile-flow ventricular assist devices: an analysis of the registry of the international society for heart and lung transplantation. J Heart Lung Transplant 30(8):854–861
99. Aaronson KD, Eppinger MJ, Dyke DB, Wright S, Pagani FD (2002) Left ventricular assist device therapy improves utilization of donor hearts. J Am Coll Cardiol 39(8):1247–1254
100. Bank AJ, Mir SH, Nguyen DQ et al (2000) Effects of left ventricular assist devices on outcomes in patients undergoing heart transplantation. Ann Thorac Surg 69(5):1369–1374; discussion 1375
101. Bhat G (2006) Predictors of clinical outcome in advanced heart failure patients on continuous intravenous milrinone therapy. ASAIO J 52(6):677–681
102. Gronda E, Bourge RC, Costanzo MR et al (2006) Heart rhythm considerations in heart transplant candidates and considerations for ventricular assist devices: international society for heart and lung transplantation guidelines for the care of cardiac transplant candidates—2006. J Heart Lung Transplant 25(9):1043–1056
103. Russell SD, Miller LW, Pagani FD (2008) Advanced heart failure: a call to action. Congest Heart Fail 14(6):316–321
104. Stewart GC, Stevenson LW (2011) Keeping left ventricular assist device acceleration on track. Circulation 123(14):1559–1568; discussion 1568
105. Mancini DM, Eisen H, Kussmaul W, Mull R, Edmunds LH Jr, Wilson JR (1991) Value of peak exercise oxygen consumption for optimal timing of cardiac transplantation in ambulatory patients with heart failure. Circulation 83(3):778–786
106. Lund LH, Aaronson KD, Mancini DM (2005) Validation of peak exercise oxygen consumption and the heart failure survival score for serial risk stratification in advanced heart failure. Am J Cardiol 95(6):734–741
107. Lund LH, Mancini DM (2008) Peak VO(2) in elderly patients with heart failure. Int J Cardiol 125:166–171
108. Goda A, Lund LH, Mancini DM (2010) Comparison across races of peak oxygen consumption and heart failure survival score for selection for cardiac transplantation. Am J Cardiol 105(10):1439–1444
109. Goda A, Williams P, Mancini D, Lund LH (2011) Selecting patients for heart transplantation: comparison of the heart failure survival score (HFSS) and the seattle heart failure model (SHFM). J Heart Lung Transplant 30(11):1236–1243
110. Parikh MN, Lund LH, Goda A, Mancini D (2009) Usefulness of peak exercise oxygen consumption and the heart failure survival score to predict survival in patients >65 years of age with heart failure. Am J Cardiol 103(7):998–1002
111. Hunt SA, Abraham WT, Chin MH et al (2005) ACC/AHA 2005 Guideline Update for the Diagnosis and Management of Chronic Heart Failure in the Adult: a report of the American College of Cardiology/American Heart Association Task Force on Practice Guidelines (Writing Committee to Update the 2001 Guidelines for the Evaluation and Management of Heart Failure): developed in collaboration with the American College of Chest Physicians and the International Society for Heart and Lung Transplantation: endorsed by the Heart Rhythm Society. Circulation 112(12):e154–e235
112. Green P, Lund LH, Mancini D (2007) Comparison of peak exercise oxygen consumption and the heart failure survival score for predicting prognosis in women versus men. Am J Cardiol 99(3):399–403
113. Lund LH, Aaronson KD, Mancini DM (2003) Predicting survival in ambulatory patients with severe heart failure on beta-blocker therapy. Am J Cardiol 92(11):1350–1354
114. Goda A, Lund LH, Mancini D (2011) The heart failure survival score outperforms the peak oxygen consumption for heart transplantation selection in the era of device therapy. J Heart Lung Transplant 30(3):315–325

115. Aaronson KD, Schwartz JS, Chen TM, Wong KL, Goin JE, Mancini DM (1997) Development and prospective validation of a clinical index to predict survival in ambulatory patients referred for cardiac transplant evaluation. Circulation 95(12):2660–2667
116. Kalogeropoulos AP, Georgiopoulou VV, Giamouzis G et al (2009) Utility of the seattle heart failure model in patients with advanced heart failure. J Am Coll Cardiol 53(4):334–342
117. Levy WC, Mozaffarian D, Linker DT, Farrar DJ, Miller LW (2009) Can the Seattle heart failure model be used to risk-stratify heart failure patients for potential left ventricular assist device therapy? J Heart Lung Transplant 28(3):231–236
118. Ketchum ES, Moorman AJ, Fishbein DP et al (2010) Predictive value of the seattle heart failure model in patients undergoing left ventricular assist device placement. J Heart Lung Transplant 29(9):1021–1025
119. Pamboukian SV, Tallaj JA, Brown RN et al (2012) Comparison of observed survival after ventricular assist device placement versus predicted survival without assist device using the Seattle heart failure model. ASAIO J 58(2):93–97
120. Gorodeski EZ, Chu EC, Chow CH, Levy WC, Hsich E, Starling RC (2010) Application of the seattle heart failure model in ambulatory patients presented to an advanced heart failure therapeutics committee. Circ Heart Fail 3(6):706–714
121. Teuteberg JJ, Lewis EF, Nohria A et al (2006) Characteristics of patients who die with heart failure and a low ejection fraction in the new millennium. J Card Fail 12(1):47–53
122. Deng MC, Loebe M, El-Banayosy A et al (2001) Mechanical circulatory support for advanced heart failure: effect of patient selection on outcome. Circulation 103(2):231–237
123. Sandner SE, Zimpfer D, Zrunek P et al (2009) Age and outcome after continuous-flow left ventricular assist device implantation as bridge to transplantation. J Heart Lung Transplant 28(4):367–372
124. Farrar DJ (1994) Preoperative predictors of survival in patients with Thoratec ventricular assist devices as a bridge to heart transplantation. Thoratec Ventricular Assist Device Principal Investigators. J Heart Lung Transplant 13(1 Pt 1):93–100; discussion 100–101
125. McCarthy PM, Smedira NO, Vargo RL et al (1998) One hundred patients with the HeartMate left ventricular assist device: evolving concepts and technology. J Thorac Cardiovasc Surg 115(4):904–912
126. Reedy JE, Swartz MT, Termuhlen DF et al (1990) Bridge to heart transplantation: importance of patient selection. J Heart Transplant 9(5):473–480; discussion 480–471
127. Butler J, Geisberg C, Howser R et al (2006) Relationship between renal function and left ventricular assist device use. Ann Thorac Surg 81(5):1745–1751
128. Sandner SE, Zimpfer D, Zrunek P et al (2009) Renal function and outcome after continuous flow left ventricular assist device implantation. Ann Thorac Surg 87(4):1072–1078
129. Alba AC, Rao V, Ivanov J, Ross HJ, Delgado DH (2009) Usefulness of the INTERMACS scale to predict outcomes after mechanical assist device implantation. J Heart Lung Transplant 28(8):827–833
130. Klotz S, Vahlhaus C, Riehl C, Reitz C, Sindermann JR, Scheld HH (2010) Pre-operative prediction of post-VAD implant mortality using easily accessible clinical parameters. J Heart Lung Transplant 29:45–52
131. Oz MC, Goldstein DJ, Pepino P et al (1995) Screening scale predicts patients successfully receiving long-term implantable left ventricular assist devices. Circulation 92(9 suppl):II169–II173
132. Rao V, Oz MC, Flannery MA, Catanese KA, Argenziano M, Naka Y (2003) Revised screening scale to predict survival after insertion of a left ventricular assist device. J Thorac Cardiovasc Surg 125(4):855–862
133. Holman WL, Kormos RL, Naftel DC et al (2009) Predictors of death and transplant in patients with a mechanical circulatory support device: a multi-institutional study. J Heart Lung Transplant 28(1):44–50
134. Matthews JC, Pagani FD, Haft JW, Koelling TM, Naftel DC, Aaronson KD (2010) Model for end-stage liver disease score predicts left ventricular assist device operative transfusion requirements, morbidity, and mortality. Circulation 121(2):214–220

135. Bonde P, Ku NC, Genovese EA et al (2012) Model for end-stage liver disease score predicts adverse events related to ventricular assist device therapy. Ann Thorac Surg 93(5):1541–1547; discussion 1547–1548
136. Potapov EV, Stepanenko A, Dandel M et al (2008) Tricuspid incompetence and geometry of the right ventricle as predictors of right ventricular function after implantation of a left ventricular assist device. J Heart Lung Transplant 27(12):1275–1281
137. Teuteberg JJ, Ewald GA, Adamson RM et al (2012) Risk assessment for continuous flow left ventricular assist devices: does the destination therapy risk score work?: An analysis of over 1,000 patients. J Am Coll Cardiol 60(1):44–51
138. Schaffer JM, Allen JG, Weiss ES et al (2009) Evaluation of risk indices in continuous-flow left ventricular assist device patients. Ann Thorac Surg 88(6):1889–1896
139. Matthews JC, Koelling TM, Pagani FD, Aaronson KD (2008) The right ventricular failure risk score a pre-operative tool for assessing the risk of right ventricular failure in left ventricular assist device candidates. J Am Coll Cardiol 51(22):2163–2172
140. Fukamachi K, McCarthy PM, Smedira NG, Vargo RL, Starling RC, Young JB (1999) Preoperative risk factors for right ventricular failure after implantable left ventricular assist device insertion. Ann Thorac Surg 68(6):2181–2184
141. Kavarana MN, Pessin-Minsley MS, Urtecho J et al (2002) Right ventricular dysfunction and organ failure in left ventricular assist device recipients: a continuing problem. Ann Thorac Surg 73(3):745–750
142. Dang NC, Topkara VK, Mercando M et al (2006) Right heart failure after left ventricular assist device implantation in patients with chronic congestive heart failure. J Heart Lung Transplant 25(1):1–6
143. Fitzpatrick JR III, Frederick JR, Hsu VM et al (2008) Risk score derived from pre-operative data analysis predicts the need for biventricular mechanical circulatory support. J Heart Lung Transplant 27(12):1286–1292
144. Kato TS, Farr M, Schulze PC et al (2012) Usefulness of two-dimensional echocardiographic parameters of the left side of the heart to predict right ventricular failure after left ventricular assist device implantation. Am J Cardiol 109(2):246–251
145. Drakos SG, Janicki L, Horne BD et al (2010) Risk factors predictive of right ventricular failure after left ventricular assist device implantation. Am J Cardiol 105(7):1030–1035
146. Wang Y, Simon MA, Bonde P et al (2012) Decision tree for adjuvant right ventricular support in patients receiving a left ventricular assist device. J Heart Lung Transplant 31:140–149
147. Brewer RJ, Morgan JA, Nemeh H et al (2009) Persistent right ventricular failure after LVAD implantation for bridge-to-transplant does not reduce survival to transplantation. J Card Fail 15(6):S47
148. Patrick JE, Miller LW, Boyce SW (2009) Improved survival with simultaneous RVAD placement in LVAD recipients at high risk for RV failure. J Heart Lung Transplant 28(2):S209
149. Fitzpatrick JR III, Frederick JR, Hiesinger W et al (2009) Early planned institution of biventricular mechanical circulatory support results in improved outcomes compared with delayed conversion of a left ventricular assist device to a biventricular assist device. J Thorac Cardiovasc Surg 137(4):971–977
150. Hill JD, Farrar DJ, Naka Y, Chen JM, Portner PM, Loisance D (2006) Positive displacement ventricular assisst devices. In: Frazier O, Kirklin J (eds) ISHLT monograph series 1, mechanical circulatory support. Maryland Heights, Missouri, USA. pp 53–75
151. Kormos RL, Gasior TA, Kawai A et al (1996) Transplant candidate's clinical status rather than right ventricular function defines need for univentricular versus biventricular support. J Thorac Cardiovasc Surg 111(4):773–782; discussion 782–773
152. Ochiai Y, McCarthy PM, Smedira NG et al (2002) Predictors of severe right ventricular failure after implantable left ventricular assist device insertion: analysis of 245 patients. Circulation 106(12 suppl 1):I198–I202
153. Santambrogio L, Bianchi T, Fuardo M et al (2006) Right ventricular failure after left ventricular assist device insertion: preoperative risk factors. Interact Cardiovasc Thorac Surg 5(4):379–382

154. Scalia GM, McCarthy PM, Savage RM, Smedira NG, Thomas JD (2000) Clinical utility of echocardiography in the management of implantable ventricular assist devices. J Am Soc Echocardiogr 13(8):754–763
155. Kormos RL, Teuteberg JJ, Pagani FD et al (2010) Right ventricular failure in patients with the HeartMate II continuous-flow left ventricular assist device: incidence, risk factors, and effect on outcomes. J Thorac Cardiovasc Surg 139(5):1316–1324
156. Farrar DJ, Hill JD, Pennington DG et al (1997) Preoperative and postoperative comparison of patients with univentricular and biventricular support with the thoratec ventricular assist device as a bridge to cardiac transplantation. J Thorac Cardiovasc Surg 113(1):202–209
157. Kormos RL, Teuteberg J, Russell SD, Massey T, Feldman D, Moazami N, Farrar C, Milano C (2008) Right ventricular failure (RVF) in patients with continuous flow left ventricular assist devices (LVAD) (abstract 203). J Heart Lung Transplant 27:S134
158. Kilic A, Ailawadi G (2012) Left ventricular assist devices in heart failure. Expert Rev Cardiovasc Ther 10(5):649–656
159. Meyns B, Klotz S, Simon A et al (2009) Proof of concept: hemodynamic response to long-term partial ventricular support with the synergy pocket micro-pump. J Am Coll Cardiol 54(1):79–86
160. Krabatsch T, Potapov E, Stepanenko A et al (2011) Biventricular circulatory support with two miniaturized implantable assist devices. Circulation 124(11 suppl):S179–S186
161. Loebe M, Bruckner B, Reardon MJ et al (2011) Initial clinical experience of total cardiac replacement with dual HeartMate-II axial flow pumps for severe biventricular heart failure. Methodist Debakey Cardiovasc J 7(1):40–44
162. Slaughter MS, Myers TJ (2010) Transcutaneous energy transmission for mechanical circulatory support systems: history, current status, and future prospects. J Card Surg 25(4):484–489
163. Kirklin JK, Naftel DC, Kormos RL et al (2011) Third INTERMACS Annual Report: the evolution of destination therapy in the United States. J Heart Lung Transplant 30(2):115–123
164. Kirklin JK, Mehra MR (2012) The dawn of the ISHLT mechanical assisted circulatory support (IMACS) registry: fulfilling our mission. J Heart Lung Transplant 31(2):115–116
165. McMurray JJ, Adamopoulos S, Anker SD et al (2012) ESC Guidelines for the diagnosis and treatment of acute and chronic heart failure 2012: the task force for the diagnosis and treatment of acute and chronic heart failure 2012 of the European Society of Cardiology. Developed in collaboration with the Heart Failure Association (HFA) of the ESC. Eur Heart J 14:803–869
166. Lindenfeld J, Albert NM, Boehmer JP et al (2010) HFSA 2010 comprehensive heart failure practice guideline. J Card Fail 16(6):e1–e194
167. Bogaev RC, Pamboukian SV, Moore SA et al (2011) Comparison of outcomes in women versus men using a continuous-flow left ventricular assist device as a bridge to transplantation. J Heart Lung Transplant 30(5):515–522
168. Morgan JA, John R, Lee BJ, Oz MC, Naka Y (2004) Is severe right ventricular failure in left ventricular assist device recipients a risk factor for unsuccessful bridging to transplant and post-transplant mortality. Ann Thorac Surg 77(3):859–863
169. Nakatani S, Thomas JD, Savage RM, Vargo RL, Smedira NG, McCarthy PM (1996) Prediction of right ventricular dysfunction after left ventricular assist device implantation. Circulation 94(9 suppl):II216–II221
170. Goda A, Takayama H, Koeckert M et al (2011) Use of ventricular assist devices in patients with mitral valve prostheses. J Card Surg 26(3):334–337
171. Krishan K, Nair A, Pinney S, Adams DH, Anyanwu AC (2012) Liberal use of tricuspid-valve annuloplasty during left-ventricular assist device implantation. Eur J Cardiothorac Surg 41:213–217
172. Puwanant S, Hamilton KK, Klodell CT et al (2008) Tricuspid annular motion as a predictor of severe right ventricular failure after left ventricular assist device implantation. J Heart Lung Transplant 27(10):1102–1107

173. Kukucka M, Stepanenko A, Potapov E et al (2011) Right-to-left ventricular end-diastolic diameter ratio and prediction of right ventricular failure with continuous-flow left ventricular assist devices. J Heart Lung Transplant 30(1):64–69
174. Acharya MN, Som R, Tsui S (2012) What is the optimum antibiotic prophylaxis in patients undergoing implantation of a left ventricular assist device? Interact Cardiovasc Thorac Surg 14(2):209–214
175. Mano A, Fujita K, Uenomachi K et al (2009) Body mass index is a useful predictor of prognosis after left ventricular assist system implantation. J Heart Lung Transplant 28(5):428–433
176. Holdy K, Dembitsky W, Eaton LL et al (2005) Nutrition assessment and management of left ventricular assist device patients. J Heart Lung Transplant 24(10):1690–1696
177. Johnsson P, Algotsson L, Ryding E, Stahl E, Messeter K (1991) Cardiopulmonary perfusion and cerebral blood flow in bilateral carotid artery disease. Ann Thorac Surg 51(4):579–584
178. Selim M (2008) Angioplasty and stenting of asymptomatic carotid stenosis before cardiac surgery: more study is needed. Arch Neurol 65(12):1672–1674
179. Lazar HL, Menzoian JO (1998) Coronary artery bypass grafting in patients with cerebrovascular disease. Ann Thorac Surg 66(3):968–974
180. Tylus-Earl N, Chillcott S (2009) Mental health and medical challenges. Management of a depressed patient with a left ventricular assist system in an inpatient psychiatric setting. J Psychosoc Nurs Ment Health Serv 47(10):43–49; quiz 51
181. Marcus P (2009) Left ventricular assist devices: psychosocial challenges in the elderly. Ann Thorac Surg 88(5):e48–e49

Chapter 16
Novel Device-Based Strategies in Treatment of Chronic Heart Failure

Gabor Toth, Marc Vanderheyden, and Jozef Bartunek

Abstract Multimodal treatments can alleviate the symptoms or reverse the progression of heart failure. Besides the lifestyle management and pharmacological therapies, various device-based interventions have been introduced. In this review, we summarize recent developments with regard to treatment of chronic heart failure as they are designed to target various components in the cascade of heart failure progression.

1 Introduction

Heart failure is a progressive but heterogeneous clinical syndrome characterized by marked pump abnormality due to either systolic or diastolic cardiac dysfunction or both that leads to the insufficient oxygenized blood supply in the periphery. Though the syndrome has a heterogeneous etiology with different mechanism, the epidemic of heart failure due to coronary artery disease is a leading cause of morbidity and mortality. The hallmark of heart failure syndrome is maladaptive ventricular remodeling that precipitates contractile dysfunction, and ultimately leads to the overt syndrome of congestive heart failure. The central feature in this cascade is the loss of cardiomyocytes, followed by replacement with fibrotic scar which ultimately leads to organ failure accelerated by hemodynamic overload, neurohumoral as well as inflammatory-oxidative stress, and/or impaired vascularization.

Implementation of state-of-the-art reperfusion strategies improved the survival of patients presenting with acute coronary disease. Yet, success of reperfusion interventions with improved survival in parallel with aging and changing patterns in the

This work has been supported by the Meijer Cardiac Research Fund, Aalst, Belgium.

G. Toth, M.D. • M. Vanderheyden, M.D., Ph.D. • J. Bartunek, M.D., Ph.D. (✉)
Cardiovascular Centre, OLV Hospital, Moorselbaan, 164, 9300 Aalst, Belgium
e-mail: jozef.bartunek@olvz-aalst.be

J. Bartunek and M. Vanderheyden (eds.), *Translational Approach to Heart Failure*, DOI 10.1007/978-1-4614-7345-9_16, © Springer Science+Business Media New York 2013

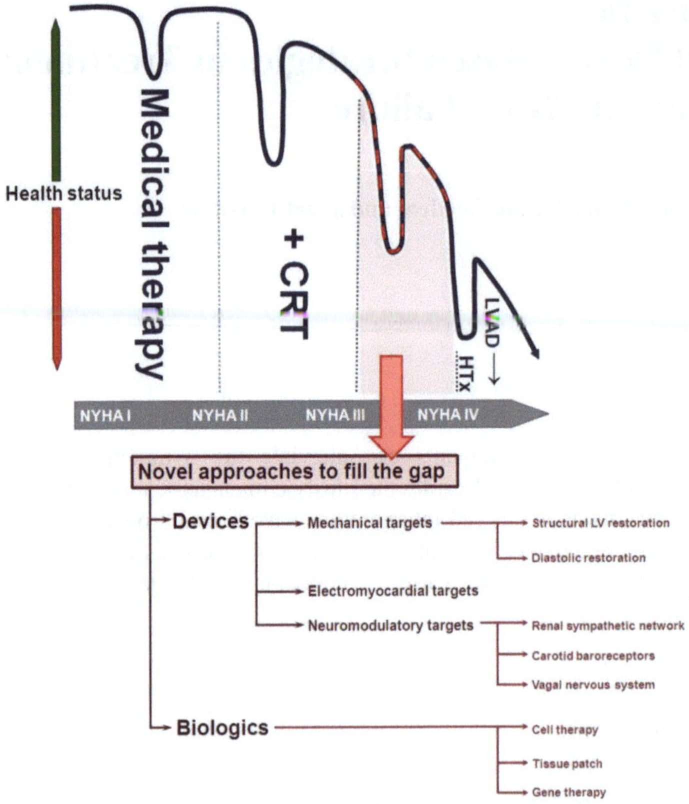

Fig. 16.1 Targets and respective devices for interventional treatment in advanced heart failure

presentation of the chronic coronary artery disease is the most important reason for increasing prevalence of heart failure. Multimodal treatments have been introduced to alleviate the symptoms or reverse the progression of heart failure. Besides the lifestyle management and pharmacological therapies, various device-based interventions have been proposed. Among them, cardiac resynchronization improved morbidity and mortality. Yet, a gap persists in therapeutic options for patients with advanced heart failure progression and a gap persists in therapeutic options for patients with advanced heart failure. Advances propelled by the translational medicine or technology development lead to novel biologic or device-based therapeutic interventions aiming to fill this therapeutic gap and halt or reverse the vicious cycle of heart failure progression (Fig. 16.1). In this review, we summarize recent developments with regard to treatment of chronic heart failure as they are designed to target various components in the cascade of heart failure progression and filling thus a gap in the therapeutic strategies of advanced heart failure (Table 16.1). For the

Table 16.1 Targets and respective devices for interventional treatment in advanced heart failure

Target	Device		Patients
Mechanical	ImCardia™	Epicardially placed metallic coils using the bow-string effect to restore diastolic function	$n = 18$
	CORolla™	Endocardially placed metallic coils using the bow-string effect to restore diastolic function	$n =$ NA
	Parachute™	Percutaneous left ventricle partitioning device for patients with big antero-apical scar	$n = 34$
	Revivent™	Percutaneous left ventricle plication device for patients with big antero-apical scar	$n = 26$
	IASD™	Interatrial shunt device for reduction of therapy-resistant increased left atrial pressure	$n = 3$
Electro-myocardial	Optimizer™	Cardiac contractility modulation with non-excitatory stimuli of the myocardium	$n = 641$
Neuro-modulatory	RDN	Renal denervation therapy for reducing baseline sympathetic activity in *systolic* CHF	$n = 7$
	BaroStim™	Continuous stimulation of the carotid baroreceptors for reducing sympathetic activity in *systolic* CHF	$n =$ NA
	CardioFit™	Chronic vagal nerve stimulation modulation of the autonomic imbalance	$n = 32$

didactic purpose, potential targets for device-based interventions can be divided into three groups: mechanical, electrical, and neuro-modulatory targets.

2 Left Ventricular Restoration

Progressive left ventricular dilation is one of the hallmarks of heart failure progression. Though serving initially as a compensatory mechanism to sustain the stroke volume and ventricular function, it is also associated with increased wall stress, thereby further precipitating progressive ventricular enlargement and failure. Specific subsets are patients with large transmural myocardial anterior infarction where transmural damage with development of akinetic- or dyskinetic-infarcted segments due to the wall thinning may precipitate infarct expansion with elongation of the affected region [1]. In accordance with Laplace Law, the altered ventricular geometry underlies increased regional wall stress and regional overload which further aggravates abnormal local mechanics, adversely affects remote myocardial segments, and perpetuates further ventricular dilation. Though initially these mechanisms may contribute to the maintenance of ventricular pump function, this self-perpetuating cycle ultimately results in spherical chamber remodeling and reduced forward stroke volume. Reduction of the wall stress by reducing the ventricular cavity has

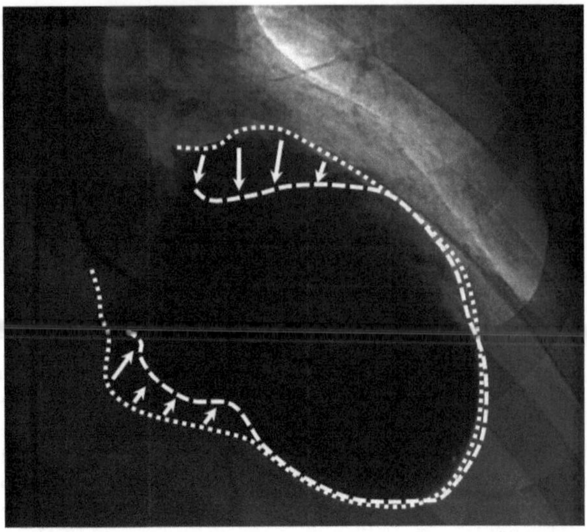

Fig. 16.2 Functional–geometrical mismatch in a patient with apical aneurysm after anterior myocardial infarct

been attempted previously surgically with aneurysma resection or using mesh-like devices to support cardiac mechanics and limit further dilation. However, none of these approaches has reached wide clinical adoption so far.

The so-called *percutaneous left ventricle partitioning* approach with Parachute™ (CardioKinetix Inc., Menlo Park, CA, USA) is an alternative percutaneous procedure to restore left ventricular geometry by partitioning dysfunctional apical segments in patients with regional apical akinesia or dyskinesia (Fig. 16.2). The device consists of an umbrella-like flexible nitinol frame, covered with poly-tetra-fluoro-ethylene surface that can be placed percutaneously using a dedicated guide catheter. Parachute™ partitions enlarged ventricle into "dynamic" and "static" chambers (Fig. 16.3). The "static" chamber is a portion of the left ventricle that is separated from the systemic circulation by the device after implantation in the apical region. After device deployment, stresses placed on the partitioned myocardium and the forces transmitted to the apical segment are decreased in diastole and systole eliminating loading forces responsible for left ventricular dilation. This leads to a regional unloading of remote segments with preserved contractility. In addition, the "dynamic" chamber with newly formed apical region consisting with the "parachute"-like device acquires more conical shape and this together with the reduced size of the "dynamic" chamber results in a decrease in myocardial wall stress. Thus, the main mechanism underlying the concept of the percutaneous partitioning is reduction of the global wall stress and ventricular unloading according to Laplace Law. The nitinol frame is also highly flexible and thanks to the newly formed shape of the dynamic chamber and exclusion of the dysfunctional apical segments, it may also hypothetically contribute to restoration of the twisting and untwisting contractile mechanics.

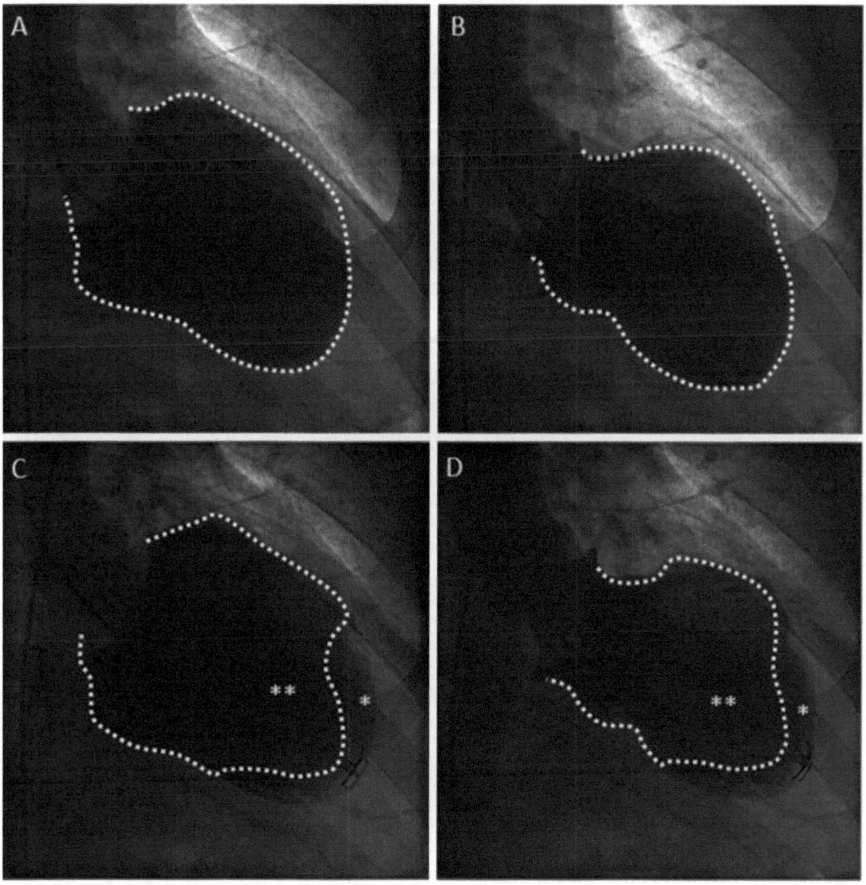

Fig. 16.3 Dilated and dysfunctional left ventricle in diastole and systole with apical dyskinesia (upper panels **a** and **b**). Parachute device partitions apical akinetic segments and creates a "new functional chamber" (**) as delineated in panel **c** (diastole) en systole (panel **d**). Partitioned ventricular volumes between Parachute device and native wall creates a "static" chamber (*)

The system implantation requires a pre-procedural planning where echocardiographic or computed tomography evaluation of the apical aneurysm and ventricular geometry should identify suitable left ventricular chamber anatomy and size of the device. It is also critical to exclude any intraventricular structure that can prevent the safe device deployment such as false chordae. The Parachute™ device is implanted through a 16Fr femoral access and assessment of appropriate peripheral access is crucial (Fig. 16.4a). Implantation is a safe and straightforward procedure performed in the following steps. Future position of the device is defined by a left-ventricular angiogram and delineation of the akinetic or dyskinetic apical regions (Fig. 16.4b, c). Then, a dedicated, preshaped 16Fr sheathless guiding catheter is advanced into the left ventricle over a diagnostic pigtail catheter aiming towards the dyskinetic apex

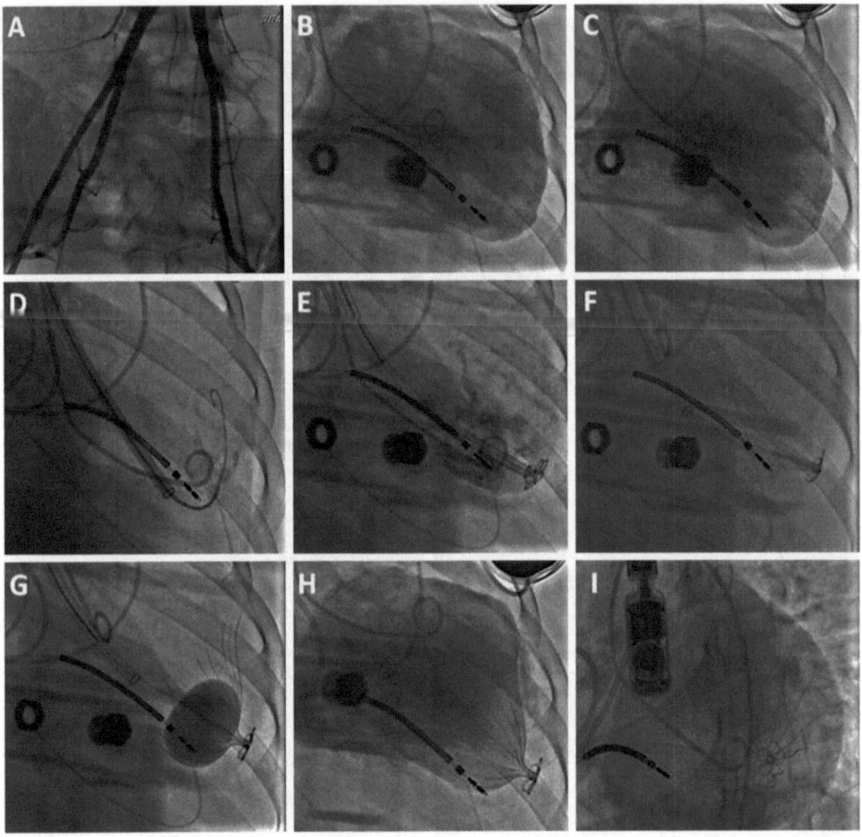

Fig. 16.4 Procedure flow of Parachute™ device implantation. (**a**) Checking of appropriate femoral access. (**b**, **c**) Defining the dyskinetic segments and identifying the aimed landing zone. (**d**) Dedicated 16Fr sheathless guiding catheter is advanced into the left ventricle over a diagnostic pigtail catheter aiming towards the dyskinetic apex. (**e**, **f**) Pulling back the guiding catheter allows the release of the nitinol frames and the opening of the Parachute™. (**g**) Inflating a balloon enhances the full deployment and the anchoring of the nitinol frame in the myocardium. (**h**, **i**) Final impact on the ventricular chamber reshaping

(Fig. 16.4d). Pigtail catheter is removed and, using an introducer tube, the device is advanced carefully into the guiding catheter while avoiding an inadvertent air bubble in the entire delivery system. The device is advanced further up to the tip of the guiding catheter. If needed the system is repositioned to achieve the desired position in the apex. The device is then advanced with its soft foot to the apex. After shouldering, the guide is slowly pulled back allowing the release of the nitinol frames and opening of the Parachute™ (Fig. 16.4e, f). This is facilitated by inflating a balloon to ensure the full deployment and anchoring of the nitinol frame in the myocardium (Fig. 16.4g). As soon as the whole frame opens up completely, the hooks are fixed in the wall of the ventricle and the Parachute™ device acquires a stable position. Final impact on the ventricular chamber reshaping is checked by a control left-ventricular angiogram (Fig. 16.4h, i).

In the feasibility and safety study with the Parachute™ [2], 39 patients were enrolled. Procedure was performed in 34 cases and implantation was performed successfully and safely in 31 patients (79 % of all patients). During the 6-month follow-up, five adverse events were observed in 34 cases with attempted implantation. In patients who completed 12 months follow-up ($n=28$), a significant improvement in functional status (New York Heart Association class 2.5±0.6 to 1.3±0.6, $p<0.001$) and in quality-of-life score (38.6±6.1 to 28.4±4.4, $p<0.002$) was observed. However no significant change in 6-min hall walk distance (from 358.5±20.4 to 374.7±25.6 m, NS) was observed. Taken together, percutaneous partitioning is an innovative approach to modify left ventricular geometry. It is a relatively safe and potentially effective treatment in well-selected patients with chronic heart failure after anterior myocardial infarction. Further randomized studies are ongoing to establish its clinical value in treatment of post-infarct heart failure.

Alternative device targeting ventricular remodeling is the Revivent™ myocardial anchoring system (BioVentrix Ltd, San Ramon, CA, USA) by applying the left ventricle plication. Left ventricular plication is performed through a minimal invasive transthoracic approach by placing anchoring stitches through the infarcted area, between the right-ventricle side of the septum, and the epicardial surface of the left ventricle. Fastening the stitches the infarcted muscle can be plicated, and so the volume of the left ventricle can be reduced. First-in-man study included 26 patients with severely reduced left ventricular systolic function (EF 13–43 %) after anterior myocardial infarction. At the 6-month follow-up, a marked reduction of the left ventricle dimensions (reduction in end-diastolic volume index and end-systolic volume index 29.9 % and 35.0 %, respectively) and moderate improvement in functional status (NYHA class 2.5 vs. 1.7) were observed (abstract presentation TCT 2012).

2.1 Diastolic Restoration

Diastolic heart failure or heart failure with preserved left ventricular ejection fraction (HFPEF) is characterized by abnormal relaxation and chamber stiffness. The main therapeutic goal achieved by either medical or device-based interventions should be to enhance diastolic relaxation by prolonged diastolic time, to reduce myocardial stiffness in tandem with afterload and volume reduction. The conventional medical therapy includes vasodilators, agents blocking the renin–angiotensin system and mainly diuretics including aldosterone blockers, which remain the mainstay in the management of HFPEF.

Recently, innovative devices emerged offering a new conceptual approach to address abnormal relaxation, namely ImCardia™ and CORolla™ (CorAssist Cardiovascular Ltd., Herzliya Pituachm, Israel). Their mechanism of action is based on the bow-string effect: the metallic frame of the device positioned in the apical region captures passively mechanical energy during systole that will be transmitted to active force during diastole through the relaxation of the tensed metal strings.

These two devices can be placed either epicardially during median sternotomy or endocardially through minimal invasive transapical approach. The clinical data with these devices are still limited. ImCardia™ first-in-human experience has been gathered in 7 unblinded patients with severe aortic stenosis and severe diastolic heart failure treated with the device at the time of aortic valve replacement. Results were compared with 7 patients undergoing aortic valve replacement since device implantation (abstract presentation TCT 2012). Device has been implanted successfully in each case and no procedural adverse event has been reported. At 24 months follow-up (14 patients), device in association with AVR led to more pronounced regression of left ventricular hypertrophy compared to aortic valve replacement only. Although these preliminary results are promising, the device efficacy has to be further investigated in larger patient cohort. The COROlla™ has just gone only through the animal testing in a renal artery ligated porcine model. Short- and long-term safety has been proven in 65 porcine models. No procedural death or device embolization has been observed. No major adverse event has been reported. Human data are not yet available.

Elevated left atrial pressures and pulmonary congestion related to backward failure belong to the hallmarks of severe HFPEF or systolic dysfunction. The resetting of the volume status in relation to pump function is the pivotal therapeutic goal in HF management. Interatrial Shunt Device (IASD™) is a pioneering concept of the palliative treatment in patients who are severely symptomatic mainly due to the backward failure. Through venous transcatheter approach, IASD™ can be implanted into the atrial septum after transseptal puncture. The device, since it looks like a kind of metallic ring, provides a controlled, "artificial atrial septal defect" and prevents closing of this preformed hole. This will relieve the pulmonary venous system from the stasis thereby improving dyspnoe. On the other hand, the deviation of the blood flow is likely increasing the right ventricular workload. Thus the device is only palliative and unlikely to affect the heart failure progression. First-in-human experience suggests the procedural safety but clinical efficacy data need to be gathered (abstract presentation TCT 2012).

3 Electro-Myocardial Targets

Devices aiming at *electro-myocardial targets* include mainly cardiac resynchronization therapy and implantable cardioverter defibrillators which represent the mainstay in the modern heart failure management. In addition, novel electrical modalities beyond pacing have been conceived for treatment of heart failure.

The concept of cardiac contractility modulation (CCM) has been under study for more than a decade. CCM is based on a delivery of low-energy stimulations during absolute refractory period of action potential or so-called non-excitatory electrical impulses on the myocardium. Preclinical experience including histological and molecular-biological analyses suggests that well-timed non-excitatory impulses can improve cardiac contractility through phosphorylation and gene expression of calcium handling proteins. In particular, in isolated myocytes obtained from canine model of chronic heart failure, non-excitatory stimulation resulted in improved contractile function in parallel with increased intracellular peak Ca^{2+} levels [3]. Likewise, in vivo assessment demonstrated improvements in indices of cardiac function and contractility.

The clinical translation has been facilitated by a pacemaker-like device called Optimizer™ III (Impulse Dynamics Germany GmbH., Willich, Germany). In the largest, randomized trial performed to investigate the clinical value of CCM in patients with CHF 164 patients were enrolled [4]. Patients received alternating active vs. sham treatment each for 3 months. Functional status was assessed by defining oxygen consumption and Minnesota Quality of Life Index before and after the active vs. the sham treatment. In this study investigators observed significant improvement in both parameters: both oxygen consumption and Minnesota Quality of Life Index ameliorated during active treatment periods as compared to the periods with sham treatment, suggesting clinical benefit related to CCM therapy in CHF.

4 Neuro-Modulatory Targets

Increased sympathetic tonus and neurohumoral dysbalance is one of the main pathophysiological mechanisms contributing to heart failure progression. Large clinical trials provided proof-of-concept that pharmacological sympathetic blockade with betablockers improves morbidity and mortality of heart failure patients. This evidence is the stepping stone for device-based interventions targeting the neurohumoral axis such as renal denervation therapies and vagal stimulation.

4.1 Renal Sympathetic Nervous System

The key role of the renal sympathetic nervous system (RSNS) in the general sympathetic activation of blood pressure, volume control, and overall homeostasis is well known. Changes in renal blood flow due to pressure drop lead to its activation and increased activity of the renin–angiotensin–aldosterone system (RAAS) resulting in compensatory efferent renal vasoconstriction, natrium retention, and rise of blood pressure. Given that RSNS is actively connected to general sympathetic nervous system, its activation stimulates the central sympathetic pathways through efferent nerves, resulting in catecholamine rise, systematic vasoconstriction, and signs of sympathetic hyperreactivity [5]. On the other hand, RSNS can be activated also through afferent renal nerves from the central sympathetic network closing the centro-renal sympathetic loop. In this loop, a minor stimulative effect can lead to marked sympathetic reaction, which is the cornerstone of diseases like hypertension and other related diseases.

The relevance of the sympathetic nervous system in heart failure progression is well established. Increased sympathetic activity is associated with worse outcome. In particular, elevated serum catecholamine levels, higher heart rate, and lower heart rate variability are hallmarks of poor prognosis and linked to higher mortality. These findings explain therapeutic benefit of beta-blockade or the RAAS-blockade. Non-pharmacological blockade by targeting the pararenal sympathetic plexus offers a possibility of a more complete and permanent disruption of hyperreactive centro-renal sympathetic loop. The concept of eradicating the pararenal sympathetic nerves has been initially attempted surgically, however, due to its invasive nature it did not gain wider application. Recently, percutaneous renal denervation therapy has been introduced to ablate the renal sympathetic plexus with the RF energy. Rapid development led to introduction of several devices including the Ardian™ (Medtronic Inc, Minneapolis, MN, USA), the Vessix™ (Boston Scientific Corp, Natick, MA, USA), or EnligHTN™ (St. Jude Medical, St. Paul, Minnesota, USA) systems. All these devices were primarily investigated in the context of uncontrolled arterial hypertension. Given the pathophysiological basis, it is attractive to hypothesize that similar interventional approach may be effective also in the setting of heart failure with primarily higher sympathetic activity such as diastolic heart failure or subsets of chronic heart failure with reduced ejection fraction. The REACH pilot-study (REnal Artery denervation in Chronic Heart failure) included 7 CHF patients, who underwent renal denervation [6]. The procedure was well tolerated and at 6 months, all patients showed lower NYHA class and improved 6-min walking test. This feasibility study is likely to be followed by a larger randomized trial with rigorous design to address potential benefits of *renal denervation therapy* in patients with CHF.

4.2 Carotid Baroreceptors

The carotid baroreceptors play a key role in the sympathetic–parasympathetic regulation and their stimulation can markedly increase the parasympathetic tone and inversely reduce the general sympathetic activity. These pathophysiological findings provided the basis for development of devices designed for continuous electrical stimulation of carotid baroreceptors to reduce sympathetic activity and modulate heart failure presentation. BaroStim™ is a novel programmable pacemaker-like device, which provides the opportunity for a personalized stimulation rate of the baroreceptors. The device has been widely tested in patients with therapy-resistant hypertension [7, 8]. Whereas, a limited experience was obtained in diastolic heart failure, no experience has been reported yet in systolic heart failure. Recently, a multicenter randomized trial has been initiated to investigate long-term efficacy of this system in 150 patients with heart failure.

4.3 Vagal Nervous System

The vagal nerve is the backbone of parasympathetic regulation and may serve as a potential target for stimulation to restore the neurohumoral imbalance towards the parasympathetic dominance. The neuro-stimulator (CardioFit 5000, BioControl Medical, Yehud, Israel) is designed for low-energy stimulation of the vagal nerve. It consists of a pacemaker-like low-energy generator, a stimulating electrode to deliver paces, and a sensor electrode for appropriate timing. The generator is implanted in the right subclavian fossa, similar to conventional pacemakers. The stimulating electrode is positioned distally to the right vagal nerve few centimeters below the carotid bifurcation. The sensing electrode is placed in the right ventricle of the heart. The device is programmable to adjust parameters for the most optimal stimulation. The timing of stimulation is set to a fixed delay (70 m s) from the R wave. First-in-man experience has been reported by De Ferrari et al. in 32 patients with NYHA II–III heart failure [9]. Implant has been associated with two procedure-related serious adverse events. During 6-month follow-up two deaths occurred due to progression of the heart failure. At 6-month follow-up, significant improvement in 6-min walking test, in Minnesota Quality of Life Index, in Left Ventricle Systolic Volume Index, and in Ejection Fraction was observed in the remaining patients, an effect that persisted up to 12-month follow-up completed in subset of patients.

The INOVATE-HF study (INcrease Of VAgal TonE in CHF) has been launched in 2011 with the aim of investigating the beneficial effect of the device in a randomized way on a large population [10].

5 Future Perspectives

Medical therapy targeting symptoms and deleterious compensatory mechanisms remains the mainstay in state-of-the-art management of heart failure. Cardiac resynchronization therapy is the first example of successful device-based interventions altering the adverse course of heart failure. Its success as well as detailed knowledge of factors and mechanisms contributing to heart failure progression facilitated the development of device-based interventions for treatment of chronic heart failure. While the assist devices are aiming at the end-stage heart failure, emerging device-based percutaneous or minimal invasive techniques comprise the wide spectrum of innovative concepts that target ventricular remodeling, cardiac contractility, or neurohumoral modulation. The clinical adoption is in the early stages of the initial feasibility and safety studies and clinical evidence needs to be gathered in the appropriately designed clinical trials.

References

1. Erlebacher J, Weiss J, Weisfeldt M et al (1984) Early dilation of the infarcted segment in acute transmural myocardial infarction: role of infarct expansion in acute ventricular enlargement. J Am Coll Cardiol 4:201–208
2. Mazzaferri EL Jr, Gradinac S, Sagic D et al (2012) Percutaneous left ventricular partitioning in patients with chronic heart failure and a prior anterior myocardial infarction: Results of the PercutAneous Ventricular RestorAtion in Chronic Heart failUre PaTiEnts Trial. Am Heart J 163:812–820
3. Rastogi IM, Gupta RC, Mishra S et al (2007) Therapy with cardiac contractility modulation electrical signals improves left ventricular function and remodeling in dogs with chronic hehart failure. J Am Coll Cardiol 49:2120–2128
4. Borggrefe MM, Lawo T, Butter C et al (2008) Randomized, double blind study of non-excitatory, cardiac contractility modulation electrical impulses for symptomatic heart failure. Eur Heart J 29:1019–1028
5. Sobotka PA, Markus F, Schlaich P et al (2011) Sympatho-renal axis in chronic disease. Clin Res Cardiol 100:1049–1057
6. Davies JE, Manisty CH, Petraco R et al (2012) First-in-man safety evaluation of renal denervation for chronic systolic heart failure: primary outcome from REACH-Pilot study. Int J Cardiol 162(3):189–192
7. Wustmann K, Kucera JP, Scheffers I et al (2009) Effects of chronic baroreceptor stimulation on the autonomic cardiovascular regulation in patients with drug-resistant arterial hypertension. Hypertension 54:530–536
8. Navaneethan SD, Lohmeier TE, Bisognano JD et al (2009) Baroreflex stimulation: a novel treatment option for resistant hypertension. J Am Soc Hypertens 3:69–74
9. De Ferrari GM, Crijns HJ, Borggrefe M et al (2011) Chronic vagus nerve stimulation: a new and promising therapeutic approach for chronic heart failure. Eur Heart J 32:847–855
10. Hauptman PJ, Schwartz PJ, Gold MR et al (2012) Rationale and study design of the increase of vagal tone in heart failure study: INOVATE-HF. Am Heart J 163:954–962

Chapter 17
Total Artificial Heart

Christof Stamm and Roland Hetzer

Abstract Given the shortage of organ donors and lack of biologic alternatives, mechanical circulatory support is gaining importance both as a bridge-to-transplantation and as destination therapy. In the majority of patients, a left ventricular assist device alone is sufficient, but some require long-term biventricular support. For those, implantation of a total artificial heart (TAH) with removal of the native heart is a drastic but reliable option. In addition, advanced intracardiac thrombosis or destruction of the heart due to infective endocarditis or myocardial infarction may leave no other option. Currently, the Syncardia TAH is the only commercially available system. In selected centers with appropriate infrastructure and surgical expertise, the Syncardia TAH and its predecessors has been implanted in more than 1,000 patients with good results. However, indications for TAH implantation and its alternatives are still being discussed with some controversy. This chapter reviews the history of TAH development and summarizes indications, implantation technique, and clinical results.

The term "Total Artificial Heart" (TAH) commonly refers to biventricular mechanical assist devices that are implanted following definitive explantation of the patients failing ventricles. This stands out against the more frequently used ventricular assist devices (VADs), where the patient's own heart is left in place, and the device may be removed should the patient's heart recover. The Dutch physician Willem Kolff (1911–2009), after developing the first clinically successful hemodialysis system, began implanting artificial hearts in dogs in the 1950s at Cleveland Clinic and later at the University of Utah. During the 1970s, Kolff refined the system together with

C. Stamm (✉) • R. Hetzer
Deutsches Herzzentrum Berlin, Klinik Fur Herz-Thorax-und Gefäßchirurgie,
Augustenburger Platz 1, Berlin, Germany
e-mail: stamm@dhzb.de

J. Bartunek and M. Vanderheyden (eds.), *Translational Approach to Heart Failure*,
DOI 10.1007/978-1-4614-7345-9_17, © Springer Science+Business Media New York 2013

Robert Jarvik, and performed a number of successful implantations of human-scale devices ("Jarvik 5") in calfs. In parallel, the Argentinean surgeon Domingo Liotta (born 1924) developed a series of left ventricular assist devices (LVADs) and TAHs in Cordoba (Argentina), Lyon (France) and later Houston, TX. Together with the Houston surgeons Michael DeBakey, Denton Cooley, and Stanley Crawford, Liotta performed the first implantations of LVAD in 1963 and 1966, before the first Liotta-Cooley TAH was implanted in a patient at Texas Heart Institute on April 4, 1969. The 47-year-old patient suffered from severe biventricular heart failure and was successfully supported by the device for nearly 3 days. He then underwent heart transplantation but died 32 h later from pulmonary infection. While the Liotta TAH is no longer available, the Jarvik TAH was developed further, and in 1982, the Jarvik 7 TAH was first implanted in a 61-year-old patient who survived 112 days on the device. In 1985, the Jarvik 7 TAH was successfully used as a bridge-to-transplantation for a period of 9 days. The original Jarvik 7 TAH had a stroke volume of 100 mL and could only be used in large patients, but development of the Jarvik 7-70 (70 mL stroke volume) made it possible to treat smaller patients, too. Between 1985 and 1990, 175 Jarvik 7 TAH were implanted world-wide. Subsequently, ownership of the technology and production facilities changed and the system was developed further into what is now known as the SynCardia TAH, formerly CardioWest TAH. In the 1990s the CardioWest TAH was mainly implanted in the context of a multi-center investigational device exemption (IDE) clinical study, until it received FDA approval in 2004 and the CE mark in 2005.

In the 1980s, similar pneumatically driven implantable TAH prototypes were also developed and implanted in patients in Berlin (Berlin TAH) and in Phoenix (Phoenix Heart), but further commercialization did not succeed. In 1996, another TAH prototype, the Phoenix-7 heart, adapted to fit into the smaller chest cavity of Asian patients, was presented in Taiwan.

A completely new development, the AbioCor TAH was first implanted in man in 2001. The AbioCor has a unique electrohydraulic design, is completely self-contained and supplied with power via wireless transcutaneous energy transmission (TET) system so that no lines traverse the skin, and produces pulsatile blood flow through two "artificial ventricles." The Abiocor TAH has so far been implanted in 14 patients who were not candidates for heart transplantation under a Humanitarian Device Exemption of the FDA, and one patient survived for 512 days before the device failed [1]. The high failure rate of the device, its large size and concerns about the stroke rate have led to the development of AbioCor II, which has not yet been tested clinically. Finally, there are reports of "custom-made" extracorporeal TAH that were used in selected patients. After excision of the native ventricles, pulsatile extracorporeal VAD chambers such as the Thoratec system [2] or the Berlin Heart EXCOR system [3] have been connected with the atrial stumps via artificial capacity chambers, and the outflow grafts were anastomosed with the great vessels while both pumping chambers remain extracorporeal. Such constructions may be helpful in selected cases when implantation of a VAD is not possible but a dedicated TAH is not available.

As mentioned above, the only currently available TAH with approval of the authorities in North America and Europe is the SynCardia TAH, formerly known as

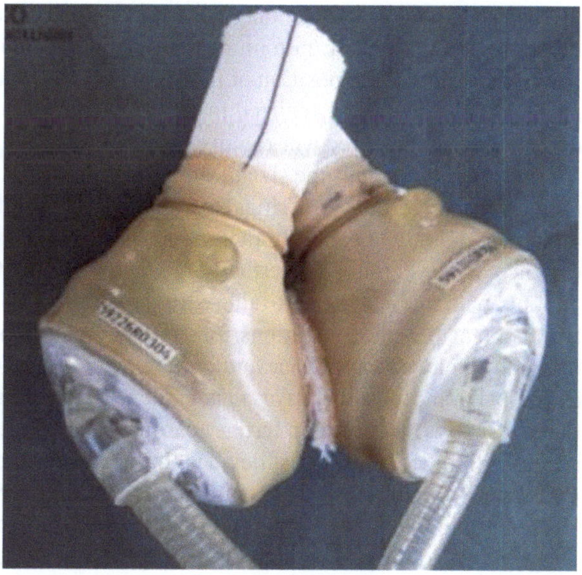

Fig. 17.1 SynCardia total artificial heart (TAH) consisting of two pneumatic pump chambers. The connecting with the great vessels are white, the drivelines for connection with the controller unit are transparent

CardioWest™ TAH. The Syncardia TAH consists of two pneumatically driven pump chambers, and once implanted, two pneumatic drivelines exit the body and are connected with one of the available driver units (Fig. 17.1). As of February 2012, it has been implanted in 1,000 patients world-wide, and this experience forms the basis of the following text.

1 Indication for TAH Implantation

As for any mechanical circulatory assist device, TAH implantation may be considered in patients who suffer from decompensated heart failure that is refractory to pharmacologic management. In the majority of candidates, extracardiac end-organ dysfunction has begun, usually in the form of renal and/or hepatic failure, and there is hemodynamic instability or manifest cardiogenic shock with progressive elevation of natriuretic peptides and acidosis. It is critical to identify patients who cannot be stabilized with traditional therapeutic means, so that VAD or TAH implantation is the only remaining option, but who still have a realistic chance of end-organ recovery. Currently, the formal indication for implantation of the SynCardia TAH includes severe biventricular failure, a risk of imminent death, and that the patient is a candidate for cardiac transplantation. The latter is a somewhat controversial issue, since there is often not enough time to conduct a complete assessment of transplant eligibility when the decision for TAH implantation must be made. Empirically, the majority of patients who received a TAH were either in INTERMACS class 1 (critical cardiogenic shock) or class 2 ("progressive decline")

[4]. These very sick patients may benefit from the fact that the TAH can provide a blood flow of up to 9.5 L/min immediately, independent from factors such as right ventricular function or position of intraventricular cannulas, so that a cardiac index of >3.0 L/min/m^2 can be realized in most patients. In consequence, both renal and hepatic function can recover rapidly. An important point regarding the indication for TAH implantation is the size of the intrapericardial cavity, which has to accommodate the large device. Critical parameters are a left ventricular end-diastolic diameter >70 mm, a cardiothoracic ratio >0.5, a body surface area >1.7 m^2, and a distance from sternum to vertebral bodies >10 cm. Given that in most of the patients with end-stage heart failure, other forms of mechanical circulatory assist are also feasible, the indications for TAH implantation ultimately depends on the individual center's experience and preference. Clearly, this kind of surgery as well as the peri- and postoperative management require manpower and infrastructure that is usually only found in tertiary cardiac referral centers with substantial experience with mechanical assist devices. In fact, only three centers world-wide have performed more than 100 TAH implantations, La Pitie Salpetrier in Paris (France), Herzzentrum Bad Oeynhausen (Germany), and the University of California, San Diego (USA). In those centers, TAH implantation is considered in every patient with biventricular failure and reasonable survival probability, when implantation of an LVAD alone would not be sufficient. Other groups prefer a more conservative approach and limit the TAH indication to situations where a VAD is clearly problematic. Those include very fragile myocardium at the ventricular implantation site in extensive myocardial infarction with a high risk of uncontrollable bleeding [4], large ventricular septal defect following acute infarction, extensive thrombus formation in the left ventricle [5], significant aortic valve regurgitation or the presence of mechanical heart valve prostheses, severe destructive endocarditis with extensive structural damage of the heart, inoperable cardiac tumor, or acute rejection of a donor heart with deleterious systemic consequences of the inflammatory processes [6].

2 TAH Indications

Definite:

- Irreparable destruction of the heart due to extensive myocardial infarction, bacterial endocarditis, or transplant graft failure
- Extensive thrombosis in the left ventricle
- Inoperable cardiac tumor

In evaluation:

- Critical cardiogenic shock (INTERMACS level 1)
- Impossibility to establish adequate cardiac output with other VAD

Controversial:

- Chronic biventricular heart failure

3 Implantation

The SynCardia TAH is available for implantation at a growing number of certified centers world-wide, which have completed the manufacturer's training and certification process. Surgery is done through a midline sternotomy, with the patient placed on cardiopulmonary bypass. First, two channels are created for the drivelines that traverse the skin in the epigastrium. Then, the ventricles are excised preserving both the mitral and tricuspid valve annulus, and the great vessels are divided just above the level of the aortic and pulmonary valve. Both atrial cuffs are now encircled with Teflon buttresses, and separate inflow connectors are sutured to the cuffs. Similarly, separate outflow connectors are sutured to the aorta as well as the pulmonary artery. The artificial ventricles are then plugged in their respective connectors; the device is carefully de-aired and started. Placement of the device so that the inflow in both pump chambers is not obstructed once the chest is closed requires great care (Fig. 17.2). Some surgeons choose to cover the device in Gore-Tex

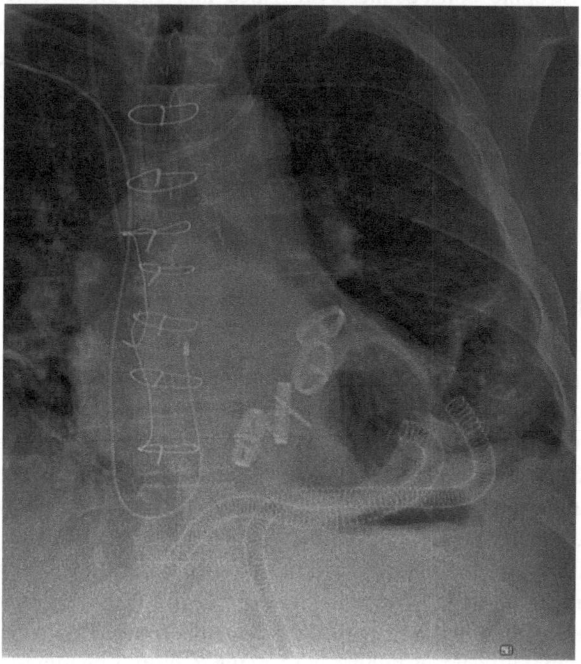

Fig. 17.2 Chest X-ray of a TAH patient. Note the four mechanical valves, two pneumatic drivelines, and the air-filled pump chambers where the apex of the heart would be

membrane to prevent adhesions and facilitate explantation at the time of heart transplantation, and sometimes silicone cushions are placed in the pericardial cavity to prevent shrinking and leave room for the transplant heart. Hemostasis is critical but may be difficult to achieve, especially in patients with compromised hepatic function.

4 Postoperative Care

In most patients, the TAH will produce sufficient "cardiac" output with a beating rate of 110–130 bpm and equal duration of filling (diastole) and ejection (systole). As in the normal heart, output will then be determined by the filling pressure, which corresponds with the available blood volume. As soon as hemostasis allows it, patients need to be placed on a stringent anticoagulation regimen including heparin, aspirin, dipyridamole, pentoxifylline, and sometimes ticoplidine or clopidogrel. Coagulation needs to be monitored closely and extensively, and activated clotting time (ACT), partial thromboplastin time (PTT), prothrombin time (PT) and INR, thrombelastography (TEG), and platelet count are among the routinely measured parameters. Greatest care must be taken regarding antisepsis of the driveline exit sites and dressings need to be changed by qualified staff on a daily basis, since ascending infections can have catastrophic consequences. Provided that end-organ function recovers, postoperative mobilization can begin shortly after surgery. The manufacturer reports that 65 % of the patients were able to leave the bed 5 days after surgery, and 60 % were able to walk more than 100 ft by postoperative day 14. Clearly, the speed of postoperative recovery very much depends on the preoperative status of the individual patient. As soon as the patient has stabilized, he can be listed for heart transplantation under UNOS status 1A and will have priority upon donor organ allocation.

5 Long-Term Care

In principle, patients on mechanical circulatory support can be discharged home, sufficient compliance provided. This also applies to TAH patients, but mobility used to be limited due to the size of the controller unit. The original "Big Blue" hospital driver of the SynCardia TAH is comparable with a dishwasher in terms of size and weight, and, although very robust and reliable, is only usable for in-hospital care. In Europe, it is currently being replaced by the more modern and smaller Companion driver that offers greater mobility within the hospital setting. Discharge of TAH patients became possible in 2006, when CE approval was granted for using the portable Berlin Heart Excor driver with the SynCardia TAH. This robust system has been used for many years in hundreds of patients with a pneumatic Berlin Heart extracorporeal assist device and has about the size of a carry-on trolley (Fig. 17.3). Very recently, the new "Freedom" discharge driver has become available, which weighs only 13.5 lb and can easily be carried in a backpack or shoulder bag [7].

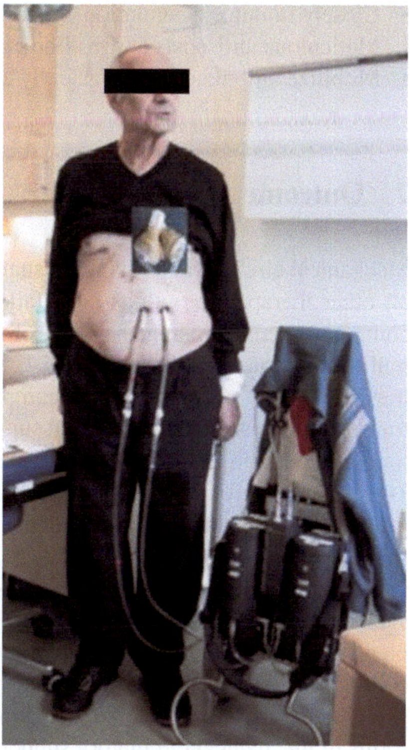

Fig. 17.3 Patient with a SynCardia TAH, connected with the mobile Berlin Heart Excor driver

Apart from those practicability issues, regular qualified exit wound care and coagulation management must be ensured. Long-term dietary recommendations for TAH patients include Vitamin C, Folic Acid, Vitamin B12, iron sulfate and Omega 3 fatty acids, and erythropoietin may be indicated to counteract hemolysis.

6 TAH Therapy Key Points

Surgery:

- Ensure adequate chest size (CT scan, AP chest X-ray)
- Excise both ventricles, preserve sufficient atrial chamber
- Meticulous hemostasis
- Adhesion prophylaxis (GoreTex membrane)
- Prevent pericardial shrinking (silicone implants)

Postoperative:

- Ensure high cardiac output
- As soon as bleeding is controlled: Stringent multiple anticoagulation (heparin/warfarine, aspirin, dipyridamole, pentoxifylline, ticoplidine, or clopidogrel)

- Closely monitor coagulation (ACT, PTT, PT, INR, TEG, platelet count)
- Meticulous antisepsis at driveline exit sites
- Mobilize/ambulate patient as early as possible.

7 Outcome

Mechanical circulatory support is usually required in extremely sick patients, when all other therapeutic options have failed. Hence, it is very difficult to assess and compare outcomes using the tools of evidence-based medicine. In a now-classic multicenter study published in 2004, 81 patients received a TAH as a bridge-to-transplantation, and outcome was compared with 35 similar patients who waited for transplantation without mechanical support [8]. Of the TAH patients, 79 % survived to transplantation, but only 46 % of the medically managed patients did. The overall 1-year survival for TAH patients was 70 %, compared with 31 % in the control group, and it was thus established that bridge-to-transplantation using TAH is indeed lifesaving. In a later risk-factor analysis, it was shown that only a history of smoking and coagulation abnormalities were risk factors, but not cardiac-related parameters such as right ventricular function [9]. This is not surprising, since the heart is completely removed. Other centers have reported less favorable results is smaller patient cohorts, with survival of approximately 50 %, but this is still a therapeutic success given the patients' extremely poor preoperative situation [10]. As with many other forms of mechanical circulatory support, results continue to improve with accumulating experience, and a survival rate of >70 % can be expected today in experienced centers [11, 12], even in patients with a relatively small chest [13].

8 Future Trends

Currently, several academic and industry research groups focus on the development of implantable TAH based on small centrifugal or axial flow pumps and experiments in vitro [14] as well as in large animals have demonstrated the feasibility of this approach [15–17]. In fact, patients have already been treated with such experimental device combinations. At the Methodist Hospital in Houston, TX, a patient with terminal failure of a transplanted heart received two non-pulsatile implantable HeartMate II VADs (Thoratec, Pleasanton, CA) [18]. Similarly, a combination of two HeartMate II VAD was implanted after excision of both ventricles in a 55-year-old patient with amyloidosis at Texas Heart Institute [19]. At Hannover Medical School, a 51-year-old patient with massive myocardial infarction and large ventricular septal defect received two HeartWare VADs (HeartWare, Framingham, MA) after excision of his irreparably destroyed heart [20]. While these life-saving interventions represent an off-label use of commercially available LVADs, the development of dedicated non-pulsatile TAHs is certainly to be expected. With ongoing miniaturization of VAD, implant size should not be a problem, but power supply, thromboembolism, hemolysis, and infection remain to be addressed as in conventional VAD. Other than the above-mentioned Syncardia and AbioCor TAH, several pulsatile implantable TAH are also in preclinical development. They include the hydraulic CARMAT heart with electrical power supply (Carmat, Velizy Villacoublay, France) and the ReinHeart System with direct linear motor and TET (RWTH Aachen, Germany). From the clinicians' point-of-view, the ultimate goal is a fully implantable TAH system with internal power supply, no skin-penetrating lines, perfect hemocompatibility, and the ability to produce a blood flow of up to 10 L/min. Whether and when this will be possible, however, cannot be foreseen, yet.

9 Alternatives

In the vast majority of patients with decompensated biventricular heart failure, TAH is not the only option regarding the choice of mechanical circulatory assist system. In the past, good results have been achieved using the Berlin Heart EXCOR VAD for biventricular support, both as bridge-to-transplantation, bridge-to-recovery, or destination therapy, but quality of life is clearly limited with such a system. Especially in small adults and children, the EXCOR system is currently the only system that has virtually no restriction in terms of patient size. In patients with unknown neurologic status and poor prognosis, it is also possible to implant EXCOR cannulas and connect those with temporary extracorporeal centrifugal pumps, which can later easily be replaced with permanent EXCOR pumps. We have also learned that many patients who present with acute biventricular failure may recover right ventricular function after implantation of an LVAD, and currently prefer to implant a permanent implantable LVAD (such as the HeartMate II, HeartWare HVAD, or Berlin Heart Incor) together with a temporary extracorporeal RVAD system (i.e., Levitronix). The latter can often be removed after some days, when pulmonary vascular resistance has decreased and RV function has recovered. In selected patients with irreversible biventricular failure, permanent intrathoracic VAD have been implanted for biventricular support (Fig. 17.4) [21]. This is possible when last generation, miniaturized pumps such as the HeartWare HVAD are used and the patient's chest is large enough to accommodate both devices in addition to the native heart [22].

There is ongoing controversy between the proponents of TAH and those of VAD, obviously also fuelled by industry. Many assume that TAH may be the best therapeutic option in patients with INTERMACS level 1, where LVAD studies have shown a particularly high risk of death, and data from the INTERMACS study group suggest better results of the Syncardia TAH than with conventional BVAD systems [23]. Although the non-pulsatile flow of modern VAD is very well tolerated, some evidence suggest that coagulation is more disturbed by blood contact with high speed VAD turbines than by the pneumatic pump chambers of a TAH [24]. The risk of infection of a TAH is believed to be higher than for VAD, but stroke rate tends to be lower with TAH. Other than that, there is hardly data that would definitively demonstrate the superiority of one concept over the other.

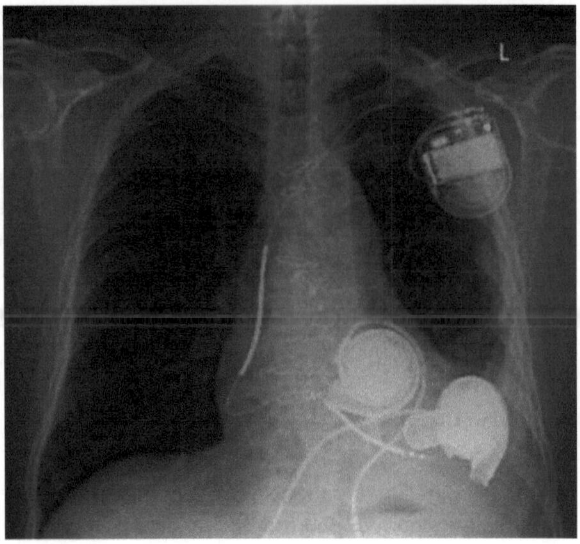

Fig. 17.4 Chest X-ray of a patient with two implantable ventricular assist devices as a biventricular assist device

There are no prospective studies that compare the TAH with the VAD approach, so that in most of the cases the surgeon will have to decide based on what he feels most comfortable with.

10 Sources of Further Information

The scientific literature that provided most of the information summarized in this chapter is listed below. Other than that, the website of the Texas Heart Institute (http://www.texasheartinstitute.org/Research/Devices/) gives a comprehensive overview of mechanical circulatory support systems and TAH and contains links to other interesting internet resources. The Syncardia website (http://www.syncardia.com/) also provides a lot of information on the history of TAH in general and the Syncardia TAH in particular. Finally, Wikipedia has a very informative page on TAH (http://en.wikipedia.org/wiki/Artificial_heart).

References

1. Samuels LE, Dowling R (2003) Total artificial heart: destination therapy. Cardiol Clin 21:115–118
2. Arusoglu L, Reiss N, Morshuis M, Schoenbrodt M, Hakim-Meibodi K, Gummert J (2010) The Thoratec system implanted as a modified total artificial heart: the Bad Oeynhausen technique. Heart Surg Forum 13:E391–E393

3. Tjan TD, Klotz S, Schmid C, Scheld HH (2008) Creation of a self-made total artificial heart using combined components of available ventricular assist devices. Thorac Cardiovasc Surg 56:51–53
4. Morshuis M, Reiss N, Arusoglu L, Tenderich G, Korfer R, El-Banayosy A (2007) Implantation of CardioWest total artificial heart for irreversible acute myocardial infarction shock. Heart Surg Forum 10:E251–E256
5. Smith MC, Arabia FA, Tsau PH, Smith RG, Bose RK, Woolley DS et al (2005) CardioWest total artificial heart in a moribund adolescent with left ventricular thrombi. Ann Thorac Surg 80:1490–1492
6. Yoda M, El-Banayosy A, Tenderich G, Koerfer R, Minami K (2009) The CardioWest total artificial heart for chronic heart transplant rejection. Circ J 73:1167–1168
7. Jaroszewski DE, Anderson EM, Pierce CN, Arabia FA (2011) The SynCardia freedom driver: a portable driver for discharge home with the total artificial heart. J Heart Lung Transplant 30:844–845
8. Copeland JG, Smith RG, Arabia FA, Nolan PE, Sethi GK, Tsau PH et al (2004) Cardiac replacement with a total artificial heart as a bridge to transplantation. N Engl J Med 351:859–867
9. Copeland JG, Smith RG, Bose RK, Tsau PH, Nolan PE, Slepian MJ (2008) Risk factor analysis for bridge to transplantation with the CardioWest total artificial heart. Ann Thorac Surg 85:1639–1644
10. El-Banayosy A, Arusoglu L, Morshuis M, Kizner L, Tenderich G, Sarnowski P et al (2005) CardioWest total artificial heart: Bad Oeynhausen experience. Ann Thorac Surg 80:548–552
11. Leprince P, Bonnet N, Rama A, Leger P, Bors V, Levasseur JP et al (2003) Bridge to transplantation with the Jarvik-7 (CardioWest) total artificial heart: a single-center 15-year experience. J Heart Lung Transplant 22:1296–1303
12. Copeland JG, Copeland H, Gustafson M, Mineburg N, Covington D, Smith RG et al (2012) Experience with more than 100 total artificial heart implants. J Thorac Cardiovasc Surg 143:727–734
13. Leprince P, Bonnet N, Varnous S, Rama A, Leger P, Ouattara A et al (2005) Patients with a body surface area less than 1.7 m2 have a good outcome with the CardioWest Total Artificial Heart. J Heart Lung Transplant 24:1501–1505
14. Khalil HA, Kerr DT, Franchek MA, Metcalfe RW, Benkowski RJ, Cohn WE et al (2008) Continuous flow total artificial heart: modeling and feedback control in a mock circulatory system. ASAIO J 54:249–255
15. Frazier OH, Cohn WE, Tuzun E, Winkler JA, Gregoric ID (2009) Continuous-flow total artificial heart supports long-term survival of a calf. Texas Heart Inst J 36:568–574
16. Frazier OH, Tuzun E, Cohn W, Tamez D, Kadipasaoglu KA (2005) Total heart replacement with dual centrifugal ventricular assist devices. ASAIO J 51:224–229
17. Frazier OH, Tuzun E, Cohn WE, Conger JL, Kadipasaoglu KA (2006) Total heart replacement using dual intracorporeal continuous-flow pumps in a chronic bovine model: a feasibility study. ASAIO J 52:145–149
18. Loebe M, Bruckner B, Reardon MJ, van Doorn E, Estep J, Gregoric I et al (2011) Initial clinical experience of total cardiac replacement with dual HeartMate-II axial flow pumps for severe biventricular heart failure. Methodist Debakey Cardiovasc J 7:40–44
19. http://www2.macleans.ca/2011/09/15/newest-artficial-heart-beats-not/
20. Strueber M, Schmitto JD, Kutschka I, Haverich A (2012) Placement of 2 implantable centrifugal pumps to serve as a total artificial heart after cardiectomy. J Thorac Cardiovasc Surg 143:507–509
21. Krabatsch T, Potapov E, Stepanenko A, Schweiger M, Kukucka M, Huebler M et al (2011) Biventricular circulatory support with two miniaturized implantable assist devices. Circulation 124:S179–S186
22. Krabatsch T, Hennig E, Stepanenko A, Schweiger M, Kukucka M, Huebler M et al (2011) Evaluation of the HeartWare HVAD centrifugal pump for right ventricular assistance in an in vitro model. ASAIO J 57:183–187

23. Stevenson LW, Pagani FD, Young JB, Jessup M, Miller L, Kormos RL et al (2009) INTERMACS profiles of advanced heart failure: the current picture. J Heart Lung Transplant 28:535–541
24. Heilmann C, Geisen U, Beyersdorf F, Nakamura L, Benk C, Berchtold-Herz M et al (2010) Acquired von Willebrand syndrome in patients with ventricular assist device or total artificial heart. Thromb Haemost 103:962–967

Chapter 18
Stem Cell Therapy for Ischemic Heart Disease

Atta Behfar, Jozef Bartunek, and Andre Terzic

Abstract Regenerative medicine aims to achieve functional and structural restoration of a failing organ. Applied to cardiovascular medicine and surgery, this emerging discipline offers a disruptive innovation poised to transform healthcare paradigms by providing the prospect of curative solutions beyond the reach of current standard-of-care. This chapter highlights recent advances fueling this promising multidisciplinary field in the context of heart failure management. Building on breakthroughs in stem cell science, the rapidly evolving regenerative armamentarium leverages natural mechanisms of heart development and lifelong innate rejuvenation. Stem cell therapies seek to boost an otherwise limited aptitude of the human adult myocardium for self-renewal by securing a tissue-specific reparative environment within the failing organ. Supported by favorable preclinical experience, translation of regenerative paradigms has been tested in the clinical setting in both acute and chronic conditions. Meta-analyses of stem cell-based clinical trials underscore the feasibility and safety of regenerative procedures in ischemic heart disease, yet commonly point to modest and variable outcome in parameters of recovery. These initial proof-of-concept trials rely on the use of purified human cells, typically delivered in their native state. Several areas of focus have developed to better establish the scope of clinical use and maximize regenerative benefit. Specifically, next generation trials aim to use the most appropriate cell sources and cell types, enhance cardiogenicity and therapeutic effectiveness, select patient populations most amenable to cell-based therapy, establish ideal timing of intervention, and optimize routes of administration. To inform early adoption in practice, the rigor of comparative effectiveness outcome analysis will ultimately be needed to empower the future

A. Behfar • A. Terzic, M.D., Ph.D. (✉)
Center for Regenerative Medicine and Division of Cardiovascular Diseases,
Department of Medicine, Mayo Clinic, 2001st Street SW #W4, Rochester, MN 55905, USA
e-mail: terzic.andre@mayo.edu

J. Bartunek
Cardiovascular Centre, OLV Hospital, Moorselbaan, Aalst, Belgium

J. Bartunek and M. Vanderheyden (eds.), *Translational Approach to Heart Failure*,
DOI 10.1007/978-1-4614-7345-9_18,

of heart failure care, enriched by regenerative strategies that address the unmet needs of a growing patient population.

1 Introduction

The World Health Organization recognizes the emergence of noncommunicable diseases, in particular heart failure, as the leading cause of morbidity and mortality [1]. The American Heart Association in the most recent Heart Disease and Stroke Report underscores that cardiovascular conditions account for 1 of every 2.9 deaths in the United States. More than 2,200 Americans die of cardiovascular disease each day, an average of 1 death every 39 s [2]. Indeed, heart failure is one of the most prominent challenges to public health. Modern management of acute myocardial infarction with rapid revascularization has reduced early mortality but has precipitated the incidence of chronic heart failure among survivors, an epidemic that is anticipated to expand worldwide accelerated by the pandemic trends of ischemic heart disease and the aging of the global population [3].

Recurrent hospitalizations and premature death, prevalent in this ever growing patient population, have imposed a major unmet need associated with the inability of current, largely palliative therapies to address massive tissue destruction post-infarction. The myocyte-deficit in infarction-induced heart failure is in the order of one billion cells with a 25 % loss of the left ventricular mass. A hallmark of this malignant pathology is the progressive maladaptive remodeling of the infarcted myocardium that perpetuates systolic and diastolic dysfunction, and ultimately leads to the overt syndrome of congestive organ failure. Repair of the failing infarcted heart is a formidable challenge, considering not only the magnitude of cardiomyocyte loss but also the requirements to reestablish optimal supply in support of functional and structural demands. Life-extending measures—such as left ventricular assist devices or heart transplantation—are often the only therapeutic option. However, a limited number of patients can benefit from such complex and costly interventions. A case in point is the United States, where an estimated 2,500 heart transplants are performed annually, yet over 100,000 additional patients wait without hope for this lifesaving procedure. Thus, a compelling clinical and societal need exists for the establishment of innovative cardiovascular therapies that will extend the reach of cardiovascular medicine and surgery of today.

Regenerative medicine aims to restore normal structure and function. Evolution of therapy towards reparative paradigms exploits the growing understanding of disease pathways and natural repair mechanisms to discover, validate, and apply therapeutics targeted to the cause of disease. The emergence of regenerative strategies, fueled by discoveries in developmental biology and stem cell science, has begun to transform the perspectives of clinical practice [4]. The U.S. Department of Health and Human Services report "2020: A new Vision" highlights that regenerative medicine is the most promising core component of modern medical practice at the vanguard of twenty-first century healthcare. Transformative practices have already been documented in multiple medical and surgical disciplines. Prototypic examples range from the treatment of previously incurable blood disorders in hematology to advances in applying bionic regenerative principles for the purpose of achieving neo-organogenesis in thoracic surgery. Without the contribution of personalized products and services emerging from regenerative medicine technology, that offer the promise of definitive solutions in patient care, experts caution that healthcare will face an escalation in inefficient treatments and a rising global cost [5].

Strategies to promote, augment, and reestablish natural repair are at the core of translating the science of stem cell biology into the practice of regenerative medicine. Aimed at addressing the root cause of disease, stem cell-based regenerative medicine offers an expanded therapeutic armamentarium that drives the evolution of medical sciences from traditional symptom mitigation to previously unreachable curative algorithms. Stem cells demonstrate a unique aptitude to differentiate into specialized cell types, and to form new tissue providing thereby the active ingredient of regenerative regimens [6]. Applied to the management of heart failure, regenerative approaches target functional restoration of damaged heart tissues not mere alleviation of disease symptomatology. Leveraging rapid advances across complementary biological, medical, and engineering disciplines, successful application of regenerative medicine principles promises significant human health benefit with tangible outcomes for an improved patient care and an increased quality of life [7].

This chapter underscores progress made in stem cell therapy for ischemic heart disease. The present overview highlights the innate mechanisms of repair which provide the rationale for regenerative approaches; targets and mechanisms of therapy delineated respectively for acute vs. chronic disease, implicating both direct and indirect modes of action; cell delivery techniques which have catalyzed early translation of stem cell-based treatment; stem cell platforms which define the spectrum of available biotherapeutics; and ultimately the clinical experience to date, providing a synopsis of cardiovascular regenerative medicine from principles to practice.

2 Innate Cardiac Rejuvenation

Developmental biology has unraveled that most cells in the adult heart are derived from the mesodermal layer during early embryogenesis [8]. Knowledge of these cell populations has helped assess the molecular cues that establish cell fate decisions. Genetic fate mapping suggests that embryonic cardiogenesis proceeds according to a stem cell-based paradigm in which lineage-restricted progenitor cells give rise to the mosaic of cells present in the adult heart. A progenitor population that persists to adulthood might in fact be involved in stimulation of cardiomyocyte division in the adult heart.

Traditionally, the human heart has been viewed as a terminally differentiated postmitotic organ in which the number of cardiomyocytes is established at birth, and these cells persist throughout the lifespan of the organ and the organism. However, the discovery that cardiac stem cells live in the heart and differentiate into the various cardiac cell lineages has changed profoundly our understanding of myocardial biology [9]. Cardiac stem cells regulate myocyte turnover and condition myocardial recovery after injury. This novel information imposes a reconsideration of the mechanisms involved in myocardial aging and regeneration.

Accordingly, stem cell-based regeneration applied to the treatment of heart failure is based on the realization that natural self-renewing processes, i.e., rejuvenation, are innate to the myocardium, yet are typically insufficient to salvage the infarcted heart muscle. The unexpected recognition that the heart is not a terminally differentiated organ as conventionally assumed, but rather harbors self-repair mechanisms to maintain tissue homeostasis has been recently documented and validated. Although the rejuvenation capacity is particularly prominent within a young heart, quantitative monitoring of innate cardiomyogenesis has established a significant renewal reserve even in the adult human heart capable of replacing both myocyte and nonmyocyte compartments (Fig. 18.1). Radio-isotope decay in the human body, a remnant of nuclear bomb testing half-a-century ago, has offered an unprecedented opportunity to quantify the birth date of single cardiomyocytes, indicating that more than half of the heart mass can be renewed over a lifespan [10]. Cardiomyocyte turnover rate has been estimated at least at about 1 % per year in young adults, and decreases to 0.5 % per year in elderly individuals. Notably, stem cell contribution to postnatal heart formation has been validated by the self/non-self chimerism characteristic of patients following allogeneic transplantation. Furthermore, within failing hearts, increase in stem cell load can contribute to the regenerative response, and involves derivation of cardiomyocytes from circulating as well as resident progenitors. Indeed, the possibility that stem cells migrate from the bone marrow to the heart and continuously repopulate the niche structures is favored by some investigators, while others consider asymmetric resident cardiac stem cell division the primary biological process controlling the number of stem cells in the myocardium [11]. In the context of large-scale destruction associated with massive ischemic injury, the native regenerative potential is typically insufficient to rescue a deteriorating myocardium. In fact, the overall efficiency for self-repair is further compromised by patient age, disease status, comorbidities or concomitant drug therapies, and defined by significant individual genetic and environmental variance. Extrapolating from the paradigms of natural heart rejuvenation and transplant-based organ replacement, activation of endogenous and/or introduction of exogenous progenitor cells into the injured infarcted heart offer legitimate strategies to ameliorate the burden of disease boosting innate reparative mechanisms [12]. Augmentation of endogenous regenerative activity is thus a compelling strategy for therapeutic cardiac repair [13].

3 Targets and Mechanisms of Regenerative Therapy

Stem cell therapy is targeted on halting or reversing progression of myocardial injury. Early after myocardial injury, the primary therapeutic goal is salvage of the jeopardized myocardium to prevent myocardial expansion and pathologic

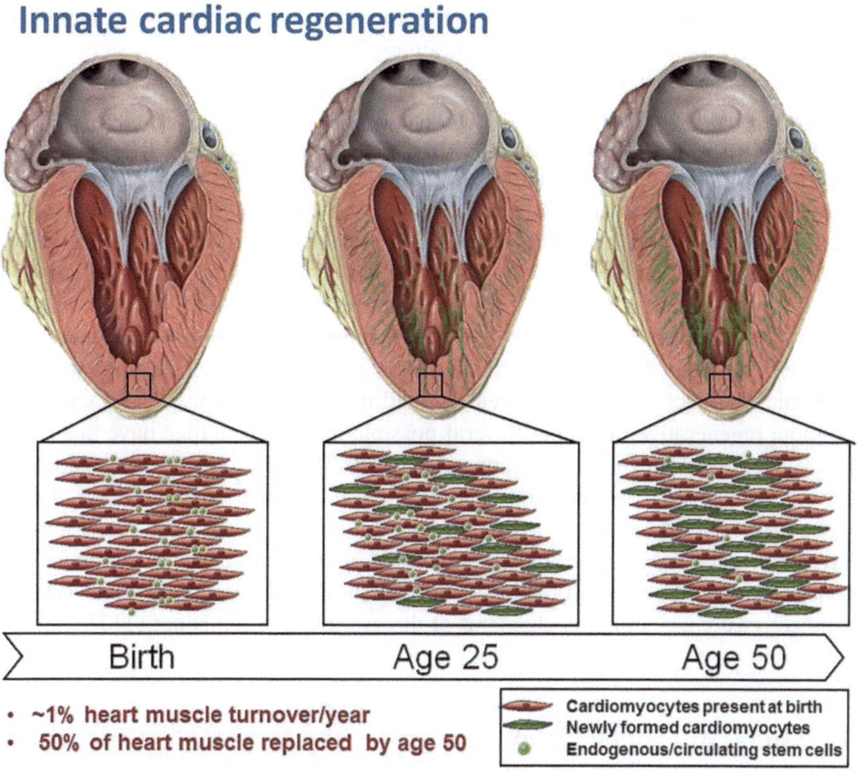

Fig. 18.1 Self-renewing processes are innate to the myocardium. The rejuvenation capacity is particularly prominent within a young heart, quantitative monitoring of innate cardiomyogenesis has established a significant renewal reserve even in the adult human heart capable of replacing both myocyte and nonmyocyte compartments. In fact, conservative estimates indicate that more than half of the heart mass can be renewed over a lifespan. The possibility that stem cells migrate from the bone marrow to the heart and continuously repopulate the niche structures is favored by some investigators, while others consider asymmetric resident cardiac stem cell division the primary biological process controlling the number of stem cells in the myocardium. In the context of large-scale destruction, the native regenerative potential is typically insufficient to rescue a deteriorating myocardium. Extrapolating from the paradigms of natural heart rejuvenation and transplant-based organ replacement, activation of endogenous, and/or introduction of exogenous progenitor cells into the injured infarcted heart offer legitimate strategies to ameliorate the burden of disease boosting innate reparative mechanisms

remodeling. At later stages of developed left ventricular dysfunction, the aim is to reverse maladaptive remodeling and ensure improved contractility [14]. In particular, excessive inflammatory response, oxidative stress, and apoptosis are the primary targets in initial stages, whereas fibrosis, loss of fiber organization, and impaired excitation–contraction coupling are key features of florid cardiomyopathy. Multidimensional interactions between cardiomyocytes, extracellular matrix, the immune system, and blood vessels determine the outcome of global remodeling and ventricular dynamics. Thus, differences in the molecular and cellular substrate during the course of disease are likely to require distinct regenerative strategies to prevent progression or treat overt heart failure.

The recognition that stem cells can differentiate into specified cell phenotypes that produce beneficial outcome when transplanted into diseased heart, often beyond that achieved with current standards of care, has initially led to the hypothesis that direct replacement of nonviable myocardium through de novo cardiogenesis is the therapeutic mode of action. Recent iterations of the regenerative paradigm move beyond the notion that transplanted cells serve per se as the sole myocardial building blocks to a more interactive model that imposes, at the molecular level, a repair process encompassing an active role for the host myocardium [15]. In this model, the interaction of delivered stem cells with the injured/diseased myocardium and its microenvironment would ensure reparative signaling to modulate inflammation, ischemic tolerance, endogenous healing, and ultimately enhanced contractility to promote regenerative outcome. Several possible indirect activities have been proposed, including activation of endogenous cardiac progenitor cells, stimulation of cardiomyocyte division, and modification of the tissue niche with increase in neovascularization and reduction in scar burden [16]. To this end, modern repair models have been amended to include augmentation of endogenous capacity for neoangiogenesis, myocardial cytoprotection, and activation of reparative resident cardiac stem cells as contributing mechanisms of the overall stem cell benefit [17].

4 Modes of Cell Delivery

Safe and efficient delivery is a prerequisite for therapeutic benefit. Indeed, ensuring a practical and reliable delivery of a sufficient amount of a stem cell-based biotherapeutics is necessary to trigger processes of repair while ensuring minimal off-target delivery and diffuse cell dissemination [18]. Distinct delivery routes have been tested (Fig. 18.2). These include systemic, i.e., intravenous injection, vs. myocardially targeted approaches, such as percutaneous intracoronary delivery, endomyocardial transplantation, and in the context of cardiothoracic surgery epicardial injections [19]. Peripheral intravenous delivery is the least invasive, but provides the lowest degree of myocardial homing and would be applicable if the mode of action solely relied upon paracrine/endocrine secretion into the circulation. Though limited, if optimized this approach would be an attractive option due to the broad accessibility in clinical practice. Recent preclinical studies have provided proof-of-concept by demonstrating benefit without the need for homing due to the bioavailability of secreted anti-inflammatory proteins from the peripheral circulation. Alternatively, intracoronary delivery is limited to facilities with established catheter-based interventions [20]. This approach has been utilized to date by most of the clinical trials capitalizing on established interventional practices carried out in the setting of acute coronary syndrome. Myocardial delivery through endocardial transplantation has been utilized in the treatment of subacute infarction or chronic heart failure. Execution of this approach is limited to centers of excellence capable of coupling

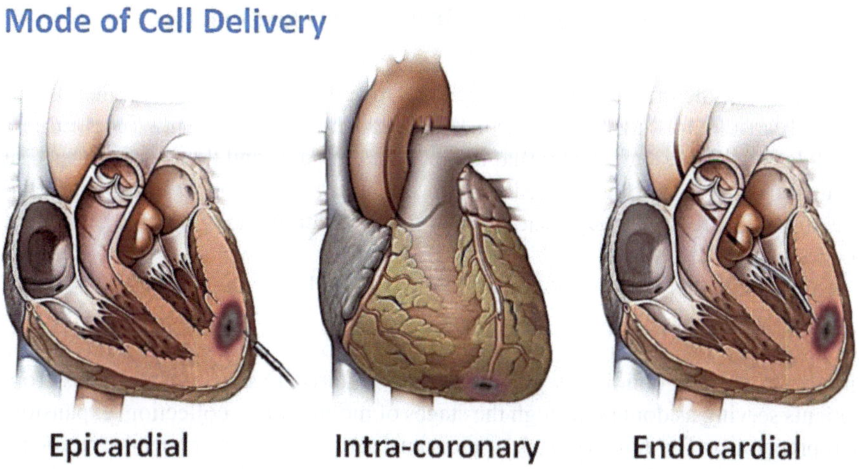

Fig. 18.2 Distinct routes for stem cell delivery have been established and applied. These include epicardial, intracoronary, and endomyocardial delivery. Epicardial cell transplantation is limited to patients with a primary indication for heart surgery. Intracoronary delivery is limited to facilities with established catheter-based interventions and is typically carried out in the setting of acute coronary syndrome. Myocardial delivery through endocardial transplantation has been utilized in the treatment of subacute infarction or chronic heart failure and is executed in centers of excellence capable of coupling cell delivery with advanced navigation and imaging to guide site-specific delivery

cell delivery with advanced navigation and imaging to guide site-specific delivery [21]. Although historically first introduced in the context of cell delivery, epicardial cell transplantation is limited to patients with a primary indication for heart surgery.

Using currently available techniques, delivery of stem cells demonstrates variable retention rates, typically not exceeding 5–10 % of the injected dose regardless of the method of administration. Progressive decrease in myocardial signals after delivery of labeled stem cells is consistent with rapid cell death or washout, within hours of administration. Although this limitation does not invalidate the efficacy of stem cells, it does suggest that reparative mechanisms involve paracrine or immunomodulatory processes that may not require local preservation of the regenerative biologics. In fact, the biodistribution of stem cells is variable, depending in part on the cell type, with cells potentially reaching remote organs such as the lungs, liver, or spleen. Although safety issues have not been raised, the consequence of extra-cardiac homing is unknown. Accordingly, long-term biovigilance has been incorporated in the development algorithm of stem cell products. Differences in the myocardial substrate and patient-specific molecular and cellular profiles governing cell retention and survival affect the choice and applicability of the technique of delivery. A concerted effort in clinical development is thus made to optimize delivery to dysfunctional but viable myocardium through increasingly optimized approaches.

5 Stem Cell Platforms and Clinical Trial Experience

Stem cells are the primary source for regenerative therapies in line with their documented capacity for self-renewal, proliferation, and differentiation [22, 23]. Multiple candidate cell types have been used in preclinical models and then further tested in clinical trials to repair the injured heart through formation of new transplanted tissue and/or indirectly through paracrine effects activating endogenous regeneration processes [24, 25].

Cell-based therapy includes autologous and allogeneic interventions [26]. Autologous stem cells are derived from noncardiac or cardiac self-sources, thereby avoiding immune intolerance. Applications for autologous stem cells are typically limited to chronic conditions given the time required to recycle stem cells from patients serving as donors through the stages of mobilization, collection, expansion, and preparation for delivery back to the same patient now serving as the recipient. In contrast, allogeneic stem cells are derived from a selected donor who is different from the recipient. In principle, allogeneic approaches can produce immune mismatch, including a host-versus-graft reaction where engrafted stem cells are recognized as non-self and attacked by the host. Yet, allogeneic tissue offers unique advantages, including the ability to generate master cell banks and store therapeutic doses to be available "off-the-shelf" for acute/subacute use or in cases where a patient has a genetically based disease that would in principle hinder the therapeutic potential of the autologous stem cell pool.

Cell-based products involve cell samples of limited amounts. This raises issues pertaining to quality-control testing. The manufacture of cell-based products must be carefully designed and validated to ensure consistency and traceability. Control and management of manufacturing and quality-control testing are carried out according to Good Manufacturing Practice requirements [27]. Screening for purity, potency, infectious contamination, and karyotype stability have become necessary elements, i.e., release criteria, in compliance with standard operating practices for production and banking of cells used as autologous or allogeneic therapy. Accordingly, regulatory agencies impose guidelines for risk assessment, quality of manufacturing, preclinical and clinical development, and postmarketing surveillance [28].

Regenerative platforms include natural vs. engineered stem cells. Examples of naturally derived stem cells range across the embryonic to adult stem cell spectrum [29]. The newest technology of nuclear reprogramming enables moreover derivation of induced pluripotent stem (iPS) cells, an example of an engineered stem cell platform [30]. Distinct stem cell types display advantages and challenges associated with availability of the source tissue from which they are derived, differentiation capacity and pluri/multipotent potential, tumorigenic tendency and immunogenic profile, and ultimately socioethical considerations [31].

Embryonic stem cells, derived from the inner mass of a developing embryo in the blastocyst stage, are considered the stem cell archetype. They harbor the capacity of self-renewal, can be clonally expanded, and are capable of differentiating into any cell type in the body, including functional cardiomyocytes [32]. Despite robust cardiomyogenic potential, significant obstacles limit their clinical translation, including risk for uncontrolled growth and immune rejection, in addition to fundamental ethical issues. In this regard, remarkable advances have been made in generating embryonic-like stem cells through dedifferentiation of somatic cells, providing an alternative and embryo-independent pluripotent source for derivation of cardiogenic lineages [33]. While applications for diagnostic and toxicology applications are already advanced [34], iPS cell-based therapeutic use faces a number of challenges, including risk of teratoma formation associated with pluripotency, time required to derive and characterize iPS cells obtained from any given patient, possible genetic instability, and ultimately low efficiency of cardiogenic differentiation [35]. Accordingly, methods to generate cardiomyocytes directly from somatic tissue, without transit through a pluripotent state, have been developed [36–39] but have not yet reached regulatory authorization for clinical translation. While in the future pluripotent stem cell platforms and their products are anticipated to be increasingly considered for human testing [40], current clinical experience has been limited to the use of multipotent adult stem cell types.

Adult skeletal myoblasts, bone marrow, or peripheral blood stem cells were in fact among first to be investigated in a clinical setting for cardiac regeneration [41]. Skeletal myoblasts, expanded from a thigh muscle biopsy, are conceptually attractive due to a potential contractile phenotype, opportunity for autologous transplantation, and resistance to ischemia [42]. Skeletal myoblasts however differentiate into multinucleated myotubes, not apparently cardiomyocytes, after injection into the heart. Myotubes lack gap junctions, resulting in possible electrical inhomogeneity that could predispose to ventricular arrhythmia. The first prospective, randomized, placebo-controlled skeletal myoblast trial (MAGIC trial) used an epicardial approach for delivery, but exhibited overall lack of functional efficacy [43]. Percutaneous intramyocardial delivery of skeletal myoblasts was alternatively applied in a subsequent trial (SEISMIC trial) which demonstrated symptomatic relief with however no significant effect on global left ventricular ejection fraction [44].

Clinical application of bone marrow and blood-derived stem cells has been catalyzed by the accessibility, and ease of cell isolation from a renewable source [45]. Case in point, the adult bone marrow contains different cell populations, including monocytes, hematopoietic, and mesenchymal stem cells. Human hematopoietic stem cells can be defined as $CD34^+$ cells capable of reconstituting blood lineages and, possibly, the ability to trans-differentiate into cardiomyocytes, endothelial cells, and smooth muscle cells in vivo. Mesenchymal stem cells can be defined as $CD105^+$ $CD90^+$ cells, isolated by preferential adherence to plastic in tissue culture, which are capable of osteogenic, chondrogenic, and adipogenic differentiation, and under guidance to cardiogenic specification [46, 47]. In the clinical setting, autologous bone marrow-derived mononuclear cells, unfractionated or enriched in progenitor subpopulations, have been most frequently used for the treatment of acute myocardial infarction typically delivered via the intracoronary mode. Experience to date highlights an excellent feasibility and safety profile, generally positive clinical outcomes, although primary endpoints have not always been met and a sustained functional benefit remains uncertain. Indeed, meta-analyses of case-controlled trials in patients with recent myocardial infarction suggest significant, albeit limited, benefit with regard to recovery of left ventricular ejection fraction beyond standard reperfusion therapy [48, 49]. Among trials based on the use of blood or bone marrow-derived stem cell populations, the double blinded, placebo controlled REPAIR-AMI (Repair of Enriched Progenitor cells And Infarct Remodeling in Acute Myocardial Infarction) trial is considered a benchmark study [50]. Furthermore, the randomized, but not placebo controlled, BOOST (Bone Marrow Transfer to Enhance ST-Elevation Infarct Regeneration) trial showed transient improvement in left ventricular function at 6 months compared to controls [51]. Conversely, the randomized controlled ASTAMI (Autologous Stem Cell Transplantation in Acute Myocardial Infarction) trial failed to demonstrate significant improvement in ejection fraction as assessed from cardiac MRI, single photon emission computed tomography or echocardiography [52]. These apparently controversial readouts may relate to different study design, heterogenous patient populations, cell number and processing, time of cell injection, or methods used to assess outcome [53, 54]. Collectively, these studies demonstrate both feasibility and safety of a stem cell approach in the setting of acute ischemic heart disease, furthermore suggesting that a stem cell source with a higher propensity to regenerate myocardium, directly and indirectly, might promote benefit [55, 56]. Bone marrow-derived cells have also been used for the treatment of refractory angina and chronic heart failure, albeit with inconsistent results in early trial experiences [57–59]. Larger trials are thus needed to dissect the true potential of stem cell therapy.

The most recent systematic review of 33 randomized controlled trials with a total of 1,765 participants indicates no statistically significant improvement in mortality with stem cell treatment or composite morbidity—which includes reinfarction, hospital readmission, restenosis, and target vessel revascularization—compared with placebo [60]. Short-term follow-up data showed that stem cell treatment can improve left ventricular ejection fraction significantly, and this improvement was sustained for 12–61 months. Also, some studies showed that the stem cell therapy improved left ventricular end systolic and end diastolic volumes as well as infarct size. The soon to be initiated large Bone Marrow Cells in Acute Myocardial Infarction (BAMI) trial will evaluate mortality benefits of bone-marrow stem cell therapy in over 3,000 reperfused myocardial infarction patients. The BAMI investigators will also develop standardized techniques for cell processing and delivery. Because the short-term mortality following successful revascularization of a culprit artery is already very low, studies looking for the benefit of stem cell therapy may have to combine mortality, reinfarction, and heart failure into a composite end point. Also, health-related quality of life should be measured to judge the full benefit.

As pointed out, trial results are not uniform owing to the current lack of standardization and optimization of cell isolation and delivery protocols. This lack of uniformity is prevalent despite newer techniques that allow point-of-care cell preparations, for example within cardiac catheterization or operating rooms, thereby providing short preparation time, facilitated logistics of cell transport, and reasonable cost-effectiveness. Beyond inter-trial variability, inter-patient variability has been increasingly recognized triggering an ongoing quest for optimization and identification of the most appropriate cell source and cell type, stratification and selection of patient populations most amenable to cell-based therapy, targeting ideal timing of intervention, and most favorable routes of administration. In this regard, it should be noted that in contrast to traditional small molecule-based medications, regenerative cell products contain life cells as the active ingredient. Moreover, cell therapy is currently limited by low rates of cell engraftment and poor cell survival. Advanced patient age, cardiovascular risk factors, and underlying heart disease appear to also have a negative impact on the functionality of delivered cells. Mechanisms of improved benefit have implicated, among other variables, a defining role for the extent of cardiovascular lineage commitment [61]. Establishing the individual efficacy profiles is thus paramount to maximize benefit of cell-based therapy in the management of cardiovascular disease.

By processing myocardial tissue excised during cardiac surgery or by endovascular biopsy, it is now possible to derive resident stem cell populations. This advance provides the prospect of anatomically matching the regenerative cell source with the target organ. Clinical evaluation of resident cardiac stem cells has been initially tested in the SCIPIO (Cardiac Stem Cell Infusion in Patients With Ischemic CardiOmyopathy) and the CADUCEUS (CArdiosphere-Derived aUtologous stem CElls to reverse ventricUlar dySfunction) trials [62, 63]. The CADUCEUS study utilizes the cell cluster or cardiosphere approach for derivation and propagation [63], while SCIPIO implements an antibody-based method to derive a homogenous C-kit$^+$ population [62]. CADUCEUS focuses on individuals with subacute myocardial infarction, with harvest of the patient's own biopsy-obtained right ventricular tissue to yield an autologous therapeutics delivered via coronary arteries [63]. The SCIPIO study utilizes right atrial tissue obtained during coronary artery bypass for autologous, intracoronary (proximal coronary artery or graft supplying the infarcted left ventricular region) delivery of derived C-kit-expressing human cardiac stem cells [62]. Both studies are first-in-man trials powered to assess safety and feasibility. Both studies reported reduction in myocardial scar mass following cell treatment, but only the SCIPIO trial reported improved left ventricular ejection fraction. The number of patients in the treatment arm of each study was 16 in SCIPIO and 17 in CADUCEUS, and neither study included a placebo group because of the invasive nature of the treatment [62, 63]. Indeed, such approaches are hampered by the invasive nature of heart tissue sampling and the limited quantity of starting material. Orienting nonresident stem cells towards cardiogenesis would eliminate the need for the patient to undergo myocardial harvest [64, 65]. Recently, hallmark traits of cardiac development were successfully triggered within bone marrow-derived mesenchymal stem cells, establishing the first human scalable lineage-specified cardiopoietic phenotype derived without heart tissue harvest [66, 67]. Preclinical testing demonstrated that cardiac-specified progenitors reliably repair the failing myocardium, providing the foundation for clinical translation [68]. The ensuing C-CURE clinical trial is a first-in-man study to address the feasibility and safety of autologous bone marrow-derived cardiopoietic stem cell therapy, and assess efficacy signals in patients with ischemic cardiomyopathy.

6 Future Trends in Regenerative Therapy

At the core of upcoming practice, state-of-the-art regenerative principles are poised to increasingly leverage the emergent understanding of multiplex parameters defining therapeutic outcome in the setting of individualized heart failure management. Individualized medicine provides a powerful engine to tailor molecular profiles of patients in order to maximize therapeutic specificity, reduce treatment variability, and minimize adverse events [69]. Insights in the regenerative basis of cell, tissue, and organ function and their interface with the environment will increasingly define disease risk, identify processes mediating disease susceptibility, or target mechanism-based therapies, providing thereby previously unanticipated opportunities for patient-specific disease management [70]. The emerging field of regenerative medicine will thus grow in conjuncture with the realization of the individualized medicine paradigm to create predictive, personalized, and preemptive solutions for tailored patient-specific strategies. Individualized treatment algorithms for regenerative medicine will require quantification of the inherent reparative potential to identify patients who would benefit from stem cell therapy. In this regard, systematic stratification of patients to match clinical traits and disease pathobiology with most adequate therapy will become integral in streamlining future evidence-based regenerative algorithms. To this end emphasis will be placed on delineating acute vs. chronic disease substrates to ensure proper target strategy, timing, and mode of intervention; separating ischemic vs. non-ischemic conditions to guide focal vs. diffuse therapy; preemptive management of comorbidities and co-therapies to limit modifiable confounding factors to regenerative regimens. Moreover, recognizing key pharmacodynamics and pharmacokinetics features of regenerative biotherapeutics will aid in the design of next generation therapies. In this context, methods to enhance the biological propensity for repair are central in processes aimed at regenerative optimization. Such ongoing efforts to translate optimized stem cell products, along with studies to clarify the duration and mechanisms of benefit as well as the implications of repeat therapy, mark the beginning of a new era in regenerative therapeutics [71–73]. While first-generation products consisted of purified, natural human cells typically used in their native state, second-generation cell products will refer to cells guided with growth factors or subpopulations selected based on tissue-specific biomarkers or genetically modified to direct cell differentiation, restrict tissue specification, and enhance the level of organ specificity. The goal with second-generation cell products is to produce derivatives with enhanced safety and efficacy profiles compared to the original stem cell source. Third-generation products would serve as delivery platforms, for example, as a gene delivery system for correction of genetic mutation or targeted therapy with recombinant protein, and/or engineered cell products with superior properties, such as enhanced stress tolerance and improved regenerative capacity. The goal with third-generation cell products is to maximize therapeutic potential beyond that inherent to the original stem cell source or the respective derivatives [74]. Furthermore, optimizing delivery procedures will entail engineering advanced methods to achieve increasingly uniform distribution of cells and limit early loss at time of administration. Indeed, efforts are under way to design and produce optimized delivery systems. These may combine utilization of biomaterials designed to solidify at the time of injection to improve long-term cell retention and engraftment [75–77]. Moreover, organ engineering based on decellularized matrix scaffolds may provide a future in tissue replacement [78–80].

7 Conclusion

Stem cell-based therapies for ischemic heart disease have significantly advanced since the inaugural procedures a decade ago. The challenge of translating regenerative principles to practice has been increasingly answered with demonstrated clinical feasibility and safety for stem cell therapeutics. Whether it is direct incorporation and function within the damaged heart and/or indirect cellular secretome-mediated benefit, stem cell-based therapy has been independently tested across numerous clinical trial designs. With further development of tools to aid successful delivery, along with advances in the dissection of mechanisms driving stem cell-based repair, regenerative medicine is poised to transit from proof-of-principle studies towards clinical validation and ultimately standardization. However, lack of consensus on cellular production, storage and identity, site and method of delivery, efficacy of autologous "sick patient" derived stem cells vs. allogeneic "healthy donor" cells, the mechanism and duration of benefit, need for adjuvant growth factors and timing of delivery provide formidable challenges that need to be systematically addressed en route to adoption. In this regard, the international multidisciplinary community of regenerative science and practice has provided an unprecedented foundation for increasingly robust trials paving the way for next generation therapies capable to address the root cause of heart failure. Beyond safety and efficacy profiles, regenerative therapies will be tested for equivalence across distinct socioeconomic and healthcare settings, as an indicator that these new management strategies can potentially reach broader populations in need. Ultimately, the rigor of comparative effectiveness outcome analysis will be needed to inform on the value of introducing a personalized regenerative therapy in standardized heart failure management.

References

1. Terzic A, Waldman SA (2011) Chronic diseases: the emerging pandemic. Clin Transl Sci 4:225–226
2. Roger VL et al (2012) Heart disease and stroke statistics—2012 update: a report from the American Heart Association. Circulation 125:188–197
3. Kovacic JC, Castellano JM, Fuster V (2012) Cardiovascular defense challenges at the basic, clinical, and population levels. Ann N Y Acad Sci 1254:1–6

4. Terzic A, Nelson TJ (2010) Regenerative medicine advancing health care 2020. J Am Coll Cardiol 55:2254–2257
5. Terzic A, Folmes CD, Martinez-Fernandez A, Behfar A (2011) Regenerative medicine: on the vanguard of health care. Mayo Clin Proc 86:600–602
6. Nelson TJ, Behfar A, Terzic A (2008) Strategies for therapeutic repair: the R^3 regenerative medicine paradigm. Clin Transl Sci 1:168–171
7. Terzic A, Edwards BS, McKee KC, Nelson TJ (2011) Regenerative medicine: a reality of stem cell technology. Minn Med 94:44–47
8. Ptaszek LM, Mansour M, Ruskin JN, Chien KR (2012) Towards regenerative therapy for cardiac disease. Lancet 379:933–942
9. Leri A, Kajstura J, Anversa P (2011) Role of cardiac stem cells in cardiac pathophysiology: a paradigm shift in human myocardial biology. Circ Res 109:941–961
10. Bergmann O, Bhardwaj RD, Bernard S, Zdunek S, Barnabé-Heider F, Walsh S, Zupicich J, Alkass K, Buchholz BA, Druid H, Jovinge S, Frisén J (2009) Evidence for cardiomyocyte renewal in humans. Science 324:98–102
11. Kajstura J, Bai Y, Cappetta D, Kim J, Arranto C, Sanada F, D'Amario D, Matsuda A, Bardelli S, Ferreira-Martins J, Hosoda T, Leri A, Rota M, Loscalzo J, Anversa P (2012) Tracking chromatid segregation to identify human cardiac stem cells that regenerate extensively the infarcted myocardium. Circ Res 111(7):894–906
12. Dimmeler S, Zeiher AM, Schneider MD (2005) Unchain my heart: the scientific foundations of cardiac repair. J Clin Invest 115:572–583
13. Malliaras K, Marbán E (2011) Cardiac cell therapy: where we've been, where we are, and where we should be headed. Br Med Bull 98:161–185
14. Bartunek J, Vanderheyden M, Hill J, Terzic A (2010) Cells as biologics for cardiac repair in ischaemic heart failure. Heart 96:792–800
15. Laflamme MA, Murry CE (2011) Heart regeneration. Nature 473:326–335
16. Loffredo FS, Steinhauser ML, Gannon J, Lee RT (2011) Bone marrow-derived cell therapy stimulates endogenous cardiomyocyte progenitors and promotes cardiac repair. Cell Stem Cell 8:389–398
17. Behfar A, Crespo-Diaz R, Nelson TJ, Terzic A, Gersh BJ (2010) Stem cells: clinical trials results the end of the beginning or the beginning of the end? Cardiovasc Hematol Disord Drug Targets 10:186–201
18. Gersh BJ, Simari RD, Behfar A, Terzic CM, Terzic A (2009) Cardiac cell repair therapy: a clinical perspective. Mayo Clin Proc 84:876–892
19. Bartunek J, Sherman W, Vanderheyden M, Fernandez-Aviles F, Wijns W, Terzic A (2009) Delivery of biologics in cardiovascular regenerative medicine. Clin Pharmacol Ther 85:548–552
20. Dib N, Menasche P, Bartunek JJ, Zeiher AM, Terzic A, Chronos NA, Henry TD, Peters NS, Fernández-Avilés F, Yacoub M, Sanborn TA, Demaria A, Schatz RA, Taylor DA, Fuchs S, Itescu S, Miller LW, Dinsmore JH, Dangas GD, Popma JJ, Hall JL, Holmes DR Jr (2010) Recommendations for successful training on methods of delivery of biologics for cardiac regeneration: a report of the International Society for Cardiovascular Translational Research. JACC Cardiovasc Interv 3:265–275
21. Psaltis PJ, Zannettino AC, Gronthos S, Worthley SG (2010) Intramyocardial navigation and mapping for stem cell delivery. J Cardiovasc Transl Res 3:135–146
22. Passier R, van Laake LW, Mummery CL (2008) Stem-cell-based therapy and lessons from the heart. Nature 453:322–329
23. Hansson EM, Lindsay ME, Chien KR (2009) Regeneration next: toward heart stem cell therapeutics. Cell Stem Cell 5:364–377
24. Segers VF, Lee RT (2008) Stem-cell therapy for cardiac disease. Nature 451:937–942
25. Steinhauser ML, Lee RT (2011) Regeneration of the heart. EMBO Mol Med 3:701–712
26. Nelson TJ, Behfar A, Yamada S, Martinez-Fernandez A, Terzic A (2009) Stem cell platforms for regenerative medicine. Clin Transl Sci 2:222–227

27. Nelson T, Behfar A, Terzic A (2008) Stem cells: biologics for regeneration. Clin Pharmacol Ther 84:620–623
28. European Medicinal Agency (2011) Reflection paper on stem cell-based medicinal products. EMA/CAT/571134/2009:1–14
29. Murry CE, Field LJ, Menasché P (2005) Cell based cardiac repair. reflections at the 10-year point. Circulation 112:3174–3183
30. Nelson TJ, Martinez-Fernandez A, Terzic A (2010) Induced pluripotent stem cells: developmental biology to regenerative medicine. Nat Rev Cardiol 7:700–710
31. Mummery CL, Davis RP, Krieger JE (2010) Challenges in using stem cells for cardiac repair. Sci Transl Med 2:27ps17
32. Shiba Y, Fernandes S, Zhu WZ, Filice D, Muskheli V, Kim J, Palpant NJ, Gantz J, Moyes KW, Reinecke H, Van Biber B, Dardas T, Mignone JL, Izawa A, Hanna R, Viswanathan M, Gold JD, Kotlikoff MI, Sarvazyan N, Kay MW, Murry CE, Laflamme MA (2012) Human ES-cell-derived cardiomyocytes electrically couple and suppress arrhythmias in injured hearts. Nature 489:322–325
33. Daley GQ (2012) The promise and perils of stem cell therapeutics. Cell Stem Cell 10:740–749
34. Nelson TJ, Terzic A (2011) Induced pluripotent stem cells: an emerging theranostics platform. Clin Pharmacol Ther 89:648–650
35. Mummery C (2011) Induced pluripotent stem cells—a cautionary note. N Engl J Med 364:2160–2162
36. Ieda M, Fu JD, Delgado-Olguin P, Vedantham V, Hayashi Y, Bruneau BG, Srivastava D (2010) Direct reprogramming of fibroblasts into functional cardiomyocytes by defined factors. Cell 142:375–386
37. Qian L, Huang Y, Spencer CI, Foley A, Vedantham V, Liu L, Conway SJ, Fu JD, Srivastava D (2012) In vivo reprogramming of murine cardiac fibroblasts into induced cardiomyocytes. Nature 485:593–598
38. Chen JX, Krane M, Deutsch MA, Wang L, Rav-Acha M, Gregoire S, Engels MC, Rajarajan K, Karra R, Abel ED, Wu JC, Milan D, Wu SM (2012) Inefficient reprogramming of fibroblasts into cardiomyocytes using Gata4, Mef2c, and Tbx5. Circ Res 110:50–55
39. Song K, Nam Y-J, Luo X, Qi X, Tan W, Huang GN, Acharya A, Smith CL, Tallquist MD, Neilson EG, Hill JA, Bassel-Duby R, Olson EN (2012) Heart repair by reprogramming non-myocytes with cardiac transcription factors. Nature 485:599–604
40. Sun N, Longaker MT, Wu JC (2010) Human iPS cell-based therapy: considerations before clinical applications. Cell Cycle 9:880–885
41. Janssens S (2010) Stem cells in the treatment of heart disease. Annu Rev Med 61:287–300
42. Menasche P (2011) Cardiac cell therapy: lessons from clinical trials. J Mol Cell Cardiol 50:258–265
43. Menasché P, Alfieri O, Janssens S, McKenna W, Reichenspurner H, Trinquart L, Vilquin JT, Marolleau JP, Seymour B, Larghero J, Lake S, Chatellier G, Solomon S, Desnos M, Hagège AA (2008) The Myoblast Autologous Grafting in Ischemic Cardiomyopathy (MAGIC) trial: first randomized placebo-controlled study of myoblast transplantation. Circulation 117:1189–1200
44. Duckers HJ, Houtgraaf J, Hehrlein C, Schofer J, Waltenberger J, Gershlick A, Bartunek J, Nienaber C, Macaya C, Peters N, Smits P, Siminiak T, van Mieghem W, Legrand V, Serruys PW (2011) Final results of a phase IIa, randomised, open-label trial to evaluate the percutaneous intramyocardial transplantation of autologous skeletal myoblasts in congestive heart failure patients: the SEISMIC trial. EuroIntervention 6:805–812
45. Wollert KC, Drexler H (2010) Cell therapy for the treatment of coronary heart disease: a critical appraisal. Nat Rev Cardiol 7:204–205
46. Bartunek J, Behfar A, Vanderheyden M, Wijns W, Terzic A (2008) Mesenchymal stem cells and cardiac repair: principles and practice. J Cardiovasc Transl Res 1:115–119

47. Williams AR, Hare JM (2011) Mesenchymal stem cells: biology, pathophysiology, translational findings, and therapeutic implications for cardiac disease. Circ Res 109:923–940
48. Abdel-Latif A, Bolli R, Tleyjeh IM, Montori VM, Perin EC, Hornung CA, Zuba-Surma EK, Al-Mallah M, Dawn B (2007) Adult bone marrow-derived cells for cardiac repair: a systematic review and meta-analysis. Arch Intern Med 167:989–997
49. Martin-Rendon E, Brunskill SJ, Hyde CJ, Stanworth SJ, Mathur A, Watt SM (2008) Autologous bone marrow stem cells to treat acute myocardial infarction: a systematic review. Eur Heart J 29:1807–18018
50. Schächinger V, Erbs S, Elsässer A, Haberbosch W, Hambrecht R, Hölschermann H, Yu J, Corti R, Mathey DG, Hamm CW, Süselbeck T, Assmus B, Tonn T, Dimmeler S, Zeiher AM, REPAIR-AMI Investigators (2006) Intracoronary bone marrow-derived progenitor cells in acute myocardial infarction. N Engl J Med 355:1210–1221
51. Wollert KC, Meyer GP, Lotz J, Ringes-Lichtenberg S, Lippolt P, Breidenbach C, Fichtner S, Korte T, Hornig B, Messinger D, Arseniev L, Hertenstein B, Ganser A, Drexler H (2004) Intracoronary autologous bone-marrow cell transfer after myocardial infarction: the BOOST randomised controlled clinical trial. Lancet 364:141–148
52. Lunde K, Solheim S, Aakhus S, Arnesen H, Abdelnoor M, Egeland T, Endresen K, Ilebekk A, Mangschau A, Fjeld JG, Smith HJ, Taraldsrud E, Grogaard HK, Bjornerheim R, Brekke M, Muller C, Hopp E, Ragnarsson A, Brinchmann JE, Forfang K (2006) Intracoronary injection of mononuclear bone marrow cells in acute myocardial infarction. N Engl J Med 355:1199–1209
53. Seeger FH, Tonn T, Krzossok N, Zeiher AM, Dimmeler S (2007) Cell isolation procedures matter: a comparison of different isolation protocols of bone marrow mononuclear cells used for cell therapy in patients with acute myocardial infarction. Eur Heart J 28:766–772
54. Malliaras K, Kreke M, Marbán E (2011) The stuttering progress of cell therapy for heart disease. Clin Pharmacol Ther 90:532–541
55. Lovell MJ, Mathur A (2010) Cardiac stem cell therapy: progress from the bench to bedside. Heart 96:1531–1537
56. Penn MS, Dong F, Klein S, Mayorga ME (2011) Stem cells for myocardial regeneration. Clin Pharmacol Ther 90:499–501
57. Strauer BE, Steinhoff G (2011) 10 years of intracoronary and intramyocardial bone marrow stem cell therapy of the heart: from the methodological origin to clinical practice. J Am Coll Cardiol 58:1095–1104
58. van Ramshorst J, Rodrigo SF, Schalij MJ, Beeres SL, Bax JJ, Atsma DE (2011) Bone marrow cell injection for chronic myocardial ischemia: the past and the future. J Cardiovasc Transl Res 4:182–191
59. Perin EC, Willerson JT, Pepine CJ, Henry TD, Ellis SG, Zhao DX, Silva GV, Lai D, Thomas JD, Kronenberg MW, Martin AD, Anderson RD, Traverse JH, Penn MS, Anwaruddin S, Hatzopoulos AK, Gee AP, Taylor DA, Cogle CR, Smith D, Westbrook L, Chen J, Handberg E, Olson RE, Geither C, Bowman S, Francescon J, Baraniuk S, Piller LB, Simpson LM, Loghin C, Aguilar D, Richman S, Zierold C, Bettencourt J, Sayre SL, Vojvodic RW, Skarlatos SI, Gordon DJ, Ebert RF, Kwak M, Moyé LA, Simari RD, Cardiovascular Cell Therapy Research Network (CCTRN) (2012) Effect of transendocardial delivery of autologous bone marrow mononuclear cells on functional capacity, left ventricular function, and perfusion in chronic heart failure: the FOCUS-CCTRN trial. JAMA 307:1717–1726
60. Clifford DM, Fisher SA, Brunskill SJ, Doree C, Mathur A, Watt S, Martin-Rendon E (2012) Stem cell treatment for acute myocardial infarction. Cochrane Database Syst Rev 2:CD006536
61. Yoon CH, Koyanagi M, Iekushi K, Seeger F, Urbich C, Zeiher AM, Dimmeler S (2010) Mechanism of improved cardiac function after bone marrow mononuclear cell therapy: role of cardiovascular lineage commitment. Circulation 121:2001–2011
62. Bolli R, Chugh AR, D'Amario D, Loughran JH, Stoddard MF, Ikram S, Beache GM, Wagner SG, Leri A, Hosoda T, Sanada F, Elmore JB, Goichberg P, Cappetta D, Solankhi NK, Fahsah I, Rokosh DG, Slaughter MS, Kajstura J, Anversa P (2011) Cardiac stem cells in patients with

ischaemic cardiomyopathy (SCIPIO): initial results of a randomised phase 1 trial. Lancet 378:1847–1857
63. Makkar RR, Smith RR, Cheng K, Malliaras K, Thomson LE, Berman D, Czer LS, Marbán L, Mendizabal A, Johnston PV, Russell SD, Schuleri KH, Lardo AC, Gerstenblith G, Marbán E (2012) Intracoronary cardiosphere-derived cells for heart regeneration after myocardial infarction (CADUCEUS): a prospective, randomised phase 1 trial. Lancet 379:895–904
64. Behfar A, Terzic A (2006) Derivation of a cardiopoietic population from human mesenchymal stem cells yields cardiac progeny. Nat Clin Pract Cardiovasc Med 3(suppl 1):S78–S82
65. Marbán E, Malliaras K (2010) Boot camp for mesenchymal stem cells. J Am Coll Cardiol 56:735–737
66. Behfar A, Faustino RS, Arrell DK, Dzeja PP, Perez-Terzic C, Terzic A (2008) Guided stem cell cardiopoiesis: discovery and translation. J Mol Cell Cardiol 45:523–529
67. Mercola M, Ruiz-Lozano P, Schneider MD (2011) Cardiac muscle regeneration: lessons from development. Genes Dev 25:299–309
68. Behfar A, Yamada S, Crespo-Diaz R, Nesbitt JJ, Rowe LA, Perez-Terzic C, Gaussin V, Homsy C, Bartunek J, Terzic A (2010) Guided cardiopoiesis enhances therapeutic benefit of bone marrow human mesenchymal stem cells in chronic myocardial infarction. J Am Coll Cardiol 56:721–734
69. Waldman SA, Terzic A (2012) Knowledge cycle transforms therapeutic innovation. Clin Pharmacol Ther 91:3–8
70. Waldman SA, Terzic A (2011) Patient-centric clinical pharmacology advances the path to personalized medicine. Biomark Med 5:697–700
71. Chavakis E, Koyanagi M, Dimmeler S (2010) Enhancing the outcome of cell therapy for cardiac repair: progress from bench to bedside and back. Circulation 121:325–335
72. Mohsin S, Siddiqi S, Collins B, Sussman MA (2011) Empowering adult stem cells for myocardial regeneration. Circ Res 109:1415–1428
73. Mirotsou M, Jayawardena TM, Schmeckpeper J, Gnecchi M, Dzau VJ (2011) Paracrine mechanisms of stem cell reparative and regenerative actions in the heart. J Mol Cell Cardiol 50:280–289
74. Nelson TJ, Behfar A, Terzic A (2009) Regenerative medicine and stem cell therapeutics. In: Waldman SA, Terzic A (eds) Pharmacology and therapeutics: principles to practice (pp 1317–1331). Saunders, Philadelphia, PA
75. Vunjak-Novakovic G, Lui KO, Tandon N, Chien KR (2011) Bioengineering heart muscle: a paradigm for regenerative medicine. Annu Rev Biomed Eng 13:245–267
76. Godier-Furnémont AF, Martens TP, Koeckert MS, Wan L, Parks J, Arai K, Zhang G, Hudson B, Homma S, Vunjak-Novakovic G (2011) Composite scaffold provides a cell delivery platform for cardiovascular repair. Proc Natl Acad Sci USA 108:7974–7979
77. Singelyn JM, Sundaramurthy P, Johnson TD, Schup-Magoffin PJ, Hu DP, Faulk DM, Wang J, Mayle KM, Bartels K, Salvatore M, Kinsey AM, Demaria AN, Dib N, Christman KL (2012) Catheter-deliverable hydrogel derived from decellularized ventricular extracellular matrix increases endogenous cardiomyocytes and preserves cardiac function post-myocardial infarction. J Am Coll Cardiol 59:751–763
78. Ott HC, Matthiesen TS, Goh SK, Black LD, Kren SM, Netoff TI, Taylor DA (2008) Perfusion-decellularized matrix: using nature's platform to engineer a bioartificial heart. Nat Med 14:213–221
79. Song JJ, Ott HC (2011) Organ engineering based on decellularized matrix scaffolds. Trends Mol Med 17:424–432
80. Weber B, Emmert MY, Schoenauer R, Brokopp C, Baumgartner L, Hoerstrup SP (2011) Tissue engineering on matrix: future of autologous tissue replacement. Semin Immunopathol 33:307–315

Chapter 19
Immunosuppressive Management of the Heart Transplant Recipient

Sofie Verstreken

Abbreviations

ACR	Acute cellular rejection
AMR	Antibody-mediated rejection
ATG	Anti-thymocyte globulin
CAV	Cardiac allograft vasculopathy
CNI	Calcineurin inhibitor
CS	Corticosteroids
CyA	Cyclosporine A
CYP3A	Cytochrome P 3A
ISHLT	International Society of Heart and Lung Transplantation
IVIG	Intravenous administration of immune globulin
MMF	Mycophenolate mofetil
PSI	Proliferation signal inhibitors
TAC	Tacrolimus

1 Introduction

Heart transplantation has become an established therapeutic option for selected patients with end-stage heart disease. However, until the advent of effective immunosuppression, allograft rejection has been the main challenge limiting survival in the early days after transplantation. Therapeutic success in cardiac transplantation evolved particularly with the introduction of the calcineurin inhibitors (CNIs),

S. Verstreken, MD (✉)
Cardiovascular Centre, OLV Hospital, Aalst, Belgium
e-mail: sofie.verstreken@olvz-aalst.be

J. Bartunek and M. Vanderheyden (eds.), *Translational Approach to Heart Failure*, 467
DOI 10.1007/978-1-4614-7345-9_19, © Springer Science+Business Media New York 2013

cyclosporin A (CyA), and Tacrolimus (TAC) [1, 2]. Not only infection but also rejection rates declined sharply and contributed to the improvement in survival noted. Although rejection rates continue to decline, the risk of rejection remains significant particularly in the early period following transplantation, necessitating routine surveillance for both acute cellular and antibody-mediated rejection (AMR).

2 Immunosuppressive Agents Used in Heart Transplantation

The different immunosuppressive drug used in heart transplantation, their dosing, therapeutic monitoring, and major toxicities are summarized in Table 19.1. The rejection cascade begins with recognition of the donor antigens by antigen presenting cells (APC). These antigens, combined with major histocompatibility complex (MHC) molecules of the APC, are recognized by the T cell receptor (TCR) CD3 complex on the surface of the T cell. When co-stimulatory signals between APC and T cells (B7-CD28, CD40-CD154) are present, T cell activation occurs, resulting in activation of the calcineurin pathway. Calcineurin dephosphorylates transcription factors, such as NF-AT, which in turn migrate to the nucleus and stimulate promoters of interleukin 2 (IL2) and other cytokines. IL2 activates cell surface receptors (IL2R), resulting in clonal expansion of T helper cells and stimulation of other immune cells. Activation of IL2R stimulates the target of rapamycin (TOR) system, which promotes translation of mRNAs to proteins that regulate the cell cycle (Fig. 19.1).

2.1 Antilymphocyte Antibody Therapy

2.1.1 Polyclonal Anti-thymocyte Antibodies

Currently, anti-thymocyte globulin (ATG) and anti-IL2 receptor antibodies are the agents most often used for induction therapy. Polyclonal antibodies are derived by immunization of horses (ATGAM^{R} also called lymphocyte immune globulin) or rabbits (Thymoglobulin^{R}) with human thymocytes. They contain antibodies directed against a wide variety of human T cell antigens, and by inducing complement-mediated cytolysis and cell-mediated opsonization in the spleen and liver, they cause rapid depletion of T lymphocytes. Therapy has evolved from a standard dosing to a dose adjustment strategy based upon CD3 or CD2 counts. In kidney transplantation, administration of Rabbit ATG for CD3 counts >50 cells/mm^3 was associated with an acceptable rejection rate and safety profile [3]. In thoracic transplantation, the CD3-guided approach has yielded similar results and has permitted a 60 % reduction in dose together with lower adverse event rates [4, 5]. Therapy with ATG typically lasts for 3–7 days.

Table 19.1 Immunosuppressive agents used in heart transplantation

		Trough levels				
Drug	Dosing	0–6 months	6–12 months	>12 months	Overall	Major toxicities
Calcineurin inhibitors						
Cyclosporine	4.8 mg/kg/day in 2 divided doses	250–350 ng/mL	200–250 ng/mL	100–200 ng/mL		Renal insufficiency, hypertension, dyslipidemia, hypokalemia and hypoMg^{2+}, hyperuricemia, neurotoxicity (encephalopathy, seizures, tremors, neuropathy), gingival hyperplasia, hirsutism
Tacrolimus	0.05–0.1 mg/kg/day in 2 divided doses	10–15 ng/mL	5–10 ng/mL	5–10 ng/mL		Renal insufficiency, hypertension, diabetes, dyslipidemia, hypoMg^{2+}, neurotoxicity (headache, tremors)
Cell cycle agents						
Azathioprine	1.5–3.0 mg/kg/day titrated to keep WBC >3,000/mm^2				None	Bone marrow suppression, hepatitis (rare), pancreatitis, malignancy
Mycophenolate Mofetil	1,000–3,000 mg/day in 2 divided doses				Mycophenolic acid (MPA): 2–5 μg/mL	Gastrointestinal disturbances, leukopenia
Proliferation signal inhibitors						
Sirolimus	1–3 mg/day				5–10 ng/mL	Oral ulcerations, hypercholesterolemia and hypertriglyceridemia, poor wound healing, lower extremity edema, pulmonary toxicities (pneumonitis, alveolar hemorrhage), potentiation of CNI nephrotoxicity, leukopenia, anemia, and thrombocytopenia

(continued)

Table 19.1 (continued)

Drug	Dosing	Trough levels				Major toxicities
		0–6 months	6–12 months	>12 months	Overall	
Corticosteroids						
Prednisone	1 mg/kg/day in 2 divided doses, tapered to 0.05 mg/kg/day by 6–12 months				None	Weight gain, hypertension, hyperlipidemia, osteopenia, hyperglycemia, poor wound healing, salt and water retention, proximal myopathy, cataracts, peptic ulcer disease, growth retardation
Antilymphocyte antibody therapy						
Polyclonal antithymocyte globulins	10–15 mg/kg/day IV over 6–8 h for 3–14 days				Requires monitoring of CD3 count. Target: 5–10 % of baseline values or <50 CD3 cells/mL	Fever, cytokine release syndrome, increased risk of CMV infection, thrombocytopenia, and neutropenia
Antithymocyte globulin	1.5 mg/kg/day IV over 6–8 h for 3–14 days				Monitoring of CD3 as above	Fever, cytokine release syndrome, increased risk of CMV infection, thrombocytopenia, and neutropenia
OKT3	2.5–5 mg/day for 3–14 days				Monitoring of CD3 as above	Cytokine release syndrome, increased risk of CMV infection, increased risk of lymphoproliferative disease
Basiliximab	20 mg IV within 6 h of surgery and 4 days postoperatively					Rare cases of hypersensitivity have been reported

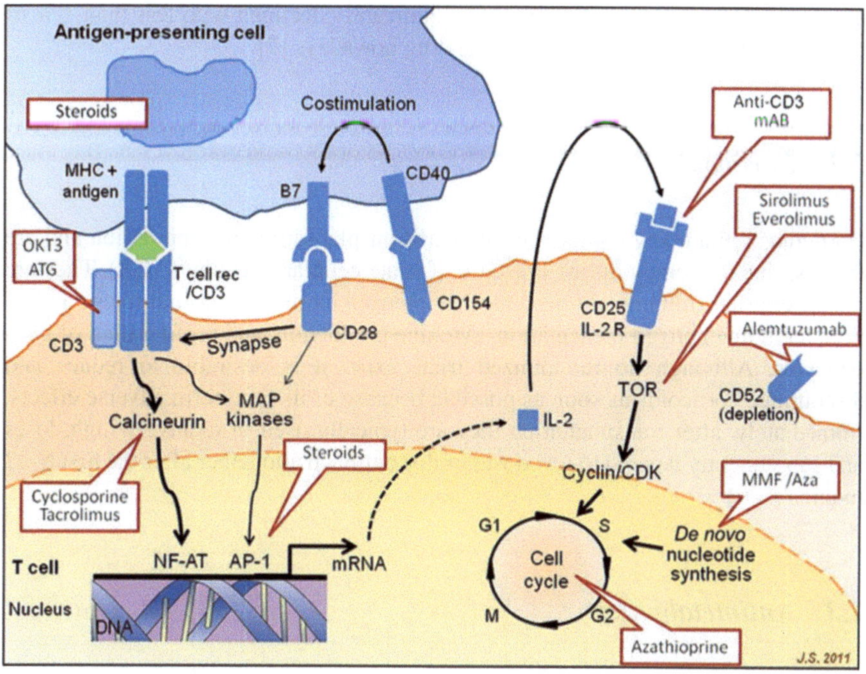

Fig. 19.1 Immunologic mechanisms involved in graft rejection and sites of action of immunosuppressive drugs (shown in *red*). *ATG* antithymocyte globulin, *Aza* azathioprine, *MMF* mycophenolate mofetil; *OKT3* muromonab, anti CD3 mAB

2.1.2 Interleukin 2 Receptor Antagonists

Basiliximab (Simulect) is a chimeric human/murine monoclonal antibody that binds to the interleukine 2 receptor on activated T cell lymphocytes and prevents their clonal expansion. It is administered at fixed doses. Compared to anti-thymocyte antibodies, this class of drugs has significantly lower incidence of drug-related adverse reactions [3].

2.1.3 Muromonab-CD3 (OKT3)

Muromonab-CD3 (OKT3) is a murine monoclonal antibody that binds to the CD3 molecule causing internalization of the T cell receptor which induces simultaneous T cell activation and depletion. The first or second drug dose induces a cytokine release syndrome characterized by fevers, rigors, hypotension, and pulmonary edema. It can be attenuated by premedication with intravenous steroids, antihistamines, antipyretics, and H2 blockers. At the long term an increased risk for life-threatening opportunistic infections and lymphoproliferative disorders has been reported [6]. Due to these adverse effects and the availability of alternate agents, the use of OKT3 as induction therapy has significantly declined with less than 1 % of heart transplant recipients receiving the drug nowadays [7].

2.2 Corticoids

Corticoids remain key component of heart transplant immunosuppression and are the first line of therapy during episodes of acute cellular rejection (ACR). They are nonspecific anti-inflammatory agents that interrupt multiple steps in immune activation, including antigen presentation, cytokine production, and proliferation of lymphocytes. Although no randomized trials exist, it is desirable to reduce and discontinue corticoids as soon as possible because of its long-term adverse effects. Immediately, after transplantation they are typically used in relatively high doses and subsequently tapered to low doses or discontinued altogether after the first 6–12 months [8, 9].

2.3 Antimetabolites

The antimetabolites azathioprine and mycophenolate mofetil (MMF) are antimetabolites or antiproliferative agents that interfere with the synthesis of nucleic acids. They exert their immunosuppressive effect by inhibiting the proliferation of both T and B lymphocytes. Both are prodrugs that are rapidly hydrolyzed in the blood to its active form. MMF has replaced azathioprine as the preferred antimetabolite agent. Despite side effects such as gastrointestinal discomfort and leucopenia, mycophenolate is associated with a significant reduction in both mortality and incidence of treatable rejection as compared to azathioprine [10].

2.4 Calcineurin Inhibitors

Tacrolimus (TAC) is a CNI that binds the FK-binding protein as opposed to Cyclosporine A (CyA), which binds cyclophilin. The net result of both drugs is similar in that calcineurin is inhibited [11]. TAC has been used extensively in solid organ transplantation and is part of immunosuppressive therapy in up to 50 % of cardiac transplant patients. It is thought to be more potent than CyA. In fact TAC has been used as a rescue therapy in patients with significant and recurrent acute rejection under CyA [12]. Several clinical trials suggest that TAC-based immunosuppression may offer an advantage over cyclosporine-based regimens with respect to decreased rates of acute rejection and an overall more favorable metabolic derangement profile with decreased incidence of hypertension and hyperlipidemia however at the cost of a higher incidence of posttransplant diabetes [13–15].

2.5 Proliferation Signal Inhibitors or Mammalian Target of Rapamycin Inhibitors

Sirolimus and everolimus, the two proliferation signal inhibitors (PSIs) registered as immunosuppressants for solid organ transplant recipients, are structurally similar to TAC. However, they exert their immunosuppressive effects via a calcineurin-independent mechanism. They inhibit the mammalian target of rapamycin (mTOR) pathway. Both drugs bind to the intracellular FK506-binding protein 12 (FKPB12) to form a complex that inhibits not only directly mTORC1 but also indirectly mTORC2 signaling pathways. mTORC1 and mTORC2 both play an important role in the transduction signals from the interleukin 2 receptor to the nucleus, causing cell cycle arrest at the G1 to S phase. As a consequence of mTOR network inhibition, various cell processes are affected including those associated with protein synthesis and cell proliferation [16, 17]. As a final result the proliferation from both T cell and B cell population in response to cytokine signals is halted. These drugs have been used in selected transplant recipients with renal insufficiency, cardiac allograft vasculopathy, or malignancies in an attempt to reverse or slow the progression of these conditions. However, due to the high incidence of drug-related adverse effects, including delayed wound healing [18], gastrointestinal symptoms, proteinuria, and even an increased risk of nephrotoxicity especially when used in conjunction with standard doses of CNI's [15, 19], their widespread use as de novo therapy is limited [42–44].

2.6 Drug–Drug Interactions

Both the Cytochrome P3A (CYP3A) and gastrointestinal P-glycoprotein system play a key role in the metabolism of many immunosuppressive agents such as CYA, TAC, sirolimus, and everolimus. In this regard drugs that either induce or inhibit CYP3A or decrease P-glycoprotein activity cause, respectively, a decrease or increase in immunosuppressive levels (Table 19.2). Clinicians involved in the care of heart transplantation should be aware of the risk for drug interactions when other agents are added or deleted from a patient's medical regimen [20]. A potential life-threatening adverse event, rhabdomyolysis, can occur with the combined use of CyA and a 3-hydroxy-3-methylglutaryl-coenzyme A (HMG-CoA) reductase inhibitor (lovastatin, simvastatin), particularly when clopidogrel is concomitantly used [21]. All three drugs are metabolized via the CYP3A4 enzyme, a process that is inhibited by CyA. The addition of clopidogrel further increases the plasma concentration of the statin due to competition for the remaining receptor sites. This effect can easily be prevented when CyA and clopidogrel are used in combination with pravastatin which is not metabolized through the CYP3A pathway. A list of possible other interactions is provided in Table 19.2.

Table 19.2 Main pharmacokinetic interactions with commonly used immunosuppressive agents

Drug	Interaction drug	Effect	Action[a]
TAC/CSA	Calcium channel blockers		
	Dihydropyridine	Increased TAC/CSA exposure	A
	No dihydropyridine	Increased TAC/CSA exposure	B
	Lipid lowering agents		
	Statins	Increased statin exposure, increased risk for myopathy/rhabdomyolysis	A
	Ezetimibe	Increased ezetimibe exposure	A
	Fibric acid derivatives	Decreased CSA/TAC exposure	B
	Antiplatelet agents (ticlopidine, clopidogrel)	Decreased CSA/TAC exposure	A
	Antifungal agents		
	Azole antifungals	Increased CSA/TAC exposure	B
	Caspofungin	Increased drugs exposure, with subsequent hepatotoxicity	B
	Amphotericin B	Increased nephrotoxic effects risk	A
	Antibiotics		
	Macrolide antibiotics	Increased CSA/TAC exposure	A
	Rifamycin derivatives	Decreased TAC/CSA exposure	B
	Anticonvulsants (carbamazepine, phenytoin, phenobarbital)	Decreased TAC/CSA exposure	B
SIR/EVE	Antifungal agents (azole antifungals)	Increased SIR/EVE exposure	B
	Calcium channel blockers (no dihydropyridine)	Increased SIR/EVE exposure	B
	CSA/TAC	Increased SIR/EVE exposure	B
	Anticonvulsants (carbamazepine, phenytoin, phenobarbital)	Decreased SIR/EVE exposure	
MMF	Cholestyramine resin	Decreased MMF exposure	B
	Iron/antacids	Decreased MMF exposure	B
	Oral contraceptives (estrogens, progestins)	Decreased contraceptives exposure, increased risk of pregnancy	B
	Rifamycin derivatives	Decreased MMF exposure	B
	CSA/TAC	Decreased MMF exposure	A
AZA	Allopurinol	Increased exposure to 6-MP with subsequent myelosuppression	C
	Vitamin K antagonists	Decreased INR	A

AZA azathioprine, *CSA* cyclosporine, *EVE* everolimus, *INR* international normalized ratio, *MMF* mycophenolate mofetil, *6-MP* 6-mercaptopurine, *SIR* sirolimus, *TAC* tacrolimus

[a]A, monitor therapy; B, consider therapy modification; C, avoid combination

3 Rejection

In histological terms, acute rejection is defined as an inflammatory response of the host to the transplanted organ. While T-cell mediated mechanisms leading to Acute cellular rejection (ACR) were initially described, there is now increasing evidence that host antibody responses play an equally important role. The diagnosis of antibody mediated rejection (AMR) remains technically more challenging and a consensus on its definition has only recently begun to evolve [22]. In addition the complications related to immunosuppressive agents such as renal insufficiency, hypertension, and hyperlipidemia contribute to posttransplant cardiac mortality and morbidity.

3.1 Acute Cellular Rejection

Younger age of recipients, female gender of both donor and recipient, higher number of human leukocyte antigen (HLA) mismatches, black recipients, and the use of induction therapy are all risk factors for ACR that have been identified [23, 24]. The development of ACR, requiring treatment, leads to a higher incidence of cardiac allograft vasculopathy [25], and patients who required treatment for ACR in the first year after transplantation and survived have a worse long-term survival compared to those without rejection during the first posttransplant year [26]. ACR is most frequently seen during the first 3–6 months posttransplant. Approximately, 40 % of adult heart transplant recipients have one or more ACR episode within the first month posttransplant and more than 60 % undergo an ACR episode (ISHLT grade ≥ 1R) within the first 6 months after transplantation [27]. Through better perioperative management with virtual cross-matching and postoperative surveillance with endomyocardial biopsies, those at elevated risk of rejection have been identified.

ACR is a T cell mediated process with myocardial cellular infiltration of CD3 reactive T lymphocytes (Fig. 19.2) and macrophages. Histologically, ACR is characterized by an inflammatory response of the recipient to the transplanted organ leading to myocyte necrosis. The diagnosis is made by endomyocardial biopsy, and a standardized grading scale was proposed by Billingham [27] and later revised in 2004 (Table 19.3) [22]. Generally, a cardiac biopsy schedule consists of endomyocardial biopsy procurement on a weekly basis during the first month, monthly until the sixth month, and then every 3 months until the end of the first year post Tx. This schedule takes into account that the highest risk of allograft rejection is generally seen during the first 3–6 months after Tx. After the first year, additional biopsies are likely not of significance because low rates of rejection are observed in this period, and biopsy procurement should only be considered when there is clinical suspicion for rejection [28].

The ISHLT established histopathologic criteria for defining and grading acute allograft rejection to grade immunosuppressive therapy (Table 19.3) [22]. Generally, Grade 0–1R are considered low grade rejection, and, in asymptomatic patients, no change in therapy is indicated. Grades 2R and 3R are compatible with significant

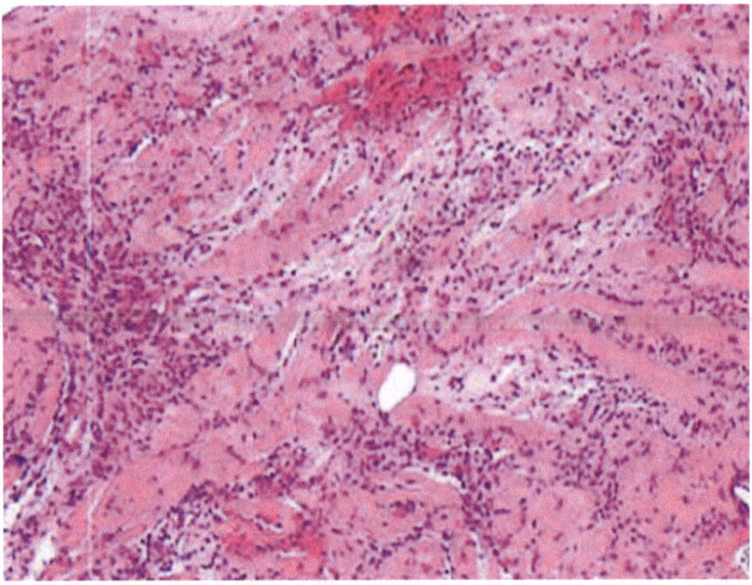

Fig. 19.2 Severe acute cellular rejection (grade 3R). Intense and diffuse polymorphic inflammatory infiltrate (including lymphocytes, macrophages, eosinophils, neutrophils, and plasma cells) with extensive myocardial necrosis and disappearance of normal myocardial architecture. Oedema, interstitial hemorrhage, and vasculitis may be present (H&E, 400×)

rejection where myocyte necrosis is present, and augmentation of immunosuppressive therapy usually is indicated.

Key Points

- Acute cellular rejection is a T cell mediated process with myocardial cellular infiltration of CD3-reactive T lymphocytes and macrophages.
- Acute cellular rejection is most frequently seen during the first 3–6 months posttransplant.
- The ISHLT established histopathologic criteria for defining and grading acute allograft rejection.

3.2 Antibody-Mediated Rejection

In a registry study, Mills and colleagues [29] confirmed that rejection associated with hemodynamic compromise was associated with a poor long-term outcome. However, those patients who had hemodynamic compromise despite a low ISHLT biopsy grade (0–1R in the present grading scale) did worse than those with a high

Table 19.3 ISHLT standardized cardiac biopsy grading: acute cellular rejection[a]

2004		1990	
Grade 0R[b]	No rejection	Grade 0	No rejection
Grade 1R, mild	Interstitial and/or perivascular infiltrate with up to 1 focus of myocyte damage	Grade 1, mild	
		A-focal	Focal perivascular and/or interstitial infiltrate without myocyte damage
		B-diffuse	Diffuse infiltrate without myocyte damage
		Grade 2 moderate	One focus of infiltrate with associated myocyte damage
Grade 2R	Two or more foci of infiltrate with associated myocyte damage	Grade 3, moderate	
		A-focal	Multifocal infiltrate with myocyte damage
Grade 3R severe	Diffuse infiltrate with multifocal myocyte damage ±edema, ±hemorrhage ±vasculitis	B-diffuse	Diffuse infiltrate with myocyte damage
		Grade 4, severe	Diffuse, polymorphous infiltrate with extensive myocyte damage ±edema, ±hemorrhage ±vasculitis

[a]The presence or absence of acute antibody-mediated rejection (AMR) may be recorded as AMR0, AMR1, as required (see Table 19.4)
[b]Where "R" denotes revised grade to avoid confusion with 1990 scheme

ISHLT biopsy grade (2R–3R). These findings suggest that immunologic mechanisms other than lymphocytic infiltration may be important. It was documented that noncellular or so-called AMR exists and should be regarded as a distinct clinical entity. AMR occurs in approximately 10–20 % of all heart transplant recipients, correlates with a poor outcome, and is associated with hemodynamic compromise, increased graft loss, cardiac allograft vasculopahy, and increased cardiovascular mortality [30–32]. Patients with a history of sensitization to HLA due to previous transplantation, transfusion, and pregnancy have an increased risk for AMR. Moreover, the proportion of allosensitized patients on cardiac transplantation list has been expanding progressively as a result of widespread use of ventricular assist devices (VAD) and the increasing number of patients undergoing retransplantation. Platelet transfusions during VAD implantation has been shown to be a risk factor associated with the development of HLA I class IgG antibodies [33]. Furthermore, VAD recipients develop prominent B-cell activation, as evidenced by increased production of anti-HLA class I and class II antibodies [33]; in this patient population not only blood and platelet transfusion but also contact with certain VAD membranes is responsible for the antibody production.

Histologically, AMR is defined by typical histopathological changes consisting of capillary endothelial changes, macrophage and neutrophil infiltration, interstitial edema, and linear accumulation of immunoglobulins and complement, especially complement component C4d (Fig. 19.3). Additional clinical and serological

Table 19.4 ISHLT recommendations for acute antibody-mediated rejection (AMR)

	2004	1990
AMR0	Negative for acute antibody-medicated rejection	
	No histologic or immunopathologic features of AMR	
AMR1	Positive for AMR	Humoral rejection (positive immunofluorescence, vaculitis or severe edema in absence of cellular infiltrate) recorded as additional required information
	Histologic features of AMR	
	Positive immunofluorescence or immunoperoxidase staining for AMR (positive CD68, C4d)	

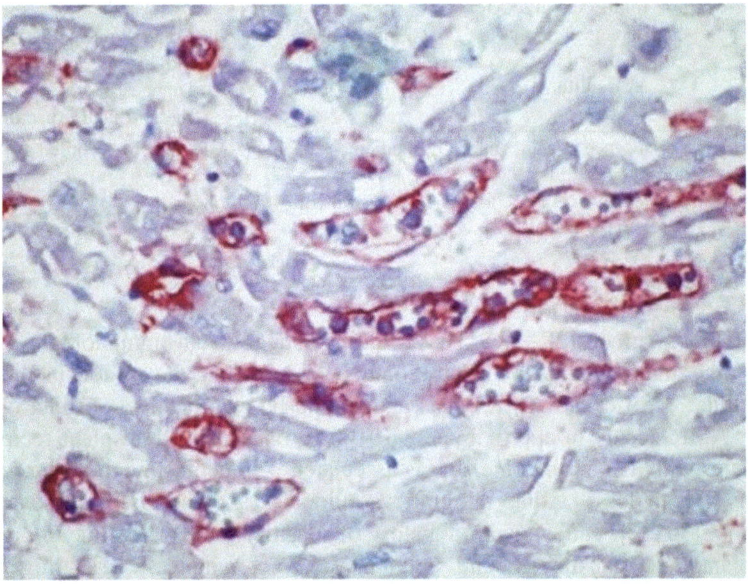

Fig. 19.3 Antibody-mediated rejection characterized by endothelial cell swelling and numerous macrophages filling vascular spaces. Immunochemistry technique staining C4d indicates diffuse, *red* linear deposits of complement C4d fragments in the wall of myocardial capillaries (600×)

findings of donor specific antibodies (DSA) support the diagnosis of AMR [34]. This has led in 2005 to a revised biopsy scale establishing immunohistochemical criteria for the reporting of AMR (Table 19.4) [22].

In its early phase AMR is usually accompanied by graft dysfunction and associated by a rise in donor-specific antibodies (DSA) [35]. When AMR occurs within the first week of transplantation, the recipient usually has evidence of pre-sensitization to donor HLA antigens [35]. It remains undetermined whether or which

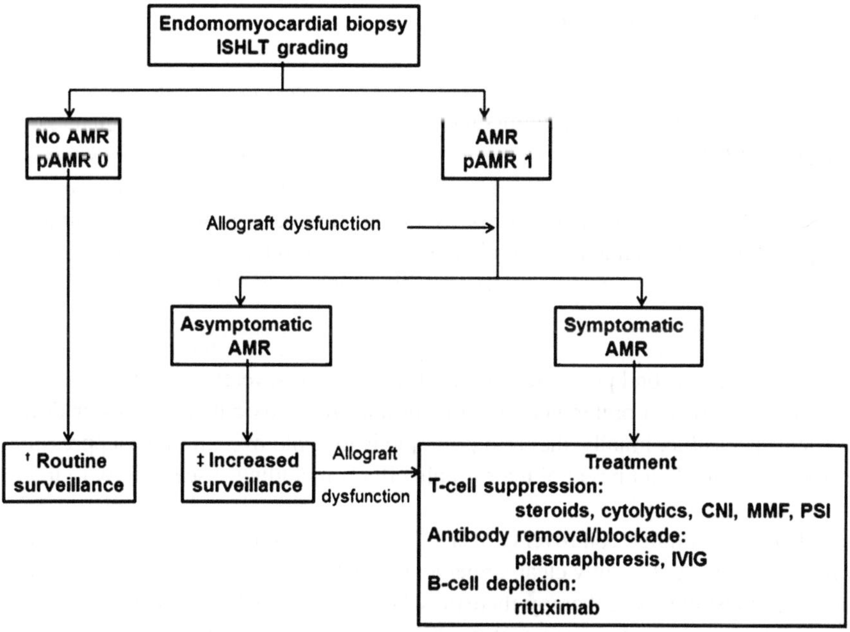

Fig. 19.4 Proposed management algorithm for AMR in heart transplantation. *AMR* indicates antibody-mediated rejection, *pAMR* pathologic AMR grade, *CNI* calcineurin inhibitors, *PSI* proliferation signal inhibitor, *IVIG* intravenous immunoglobulin's. *Dagger* DSA monitoring at week 2, months 1, 3, 6, and 12 in first year after transplant, and annually thereafter. *Double dagger* assessment of allograft function every month and DSA every 3 months until two negative or unchanged results

therapies improve the prognosis of this condition. Currently, when asymptomatic AMR is diagnosed, one should assure that baseline immunosuppression is adequate and the patient should be closely monitored [3] (Fig. 19.4).

When AMR occurs late, graft dysfunction is uncommon but poor outcome is due to hemodynamic compromised rejection and higher risk for the development of cardiac allograft vasculopathy [30, 31, 35]. As previously mentioned, risk factors associated with the development of AMR include female gender, elevated pre-transplant panel-reactive antibodies (PRAs), positive donor-specific cross-match, prior sensitization to OKT3, CMV seropositivity, prior implantation of ventricular assist device, and/or retransplantation [31, 34, 36, 37].

Key Points

- Antibody-mediated rejection (AMR) occurs in approximately 10–20 % of all heart transplant recipients and is associated with a poor outcome.
- Patients with a history of sensitization to HLA due to previous transplant and ventricular assist devices are prone to the development of AMR.
- AMR is defined by distinct histopathological findings as well as by the occurrence of donor-specific antibodies.

4 Immunosuppressive Therapy

The goal of posttransplant immunosuppressive therapy is to prevent the occurrence of allograft rejection while minimizing toxicity and infectious and malignant complications [38].

Immunosuppressive therapy can be classified as induction, maintenance, or anti-rejection therapy. Induction regimens provide intense early postoperative immunosuppression while maintenance regimens are used throughout the patient's life to prevent both acute and chronic rejection. Three general principles govern induction and immunosuppressive therapy. The first principle is that immune activation and risk for graft rejection are the highest early after heart transplantation and decrease over time. The second principle is to use low doses of several drugs with nonoverlapping toxicities in preference over higher and more toxic doses of fewer drugs, whenever feasible. Finally, the third principle is to avoid over-immunosuppression, because it leads to a myriad of undesirable effects including susceptibility to infection and malignancy.

There is still much controversy over what constitutes the optimum immunosuppressive regimen. The only clear agreement is that within the concept of low intensity immunosuppressive therapy, there must be room for flexibility and individualized approaches, according to each center's clinical experience [38].

Key Points

- Tailoring immunosuppression to the needs of each heart transplant recipient requires correct stratification of their risk and close rejection surveillance during and after minimization of immunosuppression.
- Risk stratification is based on clinical characteristics, immunological features of donor and recipient, and data from imaging techniques and cardiac biopsies.

4.1 Induction Therapy

The use of intense immunosuppression in the perioperative period is based on the empirical observation that more powerful immunosuppression is required to prevent early acute rejection. An additional advantage of induction therapy is that it may allow delayed initiation of nephrotoxic immunosuppressive drugs in patients with compromised renal function and that it may provide some flexibility with respect to early glucocorticoid weaning. Approximately, 50 % of heart transplant programs currently employ induction therapy during the early postoperative period [26]. This is achieved in 27 % of the cases with interleukin 2 receptor antagonists (basiliximab). In 23 % of patients polyclonal antithymocyte antibodies (ATGAM, Thymoglobulin) are used for this purpose. Whether induction therapy is necessary or advantageous in cardiac transplantation remains controversial, with many single-center prospective studies showing both negative and positive outcomes [39]. Of note, it remains unclear whether prophylactic monoclonal or polyclonal antibody therapy results in lower rejection and mortality rates, and long-term effects of induction agents are incompletely understood. From a clinical perspective, induction therapy may be of benefit in a subset of patients with the highest risk of acute rejection (young, pre-sensitized patients, females) and in patients with impaired renal function to delay the initiation of calcineurin inhibitors posttransplantation.

Key Points

- Induction therapy remains controversial, with many single-center prospective studies showing both negative and positive outcomes.
- Induction therapy may be of benefit in patients with a higher risk of acute rejection and in patients with impaired renal function.

4.2 Maintenance Immunosuppressive Therapy

Most maintenance immunosuppressive regimens employed in the heart transplant recipients consist of a combination of agents that affect different pathways in the activation of the T cell (Fig. 19.1). Usually, a three-drug regimen consisting of a CNI such as cyclosporin or TAC, an antimetabolite agent (MMF or less commonly azathioprine), and tapering doses of glucocorticoids is prescribed the first year post transplantation.

Although intent-to-treat analyses have shown that various immunosuppressive regimens are not associated with differential effects on survival, significant differences were reported between regimens in terms of rejection, CAV, and adverse events. Therefore, the interpretation of the randomized trials may provide valuable information that can be used by clinicians to individualize immunosuppression thereby preventing adverse effects.

It is recommended that maintenance immunosuppressive therapy should be individualized and initially consist of a CNI chosen on the basis of center-specific experience and individualized needs, MMF, and corticosteroids. MMF should be continued as part of maintenance antirejection therapy, because changing back to azathioprine is associated with an increased risk for acute rejection. Steroids are beneficial in the early posttransplant period, but efforts should be made to taper the dose to minimize adverse effects. Patients at low risk for rejection should have steroid withdrawal attempted with appropriate vigilance for rejection and CAV. Finally, sirolimus has been used for rescue therapy in refractory acute rejection, but primary use for maintenance therapy cannot be recommended pending clinical trial results [3].

TAC is currently the most widely used CNI (69 % of patients) whereas MMF remains the predominant antimetabolite agent (84 %). The use of newer antiproliferative agents such as everolimus for maintenance therapy remains low at 1 year (11 % of patients) and is typically being reserved for patients with CAV or renal insufficiency. Finally, 89 % of patients remain on low doses of glucocorticoids at 1 year posttransplantation. TAC and MMF with or without steroids is the most common immunomaintenance therapy (46 % of patients) followed by cyclosporine and MMF with or without steroids (39 % of patients).

Key Points

- The use of universal induction therapy remains controversial.
- Most modern immunosuppressive regimens consist of a two- or three-drug regimen including a CNI, an antimetabolite agent, and tapering doses of corticosteroids over the first year.
- PSI are typically used in patients with cardiac allograft vasculopathy or renal insufficiency.
- CNIs and PSIs are metabolized by the CYP3A pathway and therefore are susceptible to numerous drug interactions.

4.3 Treatment of Acute Cellular Rejection

ACR may be diagnosed in a patient presenting with symptoms and signs of graft dysfunction or the diagnosis may be made on routine surveillance endomyocardial biopsy in an asymptomatic patient. Symptoms accompanying ACR are caused by graft dysfunction and hemodynamic compromise. In this particular case prompt institution of therapy is mandatory to reverse allograft dysfunction and prevent often irreversible myocardial damage [29].

High dose of CS (1000 mg IV daily given for 3 consecutive days) should be first line therapy for symptomatic ACR of ISHLT grades 1R, 2R, and 3R. If clinical improvement does not occur within 12–24 h, cytolytic therapy with polyclonal antithymocyte antibodies or less commonly the monoclonal OKT3 has to be considered. This therapy is administered daily for 3–10 days. Premedication with corticoids, antihistamines, and antipyretics is recommended as well as antibacterial profylaxis against opportunistic infections. If noncompliance has been excluded as the likely cause for the rejection, several changes to baseline immunosuppression can be considered. These include increase in the dose of the current immunosuppressive agents, addition of new agents, or conversion to different agents. Typical antirejection therapies include the conversion to TAC if the patient was previously on CyA, conversion to MMF if previously on azathioprine, or the addition of rapamycin, cyclophosphamide, or methotrexate. An endomyocardial biopsy should be performed 1–2 weeks after initiation of therapy to assess resolution of histological changes of ACR.

The majority of ACRs occur asymptomatic and are diagnosed by surveillance endomyocardial biopsy [29]. Severe ACR ISHLT 3R should be treated even in the absence of symptoms with high dose IV CS. Moderate asymptomatic ACR (ISHLT 2R) can be treated with corticosteroids either IV or oral. In asymptomatic patients with either ISHLT 2R or ISHLT 3R ACR, maintenance therapy should be adjusted. This includes an increase of the dose of the current immunosuppressive regimen,

Table 19.5 Treatment options for ACR and AMR according to severity

	Asymptomatic	Reduced EF	Heart failure/shock
Cellular	Target higher CNI levels	Oral steroid bolus/taper	
	Oral steroid bolus ± taper	Or	
		IV pulse steroids	IV pulse steroids
			Cytolytic therapy
Humoral			Plasmapheresis
	No therapy?	Oral steroid bolus/taper	IV immune globulin
		Or	Inotropics
		IV pulse steroids	IABP or ECMO support
		w/wo immune globulin	

addition of another immunosuppressive agent, or conversion to a different immunosuppressive regimen (Table 19.5) [3].

Key Points

- The majority of acute cellular rejections occur asymptomatic.
- Severe ISHLT 3R rejection should be treated even in the absence of symptoms with high dose CS intravenously.
- In patients with ISHLT 3R or moderate ISHLT 2R maintenance therapy should be adjusted.

4.4 Treatment of Antibody-Mediated Rejection

Persisting controversy over diagnosis and a paucity of robust data to substantiate traditional therapies makes the management of AMR less clear and therefore also more challenging. Its treatment remains empiric with supporting evidence limited to small, non-randomized studies with short follow-up. The selection of individual therapies and their duration should be guided by the symptoms severity with more aggressive therapy in those with hemodynamic compromise. Treatment is only recommended for symptomatic AMR. In case AMR is asymptomatic, it is wise to assure that baseline immunosuppression is adequate and the patient should be closely monitored. In all patients routine posttransplant surveillance for AMR should include pathologic evaluation on endomyocardial biopsy, assessment of allograft dysfunction, and monitoring for donor-specific antibodies. A treatment algorithm for AMR and donor-specific antibodies (DSA) following heart transplantation is proposed in Figs. 19.4 and 19.5 [40]. Altered humoral immunity with plasma cell production of antibodies against donor antigens on the allograft is primarily responsible for myocardial injury in AMR. Plasma cells are generated by T lymphocyte-dependent activation and generation of memory B lymphocytes. Treatment strategies for AMR (Table 19.4) are directed at inhibiting the humoral response at various levels by targeting (1) removal and blockade of circulating antibodies, (2) depletion of B lymphocytes, (3) depletion of plasma cells, (4) suppression of T lymphocyte-dependent

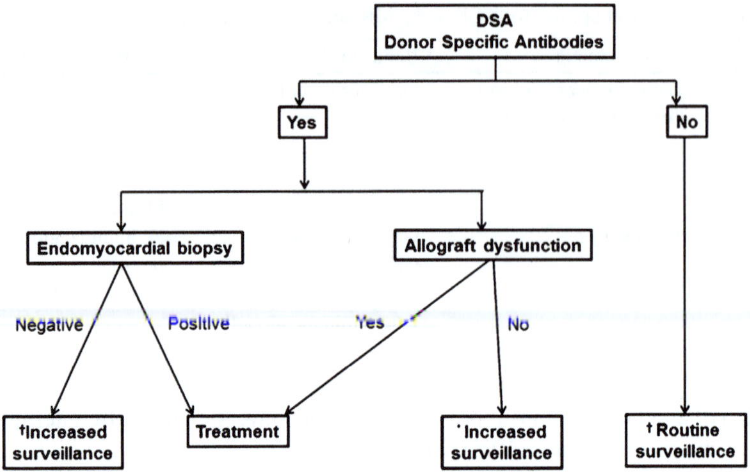

Fig. 19.5 Proposed DSA treatment algorithm. DSA indicates donor-specific antibodies, AMR antibody-mediated rejection. *Asterisk* assessment of allograft function every month and DSA every 3 months until two negative or unchanged results. *Dagger* DSA monitoring at week 2, months 1, 3, 6, and 12 in first year after transplant, and annually thereafter

antibody responses, and (5) inhibition of the complement cascade. When hemodynamic compromise is present, high dose of intravenous CS (methylprednisolone 1,000 mg daily for 3 consecutive days) together with cytolytic therapy should be administered. Polyclonal antilymphocytic antibodies are preferred to OKT3, as the latter has been associated with the development of antibodies against OKT3 with subsequent risk for AMR [41]. Plasmapheresis, which removes circulating plasma antibodies by extracorporeal separation of blood and plasma, has been proposed as therapy for AMR. As antibody production is unaffected, antibody levels may increase after discontinuation of the plasmapheresis. Although several non-randomized small studies have consistently demonstrated that plasmapheresis is an effective treatment for AMR, the variation on protocols with regard to the duration and frequency of treatment and the adjunctive treatment confounds interpretation. Nowadays, there is no consensus on the number and frequency of plasmapheresis sessions; common protocols range from 1 to 5 times per week for 1–4 weeks [32]. Immunoadsorption can also be used to remove circulating antibodies: on the one hand it is less efficient in removing circulating cytokines; on the other hand it is more specific in removal of antibodies. The big advantage of plasmapheresis is that it poses less hemodynamic stress. Nevertheless, because of limited availability it is less commonly used [42] (Fig. 19.5).

The administration of IV immunoglobulins at various doses and intervals has also been proposed as treatment of AMR. It produces a variety of immunomodulatory effects including blockade of Fc receptors, complement inhibition, and down-regulation of B lymphocyte receptors [43]. Reversal of AMR has been demonstrated following this therapy [40]. Nevertheless, data from large series are rare, and IVIG has not been systematically evaluated for the treatment of AMR after heart transplant.

Rituximab, a chimeric monoclonal IgG antibody directed against the CD20 antigen expressed on the B lymphocytes, was originally approved for the treatment of B cell lymphoma. Its efficacy for AMR treatment has only been examined in case reports and one small case study [40]. Major concerns have been raised over the increased risk of serious infections with rituximab after heart transplantation. Further studies evaluating the potential role of rituximab in the treatment of AMR are mandatory before introducing it in routine clinical practice.

While no date exist on the differential effects of various maintenance immunosuppressive regimens on the prevention or recurrence of AMR, modification of baseline immunosuppression seems reasonable. Increase of the dose of the current immunosuppressive regimen, addition of another immunosuppressant agent such as cyclophosphamide or mTOR inhibitor, or conversion to a different maintenance regimen all have been described (Table 19.4).

Key Points

- In all transplant patients routine posttransplant surveillance for AMR should include pathologic evaluation on endomyocardial biopsy, assessment of allograft dysfunction, and monitoring for donor-specific antibodies.
- Treatment strategies for AMR are directed at inhibiting the humoral response at various levels by high doses of IV CS, cytolytic therapy, plasmapheresis, immunoadsorption, or IV immune globulins.

5 Management of the Sensitized Adult Heart Transplant Candidate

There has been a steady increase in the number of sensitized patients on the waiting list for heart transplantation from 5 % in 1994 with a panel of reactive antibodies >10 % to more than 12 % in 2004 [44]. Both improvements in tissue typing and immunomodulatory therapies coupled with the growing population receiving mechanical support/VAD are responsible for this high percentage of sensitized patients on the waiting list. Following transplant these patients form a challenging subgroup of patients with a higher risk of acute rejection and graft loss and a heightened risk of cardiac allograft vasculopathy.

Desensitization strategies have evolved significantly over the last decade and typically involve a two-pronged approach in which anti-HLA antibodies are removed from circulation, and drugs are administered to halt their production. The published evidence remains scarce and the risk of infection is a significant consideration in the choice of strategy. The combined use of IVIG and plasmapheresis as therapy in reducing anti-HLA antibodies prior to heart transplantation has been proposed by the Cleveland Clinic group [44]. In this protocol IVIG at a dose of 0.4–2 g/kg every 21 days following plasmapheresis is used. Plasmapheresis is initiated when the patients become UNOS status IA and is performed 3 times a week until there is a decrease in antibody as measured by flow cytometry. Following this response the frequency of plasmapheresis is changed to weekly until transplantation. Plasmapheresis is typically continued through at least postoperative days 5–7 to ensure clinical stability and stable flow cytometry. The application of these immunomodulatory therapies, as well as the better identification of anti-HLA specificities, has allowed safe and reasonably prompt transplantation of those individuals with a positive cross-match, worrisome anti-HLA antibody specificity, AMR with hemodynamic compromise, or AMR refractory to pulse steroids. However, better understanding of B cell immunobiology and development of therapies specifically designed to ablate donor-specific antibody-producing cells remain unmet needs.

Key Points

- The growing population of patients receiving mechanical support/VAD is responsible for the growing percentage of sensitized patients on the waiting list.
- Desensitization strategies have evolved significantly and typically involve a two-pronged approach in which anti-HLA antibodies are removed from circulation, and drugs are administered to halt their production.
- The published evidence remains scarce and the risk of infection is a significant consideration in the choice of strategy.

References

1. Modry DL, Oyer PE, Jamieson SW, Stinson EB, Baldwin JC, Reitz BA, Dawkins KD, McGregor CG, Hunt SA, Moran M (1985) Cyclosporine in heart and heart-lung transplantation. Can J Surg. 28:274–280, 282
2. Armitage JM, Kormos RL, Griffith BP, Hardesty RL, Fricker FJ, Stuart RS, Marrone GC, Todo S, Fung J, Starzl TE (1991) A clinical trial of FK 506 as primary and rescue immunosuppression in cardiac transplantation. Transplant Proc 23:1149–1152
3. Costanzo MR, Dipchand A, Starling R, Anderson A, Chan M, Desai S, Fedson S, Fisher P, Gonzales-Stawinski G, Martinelli L, McGiffin D, Smith J, Taylor D, Meiser B, Webber S, Baran D, Carboni M, Dengler T, Feldman D, Frigerio M, Kfoury A, Kim D, Kobashigawa J, Shullo M, Stehlik J, Teuteberg J, Uber P, Zuckermann A, Hunt S, Burch M, Bhat G, Canter C, Chinnock R, Crespo-Leiro M, Delgado R, Dobbels F, Grady K, Kao W, Lamour J, Parry G, Patel J, Pini D, Towbin J, Wolfel G, Delgado D, Eisen H, Goldberg L, Hosenpud J, Johnson M, Keogh A, Lewis C, O'Connell J, Rogers J, Ross H, Russell S, Vanhaecke J (2010) International Society of Heart and Lung Transplantation Guidelines. The International Society of Heart and Lung Transplantation Guidelines for the care of heart transplant recipients. J Heart Lung Transplant 29:914–956
4. Uber WE, Uber LA, VanBakel AB, Crumbley AJ, Pereira NL, Ikonomidis JS, Feldman DS (2004) CD3 monitoring and thymoglobulin therapy in cardiac transplantation: clinical outcomes and pharmacoeconomic implications. Transplant Proc 36:3245–3249
5. Krasinskas AM, Kreisel D, Acker MA, Bavaria JE, Pochettino A, Kotloff RM, Arcasoy S, Blumenthal N, Kamoun M, Moore JS, Rosengard BR (2002) CD3 monitoring of antithymocyte globulin therapy in thoracic organ transplantation. Transplantation 73:1339–1341

6. Swinnen LJ, Costanzo-Nordin MR, Fisher SG, O'Sullivan EJ, Johnson MR, Heroux AL, Dizikes GJ, Pifarre R, Fisher RI (1990) Increased incidence of lymphoproliferative disorder after immunosuppression with the monoclonal antibody OKT3 in cardiac-transplant recipients. N Engl J Med 323:1723–1728
7. Stehlik J, Edwards LB, Kucheryavaya AY, Aurora P, Christie JD, Kirk R, Dobbels F, Rahmel AO, Hertz MI (2010) The Registry of the International Society for Heart and Lung Transplantation: twenty-seventh official adult heart transplant report—2010. J Heart Lung Transplant 29:1089–1103
8. Miller LW, Wolford T, McBride LR, Peigh P, Pennington DG (1992) Successful withdrawal of corticosteroids in heart transplantation. J Heart Lung Transplant 11:431–434
9. Teuteberg JJ, Shullo M, Zomak R, McNamara D, McCurry K, Kormos RL (2008) Aggressive steroid weaning after cardiac transplantation is possible without the additional risk of significant rejection. Clin Transplant 22:730–737
10. Kobashigawa J, Miller L, Renlund D, Mentzer R, Alderman E, Bourge R, Costanzo M, Eisen H, Dureau G, Ratkovec R, Hummel M, Ipe D, Johnson J, Keogh A, Mamelok R, Mancini D, Smart F, Valantine H (1998) A randomized active-controlled trial of mycophenolate mofetil in heart transplant recipients. Mycophenolate Mofetil Investigators. Transplantation 66:507–515
11. Liu J, Farmer JD, Lane WS, Friedman J, Weissman I, Schreiber SL (1991) Calcineurin is a common target of cyclophilin-cyclosporin A and FKBP-FK506 complexes. Cell 66:807–815
12. Mentzer RM, Jahania MS, Lasley RD (1998) Tacrolimus as a rescue immunosuppressant after heart and lung transplantation. The U.S. Multicenter FK506 Study Group. Transplantation 65:109–113
13. Reichart B, Meiser B, Viganò M, Rinaldi M, Martinelli L, Yacoub M, Banner NR, Gandjbakhch I, Dorent R, Hetzer R, Hummel M (1998) European Multicenter Tacrolimus (FK506) Heart Pilot Study: one-year results—European Tacrolimus Multicenter Heart Study Group. J Heart Lung Transplant 17:775–781
14. Taylor DO, Barr ML, Radovancevic B, Renlund DG, Mentzer RM, Smart FW, Tolman DE, Frazier OH, Young JB, VanVeldhuisen P (1999) A randomized, multicenter comparison of tacrolimus and cyclosporine immunosuppressive regimens in cardiac transplantation: decreased hyperlipidemia and hypertension with tacrolimus. J Heart Lung Transplant 18:336–345
15. Grimm M, Rinaldi M, Yonan NA, Arpesella G, Arizón Del Prado JM, Pulpón LA, Villemot JP, Frigerio M, Rodriguez Lambert JL, Crespo-Leiro MG, Almenar L, Duveau D, Ordonez-Fernandez A, Gandjbakhch J, Maccherini M, Laufer G (2006) Superior prevention of acute rejection by tacrolimus vs. cyclosporine in heart transplant recipients—a large European trial. Am J Transplant 6:1387–1397
16. Sarbassov DD, Ali SM, Sengupta S, Sheen J-H, Hsu PP, Bagley AF, Markhard AL, Sabatini DM (2006) Prolonged rapamycin treatment inhibits mTORC2 assembly and Akt/PKB. Mol Cell 22:159–168
17. Koehl GE, Andrassy J, Guba M, Richter S, Kroemer A, Scherer MN, Steinbauer M, Graeb C, Schlitt HJ, Jauch K-W, Geissler EK (2004) Rapamycin protects allografts from rejection while simultaneously attacking tumors in immunosuppressed mice. Transplantation 77:1319–1326
18. Mancini D, Pinney S, Burkhoff D, LaManca J, Itescu S, Burke E, Edwards N, Oz M, Marks AR (2003) Use of rapamycin slows progression of cardiac transplantation vasculopathy. Circulation 108:48–53
19. Keogh A, Richardson M, Ruygrok P, Spratt P, Galbraith A, O'Driscoll G, Macdonald P, Esmore D, Muller D, Faddy S (2004) Sirolimus in de novo heart transplant recipients reduces acute rejection and prevents coronary artery disease at 2 years: a randomized clinical trial. Circulation 110:2694–2700
20. Page RL, Miller GG, Lindenfeld J (2005) Drug therapy in the heart transplant recipient: part IV: drug-drug interactions. Circulation 111:230–239
21. Uber PA, Mehra MR, Park MH, Scott RL (2003) Clopidogrel and rhabdomyolysis after heart transplantation. J Heart Lung Transplant 22:107–108

22. Stewart S, Winters GL, Fishbein MC, Tazelaar HD, Kobashigawa J, Abrams J, Andersen CB, Angelini A, Berry GJ, Burke MM, Demetris AJ, Hammond E, Itescu S, Marboe CC, McManus B, Reed EF, Reinsmoen NL, Rodriguez ER, Rose AG, Rose M, Suciu-Focia N, Zeevi A, Billingham ME (2005) Revision of the 1990 working formulation for the standardization of nomenclature in the diagnosis of heart rejection. J Heart Lung Transplant 24:1710–1720
23. Kobashigawa JA, Kirklin JK, Naftel DC, Bourge RC, Ventura HO, Mohanty PK, Cintron GB, Bhat G (1993) Pretransplantation risk factors for acute rejection after heart transplantation: a multiinstitutional study. The Transplant Cardiologists Research Database Group. J Heart Lung Transplant 12:355–366
24. Jarcho J, Naftel DC, Shroyer TW, Kirklin JK, Bourge RC, Barr ML, Pitts DG, Starling RC (1994) Influence of HLA mismatch on rejection after heart transplantation: a multiinstitutional study. The Cardiac Transplant Research Database Group. J Heart Lung Transplant 13:583–595; discussion 595–596
25. Kobashigawa JA, Miller L, Yeung A, Hauptman P, Ventura H, Wilensky R, Valantine H, Wiedermann J (1995) Does acute rejection correlate with the development of transplant coronary artery disease? A multicenter study using intravascular ultrasound. Sandoz/CVIS Investigators. J Heart Lung Transplant 14:S221–S226
26. Stehlik J, Edwards LB, Kucheryavaya AY, Benden C, Christie JD, Dobbels F, Kirk R, Rahmel AO, Hertz MI (2011) The Registry of the International Society for Heart and Lung Transplantation: twenty-eighth adult heart transplant report–2011. J Heart Lung Transplant 30:1078–1094
27. Patel JK, Kittleson M, Kobashigawa JA (2011) Cardiac allograft rejection. Surgeon 9:160–167
28. Mehra MR, Parameshwar J (2010) Gene expression profiling and cardiac allograft rejection monitoring: is IMAGE just a mirage? J Heart Lung Transplant 29:599–602
29. Mills RM, Naftel DC, Kirklin JK, Van Bakel AB, Jaski BE, Massin EK, Eisen HJ, Lee FA, Fishbein DP, Bourge RC (1997) Heart transplant rejection with hemodynamic compromise: a multiinstitutional study of the role of endomyocardial cellular infiltrate. Cardiac Transplant Research Database. J Heart Lung Transplant 16:813–821
30. Taylor DO, Yowell RL, Kfoury AG, Hammond EH, Renlund DG (2000) Allograft coronary artery disease: clinical correlations with circulating anti-HLA antibodies and the immunohistopathologic pattern of vascular rejection. J Heart Lung Transplant 19:518–521
31. Michaels PJ, Espejo ML, Kobashigawa J, Alejos JC, Burch C, Takemoto S, Reed EF, Fishbein MC (2003) Humoral rejection in cardiac transplantation: risk factors, hemodynamic consequences and relationship to transplant coronary artery disease. J Heart Lung Transplant 22:58–69
32. Kobashigawa J, Crespo-Leiro MG, Ensminger SM, Reichenspurner H, Angelini A, Berry G, Burke M, Czer L, Hiemann N, Kfoury AG, Mancini D, Mohacsi P, Patel J, Pereira N, Platt JL, Reed EF, Reinsmoen N, Rodriguez ER, Rose ML, Russell SD, Starling R, Suciu-Foca N, Tallaj J, Taylor DO, Van Bakel A, West L, Zeevi A, Zuckermann A, Consensus Conference Participants (2011) Report from a consensus conference on antibody-mediated rejection in heart transplantation. J Heart Lung Transplant 30(3):252–269
33. Wu GD, Jin Y-S, Salazar R, Dai W-D, Barteneva N, Barr ML, Barsky LW, Starnes VA, Cramer DV (2002) Vascular endothelial cell apoptosis induced by anti-donor non-MHC antibodies: a possible injury pathway contributing to chronic allograft rejection. J Heart Lung Transplant 21:1174–1187
34. Reed EF, Demetris AJ, Hammond E, Itescu S, Kobashigawa JA, Reinsmoen NL, Rodriguez ER, Rose M, Stewart S, Suciu-Foca N, Zeevi A, Fishbein MC (2006) International Society for Heart and Lung Transplantation. Acute antibody-mediated rejection of cardiac transplants. J Heart Lung Transplant 25:153–159
35. Tambur AR, Pamboukian SV, Costanzo MR, Herrera ND, Dunlap S, Montpetit M, Heroux A (2005) The presence of HLA-directed antibodies after heart transplantation is associated with poor allograft outcome. Transplantation 80:1019–1025

36. Hammond EH, Wittwer CT, Greenwood J, Knape WA, Yowell RL, Menlove RL, Craven C, Renlund DG, Bristow MR, DeWitt CW (1990) Relationship of OKT3 sensitization and vascular rejection in cardiac transplant patients receiving OKT3 rejection prophylaxis. Transplantation 50:776–782
37. Leech SH, Rubin S, Eisen HJ, Mather PJ, Goldman BI, McClurken JB, Furukawa S (2003) Cardiac transplantation across a positive prospective lymphocyte cross-match in sensitized recipients. Clin Transplant 17(Suppl 9):17–26
38. De Maria R, Minoli L, Parolini M, Gavazzeni G, Gentile M, Grossi P, Livi U, Parisi F, Utili R (1996) Prognostic determinants of six-month morbidity and mortality in heart transplant recipients. The Italian Study Group on Infection in Heart Transplantation. J Heart Lung Transplant 15:124–135
39. Ross H, Hendry P, Dipchand A, Giannetti N, Hirsch G, Isaac D, Singh N, West L, White M, Ignaszewski A, Chung AM, Straatman L, Modry D, Tymchak W, Burton J, Warnica W, Azevedo JE, Kostuk W, Menkis A, Pflugfelder P, Quantz M, Davies R, Haddad H, Masters R, Cusimano R, Delgado D, Feindel C, Rao V, Cantarovich M, Cecere R, Carrier M, Pellerin M, Doyle D, LeBlanc M-H, Howlett J, Haddad H (2001) 2001 Canadian Cardiovascular Society Consensus Conference on cardiac transplantation. Can J Cardiol 2003:620–654
40. Chih S, Chruscinski A, Ross HJ, Tinckam K, Butany J, Rao V (2012) Antibody-mediated rejection: an evolving entity in heart transplantation. J Transplant 2012:210210
41. Hammond EA, Yowell RL, Greenwood J, Hartung L, Renlund D, Wittwer C (1993) Prevention of adverse clinical outcome by monitoring of cardiac transplant patients for murine monoclonal CD3 antibody (OKT3) sensitization. Transplantation 55:1061–1063
42. Kaczmarek I, Deutsch M-A, Sadoni S, Brenner P, Schmauss D, Daebritz SH, Weiss M, Meiser BM, Reichart B (2007) Successful management of antibody-mediated cardiac allograft rejection with combined immunoadsorption and anti-CD20 monoclonal antibody treatment: case report and literature review. J Heart Lung Transplant 26:511–515
43. Jordan SC, Toyoda M, Kahwaji J, Vo AA (2011) Clinical aspects of intravenous immunoglobulin use in solid organ transplant recipients. Am J Transplant 11:196–202
44. Eckman PM, Hanna M, Taylor DO, Starling RC, Gonzalez-Stawinski GV (2010) Management of the sensitized adult heart transplant candidate. Clin Transplant 24:726–734

Index

J. Bartunek and M. Vanderheyden (eds.), *Translational Approach to Heart Failure*,
DOI 10.1007/978-1-4614-7345-9, © Springer Science+Business Media New York 2013

D

H

I

Printed by [illegible]
in Homburg, Germany

MIX
Papier aus verantwortungsvollen Quellen
Paper from responsible sources
FSC® C105338

If you have any concerns about our products,
you can contact us on
ProductSafety@springernature.com

In case Publisher is established outside the EU,
the EU authorized representative is:
Springer Nature Customer Service Center GmbH
Europaplatz 3, 69115 Heidelberg, Germany

Printed by Libri Plureos GmbH
in Hamburg, Germany